PULMONARY MANIFESTATIONS OF PEDIATRIC DISEASES

PULMONARY MANIFESTATIONS OF PEDIATRIC DISEASES

Nelson L. Turcios, M.D., F.C.C.P.
Director, Pediatric Pulmonology &
Pediatric Asthma Institute
Somerville, New Jersey
Attending Physician
Division of Pediatric Pulmonary Medicine
University of Medicine and Dentistry of New Jersey
Robert Wood Johnson University Hospital
New Brunswick, New Jersey

Robert J. Fink, M.D.
Director, Pediatric Pulmonology
William and Hazel Gorman Newkirk Endowed Chair
Dayton Children's Medical Center
Professor of Pediatrics
Boonshoft School of Medicine
Wright State University
Dayton, Ohio

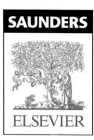

SAUNDERS

ELSEVIER

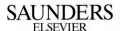

SAUNDERS
ELSEVIER

1600 John F. Kennedy Blvd.
Ste 1800
Philadelphia, PA 19103-2899

PULMONARY MANIFESTATIONS OF PEDIATRIC DISEASES   ISBN: 978-1-4160-3031-7

Notice

Knowledge and best practice in this field are constantly changing. As new research and experience broaden our knowledge, changes in practice, treatment and drug therapy may become necessary or appropriate. Readers are advised to check the most current information provided (i) on procedures featured or (ii) by the manufacturer of each product to be administered, to verify the recommended dose or formula, the method and duration of administration, and contraindications. It is the responsibility of the practitioner, relying on their own experience and knowledge of the patient, to make diagnoses, to determine dosages and the best treatment for each individual patient, and to take all appropriate safety precautions. To the fullest extent of the law, neither the Publisher nor the Editors assume any liability for any injury and/or damage to persons or property arising out of or related to any use of the material contained in this book.

The Publisher

Library of Congress Cataloging-in-Publication Data
Pulmonary manifestations of pediatric diseases / [edited by] Nelson L.
Turcios, Robert J. Fink.--1st ed.
    p. ; cm.
  Includes bibliographical references.
  ISBN 978-1-4160-3031-7
  1. Pulmonary manifestations of general diseases. 2. Pediatric respiratory diseases. I. Turcios, Nelson L.
II. Fink, Robert J., 1948-
  [DNLM: 1. Lung Diseases--etiology. 2. Adolescent. 3. Child. 4. Infant. 5. Lung Diseases--diagnosis.
6. Signs and Symptoms, Respiratory. WS 280 P9825 2009]
  RJ431.P85 2009
  618.92'2–dc22

2008032070

Acquisitions Editor: Dolores Meloni
Developmental Editor: Elena Pushaw
Project Manager: Jagannathan Varadarajan
Design Direction: Steven Stave
Publishing Services Manager: Hemamalini Rajendrababu
Marketing Manager: Courtney Ingram

Working together to grow
libraries in developing countries

www.elsevier.com | www.bookaid.org | www.sabre.org

ELSEVIER   BOOK AID International   Sabre Foundation

Printed in the United States of America

Last digit is the print number: 9 8 7 6 5 4 3 2 1

Dedication

To my loving wife, Minnie, and to our children, Nelson, Jr., and Melissa, for their love, patience, and encouragement during the preparation of "the book." To my parents, Aurora Trinidad and José Mártir, even when you are not here, I know you are always with me. I miss you. To my sisters, Olga Nelly and Lillian Marina, for their support. I also recognize that my participation in editing this book was made possible only because of the lessons learned from so many wonderful patients, families, and colleagues.

Nelson L. Turcios, M.D.

To my wife, Lois, who has always been at my side to support and encourage me throughout my career. To my mother, Mary P. Fink, who instilled in me the love of reading and academics. To my father, Dr. L. Jerome Fink, who introduced me to the joys and rewards of a career in medicine. To all the parents who have entrusted me with the care of their most precious children. And to my dream for a cure for cystic fibrosis and for a world free of lung disease and pollution, in which all children are born free, to live and breathe free.

Robert J. Fink, M.D.

Preface

Pediatric pulmonology can trace its roots to the 1940s and 1950s when early pioneers in the field recognized pediatric lung disorders as being significantly different from their adult pulmonary counterparts. In 1938, Dr. Dorothy Andersen published an autopsy series; it was the first to describe the combination of diarrhea, pancreatic abnormalities, and pneumonia seen in young infants. She coined the name, "cystic fibrosis of the pancreas."

Scarcely more than a decade later, in New York City, Dr. Paul A. di Sant'Agnese discovered the sweat defect of patients with cystic fibrosis. This landmark finding would lead to the development of the sweat test for the diagnosis of cystic fibrosis, a test which is still widely used today.

In 1967, Dr. Edwin L. Kendig published the first pediatric pulmonology textbook, *Disorders of the Respiratory Tract in Children.* This decade was marked by the development of the first comprehensive treatment program for cystic fibrosis in Cleveland, Ohio. The National Cystic Fibrosis (CF) Foundation was formed and CF Centers began to develop at most children's hospitals. The "CF Club" began to hold annual conferences in conjunction with the SPR-APS (now Pediatric Academic Societies (PAS)). The CF Club (now the North American CF Conference) and the American Thoracic Society conferences brought together physicians and researchers who shared a common interest in CF, asthma, and pediatric lung disease. Many pediatric pulmonologists today still benefit from the fellowship, intellectual stimulation, and scientific presentations at these conferences.

The 1970s saw the advent of more formalized fellowship programs in cystic fibrosis and pediatric lung disease. Major advances were made in the diagnosis and treatment of pediatric asthma during this decade. For the first time, pediatric pulmonary physiology was described, and pediatric pulmonary function testing was developed and used to assess the clinical course of lung disorders in children. Because of the tremendous advances in medical knowledge in the 1970s, pediatric pulmonology rapidly matured as a subspecialty. By the end of the decade, pediatric pulmonology was already

under discussion by the American Board of Pediatrics as to whether it should be recognized as its own, distinct subspecialty. However, pediatric pulmonology, still in its nascent stages, was seen as lacking the knowledge base to distinguish it as a unique subspecialty. With this primary criticism, the application was denied.

By the 1980s, the field had developed to such an extent that its appeal to be recognized as a boarded subspecialty was met with well-deserved success. In 1985, pediatric pulmonology became an established subspecialty of the American Board of Pediatrics. The first board examination was given on July 1, 1986, and 158 candidates were certified. Over the next 22 years, more than 500 pediatricians have become board-certified pediatric pulmonologists.

Pediatric pulmonology now has a considerable presence at all major children's hospitals, not only in the United States, but worldwide. Diseases addressed by pediatric pulmonologists include cystic fibrosis, asthma, chronic lung disease of prematurity, ventilator dependency, sleep disorders, primary ciliary dyskinesias, recurrent pneumonia, interstitial lung disease, airway and pulmonary anomalies, lung transplantation, and many other, less common conditions. Pulmonary function testing, fiberoptic laryngoscopy and bronchoscopy, genetic testing and counseling, and polysomnography are some of the tools commonly used for the diagnosis and monitoring of pediatric pulmonary disorders.

The knowledge base of pediatric pulmonology has grown dramatically since the 1970s. Annually, hundreds of clinical and research articles are published in peer-reviewed journals on various respiratory disorders that affect the entire pediatric age group. Numerous textbooks are devoted exclusively to cystic fibrosis, pediatric asthma, pediatric interstitial lung disease, sudden infant death syndrome, chronic lung disease of prematurity, sleep disorders, pediatric pulmonary function testing, and pediatric lung imaging. The "Bible" for every pediatric pulmonologist, *Disorders of the Respiratory Tract in Children,* is now in its 7th edition. Once criticized as an under-developed field with an insufficient knowledge base, after a mere 30 years it has become impossible for the modern pediatric pulmonologist to read all of the pertinent literature in the subspecialty.

As the body of medical information grows and the field of pediatric pulmonology matures, it has become increasingly evident that even disorders and conditions not primarily associated with the lung often have significant ramifications on lung function and health. It is on these effects and interactions that this textbook is focused. The first of its kind, *Pulmonary Manifestations of Pediatric Diseases* presents a fresh outlook on how the clinician can think about diseases addressed in this textbook.

Chapters contributed by some of the most distinguished and recognizable physicians in their field of expertise offer the reader the benefit of their accumulated insight and experience. The pulmonary manifestations of pediatric extrapulmonary diseases are common and often misdiagnosed. The authors of the chapters in this book hope that their efforts lead to early recognition and prompt treatment of this very variable, but important, group of respiratory manifestations.

We also hope that this textbook will become an invaluable reference for pediatric pulmonologists, pediatricians, and other health professionals not only to educate, but also to improve patient care, for this has always been our most important endeavor.

Nelson L. Turcios, MD
Robert J. Fink, MD

Acknowledgments

I am pleased to take this opportunity to acknowledge my daughter Melissa, for her invaluable contributions. She spent more hours logged onto the computer and on the telephone during the editing and proofreading of this book that I can't thank her enough. I am also grateful to Elizabeth Herron and Linda Scott for their invaluable help in finding pertinent literature.

We are particularly indebted to our many renowned and dedicated authors whose scholarly and practical contributions represent the essence of this endeavor. Additionally, the highly professional and devoted staff at Saunders/Elsevier merits our gratitude, in particular Elena Pushaw, our Editorial Assistant for her kind guidance, technical knowledge, and unrelenting support. Our thanks also go to Dolores Meloni, Senior Editor, for her extraordinary efforts towards making this project possible, and to Jagannathan Varadarajan, our Project Manager, for his diligence and attention to detail. Lastly, and most importantly, we must also thank Ginny Doyle, Health Sciences Professional Representative, for her encouragement to pursue this enterprise.

We also acknowledge the outstanding group of reviewers for their thoughtful comments: Drs. Balu Athreya, Victor Chernick, Bernard Cohen, Marc Eberhardt, Hugh E. Evans, Santiago Martinez, Seza Ozen, Arnold C. G. Platzker, Jean-Paul Praud, José Salcedo, Girish Sharma, and William W. Waring.

Nelson L. Turcios, MD

Contributors

JAMES M. ADAMS, M.D.
Professor of Pediatrics – Neonatology, Baylor College of Medicine, Attending Neonatologist, Director, Chronic Pulmonary Care Team, Texas Children's Hospital, Houston, Texas
Chronic Lung Disease of Infancy

SHERMAN J. ALTER, M.D.
Associate Professor of Pediatrics, Boonshoft School of Medicine, Wright State University, Director, Division of Pediatric Infectious Diseases, Children's Medical Center, Dayton, Ohio
Pulmonary Manifestations of Parasitic Diseases

JOHN R. BACH, M.D.
Professor of Medicine and Pediatrics, UMDNJ-New Jersey Medical School, Vice-Chairman, Department of Physical Medicine and Rehabilitation, New Jersey Medical School-University Hospital, Newark, New Jersey
Pulmonary Manifestations of Neuromuscular Diseases

KUSHAL Y. BHAKTA, M.D.
Assistant Professor of Pediatrics, Section of Neonatal/Perinatal Medicine, Baylor College of Medicine, Attending Neonatologist, Texas Children's Hospital, Houston, Texas
Chronic Lung Disease of Infancy

MICHAEL R. BYE, M.D.
Professor of Clinical Pediatrics, Columbia University, Attending, Pediatric Pulmonary Medicine, Morgan Stanley Children's Hospital, New York-Presbyterian Hospital, New York, New York
Pulmonary Manifestations of Human Immunodeficiency Virus (HIV) Infection

GUILLERMO CHANTADA, M.D.
Attending Physician, Division Pediatric Hematology and Oncology, Hospital J P Garrahan, Buenos Aires, Argentina
Pulmonary Manifestations of Hematologic and Oncologic Diseases

EDWARD FELS, M.D.
Fellow in Adult and Pediatric Rheumatology, Duke University Medical Center, Durham, North Carolina
Pulmonary Manifestations of Rheumatoid Diseases

TED M. KREMER, M.D.
Assistant Professor of Pediatrics, University of Massachusetts Memorial Medical Center, Worcester, Massachusetts
Pulmonary Manifestations of Systemic Vasculitis

JOSEPH LEVY, M.D.
Professor of Pediatrics, New York University School of Medicine, Director, Pediatric Gastroenterology and Nutrition, Children's Medical Center, New York University, New York, New York
Pulmonary Manifestations of Gastrointestinal Diseases

J. MARC MAJURE, M.D.
Associate Clinical Professor of Pediatrics, Duke University, Attending Physician, Division of Pediatric Pulmonary and Sleep Medicine, Duke University Medical Center, Durham, North Carolina
Pulmonary Manifestations of Rheumatoid Diseases

CARLOS MILLA, M.D., M.P.H
Associate Professor of Pediatrics, Stanford University, Attending Physician, Division of Pediatric Pulmonology, Children's Hospital Medical Center, Palo Alto, California
Pulmonary Manifestations of Endocrine and Metabolic Diseases

THOMAS M. MURPHY, M.D.
Professor of Pediatrics, Duke University, Director, Pediatric Pulmonary and Sleep Medicine, Duke University Medical Center, Durham, North Carolina
Pulmonary Manifestations of Rheumatoid Diseases

BRIAN P. O'SULLIVAN, M.D.
Professor of Pediatrics, University of Massachusetts, Director, Cystic Fibrosis Center, Associate Director, Pediatric Pulmonology, University of Massachusetts Memorial Children's Medical Center, Worcester, Massachusetts
Pulmonary Manifestations of Systemic Vasculitis

BETH A. PLETCHER, M.D.
Associate Professor of Pediatrics, UMDNJ-New Jersey Medical School, Attending Physician, Center for Human Genetics & Molecular Biology, New Jersey Medical School – University Hospital, Newark, New Jersey
Pulmonary Manifestations of Genetic Diseases

C.D. EGLA RABINOVICH, M.D., M.P.H
Assistant Professor of Pediatrics, Duke University, Attending Physician, Division of Pediatric Rheumatology, Duke University Medical Center, Durham, North Carolina
Pulmonary Manifestations of Rheumatoid Diseases

RAUL C. RIBEIRO, M.D.
Director, Leukemia / Lymphoma Division, Director, International Outreach Program, St Jude's Children's Research Hospital, Professor, Pediatrics, College of Medicine, University of Tennessee Health Science Center, Memphis, Tennessee
Pulmonary Manifestations of Hematologic and Oncologic Diseases

CARLOS RODRÍGUEZ-GALINDO, M.D.
Attending Physician, Division of Pediatric Hematology and Oncology, St Jude's Children's Research Hospital, Memphis, Tennessee
Pulmonary Manifestations of Hematologic and Oncologic Diseases

JOSEPH C. SHANAHAN, M.D.
Assistant Consulting Professor of Medicine, Division of Rheumatology and Immunology, Duke University Medical Center, Durham, North Carolina;
Associate, Carolina Arthritis, Wilmington, North Carolina
Pulmonary Manifestations of Rheumatoid Diseases

ROBERT SIDBURY, M.D., M.P.H.
Assistant Professor of Pediatrics, Harvard Medical School, Attending Physician, Division of Pediatric Dermatology, Children's Hospital of Boston, Boston, Massachusetts
Pulmonary Manifestations of Dermatologic Diseases

ANN R. STARK, M.D.
Professor of Pediatrics – Neonatology, Baylor College of Medicine, Chief, Neonatology Service, Texas Children's Hospital, Houston, Texas
Chronic Lung Disease of Infancy

JAMES M. STARK, M.D., PH.D.
Associate Professor of Pediatrics, Wright State University, Attending Pulmonologist, Division of Pediatric Pulmonology, The Children's Medical Center, Dayton, Ohio
Pulmonary Manifestations of Immunosuppressive Diseases other than Human Immunodeficiency Virus (HIV) Infection

JACQUELINE R. SZMUSZKOVICZ, M.D.
Assistant Professor of Pediatrics, Keck School of Medicine, University of Southern California at Los Angeles, Pediatric Cardiologist, Division of Pediatric Cardiology, Childrens Hospital Los Angeles, Los Angeles, California
Pulmonary Manifestations of Cardiac Diseases

NELSON L. TURCIOS, M.D.
Director, Pediatric Pulmonology & Asthma Institute, Somerville, New Jersey, Attending Physician, Division of Pediatric Pulmonology/Cystic Fibrosis, UMDNJ- Robert Wood Johnson University Hospital, New Brunswick, New Jersey
Pulmonary Manifestations of Dermatologic Diseases
Pulmonary Manifestations of Parasitic Diseases
Pulmonary Manifestations of Renal Diseases

MARLYN S. WOO, M.D.
Assistant Professor of Pediatrics, Keck School of Medicine, University of Southern California at Los Angeles, Attending Pulmonologist, Division of Pediatric Pulmonology, Childrens Hospital Los Angeles, Los Angeles, California
Pulmonary Manifestations of Cardiac Diseases

HEATHER J. ZAR, M.D., PH.D.
Chair of Paediatrics and Child Health, Head of Paediatric Pulmonology, School of Child and Adolescent Health, University of Cape Town, Red Cross Childrens Hospital, Cape Town, South Africa
Pulmonary Manifestations of Human Immunodeficiency Virus (HIV) Infection

Contents

Chapter 1

Chronic Lung Disease of Infancy................1

KUSHAL Y. BHAKTA, MD, JAMES M. ADAMS, MD, AND ANN R. STARK, MD

Chapter 2

Pulmonary Manifestations of Human Immunodeficiency Virus (HIV) Infection................28

HEATHER J. ZAR, MD, PHD, AND MICHAEL R. BYE, MD

Chapter 3

Pulmonary Manifestations of Immunosuppressive Diseases Other than Human Immunodeficiency Virus Infection................49

JAMES M. STARK, MD, PHD

Chapter 4

Pulmonary Manifestations of Cardiac Diseases................79

MARLYN S. WOO, MD, AND JACQUELINE R. SZMUSZKOVICZ, MD

Chapter 5

Pulmonary Manifestations of Gastrointestinal Diseases................98

JOSEPH LEVY, MD

Chapter 6

Pulmonary Manifestations of Renal Diseases................121

NELSON L. TURCIOS, MD

Chapter 7

Pulmonary Manifestations of Hematologic and Oncologic Diseases................135

RAUL C. RIBEIRO, MD, CARLOS RODRIGUEZ-GALINDO, MD, AND GUILLERMO CHANTADA, MD

Chapter 8

Pulmonary Manifestations of Endocrine and Metabolic Diseases................170

CARLOS MILLA, MD, MPH

Chapter 9

Pulmonary Manifestations of Neuromuscular Diseases................184

JOHN R. BACH, MD

Chapter 10

Pulmonary Manifestations of Rheumatoid Diseases................201

C. EGLA RABINOVICH, MD, MPH, EDWARD FELS, MD, JOSEPH SHANAHAN, MD, J. MARC MAJURE, MD, AND THOMAS M. MURPHY, MD

Chapter 11

Pulmonary Manifestations of Systemic Vasculitis................241

BRIAN P. O'SULLIVAN, MD, AND TED KREMER, MD

Chapter 12

Pulmonary Manifestations of Dermatologic Diseases................256

ROBERT SIDBURY, MD, AND NELSON L. TURCIOS, MD

Chapter 13

Pulmonary Manifestations of Parasitic Diseases................274

SHERMAN J. ALTER, MD, AND NELSON L. TURCIOS, MD

Chapter 14

Pulmonary Manifestations of Genetic Diseases................295

BETH A. PLETCHER, MD

COLOR PLATES

PLATE 1

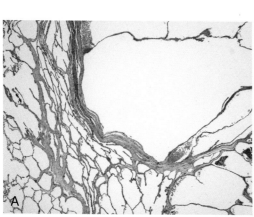

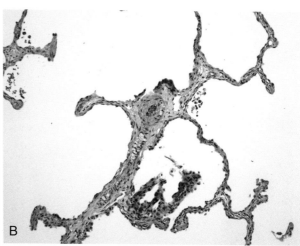

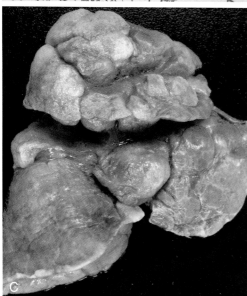

Figure 1-1. A, Classic bronchopulmonary dysplasia in a 9-month-old, former premature (25 weeks gestation) infant. Microscopically, there is marked hyperexpansion of airspaces compressing adjacent parenchyma. Focal interstitial fibrosis also is noted. (Hematoxylin and eosin, 20×.) **B**, Secondary pulmonary hypertension in the same patient is reflected microscopically by marked muscularization of the normally thin-walled intralobular arterioles. (Hematoxylin and eosin, 100×.) **C**, Classic bronchopulmonary dysplasia in a 2-year-old, former premature (26 weeks gestation) infant. The lungs grossly show hyperinflated pale areas alternating with areas of collapse and pleural retraction, producing pseudofissures. (*Courtesy of Megan K. Dishop, MD, Department of Pathology, Texas Children's Hospital and Baylor College of Medicine, Houston, TX.*)

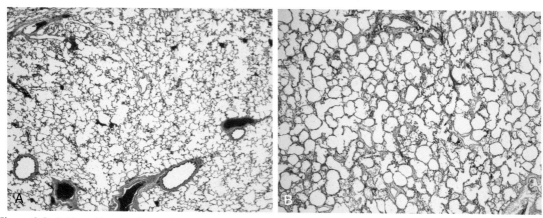

Figure 1-2. A, Normal lung in a 2-year-old, former term (38 weeks gestation) infant. (Hematoxylin and eosin, 20×.) **B**, Chronic neonatal lung disease with "new" bronchopulmonary dysplasia pattern in an 8-month-old, former premature (29 weeks gestation) infant. The lung architecture is altered with diffuse mild enlargement of airspaces with simplification and deficient septation. (Hematoxylin and eosin, 20×.) (*Courtesy of Megan K. Dishop, MD, Department of Pathology, Texas Children's Hospital and Baylor College of Medicine, Houston, TX.*)

PLATE 2

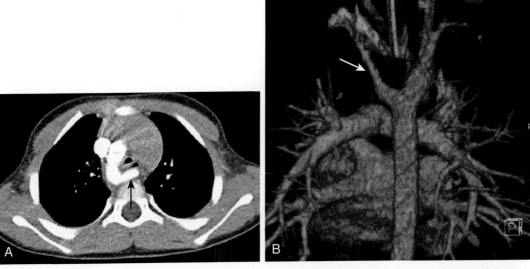

Figure 4-8 A 5-year-old boy with a right-sided aortic arch and aberrant left subclavian artery. **A,** Axial CT scan of the thorax shows compression of the trachea by the aberrant artery (*arrow*). **B,** Three-dimensional volume rendered image (posterior view) shows the right-sided aortic arch (*red arrow*) and the aberrant left subclavian artery (*white arrow*) arising from the descending aorta. (*Adapted from McLaren CA, Elliott MJ, Roebuck DJ: Vascular compression of the airway in children. Paediatr Respir Rev 9:85-94, 2008.*)

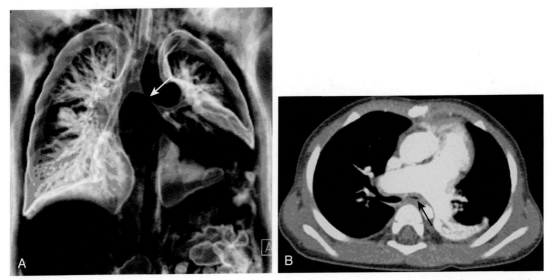

Figure 4-10 Tetralogy of Fallot and absent pulmonary valve syndrome with airway compression in a 15-month-old boy. **A,** CT volume-rendered image shows compression of the left main bronchus (*arrow*). **B,** Axial CT scan of the thorax shows severe compression of the airway between the vertebral body and the grossly enlarged pulmonary arteries. (*From McLaren CA, Elliott MJ, Roebuck DJ: Vascular compression of the airway in children. Paediatr Respir Rev 9:85-94, 2008.*)

PLATE 3

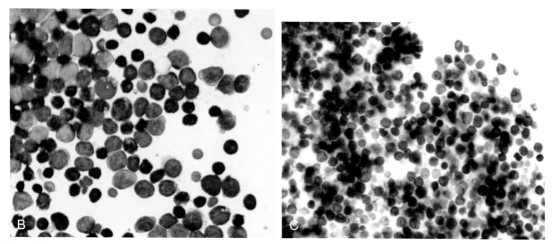

Figure 7-1 An 11-year-old boy with lymphoblastic lymphoma. **B** and **C**, Cytocentrifuge examination of the pleural effusion shows FAB L1 lymphoblasts (**B**) (Wright-Giemsa) of T cell origin (**C**) (anti-CD3 staining).

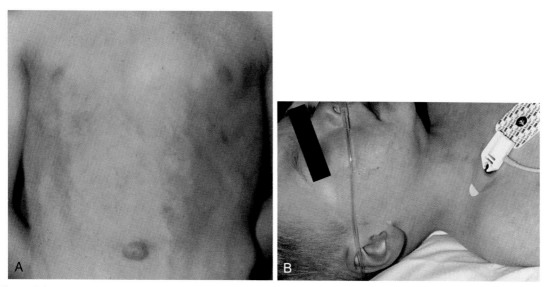

Figure 7-2 A, A 14-year-old boy with lymphoblastic lymphoma complicated by vena cava compression syndrome. The compression was predominantly vascular; the patient had no signs of respiratory distress. **B**, A 10-year-old boy with lymphoblastic lymphoma, superior vena cava syndrome, and tracheal compression. In addition to having increased collateral circulation in the frontal and cervical regions, the patient was plethoric and was experiencing respiratory distress.

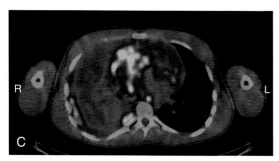

Figure 7-3 PET/CT images of a 15-year-old boy with non-Hodgkin lymphoma. **C**, Fused image of **A** and **B** overlies the anatomic image in **A** and the functional image in **B**.

PLATE 4

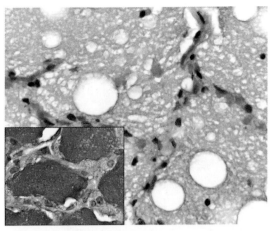

Figure 7-4 Pulmonary alveolar proteinosis (accumulation of amorphous, eosinophilic, periodic acid-Schiff-positive material) in pulmonary alveolar lumens. (Hematoxylin and eosin, 40× original magnification.) *Inset* shows PAS stain counterstained with hematoxylin.

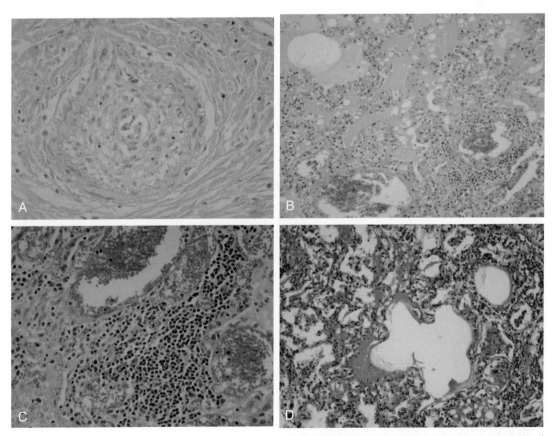

Figure 7-9 Early-onset pathologic pulmonary changes associated with treatment-induced toxicity (hematoxylin-eosin stains). **A,** Vascular changes consisting of thickening of the media and narrowing of the vascular lumen. **B,** Intra-alveolar edema and perivascular mononuclear infiltrates. **C,** Hemorrhage and interstitial mononuclear infiltrate. **D,** Hyaline membrane formation.

PLATE 5

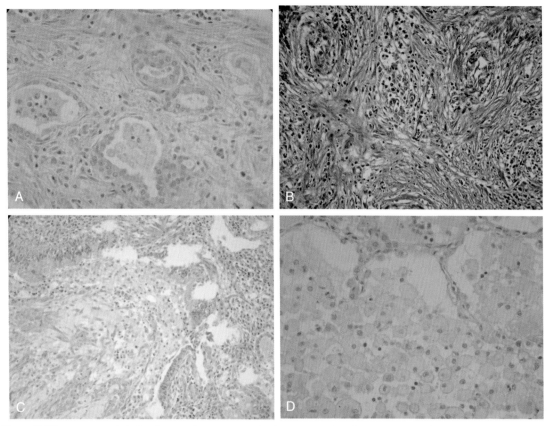

Figure 7-10 Late-onset pathologic pulmonary changes associated with treatment-induced toxicity (hematoxylin-eosin stains). **A**, Increased collagen content in the alveolar septum and epithelial hyperplasia. **B**, Interstitial fibrosis. **C**, Bronchiolitis obliterans. **D**, Organizing pneumonia.

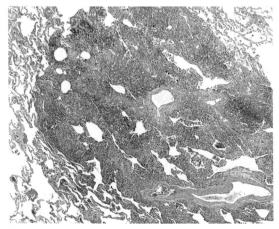

Figure 10-4 Lung biopsy histopathology specimen from a patient with Sjögren syndrome. The pattern is that of a patchy and nodular diffuse lymphoid interstitial pneumonitis.

PLATE 6

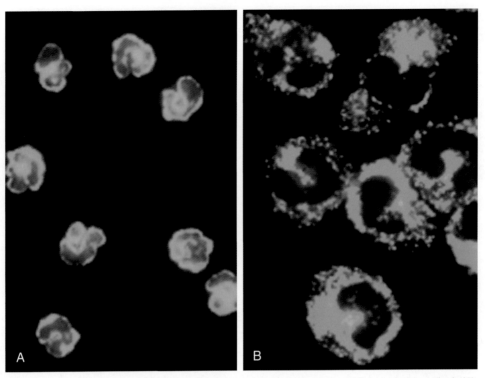

Figure 11-3. **A** and **B**, Indirect immunofluorescence staining showing perinuclear antineutrophilic cytoplasmic antibody (**A**) and cytoplasmic antineutrophilic cytoplasmic antibody (**B**) distribution.

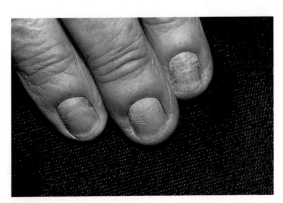

Figure 12-1. Yellowish discoloration and thickening of the nail plate.

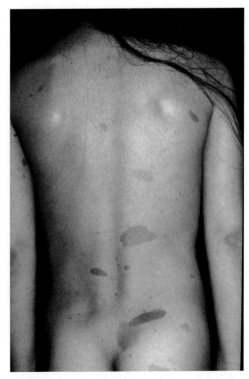

Figure 12-3. Multiple café au lait macules in a child with neurofibromatosis type 1.

PLATE 7

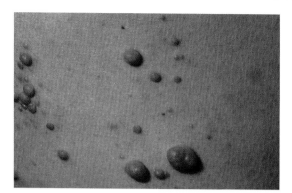

Figure 12-4. Cutaneous neurofibromas.

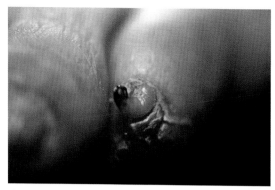

Figure 12-6. Periungual fibromas (Koenen tumors) in tuberous sclerosis.

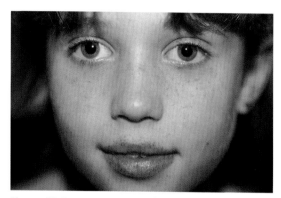

Figure 12-7. Facial angiomas in tuberous sclerosis (i.e., adenoma sebaceum).

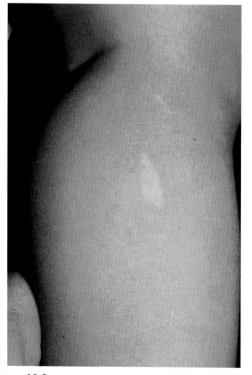

Figure 12-5. Ash-leaf macule in a child with tuberous sclerosis.

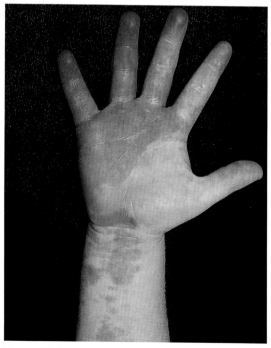

Figure 12-9. Port-wine stains clearly visible on right hand of a child affected with Klippel-Trénaunay-Weber syndrome.

PLATE 8

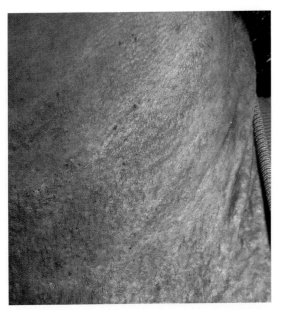

Figure 12-11. Pseudoxanthoma elasticum, showing typical "plucked chicken" grouped yellowish papules and prominent skin folds on the neck. Lesions are usually most apparent on the neck or in the axillary region; the latter may be confused with Fox-Fordyce disease, but this is confined to the axilla and does not have the soft slackness of the skin that is a feature of pseudoxanthoma elasticum.

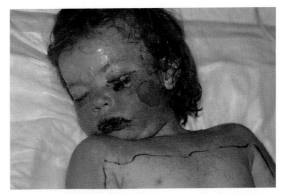

Figure 12-13. Extensive skin necrosis in Stevens-Johnson syndrome and toxic epidermal necrolysis.

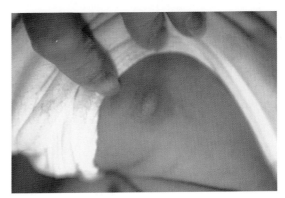

Figure 12-14. Urtication secondary to stroking of a mastocytoma (i.e., positive Darier sign).

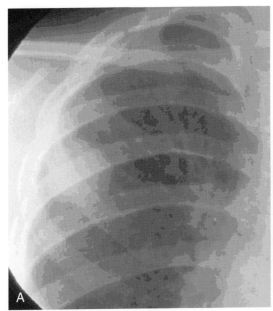

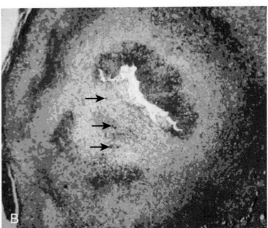

Figure 13-14 Dirofilariasis in an asymptomatic 14-year-old girl with a solitary pulmonary nodule. **A,** Chest radiograph shows a nodule with soft tissue opacity in the right upper lung. **B,** Photomicrograph obtained after surgical resection shows an infarcted peripheral vessel surrounded by necrotic lung tissue. Some remnants of the parasites are present in the lumen (*arrows*). (Masson stain, original magnification 40×.)

CHAPTER 1

Chronic Lung Disease of Infancy

KUSHAL Y. BHAKTA, JAMES M. ADAMS, AND ANN R. STARK

Historical Overview 1
Definitions of Bronchopulmonary Dysplasia 2
Epidemiology 4
Pathogenesis 4
  Prenatal Events 5
  Hyperoxia and Oxidant Stress 5
  Mechanical Ventilation and Volutrauma 6
  Infection 6
  Inflammation 7
  Bombesin-like Peptides 7
  Nutrition 7
  Genetic Factors 7
Pathology 8
  Clinical Features 9
  Physical Examination 9
  Chest Radiograph 9
  Clinical Course 9
  Cardiopulmonary Function 10
Management 11
  Respiratory Care 11
  Nutrition and Fluid Management 12
  Diuretics 12
  Bronchodilator Therapy 13
  Corticosteroids 13
Prevention 13
  Antenatal Corticosteroids 13
  Fluid Restriction 14

  Minimal Ventilation 14
  High-Frequency Oscillatory Ventilation 14
  Vitamin A 15
  Systemic Corticosteroids 15
  Inhaled Corticosteroids 16
  Inhaled Nitric Oxide 16
  Caffeine 17
  Superoxide Dismutase 17
  Summary 17
Outcome 17
  Mortality 17
  Respiratory Infections 18
  Pulmonary Function 18
  Neurodevelopment 18
  Growth 19
  Tracheobronchomalacia 19
  Glottic and Subglottic Damage 20
  Tracheal Stenosis, Bronchial Stenosis, or Granuloma Formation 20
Monitoring 21
  Cardiovascular Monitoring and Oxygenation 21
  Growth 21
  Development, Vision, and Hearing 21
Coordination of Care and Discharge Planning 21
  References 22

Historical Overview

Bronchopulmonary dysplasia (BPD) or chronic lung disease of the premature comprises a heterogeneous group of respiratory diseases of infancy that usually evolve from an acute respiratory disorder experienced by a newborn. Chronic lung disease of the premature most commonly occurs in infants with birth weights less than 1500 g, and especially in infants with birth weights less than 1000 g and who are treated for respiratory distress syndrome (RDS). This entity was first described by Northway and colleagues[1,2] in 1967 in premature infants who had severe RDS and required prolonged mechanical ventilation with high inflation pressures and inspired oxygen concentrations. The pathology was characterized by abnormalities of the terminal airways, the hallmark of which was an intense interstitial fibrosis and hyperplasia of the smooth muscle (Fig. 1-1). Affected infants experienced chronic respiratory failure, with hypoxemia and hypercapnia, and many developed cor pulmonale.

More recently, as the use of antenatal steroids and surfactant replacement therapy has resulted in increased survival of smaller preterm infants, the features of the so-called new BPD differ from the older descriptions

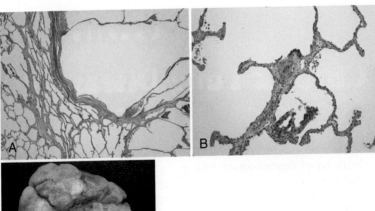

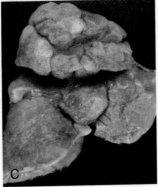

Figure 1-1. A, Classic bronchopulmonary dysplasia in a 9-month-old, former premature (25 weeks gestation) infant. Microscopically, there is marked hyperexpansion of airspaces compressing adjacent parenchyma. Focal interstitial fibrosis also is noted. (Hematoxylin and eosin, 20×.) **B**, Secondary pulmonary hypertension in the same patient is reflected microscopically by marked muscularization of the normally thin-walled intralobular arterioles. (Hematoxylin and eosin, 100×.) **C**, Classic bronchopulmonary dysplasia in a 2-year-old, former premature (26 weeks gestation) infant. The lungs grossly show hyperinflated pale areas alternating with areas of collapse and pleural retraction, producing pseudofissures. (*Courtesy of Megan K. Dishop, MD, Department of Pathology, Texas Children's Hospital and Baylor College of Medicine, Houston, TX.*) (See Color Plate)

and include milder respiratory distress that often requires minimal ventilatory support with low fractions of inspired oxygen (FiO_2) preceding the chronic condition.[3-6] Pathologic examination typically shows an arrest in pulmonary development and alveolarization, with simplification of the terminal airways (Fig. 1-2).

Definitions of Bronchopulmonary Dysplasia

The terminology used to describe chronic lung disease arising from neonatal insults is confusing. The terms "bronchopulmonary dysplasia" (BPD) and "chronic lung disease of infancy" (CLDI) are sometimes used interchangeably to describe chronic respiratory disease after treatment for RDS in preterm infants. A working definition of BPD is necessary because it is from BPD that most cases of CLDI arise. Three clinical definitions have been used to define BPD in neonates, as follows:

- Oxygen requirement at 28 days postnatal age[7,8]
- Oxygen requirement at 36 weeks postmenstrual age (PMA)[9,10]
- Diagnostic criteria proposed by a National Institute of Child Health and Human Development (NICHD) workshop based on gestational age and disease severity[11,12]

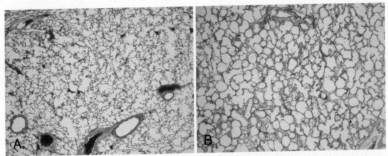

Figure 1-2. A, Normal lung in a 2-year-old, former term (38 weeks gestation) infant. (Hematoxylin and eosin, 20×.) **B**, Chronic neonatal lung disease with "new" bronchopulmonary dysplasia pattern in an 8-month-old, former premature (29 weeks gestation) infant. The lung architecture is altered with diffuse mild enlargement of airspaces with simplification and deficient septation. (Hematoxylin and eosin, 20×.) (*Courtesy of Megan K. Dishop, MD, Department of Pathology, Texas Children's Hospital and Baylor College of Medicine, Houston, TX.*) (See Color Plate)

In the 1990s, several studies showed that administration of supplemental oxygen at 36 weeks PMA rather than 28 days postnatal age more accurately predicted abnormal pulmonary outcome at 2 years of age.[9,10] In one study, the positive predictive value for abnormal outcome in very-low-birth-weight (VLBW) infants (birth weight <1,500 g) (63% versus 38%) was better for supplemental oxygen administration at 36 weeks PMA than at 28 postnatal days.[10] Outcome was normal in 90% of infants who did not receive oxygen at 36 weeks PMA. As a result, the definition of BPD as requiring administration of supplemental oxygen at 36 weeks PMA became widely used.

A precise definition of BPD is especially important when outcomes are compared among different centers or when new therapeutic interventions are tested. The increased survival of extremely-low-birth-weight (ELBW) infants (birth weight <1,000 g or gestational age <30 weeks) suggested that the definition of BPD could be refined to include infants with milder disease and account for developmental changes that occur with increasing gestational age. In 2001, the NICHD workshop proposed diagnostic criteria for BPD that included gestational age and disease severity (Table 1-1).[12] This scheme divides patients into the following two groups based on gestational age, which determines the timing of clinical assessment for BPD:

- Patients who are less than 32 weeks gestation are assessed at 36 weeks PMA or when discharged home, whichever comes first.
- Patients who are equal to or greater than 32 weeks gestation are assessed at 29 to 55 days of life or when discharged home, whichever comes first.

At the time of assessment, patients are evaluated for the severity of their disease. Infants who received treatment with supplemental oxygen for at least 28 postnatal days are classified as having mild, moderate, or severe BPD, depending on the extent of oxygen supplementation and other respiratory support.[11]

In a study from the NICHD Neonatal Research Network of infants with BPD who were born at less than 32 weeks gestational age and with birth weight less than 1000 g, these criteria predicted pulmonary and neurodevelopmental outcomes at 18 to 22 months corrected age.[11] The severity of BPD (mild, moderate, severe) was associated with use of pulmonary medications (30%, 41%, 47%) and rehospitalization for pulmonary disease (27%, 34%, 40%). The incidence of *any* neurodevelopmental impairment, including cerebral palsy, blindness, hearing deficit requiring amplification, and lower mental and psychomotor development index scores, also increased with the severity of BPD. The patients who had severe BPD often

Table 1-1	Diagnostic Criteria for Bronchopulmonary Dysplasia Proposed by National Institute of Child Health and Human Development Workshop	
	GESTATIONAL AGE <32 WEEKS PMA	**GESTATIONAL AGE ≥32 WEEKS PMA**
Time of assessment	36 wk PMA or discharge to home*	>28 days but <56 days postnatal age or discharge to home*
Mild CLD	Treatment with oxygen >21% for at least 28 days *plus* Breathing room air at 36 wk PMA or discharge*	Breathing room air by 56 days postnatal age or discharge*
Moderate CLD	Need[†] for FiO$_2$ <30% at 36 wk PMA or discharge*	Need[†] for FiO$_2$ <30% at 56 days postnatal age or discharge*
Severe CLD	Need[†] for FiO$_2$ ≥30% and/or positive pressure (IPPV or NCPAP) at 36 wk PMA or discharge*	Need[†] for FiO$_2$ ≥30% and/or positive pressure (IPPV or NCPAP) at 56 days postnatal age or discharge*

*Whichever comes first.
[†]At the time of the workshop, a physiologic test to confirm oxygen requirement had yet to be defined.
CLD, chronic lung disease of the premature; IPPV, intermittent positive-pressure ventilation; NCPAP, nasal continuous positive airway pressure; PMA, postmenstrual age.
From Jobe AH, Bancalari E: Bronchopulmonary dysplasia. Am J Respir Crit Care Med 163:1723-1729, 2001.

had substantial associated morbidity during their hospitalization at birth, such as severe intraventricular hemorrhage (25%), periventricular leukomalacia (10%), necrotizing enterocolitis (14%), late-onset infection (54%), and postdischarge deaths (5%), and were often treated with postnatal corticosteroids (78%). In this cohort, many infants who needed oxygen during the first 28 days of life no longer required oxygen at 36 weeks PMA and might not have been classified as having BPD. This study did not include an objective physiologic measure of oxygen requirement, however. These criteria, especially with the addition of a physiologic test, may improve the ability to compare therapeutic interventions in clinical trials and evaluate long-term outcomes.

In most neonatal intensive care units (NICUs), supplemental oxygen is adjusted to maintain the infant's oxygen saturation within a target range. As a result, the use of supplemental oxygen depends partly on the NICU policy for the target range, which varies among centers. To standardize the use of supplemental oxygen, the NICHD workshop also proposed that the need for oxygen less than or greater than 30% be confirmed by a physiologic test. Such a test was developed, based on oxygen administration and oxygen saturation, including a timed room air challenge in selected patients. It was found to be safe, feasible, and reliable.[13] In a prospective multicenter study of VLBW infants who remained hospitalized at 36 weeks PMA,[14] fewer infants had BPD when the physiologic definition was used (25% versus 35%) compared with the clinical definition (oxygen supplementation at 36 weeks PMA), and there was less variation among centers.

Epidemiology

The rate of BPD varies among institutions. In a report from the NICHD Neonatal Research Network (1995 to 1996), the rate of BPD ranged from 3% to 43% in the 14 participating centers.[15] Variability in incidence among centers may reflect neonatal risk factors or care practices, such as target levels for acceptable oxygen saturation.[16] The overall incidence of BPD was 23% of the VLBW infants, and increased with decreasing birth weight. Compared with the entire cohort, there were increased proportions of males with BPD and severe BPD (54% for entire cohort, 60% for males with BPD, and 67% for males with severe BPD).

In an 8-year (1994 to 2002) retrospective cohort study of six NICUs, the overall incidence of BPD remained constant at 12% for preterm infants born before 33 weeks gestation.[17] Although there has been no change in the overall incidence of BPD, there has been a significant decline in the incidence of severe BPD, from 10% in 1994 to 4% in 2002, with severe BPD defined as requiring positive-pressure respiratory support (i.e., mechanical ventilation or continuous positive airway pressure [CPAP]) at 36 weeks PMA. The risk for *any* degree BPD increases with mechanical ventilation, as described in a case-cohort study conducted at two centers (two Boston hospitals and Babies' and Children's Hospital in New York), in which the higher rate of BPD in Boston (22% versus 4%) reflected the higher rate of mechanical ventilation (75% versus 29%) and surfactant administration (45% versus 10%) as part of the initial respiratory management of VLBW infants.[16] The risk of BPD increases with decreasing birth weight. BPD is rare in infants older than 32 weeks gestation.

Pathogenesis

The etiology of BPD is multifactorial. Inflammation caused by mechanical ventilation, oxygen toxicity, or infection plays an important role. The lung seems to be most vulnerable before the saccular stage of development, which occurs at approximately 31 to 34 weeks gestation, and during which alveolar formation is initiated.[18,19] The preterm lung is especially at risk of injury because of its structural and functional immaturity. Lungs in preterm infants have poorly developed airway supporting structures, surfactant deficiency, decreased compliance, underdeveloped antioxidant mechanisms, and inadequate fluid clearance compared with term infants.[20]

Prenatal Events

Many events that occur before birth affect the development of the lung. In infants less than 27 weeks gestation—the period of highest risk for development of BPD—the human lung is in the saccular stage of development; alveolarization begins at approximately 32 weeks and proceeds through 40 weeks PMA.[21] Any factor that has an adverse effect on this process leads to disruption of lung architecture and alveolar simplification, a hallmark of the "new BPD."[22]

Inflammation, as discussed later, is considered one of the central aspects in the pathogenesis of BPD. Several studies suggest that the timing, the type, and the intensity of the inflammatory response that determine the subsequent effects on the developing preterm lung.[23] A series of studies in fetal rabbits and fetal sheep showed that intra-amniotic exposure to interleukin (IL)-1 or endotoxin accelerated lung maturation and the synthesis of surfactant proteins.[24] In these studies, repeated exposure to proinflammatory agents did not cause progressive inflammation, but rather induced tolerance and suppression of fetal monocyte function.[25] If IL-1 or endotoxin treatment was done with two doses, given 7 days apart, the fetal monocytes reacted in a manner similar to that seen in adult sheep.[25] Concomitant treatment with corticosteroids and IL-1 or endotoxin initially suppressed the inflammatory response, but caused an exaggerated inflammatory response at 5 to 15 days post-treatment.[26,27] Antenatal exposure to endotoxin and corticosteroids modulates lung injury and maturation in a time-dependent manner.

Hyperoxia and Oxidant Stress

High concentrations of inspired oxygen can damage the lungs, although the exact level or duration of exposure that is unsafe is unknown. In a study conducted in neonatal rats, exposing neonatal rat pups to moderate hyperoxia (FiO_2 0.50) for 15 days caused airway remodeling, hyperreactivity, and inflammatory alterations similar to that seen in BPD.[28] Higher degrees of hyperoxia (FiO_2 0.95) for shorter durations (≤72 hours) result in inhibition of distal airway branching with simplification of architecture in fetal mouse lung explants.[29]

The imbalance between pro-oxidant and antioxidant systems in a preterm neonate in favor of pro-oxidant processes also may contribute to the development of BPD.[30-32] Preterm infants have few antioxidant defenses and are often exposed to supplemental oxygen to treat pulmonary insufficiency. They also are prone to infection, and many of the proinflammatory cytokines activate the production of reactive oxygen species (ROS), such as superoxide free radical, hydrogen peroxide, hydroxyl free radical, and singlet oxygen, which are produced as the result of oxidative stress. In addition, preterm infants have higher plasma and tissue-free iron concentrations compared with term infants, which can promote the propagation of ROS.

The toxicity of these ROS, particularly in response to exposure to hyperoxia, has been shown in experimental animals; when exposed to equal to or greater than 0.50 FiO_2, they exhibited irreversible changes in lung growth and DNA synthesis.[32] At the cellular level, ROS cause the uncoupling of respiration from adenosine triphosphate (ATP) synthesis and disruption of the outer mitochondrial membrane. Subsequently, this disruption allows release of pro-apoptotic factors, such as cytochrome-c, apoptosis-inducing factor, and pro-caspases, from the mitochondria into the cytosol, leading to cell death.[31]

Various antioxidant defenses are available in mature human organisms to combat this oxidative stress. They include superoxide dismutase, catalase, glutathione-S-transferase (GST), and glutathione peroxidase, and nutrients such as vitamins A and E, iron, copper, zinc, and selenium, which help prevent oxygen toxicity. Preterm infants have inadequate antioxidant defenses and are at risk of oxygen free radical damage. In some species, antioxidant enzyme concentrations are lower in preterm than term animals,[33] and are poorly induced in response to oxidative stress.[34] Similarly, activities of catalase, glutathione peroxidase, and copper/zinc superoxide dismutase in human cord blood are lower in preterm than in term newborns.[35] In a small study of preterm infants (gestational age 25 to 30 weeks), copper/zinc superoxide dismutase levels were greater in infants who subsequently developed BPD; these infants also had a higher cumulative oxygen exposure.[36] These results suggest that in preterm infants with BPD, superoxide dismutase activity is upregulated and may be a marker for increased oxygen exposure and potentially increased reactive oxygen metabolites.

Mechanical Ventilation and Volutrauma

Lung injury associated with mechanical ventilation contributes to the development of BPD, and it is known that positive-pressure ventilation typically induces bronchiolar lesions.[37] Pulmonary interstitial emphysema is a result of barotrauma and is associated with a high incidence of CLDI.

Disruption of airways may occur early in the course of treatment and may be manifested by increased pulmonary resistance.[38] In one study of ventilated preterm infants in the first 5 days after birth, mean pulmonary resistance was significantly greater in infants who subsequently developed BPD compared with infants who did not.[39]

Animal studies suggest that volutrauma is more important than barotrauma in causing airway injury.[16,18,40] Distention of the airways to near-maximum lung volume causes shear injury, capillary leak, and pulmonary edema.[41,42] In studies in preterm lambs and rabbits and in adult rats, animals given large tidal volume breaths had significantly worse pulmonary mechanics and showed histologic evidence of widespread lung injury.[37,43,44] In newborn lambs, large tidal volumes seem to impair the response to subsequent surfactant administration.[44] In one study, preterm lambs ventilated with large tidal volumes (20 mL/kg) showed lower compliance, lower ventilatory efficiency, higher recovery of protein, and lower recovery of surfactant by 6 hours compared with animals ventilated

with lower tidal volumes (5 mL/kg and 10 mL/kg).[44]

In two retrospective cohort studies ($n = 235$ and $n = 188$), the authors found that increased ventilation resulting from large tidal volumes resulted in hypocarbia, a risk factor for subsequently developing BPD.[7,45] In vitro cyclic cell stretch has been shown to upregulate the expression of proinflammatory cytokines by human alveolar epithelial cells without any structural cell damage.[46,47] Tidal volumes large enough to cause similar cell stretch in vivo, without causing structural damage, may similarly initiate the cascade of proinflammatory cytokines, recruiting inflammatory cells and causing tissue damage. All of the above-described pulmonary insults occur at a time when most preterm infants have a relative adrenocortical insufficiency, which may potentiate the inflammatory effects.

Infection

Although the role of infection is incompletely understood, infants exposed to antenatal and postnatal infection seem to be at higher risk for developing BPD.[46] Antenatal chorioamnionitis may play a key role in the production of a fetal pulmonary inflammatory response to the release of proinflammatory cytokines.[48,49] This response can lead to aberrant wound healing and fibrosis, causing inhibition of alveolarization and vascular development, hallmarks of the new BPD. Similarly, infants who developed late-onset sepsis (>3 days of age) were more likely to need long-term mechanical ventilation, and were more likely to develop BPD.[50] In a retrospective study, early tracheal colonization also predisposed to the subsequent development of BPD.[51]

Nosocomial infection plays a role in some cases of CLDI, especially in association with a symptomatic patent ductus arteriosus PDA, particularly in ELBW infants. In a series of 119 ELBW infants who had mild or no initial RDS, BPD was significantly more likely to occur with patent ductus arteriosus (odds ratio [OR] 6.2) and sepsis (OR 4.4).[52] The risk of BPD increased substantially in infants with both conditions (OR 48.3).

Neither ductal ligation nor prophylactic use of low-dose indomethacin initiated in the first 24 hours has been shown to reduce significantly the incidence of CLDI, however.

Specific organisms also may play a role. In one report, development of BPD was associated with isolation of *Ureaplasma urealyticum* in tracheal aspirates performed on the first (before surfactant administration) and fourth days of mechanical ventilation in infants less than 28 weeks gestational age.[53]

Inflammation

Macrophages, lymphocytes, and platelets in the lung release multiple inflammatory mediators, including cytokines, lipid mediators, and platelet factors, which interact with endothelial and epithelial cells.[54] The airspaces of ventilated preterm infants contain many proinflammatory and chemotactic factors that are present in greater concentration in infants who subsequently develop BPD.[12,54-57] The presence of these mediators is associated with complement activation, increased vascular permeability, protein leakage, and mobilization of neutrophils into the interstitial and alveolar compartments. Release of ROS, elastase, and collagenase by activated neutrophils can damage lung structures. Interaction between macrophages and other cell types may perpetuate the production of proinflammatory mediators and sustain the cycle of lung injury. Persistence of factors such as macrophage inflammatory protein-1 and IL-8 and decreases of counter-regulatory cytokines such as IL-10 may lead to unregulated and persistent inflammation.[12]

Bombesin-like Peptides

Injury may be mediated partly by bombesin-like peptides (BLP), which are derived from pulmonary neuroendocrine cells and play an important role in normal lung growth and maturation. In one study, the number of BLP-positive cells was greater in infants who died with BPD than in controls.[58] In a baboon model, urine BLP levels were increased soon after birth in animals who developed BPD, and administration of anti-BLP antibody attenuated the disorder.[59,60] In infants ≤28 weeks gestational age, elevated urine BLP levels in the first 4 days after birth were associated with an increased risk of BPD.[61]

Nutrition

Premature infants have very poor nutritional reserves and are at high risk for being malnourished and entering a catabolic state if not provided with adequate nutrition. The goal of postnatal nutrition is to provide adequate substrate to approximate the intrauterine rate of growth. In VLBW infants, this goal can be extremely difficult to achieve for the following reasons[62]:
- Fluid restriction to prevent pulmonary edema
- Heart failure secondary to a patent ductus arteriosus
- Use of postnatal corticosteroids
- Decreased gastrointestinal absorption secondary to suspected or proven necrotizing enterocolitis
- Hypoxia and chronic respiratory acidosis
- Anemia of prematurity
- Medications that increase metabolic rate, such as methylxanthines and β-sympathomimetics

Malnutrition or undernutrition renders an infant more susceptible to injury resulting from hyperoxia, volutrauma/barotrauma, and infections, and impairs the infant's ability to recover from this injury.[63] In addition, infants with BPD are significantly more likely to have lower early protein and total energy intake.[64]

Genetic Factors

The pathogenesis of BPD is complex, with an intricate interaction of preterm birth, the *in utero* environment, inflammation/infection, fluid management, vascular maldevelopment, surfactant deficiency, mechanical ventilation, the balance of oxidative stress and antioxidant systems, and nutrition. Not all factors are required to develop BPD, and severe BPD may develop in infants who have a benign perinatal course. It had been postulated that there might be a genetic predisposition to develop BPD. Several studies have looked at the development of BPD in singleton and multiple gestation VLBW infants.[65-69] In the earliest study comparing the rate of BPD among 108 VLBW twins, it was reported that BPD in one twin significantly predicted BPD in the other twin (adjusted OR 12.3, $P < .001$), even after adjusting for birth weight, gestational age, gender, RDS, pneumothorax, and patent ductus arteriosus.[67] More recently, in a multicenter retrospective study of 450 twin pairs born at 32 weeks, the concordance of BPD was higher in monozygotic twins than predicted, after controlling for all covariates.

In addition to twin studies, many other investigators have attempted to look for candidate genes that may predispose to developing BPD. Genes involved in the differential regulation of lung development and the response to lung injury have been probed to determine whether they participate in the pathogenesis of BPD. Two separate studies looking at polymorphisms of angiotensin-converting enzyme (ACE) hypothesized that increased ACE activity, leading to increased aldosterone production and increased water retention, would increase the incidence of BPD. Kazzi and Quasney[70] found that the polymorphism that conferred increased ACE activity showed increased incidence of BPD, whereas Yanamandra and colleagues[71] did not find an association between ACE activity and incidence of BPD.

Other groups have examined the role of polymorphisms in the gene encoding for GST. GST is an innate defense mechanism against ROS and is found in various human tissues. A polymorphism of the *GST-P1* gene produces two isoforms, one of which is significantly more efficient in eliminating oxidative toxins.[72,73] In a small pilot study of 35 infants with BPD, it was shown that infants who developed BPD were more likely to have the less efficient form of the enzyme.[74] Groups that have attempted to determine the role of various polymorphisms of the anti-inflammatory cytokines IL-4 and IL-10, the anti-inflammatory transforming growth factor-β (TGF-β), and the proinflammatory chemokine monocyte chemoattractant protein-1 have found no association between allelic variants and the development of BPD.[75-77]

Finally, the role of allelic variants of various surfactant proteins in the development of RDS and BPD has been explored. Specifically, the surfactant protein A (SP-A) allele 6A-6 is more common in infants with BPD.[78] Many loss-of-function mutations of the surfactant protein B (SP-B) gene have been reported. The clinical phenotype can vary, ranging from chronic respiratory failure to refractory hypoxic respiratory failure in the neonatal period.[79-81] One group looked at polymorphisms in intron 4 of the *SP-B* gene. They found that BPD was more common in infants who had the polymorphisms in intron 4.[82] The definition of BPD that they used was that of oxygen requirement at 28 postnatal days, however; if the definition of oxygen requirement at 36 weeks PMA was used, there were no differences in the wild-type versus the intron 4 variants.

Pathology

In surfactant-treated ELBW infants, the characteristic pathologic finding of BPD is disruption of lung development.[12] Decreased septation and alveolar hypoplasia lead to fewer and larger alveoli. Reduced microvascular development also may occur. These changes have been observed in infants who died of BPD,[83] biopsy specimens from severely affected infants, and a baboon model of the disorder.[18] These findings are in contrast to BPD seen in infants before the availability of surfactant replacement therapy. The prominent pathologic findings in those cases were airway injury, inflammation, and parenchymal fibrosis.[12,83] Similar changes may be seen in surfactant-treated infants who develop severe BPD. In severely affected infants, fibrosis, bronchial smooth muscle hypertrophy, and interstitial edema may be superimposed on the characteristic reduced numbers of alveoli and capillaries. Pulmonary vascular changes, such as abnormal arterial muscularization and obliteration of vessels, may occur.

Lung injury also is associated with increased elastic tissue formation and thickening of the interstitium. These tissue deformations may compromise septation and capillary development. Disturbed elastic tissue maturation was shown in a study of 44 infants, 23 to 30 weeks gestational age, who died at 5 to 59 days of age.[84] In infants with high respiratory scores computed from supplemental oxygen concentration and mean airway pressure, the volume, density, and absolute quantity of elastic tissue were significantly greater than those of infants with low scores or control infants. Alveolar and duct diameters and septal thickness also were greater. With increased elastic tissue content and thickened interstitium, the lungs tend to collapse at end expiration and have a low functional residual capacity (FRC).

Clinical Features

BPD predominantly affects ELBW infants, and most affected infants are ventilator-dependent from birth with severe RDS requiring surfactant therapy. The evolution to BPD typically is recognized at approximately 2 weeks of age as pulmonary function deteriorates rather than improves. The infant remains ventilator-dependent, and the concentration of supplemental oxygen must be increased to maintain adequate oxygen saturation. Wide swings in oxygenation may occur, likely caused by intermittent atelectasis.

Physical Examination

The physical examination is variable. Infants usually are tachypneic, and depending on the extent of pulmonary edema or atelectasis or both, they may have mild to severe retractions, and crackles may be audible. Intermittent expiratory wheezing may be present in infants with increased airway reactivity.

Chest Radiograph

As BPD evolves, the chest radiograph becomes diffusely hazy, reflecting inflammation or pulmonary edema or both (Fig. 1-3A), with low to normal lung volumes. There may be areas of atelectasis that alternate with areas of gas trapping, related to airway obstruction from secretions or other debris. The chest radiograph in infants who develop severe BPD shows hyperinflation (Fig. 1-3B). Streaky densities or cystic areas may be prominent, corresponding to fibrotic changes. During acute exacerbations, pulmonary edema may be apparent (Fig. 1-3C).

Clinical Course

Most infants improve gradually during the next 3 to 4 months. As pulmonary function improves, infants can be weaned to CPAP,

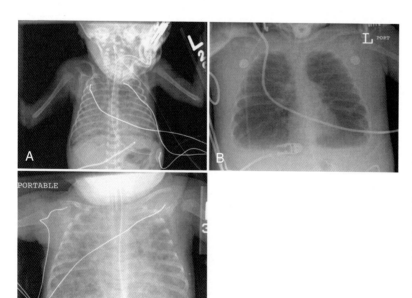

Figure 1-3. A, Chest radiograph of a former preterm (25 weeks gestation) infant on day of life (DOL) 10, with evolving lung disease. The diffuse haziness indicates pulmonary edema or inflammation or both. **B,** Chest radiograph of the same infant, now on DOL 285, with a tracheostomy tube in place. Note the extreme degree of hyperinflation and air trapping. Also evident are diffuse interstitial markings representing areas of fibrosis. **C,** Chest radiograph of the same infant, now on DOL 317. Cystic areas can be seen with hyperinflation, prominent lung markings, and areas of opacification, nearly obliterating bilateral heart borders. Significant pulmonary edema also is present, as seen by the marked diffuse bilateral haziness.

then supplemental oxygen alone, until they can maintain adequate oxygenation breathing room air. Some infants develop severe BPD that leads to prolonged ventilator dependence. The clinical course during the first few weeks after birth includes marked instability with frequent changes in oxygenation and intermittent episodes of acute deterioration requiring increased ventilator support. The marked instability typically improves after 4 to 6 weeks.

Severely affected infants may develop pulmonary hypertension and cor pulmonale.[85] Elevated pulmonary vascular resistance may impair pulmonary lymphatic drainage and exacerbate interstitial edema. In some cases, anastomoses develop between pulmonary and systemic vessels that may worsen the pulmonary hypertension.[85]

Cardiopulmonary Function

Abnormalities of pulmonary function in severe BPD include decreased tidal volume, increased airway resistance, and low dynamic lung compliance, which become frequency dependent. Uneven airway obstruction leads to air trapping and hyperinflation with abnormal distribution of ventilation.[86] Bronchomalacia can result in airway collapse during expiration, and severely affected infants can have hypoxemia and hypercapnia.

Pulmonary vascular resistance is increased because of reduced cross-sectional area of pulmonary vessels (Fig. 1-4). In addition, alveolar hypoxia in underventilated areas of the lung induces local vasoconstriction. Intact vessels in well-ventilated areas of the lung accept a disproportionate amount of

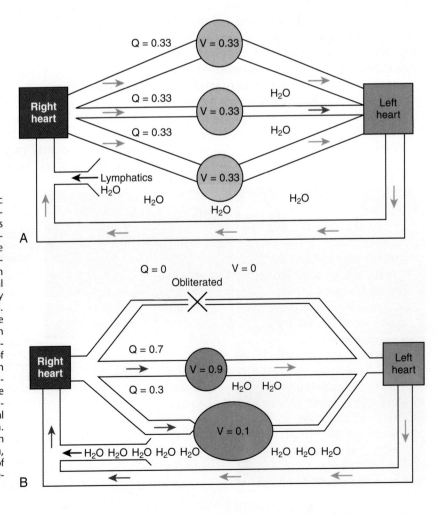

Figure 1-4. A, Schematic representation of the interaction of the heart and lungs in a normal infant. The pulmonary vascular resistance is low, and matching of ventilation (V) and perfusion (Q) is uniform. Interstitial fluid is cleared effectively by pulmonary lymphatics. **B,** Derangements of the heart-lung interaction in bronchopulmonary dysplasia. There is mismatching of ventilation (V) and perfusion (Q) with gas trapping. Pulmonary vascular resistance is elevated because of vascular obliteration and regional hypoxic vasoconstriction. Increased capillary filtration produces interstitial edema, and lymphatic drainage of the lung is impaired by elevated right heart pressures.

pulmonary blood flow. Because these vessels are already fully recruited and dilated, the additional flow results in elevated pressure and increased right ventricular afterload. The high microvascular pressure promotes increased fluid filtration into the perivascular interstitium. Elevated right atrial pressure inhibits pulmonary lymphatic drainage, further promoting pulmonary edema.

Management

The management of infants with BPD begins with prevention, attempting to avoid or minimize contributory factors.

Respiratory Care

Respiratory care of an infant with developing or established BPD is supportive and should aim to minimize additional lung injury by judicious use of mechanical ventilation and supplemental oxygen. Early use of continuous distending pressure in at-risk infants reduces the need for subsequent positive-pressure ventilation.[87] The COIN trial compared CPAP with mechanical ventilation in infants born at 25 to 28 weeks gestation. In a preliminary report, the authors found that there were no significant differences in the incidence of BPD (oxygen treatment at 36 weeks PMA), days of respiratory support, oxygen treatment, hospital stay, incidence of grade III or IV intraventricular hemorrhage, cystic periventricular leukomalacia, or home oxygen use.[88] There was an increased rate of pneumothorax in the CPAP group.

If mechanical ventilation is needed, the lowest peak airway pressure necessary to ventilate adequately should be used, and large tidal volumes should be avoided. Although this strategy is supported by few data in human neonates, the use of lower than routine tidal volumes decreased mortality and increased the number of ventilator-free days in adults with acute respiratory distress syndrome.[89] In addition, in a multicenter trial conducted by the NICHD Neonatal Research Network, the need for ventilator support at 36 weeks PMA was significantly lower in the minimal ventilation group, although this

strategy did not change the relative risk of death or BPD at 36 weeks PMA, the primary outcome.[90] Although the very low tidal volumes associated with high-frequency oscillatory ventilation (HFOV) might be expected to reduce the rate of BPD, only one of two large trials comparing HFOV and conventional ventilation in patients at the highest risk showed an effect.[91,92] This finding suggests that routine initial use of HFOV generally is not warranted.

The most appropriate range of arterial oxygenation in preterm infants with acute or chronic respiratory failure is unknown. High levels of oxygen saturation seem to offer no advantages, however, and pulmonary injury may result from the increased concentration of supplemental oxygen required to maintain higher saturations, as shown by two studies. In the STOP-ROP trial, providing supplemental oxygen to maintain higher compared with routine oxygen saturation (96% to 99% versus 89% to 94%) in infants with prethreshold retinopathy of prematurity did not reduce progression to threshold retinopathy of prematurity or the need for peripheral retinal ablation.[93] The incidence of pulmonary events, including pneumonia/exacerbation of BPD, and the need for oxygen, diuretics, and hospitalization at 3 months corrected age was higher, however, in the higher saturation group. Similarly, in the BOOST trial, in infants less than 30 weeks gestation who were oxygen dependent at 32 weeks PMA, no differences were detected in growth and neurodevelopment at 12 months corrected age—the primary outcomes—between the groups maintained at high (95% to 98%) or standard (91% to 94%) oxygen saturation ranges.[94] Infants in the high saturation group received oxygen for a longer time, however, and had higher rates of oxygen dependence at 36 weeks PMA and home oxygen therapy.

Respiratory management in infants with developing or established BPD should ensure adequate tissue oxygenation to promote growth and prevent pulmonary arterial hypertension that can result from chronic hypoxemia, and should minimize lung injury from excessive oxygen levels or mechanical ventilation. Although the safest levels are unknown, oxygen saturation is generally maintained in the 85% to 95% range, with PaO_2 greater than

50 mm Hg, and $PaCO_2$ should be allowed to increase to 50 to 60 mm Hg or possibly even higher in infants with the most severe disease as long as the pH is normal. When the infant is able to maintain adequate $PaCO_2$ and PaO_2 on the lowest ventilator settings, weaning from assisted ventilation should be attempted. Episodes of hypoxemia should be avoided because these are associated with increased airway resistance.[95,96] Supplemental oxygen may be needed for several months or longer in the most severe cases.

Nutrition and Fluid Management

Nutrition is a key component of the management of infants with BPD. Nutrition, supplied enterally or parenterally or both, must be sufficient to promote somatic growth and the development of new alveoli; this should facilitate weaning from mechanical ventilation and decrease vulnerability to infection that is associated with malnutrition.[97,98] Energy also must be sufficient to meet the demands of increased work of breathing. Plans for dietary support of infants with BPD who fail to thrive should consider that an excessive intake of carbohydrate might be associated with increased CO_2 production and impair respiratory function further. Insufficient caloric intake may potentiate oxygen toxicity and impair cell multiplication and lung growth. Deficiencies in sulfur-containing amino acids may reduce lung glutathione, an important antioxidant.[30] The adequacy of nutrition should be monitored closely, and growth charts for weight, head circumference, and length should be maintained.[97,98]

Vitamin deficiency may occur and interfere with lung healing. Vitamin A is an essential micronutrient for the normal growth and differentiation of epithelial cells. Vitamin A levels are lower in infants with severe BPD than in infants without BPD.[99,100] In animal models, low vitamin A levels contribute to airway abnormalities, such as loss of ciliated epithelium or squamous metaplasia, similar to histologic changes seen in BPD, and these changes are reversed by normalization of vitamin A levels.[101] Vitamin E is another important micronutrient and is a ubiquitous antioxidant. A small study has shown a strong correlation between low vitamin E levels in the cord blood and on the third day of life and the subsequent development of BPD,[102] but further studies are needed before the routine use of vitamin E supplementation can be recommended. Another key antioxidant that is deficient in preterm infants is vitamin C. In a pilot study with premature baboons, high-dose vitamin C treatment did not prevent pulmonary oxygen toxicity.[103] Of concern is that vitamin C in high doses can induce oxidative stress and have adverse effects on the developing lung.[31] At this time, it is recommended that specific vitamin deficiencies should be avoided in infants with BPD by providing adequate supplementation.

Inflammatory changes in the lungs of infants with BPD promote water retention. As a result, these infants tolerate excess fluid administration poorly,[97,104] and fluids should be modestly restricted (140 to 150 mL/kg/day) to avoid pulmonary edema. Further restriction may be needed in severely affected infants. Additional supplementation of human milk or formula with calories or protein or both may be required to ensure adequate nutrition in these infants.

Diuretics

Administration of the loop diuretic furosemide, hydrochlorothiazide, or spironolactone, which acts on the distal tubule, results in acute, nonsustained improvements in pulmonary mechanics.[105-107] The improvement in pulmonary mechanics seen with furosemide administration may be independent of its diuretic effect, as venous capacitance increases, and pulmonary blood flow decreases in response to furosemide administration.[108] In a Cochrane systematic review and meta-analysis, however, diuretic administration did not reduce the need for ventilator support, reduce the duration of hospital stay, or improve long-term outcomes. Long-term administration of a diuretic is often complicated by metabolic abnormalities, such as a hypokalemic, hypochloremic metabolic alkalosis, hypercalciuria leading to nephrocalcinosis, osteopenia, impaired growth, and hearing loss (with furosemide administration).

Although no evidence exists for long-term benefit, diuretics frequently are used in the management of infants with BPD to improve pulmonary function acutely. This use of diuretics may be beneficial in infants with a pulmonary exacerbation thought to be caused by pulmonary edema or to reduce the effects of circulatory overload after a packed red blood cell transfusion. Whether diuretic therapy facilitates optimal nutrition by reducing the need for fluid restriction requires further study. If diuretics are used, close monitoring of serum electrolytes is needed, and supplementation may be required to compensate for urinary losses.

Bronchodilator Therapy

Infants with severe BPD have increased baseline airway resistance that increases further with periods of hypoxemia, leading to respiratory decompensation owing to bronchoconstriction. This condition is sometimes treated with inhaled bronchodilators, a practice that has been extrapolated from the treatment of asthma. Infants with BPD treated with β-agonists respond with a short-term increase in compliance and tidal volume and decrease in airway resistance.[109,110] This treatment has not been shown to affect long-term outcome, however. In one trial in which 173 ventilator-dependent infants less than 31 weeks gestation were randomly assigned to inhaled salbutamol (albuterol), beclomethasone, combination salbutamol and beclomethasone, or placebo, treatment resulted in no difference in duration of mechanical ventilation or oxygen supplementation, diagnosis or severity of BPD at 28 days, or survival.[111] The efficacy of anticholinergic agents in the treatment of BPD has not been studied in randomized trials. Individual infants can be treated with bronchodilators to achieve short-term improvement in pulmonary mechanics. Continued use should depend on clinical response assessed by improvement in gas exchange and respiratory effort.

Corticosteroids

Administration of systemic corticosteroids to infants with evolving or established BPD reduces inflammation and improves lung mechanics, facilitating extubation.[112,113] Systemic corticosteroid use is associated with short-term adverse effects, however, such as hyperglycemia, glucosuria, and hypertension, and mortality is not reduced. In addition, outcome studies have suggested that corticosteroid treatment, especially dexamethasone, may contribute to poor neurodevelopmental outcome and cerebral palsy.[114] These concerns led the American Academy of Pediatrics Committee on Fetus and Newborn to recommend that the routine use of dexamethasone should be avoided and its use limited to extreme circumstances.[115] That the likelihood of dexamethasone treatment leading to adverse outcomes is influenced by the baseline risk of developing BPD was suggested by a meta-regression analysis.[116] Whether infants at extremely high baseline risk for developing BPD would benefit from dexamethasone remains to be established in clinical trials.

Data on the use of inhaled steroids are insufficient to recommend their routine use.[117] Corticosteroids given via a metered dose inhaler and holding chamber or nebulized budesonide have been used successfully, however, even in patients younger than 1 year.[118] The inhaled route is the preferred route for preventing side effects of systemic corticosteroids. Infants with CLDI treated with inhaled corticosteroids should be monitored for potential side effects, including delayed growth, increased blood pressure, osteoporosis, adrenal suppression, and cataracts.

Prevention

Antenatal Corticosteroids

Antenatal corticosteroids given to women at risk for preterm delivery decreases the risk of RDS, intraventricular hemorrhage, and mortality. They should be given to any pregnant woman 24 to 34 weeks gestation with intact membranes at high risk for preterm delivery within 7 days of administration. Treatment does not decrease the incidence of BPD, however, partly because increased survival has resulted in more infants at risk for the condition.

Fluid Restriction

Higher fluid intake associated with a lack of postnatal weight loss during the immediate postnatal period has been proposed as a predisposing risk factor for BPD. This hypothesis is supported by a retrospective report of premature infants (birth weight 401 to 1,000 g) from the Neonatal Research Center study that found infants who either died or developed BPD had a higher fluid intake and a lower weight loss during the first 10 days of life compared with infants who survived without BPD.[119] Small trials of fluid restriction have not shown a consistent effect on the development of BPD, although this strategy may minimize pulmonary edema.[120,121] In one study, 168 ventilated infants, gestational age 23 to 33 weeks, were randomly assigned to receive routine fluid volumes (60 mL/kg on the first day, progressing to 150 mL/kg on the seventh day) or 80% of routine volume.[120] Similar proportions in each group had BPD (26% versus 25%) and survived without oxygen dependency at 36 weeks PMA (58% versus 52%). Significantly fewer restricted infants received postnatal corticosteroid treatment (19% versus 43%), however, suggesting that their clinicians may have considered them less ill than were controls. In addition, the duration of oxygen requirement was significantly associated with colloid infusion.

Minimal Ventilation

Ventilation with high tidal volumes results in mechanical injury to the lung. Mechanical ventilation with small tidal volumes and target goals of modest permissive hypercapnia (PCO_2 50 to 55 mm Hg) may protect the lung from mechanical injury. The benefit of permissive hypercapnia has not been shown definitively in newborns at high risk for BPD, although additional studies are needed.[90,122,123] In one trial, infants with birth weight 501 to 1,000 g requiring mechanical ventilation before 12 hours of age were randomly assigned to minimal ventilation (target PCO_2 >52 mm Hg) or routine ventilation (PCO_2 <48 mm Hg) and a course of dexamethasone or placebo.[90] The trial was stopped after enrollment of 220 infants

because of excess adverse events in infants treated with dexamethasone. There was no difference between ventilator groups in the combined primary outcome of death or BPD. At 36 weeks PMA, the proportion of infants requiring mechanical ventilation was significantly less in the minimal group (16% versus 1%).

The lack of difference in lung injury between the minimal and routine ventilation groups may be due partly to an insufficient sample size. Another reason may be that target levels of PCO_2 rather than tidal volume distinguished the groups because the former usually is not measured continuously, and the difference in PCO_2 between groups was small. Because ventilated infants continued to breathe spontaneously, the measured PCO_2 reflected the selected airway pressure (which determines the tidal volume) and rate and the infant's own ventilation. Spontaneous breathing may have resulted in the modest increase in PCO_2 in the minimal ventilation group and minimized the difference between groups.

High-Frequency Oscillatory Ventilation

HFOV, a technique of rapid ventilation with very small tidal volumes, reduces lung injury in animal models compared with conventional ventilation. Nearly all trials comparing HFOV with conventional ventilation performed in preterm infants at risk for the disorder since surfactant replacement therapy has been available show no effect on the rate of BPD.[92,123-126]

In one trial in 500 preterm infants, 601 to 1,200 g birth weight, the proportion of infants who survived without BPD was slightly greater with HFOV (56% versus 47%).[91] This study was performed in centers experienced in the use of HFOV and followed strict protocols for management. Similar results may not be achieved at centers with less experience or without strict protocols.[92,127] It is recommended that conventional ventilation with low tidal volumes and modest hypercapnia, rather than HFOV, be employed as the initial mode of mechanical ventilation for most preterm infants.[127]

Vitamin A

Extremely preterm infants may have vitamin A deficiency, which may promote the development of BPD. Possible mechanisms include impaired lung healing, increased squamous cell metaplasia, reduced alveolar number, increased susceptibility to infection, and increased loss of cilia.[128] Supplementation with vitamin A reduces the risk of BPD in susceptible infants.

In the largest trial, 807 infants with birth weight 401 to 1,000 g who received mechanical ventilation or supplemental oxygen at 24 hours of age were randomly assigned to receive 5000 IU vitamin A intramuscularly three times per week for 4 weeks or a sham injection.[128] The combined outcome of death or BPD (oxygen requirement at 36 weeks PMA) occurred significantly less often in the vitamin A group compared with control group (55% versus 62%). No clinical or biochemical evidence of vitamin A toxicity was detected. In a subsequent study of the original cohort, vitamin A supplementation did not differ from placebo in reducing hospitalizations or pulmonary problems after discharge from the nursery.[129] In addition, at a corrected age of 18 to 22 months, there were no differences in mortality or neurodevelopmental impairment between the treated and nontreated infants. Some clinicians provide supplemental vitamin A (5000 IU intramuscularly three times per week for 4 weeks) to infants ≤1,000 g birth weight who require ventilatory support within 24 hours after birth. The decision to treat may depend on a balance of factors, such as the local incidence, the value of a modest decrease in BPD, and the need for repeated intramuscular injections.[130]

Systemic Corticosteroids

Administration of systemic corticosteroids reduces the risk of BPD. Routine use of corticosteroid therapy is not recommended, however, because there are concerns about significant short-term and long-term adverse effects. In systematic reviews by the Cochrane database, treatment with corticosteroids (usually dexamethasone) before 96 hours of age or at 7 to 14 days of age reduced the development of BPD at 36 weeks PMA and the need for oxygen supplementation at 28 postnatal days, and promoted earlier extubation, compared with control.[113,131] Survival did not improve with treatment, however. In addition, systemic corticosteroid use was associated with short-term adverse effects, including hypertension, hyperglycemia, poor growth, and gastrointestinal bleeding and perforation.[113,131]

Systematic reviews of long-term outcome (≤4 years of age) suggest that postnatal dexamethasone use increases neurodevelopmental delay and cerebral palsy.[115,116,132,133] A review that included nine randomized controlled trials of postnatal corticosteroids administered within the first week of life found that the risk of cerebral palsy was greater among surviving infants who were treated compared with controls (24% versus 14%, relative risk 1.75, 95% confidence interval 1.25 to 2.44).[116] A potential problem in the interpretation of these results is that many infants enrolled in trials of corticosteroids were treated with dexamethasone by their clinicians in addition to the study drug (open-label treatment).[132] Children who participated in one of the trials[134] included in the above-mentioned systematic reviews[115,116,132,133] were evaluated at school age.[135] Among the original cohort of 262 infants, 159 survived to school age, and 146 were included in follow-up (evenly distributed between treatment and control groups). Clinically significant disabilities (motor skills, coordination, visual motor integration, and IQ) were more common among children from the treatment group (39% versus 16%). Differing rates of disability persisted when the children who received open-label dexamethasone treatment were excluded from the analysis (41% versus 21%).

Even when administered in low doses or when other agents aside from dexamethasone are used, systemic corticosteroids are associated with serious adverse effects. In a multicenter trial, mechanically ventilated ELBW infants were randomly assigned to hydrocortisone therapy or placebo to determine whether prophylaxis of early adrenal insufficiency affected clinical stability and incidence of BPD.[136] Infants receiving hydrocortisone were treated with 1 mg/kg/day for 12 days and then 0.5 mg/kg/day for 3 days. Enrollment was discontinued early because of an increase of spontaneous gastrointestinal perforation in the hydrocortisone group (9% versus 2%). Overall survival without BPD did not differ between groups.

Although most of the data show the negative impact of corticosteroids, with risk of short-term and long-term adverse effects including impaired neurodevelopmental outcomes, it remains unclear whether there is a potential role for corticosteroids in selected populations. In the meta-analysis described earlier,[116] there was a significant negative correlation between the corticosteroid effect on combined outcome of death and cerebral palsy and the rate for BPD in the control groups. The rate of BPD was used as a marker for the risk for BPD and was not a variable available at trial entry. This relationship suggests that in a population of preterm infants at high risk for BPD, corticosteroid therapy may decrease the risk of death or cerebral palsy. At present, the American Academy of Pediatrics and the Canadian Pediatric Society recommend that dexamethasone should not be used routinely in VLBW infants to treat or prevent chronic lung disease because of its limited short-term benefits, no apparent long-term benefits, and substantial risk of short-term and long-term complications.[115] They further recommend that dexamethasone use should be limited to controlled trials. Outside of a trial, corticosteroids should be used only in exceptional clinical circumstances, such as an infant who requires maximal ventilatory and oxygen support. In this case, the parents should be made aware of potential risks and agree to treatment.

Inhaled Corticosteroids

In a systematic review and meta-analysis by the Cochrane database, early postnatal administration of inhaled corticosteroids did not prevent BPD, but was associated with lower rates of systemic corticosteroid treatment.[117] In the largest trial, 253 infants with gestational age less than 33 weeks and birth weight ≤1,250 g who were mechanically ventilated at 3 to 14 days of age were randomly assigned to a 4-week course of beclomethasone (tapering dose of 40 µg/kg/day to 5 µg/kg/day) or placebo.[137] The need for supplemental oxygen at 28 days (43% versus 45%) and 36 weeks PMA (18% versus 20%) was similar in the beclomethasone and placebo groups. Beclomethasone significantly reduced the rate of systemic corticosteroid use (relative risk 0.8) and mechanical ventilation (relative risk 0.8) at 28 days of age. No adverse effects were observed. In a separate report from the same trial, beclomethasone therapy was associated with slightly lower median basal cortisol levels (5 µg/dL versus 6 µg/dL) compared with placebo, but similar response to cosyntropin stimulation.[138]

Inhaled Nitric Oxide

Inhaled nitric oxide (iNO) is used in the management of term neonates with hypoxic respiratory failure, but little is known about the effects of iNO in the preterm population. Multiple physiologic effects of nitric oxide are known. Exposure to chronic hypoxemia leads to remodeling that includes increased proliferation of pulmonary vascular smooth muscle, leading to increased pulmonary vascular pressures, and eventual right ventricular hypertrophy and cor pulmonale. Several animal studies have shown that iNO prevents or ameliorates this remodeling of the pulmonary vascular bed.[139-142] Of particular concern is the effect of iNO on coagulation; iNO is known to increase bleeding time in adult patients, presumably via a cyclic guanosine monophosphate–dependent mechanism causing platelet dysfunction.[143,144] In a preterm infant already at risk for intraventricular hemorrhage, this complication would add significant long-term morbidity.

Several studies of the use of iNO in preterm neonates have been conducted, and several included BPD as an outcome.[145-149] A Cochrane systematic review and meta-analysis has shown that the use of iNO in infants less than 35 weeks of age does not show any benefit in terms of survival without BPD; there also is a trend toward an increase in the combined outcome of severe intraventricular hemorrhage or periventricular leukomalacia.[150]

Caffeine

Caffeine has been shown to reduce the frequency of apnea of prematurity and the need for mechanical ventilation.[151] A study of 1917 infants with birth weight 500 to 1,250 g showed that the rate of BPD (a secondary outcome) in infants treated with caffeine was significantly lower than in the placebo group (36% versus 47%).[151] The rates of adverse outcomes—specifically death, brain abnormalities by head ultrasonography, and necrotizing enterocolitis—were not different between the two groups. This cohort has been followed to assess the primary outcome measure, which is the combined rate of mortality and neurodevelopmental disability in survivors at a corrected age of 18 to 21 months, and the authors more recently reported improved survival without neurodevelopmental disability in the caffeine-treated group.[152] Neurodevelopmental outcomes in this cohort also will be followed up at 5 years of age.

Superoxide Dismutase

Preterm infants may have inadequate antioxidant defense because of nutrient deficiencies or immature enzyme development. Postnatal administration of antioxidants such as superoxide dismutase may protect against oxidant injury, although additional evidence is needed. In one study performed after replacement surfactant became available, 33 infants with birth weight 700 to 1,300 g who were mechanically ventilated for RDS were randomly assigned to intratracheal administration of recombinant human copper/zinc superoxide dismutase (rhSOD) (2.5 mg/kg or 5 mg/kg) or saline every 48 hours while they remained intubated, for up to seven doses.[153] Clinical outcomes did not differ between groups. Tracheal aspirate inflammatory markers (neutrophil chemotactic activity, albumin concentration) were lower, however, in the rhSOD groups than in the control group. In a larger multicenter trial, no difference was found in the rate of oxygen dependence at 28 postnatal days or 36 weeks PMA.[154] At 1 year of age, infants who received rhSOD had less respiratory illness, however. Growth and neurodevelopmental status were similar.

Summary

Multiple strategies are needed to prevent BPD in high-risk patients.
- Although antenatal corticosteroids do not affect the incidence of BPD, they reduce the risk of RDS and intraventricular hemorrhage, and improve survival in preterm infants. Antenatal corticosteroids should be given to pregnant women at high risk for preterm delivery.
- Excessive fluid administration should be avoided in ELBW infants, and fluids should be restricted to minimize the development of pulmonary edema. Use of colloid infusions should be avoided.
- Conventional ventilation with low tidal volumes and reasonable ventilation goals (initially, $PaCO_2$ 50 to 55 mm Hg) should be used in preterm infants with respiratory failure in most cases. In centers experienced with the technique, HFOV may be an appropriate alternative.
- Optimal nutrition should be provided to promote somatic and lung growth. Administration of supplemental vitamin A (5000 IU intramuscularly three times per week for 4 weeks) to ELBW infants who require early respiratory support should be considered.
- Routine use of postnatal dexamethasone should be avoided.
- Use of iNO to prevent BPD should await publication of follow-up studies.
- Caffeine decreases the rate of BPD in infants 500 to 1,250 g, without neurodevelopmental sequelae at 18 to 21 months of age.

Outcome

Mortality

Infants with severe BPD have a higher risk of mortality than unaffected infants or infants with mild disease. Death usually is caused by respiratory failure, unremitting pulmonary hypertension with cor pulmonale, or sepsis. The risk of mortality increases with the duration of mechanical ventilation. In one report, among 47 infants mechanically ventilated for more than 27 days, 20 died.[155] In another study of 144 newborns who required prolonged mechanical ventilation after birth, death occurred in 35% and 90% of infants ventilated for 2 months and more than 4 months.[156] At 30 days of age, the mean airway pressure and a diagnosis of bacterial sepsis during the previous month were significant predictors of mortality. In patients who still required ventilation at 60 days of age, mean airway pressure and oxygen concentration were the best predictors.

Respiratory Infections

Infants with BPD are at increased risk for respiratory infections, including respiratory syncytial virus (RSV), which may be life-threatening.[157] Episodes of wheezing that suggest bronchiolitis or asthma also are common before 2 years of age.[158] Respiratory illnesses contribute to high rates of rehospitalization, especially in the first year of life.[159-161] In one report, infants with BPD were rehospitalized more often during the first year (58% versus 35%) and more likely to be readmitted for respiratory illness (39% versus 20%) than controls.[159]

Pulmonary Function

Early Childhood
Infants with severe BPD may have abnormal pulmonary function tests for many years, even though some are asymptomatic.[158] Pulmonary function normalizes in early childhood in most cases, however, especially in infants with milder disease. In one study, 28 children (<3 years old) with a history of prematurity (mean gestational age 26.4 weeks, mean birth weight 898 g) and BPD underwent routinely scheduled infant lung testing at a mean age of 68 weeks.[162] Compared with a previously studied group of healthy term infants, infants with a

history of BPD had findings consistent with airflow obstruction and air trapping. In another study, 39 preterm infants (mean gestational age 29.8 weeks) with BPD had serial measurements of pulmonary function from 1 to 36 months of age.[163] Compared with normal controls, infants with BPD had evidence of decreased pulmonary function that remained fairly constant up to 6 months of age, and steadily improved by the 36-month follow-up. All of these infants still had mildly reduced pulmonary function parameters (approximately 85% of normal) at the 36-month follow-up. These findings are consistent with formation of new alveoli in early infancy, leading to improved compliance. Airway growth is slow during the first 6 months after birth, but subsequent faster growth results in improved conductance.

Late Childhood
In some patients, abnormal pulmonary function persists through later childhood. In one study, children 11 years old who had BPD had diminished airflow and higher residual volume compared with controls, but few had abnormalities that were clinically significant.[164] Similar findings were noted in a small but more contemporary series of patients with moderate to severe BPD, of whom most had pulmonary function testing at 24 months of age and at a mean of 8.8 years.[165,166] Among 18 children, 15 had mild to severe airflow limitation, with mean forced expiratory volume in 1 second (FEV_1) and forced mid-expiratory flow (FEF 25%-75%) less than 60% of predicted in 4 and 9 children. Abnormalities in childhood correlated with reduced maximal airflow values at functional residual capacity (FRC) measured in infancy. Most children had no signs of airway obstruction, although three had reduced exercise tolerance, and one used medication for asthma-like symptoms.

Neurodevelopment

Infants with severe BPD are at increased risk for neurodevelopmental sequelae. In a large cohort of ELBW infants cared for in the centers of the NICHD Neonatal Research

Network and evaluated at 18 to 22 months corrected age, BPD was a significant risk factor for abnormal neurologic examination and scores less than 70 (>2 standard deviations below the mean) on the mental development index and psychomotor development index scales of the Bayley Scales of Infant Development.[167] In a separate study, follow-up at 3 years of age showed that significantly more VLBW infants with BPD had scores less than 70 for the mental development index (21% versus 11% and 4%) and psychomotor development index (20% versus 9% and 1%) compared with control groups of unaffected VLBW infants and term infants.[168] In another report from the same center, children with BPD had poorer receptive and expressive language skills at 3 years old compared with controls.[169]

The effect of BPD on outcome persists through school age. In one study, VLBW infants with BPD tested at 8 to 10 years old scored poorest on all eight measures of cognitive performance compared with control groups of term and unaffected VLBW infants.[170] In another report, neuromotor outcome was evaluated at approximately 10 years of age in children who had severe BPD and required home oxygen therapy and was compared with neuromotor outcome of unaffected preterm controls.[171] Neurologic abnormalities, including subtle neurologic signs, cerebral palsy, microcephaly, and behavioral problems, were significantly more prevalent in the BPD group (71% versus 19%). More than half of the BPD group had abnormalities of gross or fine motor skills or both.

When interpreting follow-up studies such as the above-cited studies, many factors influence outcome, including incidence of neurologic risk factors (e.g., cranial ultrasound abnormalities), neurosensory problems (e.g., retinopathy of prematurity, hearing impairment), hospital course, and poor social environment. In one study, infants with BPD evaluated at 8 years had significantly poorer psychoeducational and school performance test scores than controls.[172] Most variance in academic achievement was attributed to the lowest recorded pH or PaO_2 and the father's socioeconomic status.

Growth

The effect of BPD on long-term growth is uncertain. Poor growth of infants with BPD was seen in some follow-up studies, although others have shown no difference from unaffected infants. One study followed 20 preterm infants with BPD for 2 years after term PMA.[173] The infants were severely growth restricted at term, with the average weight and height less than or equal to the 3rd percentile. Growth accelerated as respiratory symptoms improved. At 2 years, weight for boys and girls was 3rd to 10th percentile, and height was 10th to 25th percentiles for boys and girls respectively. In another series of 16 affected children evaluated at 2 years, height and weight were less than 10th percentile in 37% and 25%, respectively.[174]

In other reports, BPD does not seem to affect growth at 8 to 10 years of age, which might be influenced more by factors other than respiratory disease, such as low birth weight.[172,175] In one report, infants with BPD were significantly smaller than unaffected infants.[175] After adjustment for confounding variables, however, no significant differences were detected.

Tracheobronchomalacia

Abnormalities of the trachea and bronchi always must be considered in infants with BPD who remain persistently ventilator-dependent.[176] Depending on the series, 16% to 50% of infants with BPD show evidence of tracheobronchomalacia at bronchoscopy.[177-180] Owing to acute collapse of the airways, leading to a marked increase in total airway resistance and decreased airflow, infants can experience life-threatening episodes that are characterized by extreme difficulty in ventilation.[176] The use of bronchodilators generally worsens or prolongs these episodes.

Acquired tracheobronchomalacia is differentiated clinically from congenital tracheobronchomalacia by a history of airway intubation and mechanical ventilation. Other lesions that cause airway compression, such as vascular rings, hypertensive enlarged pulmonary arteries, and hyperinflated lobes, must be ruled out. Acquired tracheobronchomalacia in CLDI has been attributed to barotrauma, chronic or recurrent infection, and local effects of artificial airways. The immature trachea is a highly compliant structure that undergoes progressive stiffening with age.[181] These changes seem to parallel changes in cartilage mechanics, rather than passive properties of tracheal smooth muscle.

Infants with abnormal central airway collapse may be asymptomatic at rest or have wheezing, often unresponsive to bronchodilator therapy. Wheezing becomes prominent with increased expiratory effort, and cyanotic spells may result.

One treatment modality available after this diagnosis is made is CPAP via nasopharyngeal, endotracheal, or tracheostomy tube.[182] Zinman has shown that by providing sufficient CPAP to prevent collapse of the affected segment, dynamic lung compliance is increased, and airway resistance is decreased.[183]

Glottic and Subglottic Damage

Endotracheal intubation has been associated with injury to supraglottic, glottic, subglottic, and tracheal tissues in newborns.[184-185] Some degree of epithelial damage after endotracheal intubation is common, ranging from focal epithelial necrosis over the arytenoid or cricoid cartilages or vocal cords to extensive mucosal necrosis of the trachea. Because superficial lesions seen at the time of extubation often resolve without sequelae, early endoscopy after tracheal extubation overestimates the possibility of long-term damage. The relationship between acute laryngeal or subglottic damage and development of acquired subglottic stenosis is unclear.

Acquired subglottic stenosis has been reported to occur in about 10% of previously intubated neonates. Clinical manifestations include postextubation stridor, hoarseness, apnea, and bradycardia; failure to tolerate extubation; and cyanosis or pallor. Similar manifestations can result from vocal cord injuries, glottic or subglottic cysts or webs, laryngomalacia, or extrathoracic tracheomalacia. Fixed lesions of the glottis and subglottis often produce biphasic stridor, whereas variable lesions usually cause only inspiratory stridor. Postextubation stridor is a significant marker for the presence of moderate to severe subglottic stenosis or laryngeal injury.

Risk factors for laryngeal injury include intubation for 7 days or more and three or more intubations.[186] These same factors also are associated with acquired subglottic stenosis. Use of inappropriately large endotracheal tubes also is an important risk factor for the development of subglottic stenosis. A tube size-to-gestational age (in weeks) ratio greater than 0.1 has been correlated with acquired airway obstruction.[187]

Tracheal Stenosis, Bronchial Stenosis, or Granuloma Formation

Acquired tracheal and bronchial stenosis or granuloma formation has been reported in infants with CLDI 3 weeks to 17 months old.[180] Endoscopic findings consist of airway narrowing or obstruction by thickened respiratory mucosa or circumferential nodular or polypoid granulations in the distal trachea, often extending into main bronchi.[188]

Stenosis and granulation formation may not be complications of CLDI per se, but instead may be the result of extended endotracheal intubation and vigorous suctioning techniques. Because these lesions tend to occur in the distal trachea and right-sided bronchi, repeated mucosal injury from suction catheters has been implicated as the likely mechanism.

Acute mucosal injury to the carina and main bronchi occurs from unrestricted or "deep" suctioning.[189] The size of the catheter should be small enough (usually 5F to 6F in newborns) so as not to occlude the artificial airway completely, avoiding excessive negative pressure.[190] Catheters with multiple side holes on several planes are less likely to cause invagination of airway mucosa into the catheter than catheters with single side or end holes. Use of negative pressures greater than 50 to 80 cm H_2O increases the likelihood of mucosal damage and does not increase the efficiency of secretions removal.[191] The most important preventive measure is to limit passage of the suction catheter to the distal tip of the artificial airway, so that the airway mucosa is protected from injury.[192]

Monitoring

Infants with BPD need close monitoring to minimize further lung injury, reduce the risks of pulmonary and systemic hypertension, and promote adequate growth and development. This monitoring should begin during hospitalization and continue after discharge.

Cardiovascular Monitoring and Oxygenation

The pulmonary circulation in infants with BPD has structural, functional, and anatomic abnormalities.[189,190] Structural alterations include smooth muscle hyperplasia, increased fibroblast incorporation, and adventitial thickening. Functional abnormalities include impaired vasodilation and increased hypoxic vasoconstriction. Anatomic changes include decreased total blood vessel mass and decreased total surface area. These changes can result in pulmonary arterial and systemic arterial hypertension, eventually leading to right and left ventricular hypertrophy.[193] The major approach to avoid or treat pulmonary hypertension is maintaining adequate oxygenation, although pharmacologic treatment may be required in severe cases.[189,190] Generally, in infants with severe BPD who do not have pulmonary hypertension, oxygen saturations are maintained greater than 92%; in infants with pulmonary hypertension, saturations are maintained higher (94% to 96%).[194]

Serial echocardiographic screening for pulmonary arterial hypertension is recommended in premature infants with BPD who have gestational age at birth of less than or equal to 25 weeks or birth weight less than or equal to 600 g, small for gestational age, requirement for prolonged mechanical ventilation, oxygen requirement out of proportion to the severity of lung disease, or persistent poor growth despite adequate caloric intake.[195] A pediatric cardiologist should follow patients with pulmonary arterial hypertension. Cardiac catheterization may be recommended for patients with severe pulmonary hypertension to rule out anatomic cardiac disease, pulmonary vein stenosis, or pulmonary vein

occlusion, to assess the severity of pulmonary hypertension, to test the reactivity to oxygen or vasodilators, and to assess for development of large systemic-pulmonary collaterals.[196] Systemic blood pressure should be monitored routinely because of the risk of systemic hypertension.[191,192] Systemic hypertension should be treated if it is detected.

Growth

As previously noted, nutrition is an important component of the care of infants with CLD. Hospitalized infants should be weighed two to three times per week, and length and head circumference should be measured weekly. Biochemical monitoring, including measurement of blood urea nitrogen, albumin, calcium, phosphorus, and alkaline phosphatase, may assist with nutritional assessment. Serum electrolytes should be followed in infants on diuretic therapy, and supplements should be provided as needed. Infants who exhibit oromotor dysfunction or other feeding disorders inhibiting growth should be evaluated and receive specific intervention.

Development, Vision, and Hearing

As discussed previously, infants with BPD generally have poorer neurodevelopmental outcomes than unaffected infants.[168] Developmental assessment should begin while the infant is still hospitalized and continue on a regular basis after discharge. Infants should have serial eye examinations to detect retinopathy of prematurity or other eye disorders, and receive appropriate intervention. Routine hearing screening should be done to detect impairment, with early intervention by an audiologist if needed.

Coordination of Care and Discharge Planning

Infants with severe BPD usually have a prolonged hospitalization and require substantial planning for discharge to home and postdischarge care. Discharge should be planned by a multidisciplinary care team that ideally includes individuals with skills in neonatology, pulmonology, nursing, respiratory therapy, social work, child life, nutrition, physical and occupational therapy, and, if needed, audiology. This team can ease the transition from the hospital to the home environment for the infant and the rest of the family. Depending on the severity of CLDI, some infants may be discharged home on supplemental oxygen or, rarely, on mechanical ventilation. Parents and other potential caregivers need to be instructed in the administration of medications, preparation of any special nutritional formulas, and cardiopulmonary resuscitation. Finally, infants with severe BPD may develop respiratory failure after infection with respiratory syncytial virus, and infants younger than 2 years who required treatment for BPD within 6 months of the respiratory syncytial virus season should receive prophylaxis with palivizumab.

References

1. Northway WH Jr, Rosan RC, Porter DY: Pulmonary disease following respirator therapy of hyaline-membrane disease: Bronchopulmonary dysplasia. N Engl J Med 276:357-368, 1967.
2. Northway WH Jr, Rosan RC: Radiographic features of pulmonary oxygen toxicity in the newborn: Bronchopulmonary dysplasia. Radiology 91:49-58, 1968.
3. Bancalari E: Epidemiology and risk factors for the "new" bronchopulmonary dysplasia. NeoReviews 1:2-5, 2000.
4. Bancalari E: Changes in the pathogenesis and prevention of chronic lung disease of prematurity. Am J Perinatol 18:1-9, 2001.
5. Bancalari E: Bronchopulmonary dysplasia: Old problem, new presentation. J Pediatr 82:2-3, 2006.
6. Bancalari E, Claure N, Sosenko IR: Bronchopulmonary dysplasia: Changes in pathogenesis, epidemiology and definition. Semin Neonatol 8:63-71, 2003.
7. Kraybill EN, et al: Risk factors for chronic lung disease in infants with birth weights of 751 to 1000 grams. J Pediatr 115:115-120, 1989.
8. Sinkin RA, Cox C, Phelps DL: Predicting risk for bronchopulmonary dysplasia: Selection criteria for clinical trials. Pediatrics 86:728-736, 1990.
9. Marshall DD, et al: Risk factors for chronic lung disease in the surfactant era: A North Carolina population-based study of very low birth weight infants. North Carolina Neonatologists Association. Pediatrics 104:1345-1350, 1999.
10. Shennan AT, et al: Abnormal pulmonary outcomes in premature infants: Prediction from oxygen requirement in the neonatal period. Pediatrics 82:527-532, 1988.
11. Ehrenkranz RA, et al: Validation of the National Institutes of Health consensus definition of bronchopulmonary dysplasia. Pediatrics 116:1353-1360, 2005.
12. Jobe AH, Bancalari E: Bronchopulmonary dysplasia. Am J Respir Crit Care Med 163:1723-1729, 2001.
13. Walsh MC, et al: Safety, reliability, and validity of a physiologic definition of bronchopulmonary dysplasia. J Perinatol 23:451-456, 2003.
14. Walsh MC, et al: Impact of a physiologic definition on bronchopulmonary dysplasia rates. Pediatrics 114:1305-1311, 2004.
15. Lemons JA, et al: Very low birth weight outcomes of the National Institute of Child Health and Human Development Neonatal Research Network, January 1995 through December 1996. NICHD Neonatal Research Network. Pediatrics 107:E1, 2001.
16. Van Marter LJ, et al: Do clinical markers of barotrauma and oxygen toxicity explain interhospital variation in rates of chronic lung disease? The Neonatology Committee for the Developmental Network. Pediatrics 105:1194-1201, 2000.
17. Smith VC, et al: Trends in severe bronchopulmonary dysplasia rates between 1994 and 2002. J Pediatr 146:469-473, 2005.
18. Coalson JJ, et al: Neonatal chronic lung disease in extremely immature baboons. Am J Respir Crit Care Med 160:1333-1346, 1999.
19. Langston C, et al: Human lung growth in late gestation and in the neonate. Am Rev Respir Dis 129:607-613, 1984.
20. Randell SH, Young SI: Unique features of the immature lung that make it vulnerable to injury. In Nehgme RA Bland RD and Coalson JJ, eds: Chronic Lung Disease in Early Infancy. New York, Marcel Dekker, 2000, p 377.
21. Burri PH: Structural aspects of prenatal and postnatal development and growth of the lung. In McDonald JA, ed: Lung Growth and Development. New York, Marcel Dekker, 1997, p 1.
22. Jobe AH: Antenatal factors and the development of bronchopulmonary dysplasia. Semin Neonatol 8:9-17, 2003.
23. Jobe AH: Antenatal associations with lung maturation and infection. J Perinatol 25(Suppl 2):S31-S35, 2005.
24. Bry K, Lappalainen U, Hallman M: Intraamniotic interleukin-1 accelerates surfactant protein synthesis in fetal rabbits and improves lung stability after premature birth. J Clin Invest 99:2992-2999, 1997.
25. Kramer BW, et al: Endotoxin-induced chorioamnionitis modulates innate immunity of monocytes in preterm sheep. Am J Respir Crit Care Med 171:73-77, 2005.
26. Kallapur SG, Jobe AH: Contribution of inflammation to lung injury and development. Arch Dis Child Fetal Neonatal Ed 91:F132-F135, 2006.
27. Kallapur SG, et al: Maternal glucocorticoids increase endotoxin-induced lung inflammation in preterm lambs. Am J Physiol Lung Cell Mol Physiol 284:L633-L642, 2003.
28. Denis D, et al: Prolonged moderate hyperoxia induces hyperresponsiveness and airway inflammation in newborn rats. Pediatr Res 50:515-519, 2001.
29. Dieperink HI, Blackwell TS, Prince LS: Hyperoxia and apoptosis in developing mouse lung mesenchyme. Pediatr Res 59:185-190, 2006.

30. Asikainen TM, White CW: Antioxidant defenses in the preterm lung: Role for hypoxia-inducible factors in BPD? Toxicol Appl Pharmacol 203: 177-188, 2005.
31. Saugstad OD: Bronchopulmonary dysplasia—oxidative stress and antioxidants. Semin Neonatol 8:39-49, 2003.
32. Wilborn AM, Evers LB, Canada AT: Oxygen toxicity to the developing lung of the mouse: Role of reactive oxygen species. Pediatr Res 40:225-232, 1996.
33. Frank L, Sosenko IR: Development of lung antioxidant enzyme system in late gestation: Possible implications for the prematurely born infant. J Pediatr 110:9-14, 1987.
34. Frank L, Sosenko IR: Failure of premature rabbits to increase antioxidant enzymes during hyperoxic exposure: Increased susceptibility to pulmonary oxygen toxicity compared with term rabbits. Pediatr Res 29:292-296, 1991.
35. Georgeson GD, et al: Antioxidant enzyme activities are decreased in preterm infants and in neonates born via caesarean section. Eur J Obstet Gynecol Reprod Biol 103:136-139, 2002.
36. Fu RH, et al: Erythrocyte Cu/Zn superoxide dismutase activity in preterm infants with and without bronchopulmonary dysplasia. Biol Neonate 88:35-41, 2005.
37. Nilsson R, Grossmann G, Robertson B: Lung surfactant and the pathogenesis of neonatal bronchiolar lesions induced by artificial ventilation. Pediatr Res 12(4 Pt 1):249-255, 1978.
38. Robertson B: The evolution of neonatal respiratory distress syndrome into chronic lung disease. Eur Respir J Suppl 3:33s-37s, 1989.
39. Goldman SL, et al: Early prediction of chronic lung disease by pulmonary function testing. J Pediatr 102:613-617, 1983.
40. Hernandez LA, et al: Chest wall restriction limits high airway pressure-induced lung injury in young rabbits. J Appl Physiol 66:2364-2368, 1989.
41. Carlton DP, et al: Lung overexpansion increases pulmonary microvascular protein permeability in young lambs. J Appl Physiol 69:577-583, 1990.
42. Dreyfuss D, Saumon G: Role of tidal volume, FRC, and end-inspiratory volume in the development of pulmonary edema following mechanical ventilation. Am Rev Respir Dis 148:1194-1203, 1993.
43. Bjorklund LJ, et al: Manual ventilation with a few large breaths at birth compromises the therapeutic effect of subsequent surfactant replacement in immature lambs. Pediatr Res 42:348-355, 1997.
44. Wada K, Jobe AH, Ikegami M: Tidal volume effects on surfactant treatment responses with the initiation of ventilation in preterm lambs. J Appl Physiol 83:1054-1061, 1997.
45. Garland JS, et al: Hypocarbia before surfactant therapy appears to increase bronchopulmonary dysplasia risk in infants with respiratory distress syndrome. Arch Pediatr Adolesc Med 149: 617-622, 1995.
46. Speer CP: Inflammation and bronchopulmonary dysplasia. Semin Neonatol 8:29-38, 2003.
47. Vlahakis NE, et al: Stretch induces cytokine release by alveolar epithelial cells in vitro. Am J Physiol 277(1 Pt 1):L167-L173, 1999.
48. Ben-Ari J, et al: Cytokine response during hyperoxia: Sequential production of pulmonary tumor necrosis factor and interleukin-6 in neonatal rats. Isr Med Assoc J 2:365-369, 2000.
49. Yoon BH, et al: Amniotic fluid cytokines (interleukin-6, tumor necrosis factor-alpha, interleukin-1 beta, and interleukin-8) and the risk for the development of bronchopulmonary dysplasia. Am J Obstet Gynecol 177:825-830, 1997.
50. Stoll BJ, et al: Late-onset sepsis in very low birth weight neonates: The experience of the NICHD Neonatal Research Network. Pediatrics 110(2 Pt 1):285-291, 2002.
51. Young KC, et al: The association between early tracheal colonization and bronchopulmonary dysplasia. J Perinatol 25:403-407, 2005.
52. Rojas MA, et al: Changing trends in the epidemiology and pathogenesis of neonatal chronic lung disease. J Pediatr 126:605-610, 1995.
53. Hannaford K, et al: Role of *Ureaplasma urealyticum* in lung disease of prematurity. Arch Dis Child Fetal Neonatal Ed 81:F162-F167, 1999.
54. Ozdemir A, Brown MA, Morgan WJ: Markers and mediators of inflammation in neonatal lung disease. Pediatr Pulmonol 23:292-306, 1997.
55. Groneck P, et al: Association of pulmonary inflammation and increased microvascular permeability during the development of bronchopulmonary dysplasia: A sequential analysis of inflammatory mediators in respiratory fluids of high-risk preterm neonates. Pediatrics 93:712-718, 1994.
56. Groneck P, et al: Bronchoalveolar inflammation following airway infection in preterm infants with chronic lung disease. Pediatr Pulmonol 31: 331-338, 2001.
57. Groneck P, Speer CP: Inflammatory mediators and bronchopulmonary dysplasia. Arch Dis Child Fetal Neonatal Ed 73:F1-F3, 1995.
58. Johnson DE, et al: Pulmonary neuroendocrine cells in hyaline membrane disease and bronchopulmonary dysplasia. Pediatr Res 16:446-454, 1982.
59. Sunday ME, Shan L, Subramaniam M: Immunomodulatory functions of the diffuse neuroendocrine system: Implications for bronchopulmonary dysplasia. Endocr Pathol 15:91-106, 2004.
60. Sunday ME, et al: Bombesin-like peptide mediates lung injury in a baboon model of bronchopulmonary dysplasia. J Clin Invest 102:584-594, 1998.
61. Cullen A, et al: Urine bombesin-like peptide elevation precedes clinical evidence of bronchopulmonary dysplasia. Am J Respir Crit Care Med 165:1093-1097, 2002.
62. Biniwale MA, Ehrenkranz RA: The role of nutrition in the prevention and management of bronchopulmonary dysplasia. Semin Perinatol 30:200-208, 2006.
63. Frank L, Sosenko IR: Undernutrition as a major contributing factor in the pathogenesis of bronchopulmonary dysplasia. Am Rev Respir Dis 138: 725-729, 1988.
64. Radmacher PG, Rafail ST, Adamkin DH: Nutrition and growth in VVLBW infants with and without bronchopulmonary dysplasia. Neonatal Intensive Care 16:22-26, 2004.
65. Chen SJ, Vohr BR, Oh W: Effects of birth order, gender, and intrauterine growth retardation on the outcome of very low birth weight in twins. J Pediatr 123:132-136, 1993.
66. Nielsen HC, et al: Neonatal outcome of very premature infants from multiple and singleton gestations. Am J Obstet Gynecol 177:653-659, 1997.
67. Parker RA, Lindstrom DP, Cotton RB: Evidence from twin study implies possible genetic

susceptibility to bronchopulmonary dysplasia. Semin Perinatol 20:206-209, 1996.

68. Parton LA, et al: The genetic basis for bronchopulmonary dysplasia. Front Biosci 11:1854-1860, 2006.

69. Shinwell ES, et al: Effect of birth order on neonatal morbidity and mortality among very low birth-weight twins: A population based study. Arch Dis Child Fetal Neonatal Ed 89:F145-F148, 2004.

70. Kazzi SN, Quasney MW: Deletion allele of angiotensin-converting enzyme is associated with increased risk and severity of bronchopulmonary dysplasia. J Pediatr 147:818-822, 2005.

71. Yanamandra K, Loggins J, Baier RJ: The angiotensin converting enzyme insertion/deletion polymorphism is not associated with an increased risk of death or bronchopulmonary dysplasia in ventilated very low birth weight infants. BMC Pediatr 4:26, 2004.

72. Hayes JD, Strange RC: Glutathione S-transferase polymorphisms and their biological consequences. Pharmacology 61:154-166, 2000.

73. Spiteri MA, et al: Polymorphisms at the glutathione S-transferase, GSTP1 locus: A novel mechanism for susceptibility and development of atopic airway inflammation. Allergy 55(Suppl 61):15-20, 2000.

74. Manar MH, et al: Association of glutathione-S-transferase-P1 (GST-P1) polymorphisms with bronchopulmonary dysplasia. J Perinatol 24: 30-35, 2004.

75. Lin HC, et al: Nonassociation of interleukin 4 intron 3 and 590 promoter polymorphisms with bronchopulmonary dysplasia for ventilated preterm infants. Biol Neonate 87:181-186, 2005.

76. Yanamandra K, et al: Interleukin-10-1082 G/A polymorphism and risk of death or bronchopulmonary dysplasia in ventilated very low birth weight infants. Pediatr Pulmonol 39:426-432, 2005.

77. Adcock K, et al: The TNF-alpha-308, MCP-1-2518 and TGF-beta1 +915 polymorphisms are not associated with the development of chronic lung disease in very low birth weight infants. Genes Immun 4:420-426, 2003.

78. Weber B, et al: Polymorphisms of surfactant protein A genes and the risk of bronchopulmonary dysplasia in preterm infants. Turk J Pediatr 42:181-185, 2000.

79. Clark JC, et al: Decreased lung compliance and air trapping in heterozygous SP-B-deficient mice. Am J Respir Cell Mol Biol 16:46-52, 1997.

80. Dunbar AE 3rd, et al: Prolonged survival in hereditary surfactant protein B (SP-B) deficiency associated with a novel splicing mutation. Pediatr Res 48:275-282, 2000.

81. Whitsett JA, et al: Human surfactant protein B: Structure, function, regulation, and genetic disease. Physiol Rev 75:749-757, 1995.

82. Makri V, et al: Polymorphisms of surfactant protein B encoding gene: Modifiers of the course of neonatal respiratory distress syndrome? Eur J Pediatr 161:604-608, 2002.

83. Husain AN, Siddiqui NH, Stocker JT: Pathology of arrested acinar development in postsurfactant bronchopulmonary dysplasia. Hum Pathol 29:710-717, 1998.

84. Thibeault DW, et al: Lung elastic tissue maturation and perturbations during the evolution of chronic lung disease. Pediatrics 106:1452-1459, 2000.

85. Goodman G, et al: Pulmonary hypertension in infants with bronchopulmonary dysplasia. J Pediatr 112:67-72, 1988.

86. Watts JL, Ariagno RL, Brady JP: Chronic pulmonary disease in neonates after artificial ventilation: Distribution of ventilation and pulmonary interstitial emphysema. Pediatrics 60:273-281, 1977.

87. Ho JJ, Henderson-Smart DJ, Davis PG: Early versus delayed initiation of continuous distending pressure for respiratory distress syndrome in preterm infants. Cochrane Database Syst Rev 2:CD002975, 2002.

88. Morley CJ, Davis PG, et al: N Engl J Med, 358(7):700-708, 2008.

89. Ventilation with lower tidal volumes as compared with traditional tidal volumes for acute lung injury and the acute respiratory distress syndrome. The Acute Respiratory Distress Syndrome Network. N Engl J Med 342:1301-1308, 2000.

90. Carlo WA, et al: Minimal ventilation to prevent bronchopulmonary dysplasia in extremely-low-birth-weight infants. J Pediatr 141:370-374, 2002.

91. Courtney SE, et al: High-frequency oscillatory ventilation versus conventional mechanical ventilation for very-low-birth-weight infants. N Engl J Med 347:643-652, 2002.

92. Johnson AH, et al: High-frequency oscillatory ventilation for the prevention of chronic lung disease of prematurity. N Engl J Med 347:633-642, 2002.

93. Supplemental Therapeutic Oxygen for Prethreshold Retinopathy Of Prematurity (STOP-ROP), a randomized, controlled trial, I: Primary outcomes. Pediatrics 105:295-310, 2000.

94. Askie LM, et al: Oxygen-saturation targets and outcomes in extremely preterm infants. N Engl J Med 349:959-967, 2003.

95. Tay-Uyboco JS, et al: Hypoxic airway constriction in infants of very low birth weight recovering from moderate to severe bronchopulmonary dysplasia. J Pediatr 115:456-459, 1989.

96. Teague WG, et al: An acute reduction in the fraction of inspired oxygen increases airway constriction in infants with chronic lung disease. Am Rev Respir Dis 137:861-865, 1988.

97. Bancalari EH: Neonatal chronic lung disease. In Fanaroff AA, Martin RJ, eds: Neonatal-Perinatal Medicine: Diseases of the Fetus and Infant. St Louis, Mosby, 2002, p 1057.

98. Huysman WA, et al: Growth and body composition in preterm infants with bronchopulmonary dysplasia. Arch Dis Child Fetal Neonatal Ed 88: F46-F51, 2003.

99. Mactier H, et al: Inadequacy of IV vitamin A supplementation of extremely preterm infants? J Pediatr 146:846-847, author reply 847-848, 2005.

100. Mactier H, Weaver LT: Vitamin A and preterm infants: What we know, what we don't know, and what we need to know. Arch Dis Child Fetal Neonatal Ed 90:F103-F108, 2005.

101. Shenai JP: Vitamin A supplementation in very low birth weight neonates: Rationale and evidence. Pediatrics 104:1369-1374, 1999.

102. Falciglia HS, et al: Role of antioxidant nutrients and lipid peroxidation in premature infants with respiratory distress syndrome and bronchopulmonary dysplasia. Am J Perinatol 20:97-107, 2003.

103. Berger TM, et al: Early high dose antioxidant vitamins do not prevent bronchopulmonary dysplasia in premature baboons exposed to prolonged

hyperoxia: A pilot study. Pediatr Res 43:719-726, 1998.

104. Adams JM, Stark AR: Management of bronchopulmonary dysplasia. UpToDate Online 13.2 2005 March 24, 2005.

105. Kao LC, et al: Effect of oral diuretics on pulmonary mechanics in infants with chronic bronchopulmonary dysplasia: Results of a double-blind crossover sequential trial. Pediatrics 74:37-44, 1984.

106. Kao LC, et al: Furosemide acutely decreases airways resistance in chronic bronchopulmonary dysplasia. J Pediatr 103:624-629, 1983.

107. Rush MG, et al: Double-blind, placebo-controlled trial of alternate-day furosemide therapy in infants with chronic bronchopulmonary dysplasia. J Pediatr 117(1 Pt 1):112-118, 1990.

108. Bancalari E, Wilson-Costello D, Iben SC: Management of infants with bronchopulmonary dysplasia in North America. Early Hum Dev 81:171-179, 2005.

109. Sosulski R, et al: Physiologic effects of terbutaline on pulmonary function of infants with bronchopulmonary dysplasia. Pediatr Pulmonol 2:269-273, 1986.

110. Wilkie RA, Bryan MH: Effect of bronchodilators on airway resistance in ventilator-dependent neonates with chronic lung disease. J Pediatr 111:278-282, 1987.

111. Denjean A, et al: Inhaled salbutamol and beclomethasone for preventing broncho-pulmonary dysplasia: A randomised double-blind study. Eur J Pediatr 157:926-931, 1998.

112. Halliday HL, Ehrenkranz RA, Doyle LW: Delayed (>3 weeks) postnatal corticosteroids for chronic lung disease in preterm infants. Cochrane Database Syst Rev 1:CD001145, 2003.

113. Halliday HL, Ehrenkranz RA, Doyle LW: Moderately early (7-14 days) postnatal corticosteroids for preventing chronic lung disease in preterm infants. Cochrane Database Syst Rev 1:CD001144, 2003.

114. O'Shea TM, et al: Randomized placebo-controlled trial of a 42-day tapering course of dexamethasone to reduce the duration of ventilator dependency in very low birth weight infants: Outcome of study participants at 1-year adjusted age. Pediatrics 104(1 Pt 1):15-21, 1999.

115. Committee on Newborn and Fetus: Postnatal corticosteroids to treat or prevent chronic lung disease in preterm infants. Pediatrics 109:330-338, 2002.

116. Doyle LW, et al: Impact of postnatal systemic corticosteroids on mortality and cerebral palsy in preterm infants: Effect modification by risk for chronic lung disease. Pediatrics 115:655-661, 2005.

117. Shah V, et al: Early administration of inhaled corticosteroids for preventing chronic lung disease in ventilated very low birth weight preterm neonates. Cochrane Database Syst Rev 2:CD001969, 2000.

118. Yuksel B, Greenough A. Randomised trial of inhaled steroids in preterm infants with respiratory symptoms of follow up. Thorax 47:910-913, 1992.

119. Oh W, et al: Association between fluid intake and weight loss during the first ten days of life and risk of bronchopulmonary dysplasia in extremely low birth weight infants. J Pediatr 147:786-790, 2005.

120. Kavvadia V, et al: Randomised trial of fluid restriction in ventilated very low birthweight infants. Arch Dis Child Fetal Neonatal Ed 83:F91-F96, 2000.

121. Tammela OK, Lanning FP, Koivisto ME: The relationship of fluid restriction during the 1st month of life to the occurrence and severity of bronchopulmonary dysplasia in low birth weight infants: A 1-year radiological follow up. Eur J Pediatr 151:367-371, 1992.

122. Mariani G, Cifuentes J, Carlo WA: Randomized trial of permissive hypercapnia in preterm infants. Pediatrics 104(5 Pt 1):1082-1088, 1999.

123. Woodgate PG, Davies MW: Permissive hypercapnia for the prevention of morbidity and mortality in mechanically ventilated newborn infants. Cochrane Database Syst Rev 2:CD002061, 2002.

124. Moriette G, et al: Prospective randomized multicenter comparison of high-frequency oscillatory ventilation and conventional ventilation in preterm infants of less than 30 weeks with respiratory distress syndrome. Pediatrics 107:363-372, 2001.

125. Ogawa Y, et al: A multicenter randomized trial of high frequency oscillatory ventilation as compared with conventional mechanical ventilation in preterm infants with respiratory failure. Early Hum Dev 32:1-10, 1993.

126. Thome U, et al: Randomized comparison of high-frequency ventilation with high-rate intermittent positive pressure ventilation in preterm infants with respiratory failure. J Pediatr 135:39-46, 1999.

127. Stark AR: High-frequency oscillatory ventilation to prevent bronchopulmonary dysplasia—are we there yet? N Engl J Med 347:682-684, 2002.

128. Tyson JE, et al: Vitamin A supplementation for extremely-low-birth-weight infants. National Institute of Child Health and Human Development Neonatal Research Network. N Engl J Med 340:1962-1968, 1999.

129. Ambalavanan N, et al: Vitamin A supplementation for extremely low birth weight infants: Outcome at 18 to 22 months. Pediatrics 115: e249-e254, 2005.

130. Darlow BA, Graham PJ: Vitamin A supplementation for preventing morbidity and mortality in very low birthweight infants. Cochrane Database Syst Rev 2:CD000501, 2000.

131. Halliday HL, Ehrenkranz RA, Doyle LW: Early postnatal (<96 hours) corticosteroids for preventing chronic lung disease in preterm infants. Cochrane Database Syst Rev 1:CD001146, 2003.

132. Barrington KJ: The adverse neuro-developmental effects of postnatal steroids in the preterm infant: A systematic review of RCTs. BMC Pediatr 1:1, 2001.

133. Doyle L, Davis P: Postnatal corticosteroids in preterm infants: Systematic review of effects on mortality and motor function. J Paediatr Child Health 36:101-107, 2000.

134. Yeh TF, et al: Early postnatal dexamethasone therapy for the prevention of chronic lung disease in preterm infants with respiratory distress syndrome: A multicenter clinical trial. Pediatrics 100:E3, 1997.

135. Yeh TF, et al: Outcomes at school age after postnatal dexamethasone therapy for lung disease of prematurity. N Engl J Med 350:1304-1313, 2004.

136. Watterberg KL, et al: Prophylaxis of early adrenal insufficiency to prevent bronchopulmonary dysplasia: A multicenter trial. Pediatrics 114:1649-1657, 2004.

137. Cole CH, et al: Early inhaled glucocorticoid therapy to prevent bronchopulmonary dysplasia. N Engl J Med 340:1005-1010, 1999.

138. Cole CH, et al: Adrenal function in premature infants during inhaled beclomethasone therapy. J Pediatr 135:65-70, 1999.

139. Garg UC, Hassid A: Nitric oxide-generating vasodilators and 8-bromo-cyclic guanosine monophosphate inhibit mitogenesis and proliferation of cultured rat vascular smooth muscle cells. J Clin Invest 83:1774-1777, 1989.

140. Kouyoumdjian C, et al: Continuous inhalation of nitric oxide protects against development of pulmonary hypertension in chronically hypoxic rats. J Clin Invest 94:578-584, 1994.

141. Roberts JD Jr, et al: Continuous nitric oxide inhalation reduces pulmonary arterial structural changes, right ventricular hypertrophy, and growth retardation in the hypoxic newborn rat. Circ Res 76:215-222, 1995.

142. Scott-Burden T, et al: Growth factor regulation of interleukin-1 beta-induced nitric oxide synthase and GTP:cyclohydrolase expression in cultured smooth muscle cells. Biochem Biophys Res Commun 196:1261-1266, 1993.

143. Hogman M, et al: Bleeding time prolongation and NO inhalation. Lancet 341:1664-1665, 1993.

144. Samama CM, et al: Inhibition of platelet aggregation by inhaled nitric oxide in patients with acute respiratory distress syndrome. Anesthesiology 83:56-65, 1995.

145. Ballard RA, et al: Inhaled nitric oxide in preterm infants undergoing mechanical ventilation. N Engl J Med 355:343-353, 2006.

146. Kinsella JP, et al: Early inhaled nitric oxide therapy in premature newborns with respiratory failure. N Engl J Med 355:354-364, 2006.

147. Schreiber MD, et al: Inhaled nitric oxide in premature infants with the respiratory distress syndrome. N Engl J Med 349:2099-2107, 2003.

148. Subhedar NV, Shaw NJ: Changes in oxygenation and pulmonary haemodynamics in preterm infants treated with inhaled nitric oxide. Arch Dis Child Fetal Neonatal Ed 77:F191-F197, 1997.

149. Van Meurs KP, et al: Inhaled nitric oxide for premature infants with severe respiratory failure. N Engl J Med 353:13-22, 2005.

150. Barrington KJ, Finer NN: Inhaled nitric oxide for respiratory failure in preterm infants. Cochrane Database Syst Rev 3:CD000509, 2007.

151. Schmidt B, et al: Caffeine therapy for apnea of prematurity. N Engl J Med 354:2112-2121, 2006.

152. Schmidt B, et al: Long-term effects of caffeine therapy for apnea of prematurity. N Engl J Med 357:1893-1902, 2007.

153. Davis JM, et al: Safety and pharmacokinetics of multiple doses of recombinant human CuZn superoxide dismutase administered intratracheally to premature neonates with respiratory distress syndrome. Pediatrics 100:24-30, 1997.

154. Davis JM, et al: Pulmonary outcome at 1 year corrected age in premature infants treated at birth with recombinant human CuZn superoxide dismutase. Pediatrics 111:469-476, 2003.

155. Wheater M, Rennie JM: Poor prognosis after prolonged ventilation for bronchopulmonary dysplasia. Arch Dis Child Fetal Neonatal Ed 71:F210-F211, 1994.

156. Overstreet DW, et al: Estimation of mortality risk in chronically ventilated infants with bronchopulmonary dysplasia. Pediatrics 88:1153-1160, 1991.

157. Groothuis JR, Gutierrez KM, Lauer BA: Respiratory syncytial virus infection in children with bronchopulmonary dysplasia. Pediatrics 82:199-203, 1988.

158. Bancalari E: Neonatal chronic lung disease. In Fanaroff AA, Martin RJ, eds: Neonatal-Perinatal Medicine: Diseases of the Fetus and Infant, 8th ed. Philadelphia, Elsevier, 2006.

159. Chye JK, Gray PH: Rehospitalization and growth of infants with bronchopulmonary dysplasia: A matched control study. J Paediatr Child Health 31:105-111, 1995.

160. Gross SJ, et al: Effect of preterm birth on pulmonary function at school age: A prospective controlled study. J Pediatr 133:188-192, 1998.

161. Smith VC, et al: Rehospitalization in the first year of life among infants with bronchopulmonary dysplasia. J Pediatr 144:799-803, 2004.

162. Robin B, et al: Pulmonary function in bronchopulmonary dysplasia. Pediatr Pulmonol 37:236-242, 2004.

163. Gerhardt T, et al: Serial determination of pulmonary function in infants with chronic lung disease. J Pediatr 110:448-456, 1987.

164. Blayney M, et al: Bronchopulmonary dysplasia: Improvement in lung function between 7 and 10 years of age. J Pediatr 118:201-206, 1991.

165. Baraldi E, et al: Pulmonary function until two years of life in infants with bronchopulmonary dysplasia. Am J Respir Crit Care Med 155:149-155, 1997.

166. Filippone M, et al: Flow limitation in infants with bronchopulmonary dysplasia and respiratory function at school age. Lancet 361:753-754, 2003.

167. Vohr BR, et al: Neurodevelopmental and functional outcomes of extremely low birth weight infants in the National Institute of Child Health and Human Development Neonatal Research Network, 1993-1994. Pediatrics 105:1216-1226, 2000.

168. Singer L, et al: A longitudinal study of developmental outcome of infants with bronchopulmonary dysplasia and very low birth weight. Pediatrics 100:987-993, 1997.

169. Singer LT, et al: Preschool language outcomes of children with history of bronchopulmonary dysplasia and very low birth weight. J Dev Behav Pediatr 22:19-26, 2001.

170. Hughes CA, et al: Cognitive performance at school age of very low birth weight infants with bronchopulmonary dysplasia. J Dev Behav Pediatr 20:1-8, 1999.

171. Majnemer A, et al: Severe bronchopulmonary dysplasia increases risk for later neurological and motor sequelae in preterm survivors. Dev Med Child Neurol 42:53-60, 2000.

172. Robertson CM, et al: Eight-year school performance, neurodevelopmental, and growth outcome of neonates with bronchopulmonary dysplasia: A comparative study. Pediatrics 89:365-372, 1992.

173. Markestad T, Fitzhardinge PM: Growth and development in children recovering from bronchopulmonary dysplasia. J Pediatr 98:597-602, 1981.

174. Yu VY, et al: Growth and development of very low birthweight infants recovering from bronchopulmonary dysplasia. Arch Dis Child 58:791-794, 1983.

175. Vrlenich LA, et al: The effect of bronchopulmonary dysplasia on growth at school age. Pediatrics 95:855-859, 1995.
176. Doull IJM, Mok Q, Tasker RC: Tracheobronchomalacia in preterm infants with chronic lung disease. Arch Dis Child Fetal Neonatal Ed 76:F203-F205, 1997.
177. Downing GJ, Kilbride HW: Evaluation of airway complications in high-risk preterm infants: application of flexible fiberoptic airway endoscopy. Pediatrics 95(4):567-572, 1995.
178. Greenholz SK, et al: Surgical implications of bronchopulmonary dysplasia. J Pediatr Surg 22(12):1132-1136, 1987.
179. Lindahl H, et al: Bronchoscopy during the first month of life. J Pediatr Surg 27(5):548-550, 1992.
180. Miller RW, et al: Tracheobronchial abnormalities in infants with bronchopulmonary dysplasia. J Pediatr 111(5):779-782, 1987.
181. Shaffer TH, Bhutani VK, Wolfson MR, et al: *In vivo* mechanical properties of the developing airway. Pediatr Res 25:143-146, 1989.
182. Panitch HB, Allen JL, et al: Effects of CPAP on lung mechanics in infants with acquired tracheobronchomalacia. Am J Resp Crit Care Med 150:1341-1346, 1994.
183. Zinman R: Tracheal stenting improves airway mechanics in infants with tracheobronchomalacia. Pediatr Pulmonol 19(5):275-281, 1995.
184. Strong RM, Passy V: Endotracheal intubation: complications in neonates. Arch Otolaryngol 103:329-335, 1977.
185. Fan LL, Flynn JW, et al: Predictive value of stridor in detecting laryngeal injury in extubated neonates. Crit Care Med 10:453-455, 1982.
186. Fan LL, Flynn JW, et al: Risk factors predicting laryngeal injury in intubated neonates. Crit Care Med 11:431-433, 1983.
187. Sherman JM, Lowitt S, et al: Factors influencing acquired subglottic stenosis in infants. J Pediatr 109:322-327, 1986.
188. Grylack LJ, Anderson KD: Diagnosis and treatment of traumatic granuloma in tracheobronchial tree of newborn with history of chronic intubation. J Pediatr Surg 19:200-201, 1984.
189. Brodsky L, Reidy M, Stanievich JF: The effects of suctioning techniques on the distal tracheal mucosa in intubated low birth weight infants. Int Ped Otorrrhinolaryngol, 14:1-14, 1987.
190. Hodge D: Endotracheal suctioning and the infant: a nursing care protocol to decrease complications. Neonatal Netw, 77:202-207, 1991.
191. Kuzenski BM: Effect of negative pressure on tracheobronchial trauma. Nurs Res, 27:260-263, 1978.
192. Runton N: Suctioning artificial airways in children: appropriate technique. Pediatr Nurs 18:115-118, 1992.
193. Malnick G, et al: Normal pulmonary vascular resistance and left ventricular hypertrophy in young infants with bronchopulmonary dysplasia: an echocardiographic and pathologic study. Pediatrics 66(4):589-596, 1980.
194. Kotecha S, Allen J: Oxygen therapy for infants with chronic lung disease. Arch Dis Child Fetal Neonatal Ed 87:F11-4, 2002.
195. Abman SH: Monitoring cardiovascular function in infants with chronic lung disease of prematurity. Arch Dis Child Fetal Neonatal Ed 87(1):F15-8, 2002.
196. Apkon MNR, Lister G: Cardiovascular abnormalities in BPD, in Chronic Lung Disease of Infancy. Bland RD, Coalson JJ, Eds. Marcel Dekker: New York p. 321-356, 2000.

CHAPTER 2

Pulmonary Manifestations of Human Immunodeficiency Virus (HIV) Infection

HEATHER J. ZAR AND MICHAEL R. BYE

Epidemiology 28
Pathogenesis 29
Acute Respiratory Infections 29
  Bacterial Pneumonia 30
  Mycobacterial Infection 32
  Viral Infection 35
  Pneumocystis Infection 37
  Fungal Infection 40
Chronic Lung Disease 41
  Lymphocytic Interstitial Pneumonia 41
  Interstitial Pneumonitis 42

Chronic Pulmonary Infections 42
Immune Reconstitution Inflammatory
  Syndrome 42
Bronchiectasis 43
Malignancy 43
**Diagnostic Evaluation of an HIV-1-
  Infected Child with Pulmonary
  Manifestations** 43
Summary 44
  References 44

Respiratory complications in children infected with human immunodeficiency virus (HIV) are common and responsible for substantial morbidity and mortality.[1] With advances in diagnostic, therapeutic, and preventive strategies for HIV, the spectrum of childhood respiratory disease has changed. In developed countries, programs to prevent perinatal HIV-1 transmission, early diagnosis of HIV-1 infection in infants, and use of *Pneumocystis* prophylaxis and highly active antiretroviral therapy (HAART) have led to a substantial decline in pediatric HIV incidence and associated respiratory infections.[2] In contrast, the major burden of pediatric HIV now exists in developing countries.[3] In these areas, acute and chronic HIV-associated respiratory disease remain a major cause of childhood morbidity and mortality.[1,4] This situation is compounded by limited access to appropriate health care and antiretroviral therapy. In the absence of HAART, 90% of HIV-1-infected children may develop a severe respiratory illness sometime in the course of their HIV disease.[1,4] Pneumonia is the most common cause of hospitalization in African HIV-1-infected children;

pneumonia-specific mortality rates are three to six times higher than the rates of HIV-1-negative patients.[4]

The burden of HIV-associated respiratory disease in developing countries often occurs in the context of existing high rates of childhood pneumonia, poverty, coexisting malnutrition, suboptimal immunization coverage, and under-resourced or inaccessible health care facilities. HIV-infected children have a higher risk of respiratory infections and diseases and of more severe illness compared with immunocompetent children. Increasing evidence also suggests, however, that HIV-exposed but uninfected children also are at greater risk of respiratory infections and illnesses compared with children born to uninfected mothers.

Epidemiology

Globally, there are approximately 33.2 million HIV-1-infected individuals, of whom 2.5 million are children younger than 15 years old.[3] Most of these HIV-1-infected children—almost 2.2 million—reside in sub-Saharan

Africa.[3] In 2006, there were an estimated 420,000 new HIV-1 infections in children (370,000 in sub-Saharan Africa) and approximately 330,000 childhood deaths from HIV-1 (290,000 in sub-Saharan Africa).[3] Conversely, in the last decade in developed countries, the number of HIV-infected children has greatly declined because of a dramatic reduction in perinatal HIV transmission.[2] New cases of HIV-1 infection in children in developed countries occur predominantly in adolescents secondary to sexual transmission; most adolescents remain asymptomatic until adulthood.[2] HIV-1 infection and AIDS have disproportionately affected minority populations in the United States.

Most new HIV-1 infections in children occur through perinatal transmission *in utero*, intrapartum, or through breastfeeding. Breastfeeding may account for 40% of infants becoming infected after delivery, especially in developing countries, where mothers continue to breastfeed for prolonged periods or mixed feeding is introduced early.

The impact of HIV-1 on children is compounded by maternal HIV-1 infection. Infection rates in African women are two to five fold higher than in men, with women of childbearing age most affected.[3] In many countries in sub-Saharan Africa, more than 20% of pregnant women are HIV-1-infected. As a result, many HIV-1-exposed children may be cared for by ill mothers, and other caregivers, or be orphaned. Maternal illness and inability to work exacerbates the cycle of poverty and child illness. Children living in sub-Saharan Africa are particularly vulnerable to HIV-1-associated illness because access to antiretroviral therapy and appropriate medical care may be very limited or unaffordable.

Pathogenesis

HIV-1 is a retrovirus, belonging to a group of heterogeneous, lipid-enveloped RNA viruses. Another retrovirus, HIV-2, is relatively rare and causes a less severe AIDS-like syndrome. HIV-1 has two major viral envelope proteins—the external glycoprotein gp120 and the transmembrane glycoprotein gp41.

The primary target cell of HIV-1 is the human $CD4^+$ lymphocyte. The HIV-1 gp120 envelope protein binds to the $CD4^+$ molecule on the host cell membrane with high affinity. This binding allows the virus to enter the T cell and to integrate its genome into the host DNA. HIV-1 also infects monocytes and macrophages but with less marked cytopathic effects. Infected monocytes serve as a reservoir for HIV-1, allowing further spread of the virus throughout the body.[5] Infection with HIV-1 results in progressive depletion of the $CD4^+$ helper lymphocytes. This depletion serves as a marker of the severity of HIV-1 infection because the incidence of opportunistic infections and other complications correlates with the number and percentage of $CD4^+$ lymphocytes, particularly in children older than 1 year.[6]

The ability to produce cytokines, such as interleukin-2 and interferon-γ, is progressively lost in HIV-1-infected children. Natural killer cell–mediated cytotoxicity also is reduced in HIV-1-infected children. In addition, B cell dysfunction with defective humoral immunity further predisposes to severe infection.[7]

Acute Respiratory Infections

Respiratory infection was the most common cause of death in children younger than 6 years of age in a U.S. cohort of HIV-1-infected children in the pre-HAART era; the frequency of pulmonary disease as a cause of death was greatest in infants, with 56% of respiratory-related deaths occurring within the first year of life.[8] The rate of acute respiratory infections and opportunistic infections has decreased dramatically with the use of HAART (Table 2-1).[5-9] Before HAART, bacterial pneumonia, *Pneumocystis* pneumonia (PCP), disseminated *Mycobacterium avium-intracellulare* complex (MAC), and tracheobronchial candidiasis were the most frequent respiratory infections, occurring at an event rate of more than 1 per 100 child-years; these all have declined substantially with HAART (see Table 2-1).[5,9] Although the frequency of bacterial infections has declined substantially, pneumonia or secondary respiratory failure remains the

Table 2-1	Impact of HAART on Opportunistic Respiratory Infections			
INFECTION	**PRE-HAART RATE[9]**		**POST-HAART RATE[5]**	
	Incidence Rate per 100 Child-Years	95% CI	Incidence Rate per 100 Child-Years	95% CI
PCP	1.3	1.1-1.6	0.1	0.04-0.2
Bacterial pneumonia	11.1	10.3-12.0	2.2	1.8-2.6
Bacteremia	3.3	2.9-3.8	0.4	0.2-0.5
Disseminated MAC	1.8	1.5-2.1	0.1	0.1-0.3
Tracheobronchial or esophageal candidiasis	1.2	1.0-1.5	0.1	0.03-0.2

CI, confidence interval; HAART, highly active antiretroviral therapy; MAC, *Mycobacterium avium-intracellulare* complex; PCP, *Pneumocystis* pneumonia.

predominant cause of death in children receiving HAART, accounting for 27% of deaths.[5] In children not receiving HAART or children resistant to antiretroviral therapy, acute respiratory infections are common, often severe, and the most frequent cause of hospitalization or death. Bacteria, mycobacteria, viruses, *Pneumocystis,* or fungi may cause respiratory infections; mixed infections also commonly occur (Table 2-2).

Bacterial Pneumonia

Before HAART, bacterial pneumonia was the most common serious infection in HIV-1-infected children with an event rate of 11 per 100 child-years[9]; this rate has declined to 2.2 in the HAART era (see Table 2-1).[5] Pneumonia, particularly caused by *Streptococcus pneumoniae, Haemophilus influenzae* type b, and *Staphylococcus aureus,* is a major cause of hospitalization and death in children in developing countries.[10-12] *S. pneumoniae* is the most important bacterial pathogen in HIV-1-infected and uninfected children.[11-16] HIV-1-infected children also are at increased risk for recurrent infections.

S. aureus is an increasingly important cause of pneumonia in HIV-1-infected children and is the most common pathogen in catheter-associated bacteremia.[16,18] Staphylococcal pneumonia may be complicated by empyema, pneumatoceles, or lung abscess (Fig. 2-1). A wider range of bacteria, including gram negative pathogens such as *Klebsiella pneumoniae, Pseudomonas aeruginosa, H. influenzae,* nontyphoid salmonella, and *Escherichia coli,* cause pneumonia with or without bacteremia in HIV-1-infected children.[11,12,16,19,20]

HIV-1 infection has been associated with an increase in the antimicrobial resistance patterns of bacterial pneumonia, with implications for empiric antibiotic therapy.[11] Methicillin-resistant *S. aureus* (MRSA) has increasingly emerged as a pathogen in HIV-1-infected children.[16] Data on the prevalence of penicillin-resistant pneumococcal infection are variable, but no clear differences in clinical outcome for susceptible and resistant strains have been shown except for isolates with high-level resistance.[21]

Etiologic diagnosis of bacterial pneumonia is difficult because signs are nonspecific, coinfection with more than one organism occurs frequently, and culture of upper respiratory tract secretions or sputum may reflect colonization rather than pathogenic organisms. Blood culture, may be useful because of higher rates of bacteremia, occurring in approximately 15% of HIV-1-infected children hospitalized for pneumonia.[11,16] Empiric therapy for pneumonia should include broad-spectrum antibiotics, based on the local prevalence of antimicrobial resistance and recent use of prophylactic or therapeutic antibiotics (see Table 2-2).[1,6] A combination of a β-lactam with an aminoglycoside or a second-generation or third-generation cephalosporin alone is appropriate empiric therapy. The choice of antimicrobial agent should be modified according to culture results and susceptibility testing.

The outcome of HIV-1-infected children with bacterial pneumonia is worse than the outcome for immunocompetent children with more severe disease and higher case-fatality rates.[1,4] In addition, HIV-1-exposed but uninfected children have higher rates of

Table 2-2	Etiology and Therapy of Lower Respiratory Infections in HIV-Infected Children	
INFECTION	**PATHOGENS**	**FIRST-LINE THERAPY**
Bacterial pneumonia	*Streptococcus pneumoniae*	Broad-spectrum antibiotic—β-lactam with an aminoglycoside *or* a second- or third-generation cephalosporin
	Haemophilus influenzae	Add antistaphylococcal antibiotics if *S. aureus* suspected or vancomycin if methicillin-resistant *S. aureus* suspected
	Staphylococcus aureus	
	Nontyphoid salmonella	
	Klebsiella pneumoniae	
	Streptococcus milleri	
	Escherichia coli	
	Moraxella catarrhalis	
PCP	*Pneumocystis jiroveci*	Trimethoprim-sulfamethoxazole
		Corticosteroids if hypoxic
Mycobacterial	*Mycobacterium tuberculosis*	Isoniazid, rifampin, pyrazinamide as induction for 2 mo (add fourth drug if suspected drug resistance *or* smear-positive pulmonary TB *or* smear-negative pulmonary TB with extensive parenchymal involvement *or* severe extrapulmonary TB *or* severe concomitant HIV disease); then maintenance with isoniazid, rifampin for 4-7 mo for pulmonary TB
		Corticosteroids if endobronchial disease, pericardial effusion, meningitis
	Mycobacterium bovis	Surgical excision of localized disease; 4-drug therapy for disseminated disease (isoniazid, rifampin, ethambutol, ofloxacin or ciprofloxacin)
	Mycobacterium avium-intracellulare complex	Clarithromycin plus ethambutol
Viral pneumonia	Respiratory syncytial virus	
	CMV	Ganciclovir for CMV
	Human metapneumovirus	
	Parainfluenza viruses 1 and 3	
	Adenovirus	
	Influenza viruses A and B	Neuraminidase inhibitor for influenza A or B
	Measles virus	High-dose vitamin A for measles
	HSV	Acyclovir for HSV
	Varicella-zoster virus	Acyclovir for varicella-zoster virus
	HPV types 6 and 11	Laser or surgery, topical therapy for HPV
Fungal	*Candida* species	Topical nystatin or oral itraconazole, fluconazole
	Aspergillus species	Amphotericin B
	Histoplasma capsulatum	Amphotericin B, itraconazole, fluconazole for mild illness
	Cryptococcus neoformans	Amphotericin B, itraconazole, fluconazole
	Coccidioides immitis	Amphotericin B, itraconazole, fluconazole for mild illness

CMV, cytomegalovirus; HPV, human papillomavirus; HSV, herpes simplex virus; PCP, *Pneumocystis* pneumonia; TB, tuberculosis.

treatment failure and mortality compared with children born to uninfected mothers.[16]

Prevention of bacterial pneumonia through immunization is an important strategy, although the efficacy may be reduced in HIV-1-infected children. Immunization with inactivated vaccines (diphtheria, pertussis, tetanus toxoid; inactivated poliovirus; *H. influenzae* type b; hepatitis B; and pneumococcal conjugate vaccine) should be given to HIV-1-infected children at the usual recommended age.[22] Use of the *H. influenzae*

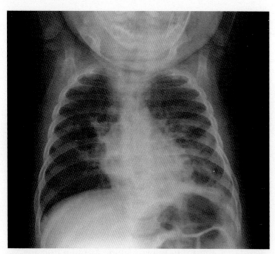

Figure 2-1. Chest x-ray of a young child with *S. aureus* infection showing a large pneumatocele.

type b conjugate vaccine potentially may reduce Hib invasive disease by 46% to 93% in immunocompetent vaccine recipients.[23,24] The efficacy of this vaccine against invasive disease is reduced, however, in HIV-1-infected children not receiving antiretroviral therapy (44% in HIV-infected compared with 96% in uninfected children).[19] The pneumococcal conjugate vaccine has lower efficacy in HIV-1-infected children[25-27]; nevertheless, it reduces the incidence of invasive disease caused by vaccine strains by 65% and prevents 13% of radiologically confirmed pneumonia in HIV-1-infected children not receiving HAART.[25] Immunization also reduces the incidence of infection with drug-resistant pneumococcal strains.[25] Reimmunization after 3 to 5 years is recommended. Adolescents should receive the 23-valent polysaccharide vaccine.[9]

Intravenous immunoglobulin (IVIG) is currently recommended in HIV-1-infected children with hypogammaglobulinemia (IgG <4 g/L); two or more severe bacterial infections in a 1-year period; failure to form antibodies to common antigens; or chronic parvovirus B19 infections.[14,22,28] IVIG may not offer additional protection, however, if children are taking trimethoprim-sulfamethoxazole (TMP-SMX) prophylaxis.[14] Moreover there is no evidence to suggest that IVIG therapy offers additional protection for children receiving HAART. Children with bronchiectasis may benefit from monthly immunoglobulin infusions.[22]

Mycobacterial Infection

Respiratory disease also may result from infection with numerous mycobacteria. *Mycobacterium tuberculosis* is the most common cause of respiratory infection, but localized or disseminated disease from *Mycobacterium bovis* or the nontuberculous mycobacteria (NTM), particularly MAC may occur (see Table 2-2).

In high tuberculosis (TB) prevalence areas, *M. tuberculosis* is an important cause of acute pneumonia and of chronic respiratory infection in HIV-1-infected children. Culture-confirmed pulmonary TB has been reported in approximately 8% to 15% of children hospitalized with acute pneumonia in these areas.[11,12,16,29] The incidence of TB usually primary infection, than in non-HIV infected children is higher in HIV-1-infected children.[29-32] Coinfection with *M. tuberculosis* and HIV-1 results in more rapid deterioration of immune dysfunction, viral replication, and HIV-1 progression, and other more frequent and severe infections.[33-36]

HIV-1-infected children with TB may present with nonspecific signs, such as weight loss, failure to thrive, or fever; with signs and symptoms of acute pneumonia or airway obstruction (Fig. 2-2); or with chronic, persistent respiratory symptoms.[29,33-36] Cavitary lung disease, or extrapulmonary spread. (Fig. 2-3) occurs more commonly in HIV-1-infected children. Multidrug-resistant TB is increasingly prevalent in TB-endemic areas and has a poor prognosis.[37] In the United States, multidrug-resistant TB is

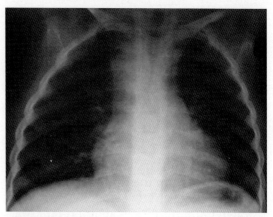

Figure 2-2. Chest x-ray of a child with culture-confirmed tuberculosis showing compression of the trachea by lymph nodes.

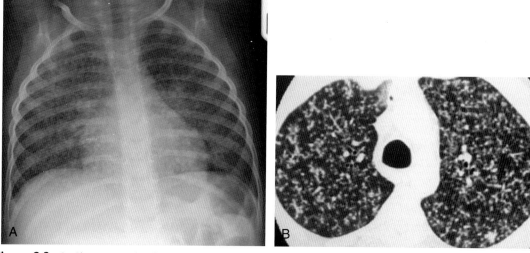

Figure 2-3. A, Chest x-ray of a child with miliary tuberculosis with diffuse nodules, producing a "snowstorm" appearance. **B,** Chest CT scan of a child with miliary tuberculosis showing multiple diffuse small nodules.

uncommon, reported in 2.8% of foreign-born and 1.4% of U.S.-born cases.[32]

Localized or disseminated *M. bovis* infection, including pneumonia, has been reported in HIV-1-infected children occurring weeks to years after receiving bacille Calmette-Guérin (BCG) immunization.[38-40] The most common manifestation of *M. bovis* disease is ulceration at the site of vaccination or localized lymphadenopathy; systemic dissemination occurs more rarely. The risk of disseminated BCG disease is greatly increased in HIV-1-infected infants.[38] The clinical presentation of disseminated *M. bovis* may be indistinguishable from *M. tuberculosis* infection.[40] Disseminated *M. bovis* infection has a poor prognosis with a case-fatality rate of approximately 50%.

NTM, particularly MAC, may cause disseminated disease, including pulmonary infection, in severely immunosuppressed HIV-1-infected children; isolated pulmonary disease is rare.[41] The incidence of NTM disease has declined significantly from a rate of 1.8 per 100 child-years before HAART to 0.1 after HAART (see Table 2-1).[5,9] Children with pulmonary disease are at high risk for dissemination; 72% may develop systemic disease within 8 months.[6] Disseminated MAC seems to be more common in children who have transfusion-acquired HIV-1 rather than perinatal acquisition.[42] Disease occurs in adults with CD4$^+$ counts less than 50 cells/µL; however, the threshold is less well established in

young children.[6,43] Primary and secondary prophylaxis is recommended for severely immunosuppressed children based on CD4$^+$ counts.[43,44]

Establishing the diagnosis of pulmonary TB is difficult in HIV-1-infected children, for whom clinical scoring systems have not been developed, and in whom anergy may reduce the reliability of the tuberculin skin test. A tuberculin skin test of 5mm or more of induration is regarded as positive.[7] Tests of T lymphocyte interferon-ɣ production are promising. A study of children with suspected TB reported that the T cell–based enzyme-linked immunospot assay (ELISPOT) had a higher sensitivity than the tuberculin skin test. In HIV-1-infected children, the ELISPOT sensitivity was 73% compared with 36% for the skin test.[45] Definitive diagnosis and drug resistance testing require culture confirmation of *M. tuberculosis*.[46] Sputum induction was reported more recently to be effective and safe for culture confirmation in infants and children, with the yield from a single induced sputum equivalent to that obtained from three gastric lavages.[47] Induced sputum should be the primary diagnostic procedure in a child with suspected pulmonary TB. In contrast, the culture yield from a single bronchoalveolar lavage (BAL) is lower than that from three properly performed consecutive gastric lavages.[48] The efficacy of polymerase chain reaction has been disappointing, with sensitivity on gastric aspirates ranging from 45% to 83% in HIV-1-negative children.[46]

Definitive diagnosis of *M. bovis* or MAC relies on isolation of the organism from the blood or biopsy specimens.[6] If lymphadenopathy is present, an aspirate and culture can be diagnostic. Multiple mycobacterial blood cultures may be necessary to improve the yield. Culture is essential to differentiate NTM from *M. tuberculosis* and to determine drug susceptibilities.

The response to standard TB therapy in HIV-1-infected children is poorer than in HIV-1-negative children, with lower cure rates and higher mortality.[36,37] Optimal therapy for HIV-1-infected children has not been tested in well-designed clinical studies. Empiric therapy for pulmonary TB in HIV-1-infected children should include three drugs (isoniazid, rifampin, pyrazinamide) daily for a 2-month induction period; a fourth drug (ethambutol, ethionamide, or streptomycin) should be added if drug resistance is suspected or if there is smear-positive pulmonary TB, smear-negative pulmonary TB with extensive parenchymal involvement, severe extrapulmonary TB, or severe concomitant HIV-1 disease.[6,35,37,49]

After the induction phase, therapy with two drugs (isoniazid, rifampin) should be continued either daily or three times a week.[22,49] Directly observed therapy (DOT) is advised to promote adherence and reduce the rate of treatment relapse or failure. Because high rates of treatment failure occur in children treated for 6 months, some guidelines recommend 9 months.[6,49,50] For extrapulmonary TB, the duration of therapy may be increased to 12 months.[6,49] Therapy for drug-resistant TB should be individualized, using a minimum of three drugs, at least two of which are bactericidal. Adjunctive corticosteroids may be beneficial in children with complicated TB, including pericardial disease, meningitis, or an endobronchial lesion with airway obstruction; a suggested regimen is 1 to 2mg/kg/day of prednisone tapered over 6 to 8 weeks. A chest radiograph should be obtained at baseline and repeated 2 to 3 months into therapy to evaluate response; however, the chest radiograph may remain abnormal for

months even years, and a normal radiograph is not a criterion for discontinuing therapy.[6]

For children receiving HAART, the antiretroviral regimen should provide optimal TB and HIV-1 therapy and minimize potential toxicity and drug interactions.[35,49] Rifampin induces hepatic cytochrome P-450 enzymes and may reduce levels of antiretroviral agents, particularly protease inhibitors (PIs) and non-nucleoside reverse transcriptase inhibitors (NNRTIs). Rifampin should not be used in conjunction with single protease inhibitors except for ritonavir.[6] Alternatively, rifampin may be used in conjunction with ritonavir-boosted saquinavir, provided that high-dose ritonavir boosting (400mg) is used.[6] Concurrent rifampin with the non-nucleoside reverse transcriptase inhibitor delavirdine is not recommended; however, use with efavirenz is possible. Use with nevirapine is recommended only when there are no other options because of the potential decrease in nevirapine levels. Rifabutin is a less potent inducer of the P-450 enzymes, and is a suitable alternative to rifampin, but there is limited experience with its use in children. Adjustments in dosage of rifabutin and coadministered antiretroviral drugs may be necessary because some drugs decrease rifabutin levels, whereas others increase levels. For antiretroviral-naïve children, the timing of HAART after initiation of TB therapy depends on the clinical and immunologic severity of disease. In children with severe clinical illness or advanced HIV-1 infection, HAART should be started 2 to 8 weeks after TB therapy to minimize the risk of immune reconstitution inflammatory syndrome (IRIS), to optimize adherence, and to differentiate potential side effects secondary to TB or antiretroviral drugs.[49,51-54]

Management of BCG disease is difficult. The inherent resistance of *M. bovis* to pyrazinamide, inherent intermediate resistance of some strains to isoniazid, and the emergence of resistance owing to inappropriate therapy complicate treatment.[55] Although localized BCG disease is usually self-limited in immunocompetent children, in HIV-1-infected children, treatment is warranted because of the risk of dissemination and poor outcome.[40] Surgical excision of localized lymphadenopathy is one option.

Alternatively, therapy with four drugs (isoniazid, rifampin, ethambutol, ofloxacin, or ciprofloxacin) in high doses is recommended. The optimal duration of therapy is unknown, but at least 9 months of treatment is recommended, based on experience with adults.[56]

Treatment of MAC should consist of combination therapy with a minimum of two drugs because monotherapy with a macrolide leads rapidly to resistance.[6] Initial recommended therapy is clarithromycin or azithromycin with ethambutol. Rifabutin may be added as a third drug in patients with severe disseminated infection; addition to ciprofloxacin, amikacin, or streptomycin may be considered depending on the severity of illness.

For prevention of mycobacterial disease, the BCG vaccine may be beneficial for HIV-1-exposed but uninfected children in areas of high TB prevalence. Chemoprophylaxis with isoniazid is recommended for a child who has been exposed to a household contact with TB after active TB disease has been excluded or for a child with evidence of TB infection (tuberculin skin test >5mm induration but asymptomatic with a normal chest radiograph).[6,22,49] A study in a high TB prevalence area found that isoniazid prophylaxis given to HIV-1-infected children regardless of tuberculin skin reactivity or a household TB contact substantially reduced TB incidence by almost 70% and mortality by more than 50%. The effect of isoniazid occurred in all categories of clinical HIV-1 illness and in children of all ages. Isoniazid prophylaxis should be considered for HIV-1-infected children living in TB endemic areas, especially children who are not taking HAART.[57]

Primary prophylaxis for NTM with azithromycin or clarithromycin should be considered for severely immunosuppressed children (Table 2-3) as follows: children younger than 1 year, CD4$^+$ less than 750/μL; children 1 to 2 years old, CD4$^+$ less than 500/μL; children 2 to 6 years old, CD4$^+$ less than 75/μL; children 6 years or older, CD4$^+$ less than 50/μL.[22] Rifabutin may be an alternative agent in children older than 6 years. Secondary prophylaxis should be given to children with a history of disseminated MAC to

Table 2-3	Indications for *Pneumocystis* Pneumonia Prophylaxis in HIV-Infected Children
AGE	**CD4$^+$T LYMPHOCYTE COUNT***
4-6 wk to 12 mo†	All patients regardless of CD4$^+$count
1-5 yr	<500/mm³ *or* <15%
>5 yr	<200/mm³ *or* <15%

*If CD4$^+$ counts are unavailable, prophylaxis should be given to all symptomatic children indefinitely.[100]
†HIV-exposed children should receive prophylaxis from 4-6 weeks to 4 months; thereafter, prophylaxis may be discontinued if HIV infection has been excluded, and the mother is not breastfeeding.
Data from references 22 and 100.

prevent recurrence. Lifelong prophylaxis is indicated; the safety of discontinuing secondary prophylaxis in the context of sustained immune restoration after HAART has not been well studied in children.

Viral Infection

Although respiratory viruses are identified less frequently in HIV-1-infected children hospitalized for pneumonia (approximately 15%) compared with HIV-1-negative children (45%), the absolute burden of hospitalization for viral-associated pneumonia is twofold to eightfold greater in HIV-1-infected children.[58] HIV-1-infected children in whom respiratory viruses are identified are more likely to develop pneumonia, to have a more prolonged hospital stay, and to have a higher case-fatality rate than HIV-1-uninfected children. Respiratory syncytial virus (RSV) is the most common cause of viral pneumonia, although human metapneumovirus is emerging as an important respiratory pathogen with a spectrum of disease similar to RSV.[59] Other respiratory viruses causing lower respiratory tract infection include cytomegalovirus (CMV), adenovirus, influenza, parainfluenza, and measles (see Table 2-2).[58] Treatment may be beneficial for specific viral pathogens. For influenza A or B, a neuraminidase inhibitor, such as oseltamivir or zanamivir, can reduce the severity of illness and complications.[22]

Concurrent bacterial infection has been reported in 30% to 50% of children hospitalized with viral pneumonia.[16] Pneumococcal conjugate vaccine reduces the incidence of hospitalization for viral-associated pneumonia, suggesting that more severe pneumonia requiring hospitalization may be the result of viral and *S. pneumoniae* coinfection.[60] Influenza vaccine should be given annually to all HIV-1-infected children at the start of the influenza season.[22] The efficacy of the humanized monoclonal specific antibody against RSV (palivizumab) or RSV IVIG has not been well evaluated in HIV-1-infected children. Nevertheless, children at risk for severe RSV infection, such as HIV-1-infected infants born prematurely, children younger than 2 years with chronic lung disease, or severely immunosuppressed children, may benefit from palivizumab prophylaxis. A dose should be given monthly for the duration of the RSV season.

CMV is a herpesvirus that can cause primary pneumonitis or severe, disseminated disease in HIV-1-infected children.[6] CMV infection is more likely to occur in children with low $CD4^+$ counts. Coinfection with CMV and HIV-1 results in more rapid progression of HIV-1 disease.[6,61] The incidence of CMV infection has decreased with the use of HAART.[5,9] CMV may occur in association with other pathogens, especially *Pneumocystis*.[62] Treatment of CMV disease focuses on preventing disease progression and not on cure. Ganciclovir is most widely used, with drug dosing separated into induction and maintenance dosage.[6,22] Prophylaxis against CMV with oral ganciclovir or valganciclovir should be given to severely immunosuppressed children or children with a history of disseminated CMV disease to prevent recurrence.[63] There are few data on the safety of discontinuing prophylaxis after sustained immune reconstitution on HAART has occurred.

Other herpesvirus infections may also involve the respiratory tract in HIV-1-infected children. Oral herpes simplex virus lesions may spread to involve the upper airways and the larynx, resulting in croup[64]; disseminated disease including pneumonia also may occur. Pneumonia may occur as a complication of varicella-zoster virus infection.[65] Intravenous acyclovir is recommended for therapy; high-dose oral acyclovir or valacyclovir may be

considered in children with mild immunosuppression.[22] Varicella vaccine should be considered at 12 to 15 months for asymptomatic or mildly symptomatic HIV-1-infected children without immunosuppression (Centers for Disease Control and Prevention categories N1 and A1); vaccine should not be administered to symptomatic immunosuppressed children because of the potential for disseminated disease. Administration of varicella-zoster globulin should be considered for HIV-1-infected children exposed to varicella or zoster who have no prior history of varicella infection or immunization and who have not received immunoglobulin within 2 weeks of exposure.

Measles may result in severe pneumonia in HIV-1-infected children; measles may present without the typical skin rash, making the diagnosis particularly difficult.[66] Children with suspected measles should be given a single high dose of vitamin A because studies in HIV-1-negative children have shown that vitamin A reduces morbidity and mortality from measles-associated pneumonia.[67] Measles, mumps, rubella vaccine (MMR), a live attenuated vaccine, should be given to HIV-1-infected children at 12 months of age, unless they are severely immunocompromised.[22] HIV-1-infected children exposed to measles should receive a dose of intramuscular immunoglobulin regardless of immunization status.

Human papillomavirus (HPV) type 6 or type 11 may produce lesions in the oral cavity, pharynx, and larynx and rarely in the lower airways or lungs; the disease has a tendency to recur.[68] Clinically, the disease may manifest as progressive hoarseness, stridor, wheezing, and respiratory distress.[69] Rarely, lung nodules, cysts, recurrent pneumonia, emphysema, or atelectasis occurs in immunocompetent children.[68,69] Little is known about the epidemiologic risk of disease in HIV-1-infected children. An increased prevalence of HPV in HIV-1-infected compared with HIV-1-uninfected women has been reported; however, the rate of HPV transmission to children has not been associated with the HIV-1 status of the mother or child.[70,71] Laryngeal HPV lesions are difficult to treat. Therapy is directed at maintaining airway patency, so obstructing papillomas should be removed. Adjuvant therapy using intralesional cidofovir has been reported to result in regression and reduced need for surgery in HIV-1-uninfected children.[72]

Pneumocystis Infection

Children with HIV-1 who are not taking HAART or TMP-SMX prophylaxis are at high risk of developing PCP. *Pneumocystis jiroveci* (formerly *Pneumocystis carinii*) originally was classified as a protozoan. Studies of RNA sequences show a similarity between fungi and *P. jiroveci,* and the organism is now classified as a fungus. Two morphologic forms of the organism are found in infected lungs: thin-walled, single-nucleated trophozoites adherent to type I pneumocytes, and thick-walled cysts containing four to eight single-nucleated sporozoites. The organism attaches to the alveolar epithelium, resulting in desquamation of alveolar cells. As the infection progresses, a diffuse desquamative alveolitis ensues, and alveoli become filled with a foamy exudate consisting of alveolar macrophages and cysts. Interstitial inflammation develops.

PCP was the most common opportunistic infection in HIV-1-infected infants before widespread prenatal HIV-1 screening, TMP-SMX prophylaxis, and HAART.[9] In the United States, the incidence of PCP has declined substantially from 1.3 per 100 child-years before HAART to 0.1 after HAART.[5,9] In developed countries, PCP occurs most commonly in infants born to women with unrecognized HIV-1 infection.[73] In developing countries, PCP remains a frequent presentation of HIV-1 infection in infants and a major cause of severe pneumonia and death.[10,16,74-76] The incidence of PCP ranges from 8% to 49% among HIV-1-infected African children hospitalized for pneumonia.[16,74-76] Increasingly, PCP also has been reported in older HIV-1-infected children; 25% of cases in a Zambian postmortem study occurred in children older than 6 months.[10] Moreover, HIV-1-exposed but uninfected children have been described to have a higher risk of PCP compared with children born to HIV-1-uninfected mothers.[16]

Children with PCP most commonly have acute onset of cough, fever, tachypnea, and chest retractions.[77] Infants younger than 6 months are especially at risk for PCP and have an acute, severe illness characterized by rapidly prominent and progressive hypoxia and increasing respiratory distress.[77] In HIV-1-infected children not taking HAART, four clinical variables have been reported to be associated with PCP: age younger than 6 months, respiratory rate greater than 59 breaths/min, arterial hemoglobin saturation less than 92%, and absence of a history of vomiting.[78] Clinical signs may be compounded by coinfection with bacterial or viral pathogens.[16,62,79] Most children have significant hypoxemia with an alveolar-arterial oxygen gradient greater than 30mmHg.

Laboratory findings include a normal white blood cell count, elevated serum lactate dehydrogenase (LDH), and normal IgG level. LDH values greater than 1000 IU/L are associated with PCP, but they are nonspecific and may reflect the extent of lung involvement.[80,81] The chest radiograph usually shows a diffuse pattern, which progresses to alveolar opacification (Fig. 2-4); however, hyperinflation, focal infiltrates, cavities, a miliary pattern, pneumothoraces, pleural effusion, or even a normal appearance also may occur.[82,83] Less commonly, PCP may manifest with a pneumothorax, cyst, pneumatoceles, or a bronchiolitis-like picture.[83,84]

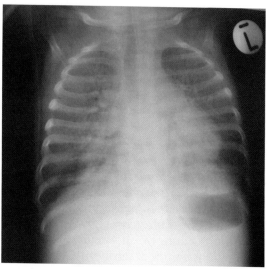

Figure 2-4. Chest x-ray of an infant with *Pneumocystis* pneumonia showing diffuse interstitial infiltrates.

PCP is associated with high mortality ranging from 35% to 87% with higher rates in children with respiratory failure requiring mechanical ventilation.[74-76,85,86] Timely anti-*Pneumocystis* therapy may improve the outcome, as suggested by historical comparisons and adult studies in which early use of corticosteroids has been associated with improved survival.[87-89] Mutations in *P. jiroveci* dihydropteroate synthetase genes—a key enzyme target of TMP-SMX—have been described in HIV-1-infected patients with PCP, especially with widespread use of TMP-SMX prophylaxis.[87] The clinical importance of mutant strains is unclear, however, and the response to TMP-SMX treatment varies.

HIV-1-exposed but uninfected children may also be at increased risk of PCP.[16] Transmission of *P. jiroveci* from an HIV-1-infected mother to her HIV-1-uninfected infant has been reported in a few cases.[90-92] HIV-1-exposed children may be at risk for PCP as a result of close and early exposure to the organism from the mother, reduced passage of functional maternal antibody, impaired cell-mediated immunity, or concomitant malnutrition.

Definitive diagnosis requires identification of *P. jiroveci* from sputum, bronchial washings, or lung tissue. Induced sputum using nebulized hypertonic saline has been used to diagnose PCP in children; a positive yield has been reported in infants 1 month of age.[75] In this procedure, the child inhales a mist of 3% to 5% saline generated by a jet nebulizer for 10 to 15 minutes. The diagnostic yield using this technique depends on collection of an adequate specimen. Nasopharyngeal aspirates have been used to identify *P. jiroveci*, but the yield is lower than with induced sputum.[74-76] Induced sputum combined with nasopharyngeal aspirates may provide a higher yield than either technique alone; the sensitivity and specificity for induced sputum and nasopharyngeal aspirates for diagnosis of PCP compared with the yield on autopsy have been reported to be 75% and 80%.[76] BAL with fiberoptic bronchoscopy is the diagnostic procedure of choice in young children, with reported sensitivity of 55% to 97%.[6] Transbronchial biopsy is not recommended unless BAL is nondiagnostic.[6]

Transbronchial biopsy may be positive 10 days after starting therapy; the sensitivity of biopsy is 87% to 95%.[6,8]

Because *P. jiroveci* cannot be cultured, identification requires special stains.[77] Silver methenamine, toluidine blue O, and calcofluor white are useful for staining cyst forms, whereas Giemsa, modified Wright-Giemsa, and modified Papanicolaou stains identify trophozoites.[77,87] Fluorescein-conjugated monoclonal antibodies provide greater sensitivity, detecting the cyst and trophozoite forms.[87] Polymerase chain reaction techniques with a high sensitivity and specificity and potential to improve diagnostic accuracy are promising, but currently are used mainly as a research tool.

Empiric therapy for *Pneumocystis* should be given to any HIV-1-infected child with suspected PCP because untreated infection is usually fatal.[77] The most effective therapy is TMP-SMX (15 to 20mg/kg/day of TMP) intravenously three to four times a day for 21 days (see Table 2-4).[6,22,77,87] Oral treatment can be used if intravenous therapy is not feasible, if disease is mild, or after clinical improvement occurs. The response to therapy may be slow with clinical improvement observed by 5 to 7 days.[77] Adverse reactions to TMP-SMX occur in approximately 15% of cases, but treatment should be discontinued only if reactions are severe, such as neutropenia or a severe skin rash.[22,77,93]

Intravenous pentamidine (4mg/kg/once daily) may be an alternative treatment for children who cannot tolerate TMP-SMX, or who have not responded after 5 to 7 days of TMP-SMX (see Table 2-4).[6,22] Pentamidine is associated with a high incidence of adverse reactions, including pancreatitis, hyperglycemia and hypoglycemia, renal dysfunction, cardiac dysrhythmias, fever, neutropenia, and hypotension.[94] Patients who show clinical improvement after 7 to 10 days of intravenous pentamidine may be switched to an oral drug to complete 21 days of therapy. Other alternative anti-*Pneumocystis* agents include atovaquone, dapsone with trimethoprim, trimetrexate glucuronate with leucovorin, and clindamycin with primaquine, but there is little information on the efficacy or tolerability of these regimens in children (see Table 2-4).[6,22]

Table 2-4	Treatment of *Pneumocystis* Pneumonia in Children*		
DRUG	**DOSE**	**ROUTE**	**COMMENTS**
TMP-SMX	15-20mg/kg TMP/75-100mg/kg SMX per day q6h	Intravenous *or* oral	First choice. Oral therapy only if mild disease or after clinical improvement occurs
Pentamidine	4 mg/kg once daily	Intravenous	Use in children who cannot tolerate TMP-SMX or when no response after 5-7 days. High incidence of side effects. Should not be administered with didanosine owing to risk of pancreatitis
Atovaquone	30-45 mg/kg/day	Oral	Limited experience in children
Trimetrexate glucuronate with leucovorin	No studies in children of established doses. Adult dose 45mg/m^2/day trimetrexate glucuronate with 20mg/m^2 leucovorin q6h	Intravenous	Limited experience in children
Dapsone and trimethoprim	No studies in children of established doses. Adult dose 100mg dapsone daily (pediatric equivalent 2mg/kg) and 15mg/kg trimethoprim	Oral	Limited experience in children
Primaquine and clindamycin	No studies in children of established doses. Primaquine adult dose 30mg daily orally (pediatric equivalent 0.3mg/kg daily orally). Clindamycin adult dose 600mg intravenously q6h for 10 days, then 300-450mg orally q6h for 11 days (pediatric equivalent 10mg/kg q6h orally or intravenously)	Oral/intravenous	Limited experience in children. Most effective alternative therapy for adults with PCP unresponsive to primary therapy

*Corticosteroids should be added for children with hypoxia.
PCP, *Pneumocystis* pneumonia; TMP-SMX, trimethoprim-sulfamethoxazole

Corticosteroids are recommended in hypoxemic children. Although no controlled trials on the use of corticosteroids in children have been performed, corticosteroid use has been reported to reduce the need for mechanical ventilation and to improve survival compared with historical controls.[88,89,95] Studies of hypoxemic HIV-1-infected adults with PCP found that corticosteroids improve oxygenation and reduce the incidence of respiratory failure when used within 72 hours of starting anti-*Pneumocystis* therapy.[87,89] Corticosteroids are recommended for patients with a PaO_2 less than 70mmHg or an alveolar-arterial oxygen gradient greater than 35mmHg.[6] The optimal dose and duration have not been determined, but a recommended regimen is prednisone, 2mg/kg/day for 7 to 10 days with tapering doses over the next 10 to 14 days.[88]

A few case reports have described the use of surfactant to improve pulmonary function in children with severe PCP.[96,97] Children with PCP may be co-infected with bacterial or viral pathogens[16,62,79]; additional antimicrobial therapy for these should be used when appropriate. Specifically, CMV co-infection has been associated with more severe disease requiring mechanical ventilation and a poor outcome. The effect of corticosteroid therapy for PCP on CMV pneumonitis is unclear.

Because of the high mortality and morbidity associated with PCP, prevention should be the primary objective. Prevention of PCP is an important and effective intervention, if initiated in HIV-1-exposed infants within the first weeks of life.[98] Oral TMP-SMX is the most effective prophylactic agent.[17,22] In the only randomized controlled study of TMP-SMX prophylaxis in HIV-1-infected children, mortality was reduced by 43% and morbidity, including hospitalization, was reduced by 23% in Zambia.[99] The impact on mortality occurred in children of all ages, suggesting that prophylaxis may also provide protection against bacterial infections.[99] TMP-SMX prophylaxis ($150mg/m^2$/day of TMP) may be given three times a week (single dose on 3 consecutive days, or two divided doses on consecutive or alternate days).

Current recommendations for PCP prophylaxis include the following (see Table 2-3)[22,100]:
- All infants born to HIV-1-infected mothers from 6 weeks of age until HIV-1 infection has been excluded in the child and the mother is no longer breastfeeding.
- All HIV-1-infected children from 6 weeks of age until 1 year. HIV-1-infected children older than 1 year should receive prophylaxis if their $CD4^+$ counts are less than 15% of lymphocytes or if they have symptomatic HIV-1 disease. A higher $CD4^+$ threshold for providing prophylaxis may be applicable in developing countries, however, as evidenced by a trial in Zambia where prophylaxis reduced mortality in children, even in children with higher $CD4^+$ counts.[99] Prophylaxis should be continued indefinitely regardless of age or $CD4^+$ counts when HAART is unavailable.[100]
- Prophylaxis should be continued in children taking HAART for at least 6 months. There is little information on the safety of discontinuing prophylaxis after immune reconstitution has occurred. Discontinuation of prophylaxis may be considered in children with confirmed immune restoration for 6 months or more as indicated by two measurements of $CD4^+$ greater than 25% at least 3 to 6 months apart in children 2 to 6 years old.[101]

Lifelong prophylaxis should be given to all children who have had an episode of PCP; the safety of discontinuing secondary prophylaxis in the context of immune reconstitution has not been established. If TMP-SMX is not tolerated or cannot be used, alternatives include dapsone (2mg/kg once daily), parenteral pentamidine (4mg/kg every 2 to 4 weeks), or aerosolized pentamidine (300mg via Respigard II inhaler every 4 weeks) if the child is older than 5 years.[6,22,102-105] Safety and efficacy concerns regarding aerosolized

pentamidine preclude its use in younger children.

Fungal Infection

Chronic *Candida* infection is common in HIV-1-infected children and may produce oropharyngeal, laryngeal, or esophageal candidiasis and promote the development of gastroesophageal reflux disease.[5,6,9,106] The incidence of tracheobronchial or esophageal candidiasis has declined substantially with HAART (see Table 2-1).[5,9] Infection of the upper airways may result in *Candida* supraglottitis, epiglottitis, and a croup-like picture.[107,108] Laryngeal candidiasis may manifest as severe acute airway obstruction.[107] Pulmonary disease may also occur in the context of severe disseminated disease. Uncomplicated oropharyngeal candidiasis can be treated with topical therapy (see Table 2-2).[109] Oral fluconazole, itraconazole, or ketoconazole are effective alternative agents.[6,22,110] For esophageal disease, fluconazole or itraconazole is recommended.[6,22]

Other fungal infections, including aspergillosis, histoplasmosis, cryptococcosis, and coccidioidomycosis, may produce respiratory illness usually in the context of severe immunosuppression and disseminated disease (see Table 2-2). Pulmonary cryptococcosis without dissemination may manifest with fever, intrathoracic adenopathy, and pulmonary infiltrates.[6] Occasionally, pulmonary cryptococcosis may be asymptomatic and manifest on routine chest x-rays as pulmonary nodules. Pulmonary coccidioidomycosis may produce nodules, cavities, or diffuse reticulonodular infiltrates associated with fungemia and systemic disease. Children with severe pulmonary cryptococcosis should be treated with amphotericin B; maintenance therapy with fluconazole or itraconazole can be substituted after improvement has occurred.[6,8,22] Mild or moderate pulmonary cryptococcosis can be treated with oral fluconazole or itraconazole.[6,22] Lifelong suppressive therapy with fluconazole or itraconazole is necessary to prevent relapse.[6] There are few data on treatment of pulmonary coccidioidomycosis in children, and recommendations are based on adult data, with amphotericin B recommended for the acute illness followed by long-term suppressive therapy with fluconazole or itraconazole.[6,111] Alternatively, in mild disease therapy may be initiated with fluconazole or itraconazole.[6]

Chronic Lung Disease

Chronic lung disease was reported as common in HIV-1-infected children before HAART.[112,113] A longitudinal birth-cohort study before widespread HAART usage reported a cumulative incidence of chronic radiographic lung changes in HIV-1-infected children of 33% by 4 years of age.[112] The most common chronic radiologic changes were increased bronchovascular markings, reticular densities, or bronchiectasis (Fig. 2-5).[112,113] These radiographic findings were associated with an increased frequency of tachypnea, crackles and clubbing, and a decreased oxygen saturation. Resolution of these chronic changes was associated with reduced CD4+ cell counts and higher viral loads, and thus may be an indication of progression of HIV-1 infection.[112]

The spectrum of chronic lung disease in HIV-1-infected children includes lymphocytic interstitial pneumonia (LIP), interstitial pneumonitis, immune reconstitution inflammatory syndrome (IRIS), bronchiectasis, malignancies, and bronchiolitis obliterans.

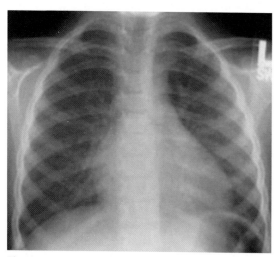

Figure 2-5. Early radiologic evidence of chronic HIV-associated lung disease showing increased bronchovascular markings.

Persistent or recurrent pneumonia is an important cause of chronic lung disease. In African children, TB commonly produces chronic lung disease.[30,32-35]

Lymphocytic Interstitial Pneumonia

LIP, resulting from diffuse interstitial lymphocytic infiltration of the lungs, is common in HIV-1-infected children. The etiology is unknown, but evidence suggests that infection with Epstein-Barr virus may initiate a lymphoproliferative response in the presence of HIV-1 infection.[114] Clinically, children develop chronic respiratory symptoms, principally cough and mild tachypnea.[115] Lymphoproliferation occurring in other organs may produce generalized lymphadenopathy, bilateral nontender parotid enlargement, and hepatosplenomegaly.[115-117] Digital clubbing frequently occurs. Hypoxia, if present, is usually mild. Children may survive for years with a course characterized by recurrent episodes of acute lower respiratory tract infections.[118] Cor pulmonale or bronchiectasis may develop.[119]

Children with LIP have moderately elevated serum IgG and LDH levels and titers to viral capsid antigen of Epstein-Barr virus.[114] Chest radiographs often show a diffuse reticulonodular pattern, more pronounced centrally (Fig. 2-6A), which may be difficult to distinguish from pulmonary or miliary TB (see Fig. 2-3A).[117] Clinically, mild respiratory illness, the presence of parotid enlargement, and a reticulonodular pattern on chest x-ray or computed tomography (CT) scan may help to distinguish children with LIP from children with miliary TB.[117] Peribronchiolar thickening alone or normal chest radiographs also may occur.[116,117] Radiographic lesions may resolve in association with worsening immune status.[120,121] Respiratory status may improve with the use of HAART[122]; among HIV-1-infected adults with LIP, HAART has been reported to result in resolution of radiographic abnormalities.[122]

High-resolution CT may improve diagnostic certainty; typical features include micronodules of 1 to 3mm in diameter, with a perilymphatic distribution, and subpleural nodules (see Fig. 2-6B).[123] The role of nuclear scanning in confirming the diagnosis has not

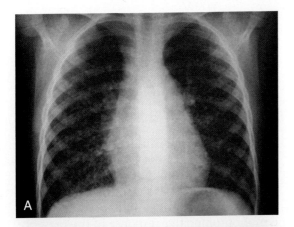

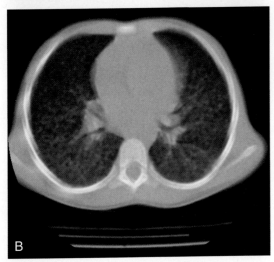

Figure 2-6. A, Chest x-ray of a child with lymphocytic interstitial pneumonia showing multiple nodular densities throughout the lung fields. **B,** High-resolution chest CT scan of a child with lymphocytic interstitial pneumonia showing a diffuse micronodular pattern.

been well studied, but diffuse pulmonary gallium uptake has been reported in an HIV-1-infected child with LIP.[124] Definitive diagnosis requires lung biopsy.[116] Lung biopsies reveal collections of lymphoid aggregates, often with germinal centers, surrounding the airways and a significant interstitial infiltrate composed primarily of lymphocytes.

Treatment is symptomatic, including antibiotics for acute infections and inhaled bronchodilators. Oxygen is administered for hypoxia as needed. Although there are no trials of efficacy, case reports indicate a response to systemic corticosteroids.[125-127] Oral corticosteroids are recommended for children with hypoxia.[127] A suggested regimen is prednisone, 2mg/kg/day for 2 to 4 weeks, until the arterial oxygen saturation

increases. Corticosteroids are tapered to 0.5 to 0.75mg/kg on alternate days, provided that the arterial oxygen saturation remains adequate.[127] Further tapering may be possible as long as adequate oxygenation is maintained. No data exist on the use of inhaled corticosteroids.

LIP is categorized as a World Health Organization stage 3 AIDS-defining illness and is an indication for initiating HAART in children who are not yet receiving antiretroviral therapy.[128]

Interstitial Pneumonitis

Non-specific interstitial pneumonitis may occur in children with AIDS. The clinical manifestations are cough, progressive dyspnea, and hypoxemia; chest radiographs show interstitial pneumonitis. Interstitial pneumonitis may be difficult to distinguish from LIP or TB without open lung biopsy,[117] which is required for definitive diagnosis.

Chronic Pulmonary Infections

Chronic infection, resulting from recurrent or persistent pneumonia, may produce chronic lung disease. Infection with *M. tuberculosis* is a particularly important and prevalent cause of chronic lung disease in developing countries.[29,30,33-35,117] Distinguishing pulmonary or miliary *M. tuberculosis* from LIP may be difficult; generally, children with LIP are older and less severely ill, enlarged parotid glands may occur, and chest radiograph shows a reticulonodular pattern.[117] A few case reports have described chronic *P. jiroveci* infection occurring in HIV-1-infected children, usually manifesting with cystic disease or with pneumatocele formation.[84,129]

Immune Reconstitution Inflammatory Syndrome

With increasing use of HAART, IRIS associated with mycobacterial infection and with other opportunistic infections such as CMV has been reported.[130] IRIS may occur weeks to months after initiation of HAART and may result either from unrecognized mycobacterial infection or from a florid immune response directed against a mycobacterial antigen in patients already receiving therapy for mycobacterial infection.[130] IRIS has been described with different mycobacterial species, including *M. tuberculosis, M. bovis,* or MAC infection.[51,131,132] Most cases of IRIS have been described in HIV-1-infected adults,[52,53] but IRIS is increasingly being recognized in HIV-1-infected children from high TB prevalence areas.[51,54]

Clinically, IRIS is characterized by a seemingly paradoxical worsening in signs with increasing lymphadenopathy, new clinical and radiologic respiratory signs, and fever.[51,53,54,132] The tuberculin skin test may become positive, and chest radiographs may show development of lymphadenopathy or new infiltrates.[53,54] IRIS must be distinguished from other infections, multidrug-resistant TB, or secondary to nonadherence to TB therapy.[53] To minimize the risk of IRIS, HIV-1-infected children with confirmed or probable TB should be treated with antituberculous drugs for 2 to 8 weeks before starting HAART.[49,53] When IRIS develops in a child who was unknown to have TB, therapy for TB should be initiated. If lymphadenopathy or respiratory manifestations are particularly severe, oral corticosteroids may be beneficial, although there are no controlled trials in children.[53]

Bronchiectasis

Bronchiectasis may occur secondary to acute or chronic infection, including *M. tuberculosis*; after recurrent bacterial infections; after a severe viral lower respiratory tract infection; or as a consequence of LIP.[119,133] Development of bronchiectasis may be associated with the severity of immunosuppression; of 23 HIV-infected children (median age 7.5 years) with bronchiectasis, all had CD4$^+$ cell counts less than 100cells/mm^3.[133] Clinical manifestations include increased sputum production, halitosis, abnormalities on chest auscultation, and digital clubbing. Bronchiectasis should be suspected radiologically when there are persistent infiltrates or atelectasis in the same anatomic area for longer than 6 months. High-resolution CT is useful to confirm the diagnosis. Therapy includes physiotherapy and aggressive treatment of intercurrent infections. Use of IVIG therapy at 600mg/kg per dose at monthly intervals may be beneficial.

Malignancy

HIV-1-infected children have an increased risk of malignancy; malignant tumors occur in 2.5% of children with AIDS in the United States.[134] Non-Hodgkin lymphoma is most common, followed by Kaposi sarcoma, leiomyosarcoma, and Hodgkin lymphoma.[135,138] Infection with Epstein-Barr virus has been associated with the development of non-Hodgkin lymphoma in HIV-1-infected children, including children with mild immunosuppression.[135] Primary non-Hodgkin lymphoma may arise in a lymph node or be extranodal.[134,135] AIDS-related non-Hodgkin lymphoma may occur in almost any extranodal site, including the lungs; in addition, pulmonary disease may result from dissemination from a primary focus.

In African HIV-1-infected children, Kaposi sarcoma is the most common AIDS-defining malignancy, probably because of the prevalence of human herpes virus-8 infection.[136-138] Human herpesvirus-8 may be transmitted to a child from an infected mother.[138] The most common clinical presentation is of violaceous plaques on the skin.[139] Kaposi sarcoma lesions may produce upper airway obstruction. Pulmonary dissemination may result in persistent cough, chronic progressive dyspnea, and fever; hemoptysis may occur with endobronchial lesions.[137-139] Abnormalities on chest radiograph include bilateral adenopathy; perihilar infiltrates; pleural effusion; or combinations of interstitial, alveolar, or nodular patterns. The finding of poorly marginated discrete lesions on CT scan might be specific for Kaposi sarcoma.[140] Definitive diagnosis is made by lung biopsy.

Diagnostic Evaluation of an HIV-1-Infected Child with Pulmonary Manifestations

An HIV-1-infected child often presents with fever and tachypnea. The differential diagnosis is extensive, and a systematic approach based on the clinical course of HIV-1 infection and epidemiologic context is useful. Most severe complications are infectious, and the likelihood increases with decreasing CD4$^+$ cell counts. Many lower respiratory tract infections are due to coinfections, such as bacterial-viral, bacterial-bacterial, viral-*Pneumocystis,* or bacterial-*Pneumocystis.*[16] Progressive ventricular dysfunction and cardiomyopathy also occur in HIV-1-infected children, associated with immunocompromise.[141,142] It is important to exclude cardiac involvement with congestive heart failure as a cause of respiratory manifestations.

If a child has acute severe respiratory symptoms, chest x-ray, oxygen saturation, complete blood count, and blood cultures should be obtained. Hypoxia with a diffuse interstitial infiltrate may suggest PCP. A diffuse miliary pattern may suggest TB, but this also can be confused with LIP. For etiologic identification, a blood culture may be helpful. A nasopharyngeal aspirate for identification of respiratory viruses, including RSV, may be indicated. Serum immunoglobulin levels and LDH may be helpful to distinguish PCP from LIP. Sputum or a BAL may be useful for identifying PCP or *M. tuberculosis.* The predominance of neutrophils in BAL and a positive bacterial culture that does not reflect usual oral flora is evidence for bacterial pneumonia. Viral studies from sputum, BAL, or a nasopharyngeal aspirate also may be helpful for detecting a viral pathogen, although for some viruses, such as CMV, this may reflect shedding from the respiratory tract and not disease. If sputum induction or BAL is negative, an open lung biopsy may be necessary to establish the diagnosis. Persistent infiltrates of more than 6 months' duration may suggest bronchiectasis, for which high-resolution CT of the chest is useful. A diffuse nodular infiltrate with hilar adenopathy and normal oxygen saturation suggests LIP.

Empiric treatment should be initiated based on the age of the child, severity of illness, and degree of immunosuppression. Children with acute respiratory signs who are hypoxic and children with severe illness should be treated empirically with antibiotics and oxygen and admitted to the hospital. Infants and children who are not receiving TMP-SMX also should be empirically treated for *Pneumocystis.* For children with milder illness, oral antibiotics may be indicated, or specific treatment may be given according to the etiology (see Table 2-2).

Summary

Acute and chronic respiratory diseases are an important cause of morbidity and mortality in HIV-1-infected children. The burden of childhood HIV and associated respiratory illness occurs predominantly in developing countries. Antiretroviral therapy has changed the spectrum of pulmonary diseases in HIV-1-infected children, resulting in a marked reduction in opportunistic respiratory infections.

References

1. Zar HJ: Pneumonia in HIV-infected and uninfected children in developing countries—epidemiology, clinical features and management. Curr Opin Pulm Med 10:176-182, 2004.
2. Steinbrook R: The AIDS epidemic in 2004. N Engl J Med 351:115-117, 2004.
3. UNAIDS: AIDS epidemic update: Special report on HIV/AIDS. Accessed March 5, 2008. Available at: www.unaids.org.
4. Graham SM: HIV and respiratory infections in children. Curr Opin Pulm Med 9:215-220, 2003.
5. Gona P, et al: Incidence of opportunistic and other infections in HIV-infected children in the HAART era. JAMA 296:292-300, 2006.
6. Mofenson LM, et al: Treating opportunistic infections among HIV-exposed and infected children: Recommendations from CDC, the National Institutes of Health, and the Infectious Diseases Society of America. Clin Infect Dis 40:S1-S84, 2005.
7. Lindegren ML, Steinberg S, Byers RH Jr: Epidemiology of HIV/AIDS in children. Pediatr Clin North Am 47:1-20, 2000.
8. Langston C, et al: Human immunodeficiency virus-related mortality in infants and children: Data from the pediatric pulmonary and cardiovascular complications of vertically transmitted HIV (P(2)C(2)) Study. Pediatrics 107:328-338, 2001.
9. Dankner WM, Lindsey JC, Levin MJ; Pediatric AIDS Clinical Trials Group Protocol Teams 051, 128, 138, 144, 152, 179, 190, 220, 240, 245, 254, 300 and 327: Correlates of opportunistic infections in children infected with the human immunodeficiency virus managed before highly active antiretroviral therapy. Pediatr Infect Dis J 20:40-48, 2001.
10. Chintu C, et al: Lung disease at necropsy in African children dying from respiratory illnesses: A descriptive necropsy study. Lancet 360:985-990, 2002.
11. Madhi SA, et al: Increased disease burden and antibiotic resistance of bacteria causing severe community-acquired lower respiratory tract infections in human immunodeficiency type 1-infected children. Clin Infect Dis 31:170-176, 2000.

12. Zar HJ, et al: Aetiology and outcome of pneumonia in human immunodeficiency virus-infected children hospitalized in South Africa. Acta Paediatr 90:119-125, 2001.
13. National Institute of Child Health and Human Development Intravenous Immunoglobulin Study Group: Intravenous immune globulin for the prevention of bacterial infections in children with symptomatic human immunodeficiency virus infections. N Engl J Med 325:73-80, 1991.
14. Spector SA, et al: A controlled trial of intravenous immune globulin for the prevention of serious bacterial infections in children receiving zidovudine for advanced human immunodeficiency virus infection. N Engl J Med 331:1181-1187, 1994.
15. Madhi SA, et al: Impact of human immunodeficiency virus type 1 on the disease spectrum of *Streptococcus pneumoniae* in South African children. Pediatr Infect Dis J 19:1141-1147, 2000.
16. McNally L, et al: Effect of age, polymicrobial disease and maternal HIV status on treatment response and cause of severe pneumonia in South African children: A prospective descriptive study. Lancet 369:1440-1451, 2007.
17. Zar HJ, Hanslo D, Hussey G: The impact of HIV infection and trimethoprim-sulphamethoxazole prophylaxis on bacterial isolates from children with community-acquired pneumonia in South Africa. J Trop Pediatr 49:78-83, 2003.
18. Roilides E, et al: Bacterial infections in human immunodeficiency virus type 1-infected children: The impact of central venous catheters and antiretroviral agents. Pediatr Infect Dis J 10:813-819, 1991.
19. Madhi SA, et al: Reduced effectiveness of *Hemophilus influenzae* type b conjugate vaccine in children with a high prevalence of human immunodeficiency virus type 1 infection. Pediatr Infect Dis J 21:315-321, 2002.
20. Rongkavilit C, et al: Gram-negative bacillary bacteremia in human immunodeficiency virus type 1-infected children. Pediatr Infect Dis J 19:122-128, 2000.
21. Tan TQ: Antibiotic resistant infections due to *Streptococcus pneumoniae*: Impact on therapeutic options and clinical outcome. Curr Opin Infect Dis 16:271-277, 2003.
22. Pickering LK, ed: Red Book: 2006 Report of the Committee on Infectious Diseases, 27th ed. Elk Grove Village, IL, American Academy of Pediatrics, 2006.
23. Mulholland K, et al: Randomised trial of *Hemophilus influenzae* type-b tetanus protein conjugate vaccine for prevention of pneumonia and meningitis in Gambian infants. Lancet 349:1191-1197, 1997.
24. Swingler G, Fransman D, Hussey G: Conjugate vaccines for preventing *Hemophilus influenzae* type b infections. Cochrane Database Syst Rev 4: CD001729, 2003.
25. Klugman KP, et al: A trial of 9-valent pneumococcal conjugate vaccine in children with and without HIV infection. N Engl J Med 349:1341, 2003.
26. Cutts FT, et al: Efficacy of nine-valent pneumococcal conjugate vaccine against pneumonia and invasive pneumococcal disease in The Gambia: Randomised, double-blind, placebo-controlled trial. Lancet 365:1139-1146, 2005.
27. Black S, et al: Efficacy, safety and immunogenicity of heptavalent pneumococcal conjugate vaccine in children. Pediatr Infect Dis J 19:187-195, 2000.
28. Crow ME: Intravenous immune globulin for prevention of bacterial infections in pediatric AIDS patients. Am J Health Syst Pharm 52:803-811, 1995.
29. Jeena PM, et al: Impact of HIV-1 co-infection on presentation and hospital related mortality in children with pulmonary tuberculosis in Durban, South Africa. Int J Tuberc Lung Dis 6:672-678, 2002.
30. Coovadia HM, Jeena P, Wilkinson D: Childhood human immunodeficiency virus and tuberculosis co-infection: Reconciling conflicting data. Int J Tuberc Lung Dis 2:844-851, 1998.
31. Thomas P, et al: Tuberculosis in human immunodeficiency virus-infected and human immunodeficiency virus-exposed children in New York City. Pediatr Infect Dis J 19:700-706, 2000.
32. Gutman LT, et al: Tuberculosis in human immunodeficiency virus-exposed or infected United States children. Pediatr Infect Dis J 13:963-968, 1994.
33. Palme IB, et al: Impact of human immunodeficiency virus 1 infection on clinical presentation, treatment outcome and survival in a cohort of Ethiopian children with tuberculosis. Pediatr Infect Dis J 21:1053-1061, 2002.
34. Mukadi YD, et al: Impact of HIV infection on the development, clinical presentation, and outcome of tuberculosis among children in Abidjan, Cote d'Ivoire. AIDS 11:1151-1158, 1997.
35. Chintu C: Tuberculosis and human immunodeficiency virus co-infection in children: Management challenges. Paediatr Respir Rev 8:142-147, 2007.
36. Hesseling AC, et al: Outcome of HIV-infected children with culture-confirmed tuberculosis. Arch Dis Child 90:1171-1174, 2005.
37. Soeters M, et al: Clinical features and outcome in children admitted to a TB hospital in the Western Cape—the influence of HIV infection and drug resistance. S Afr Med J 95:602-606, 2005.
38. Hesseling AC, et al: The risk of disseminated bacille Calmette-Guerin (BCG) disease in HIV-infected children. Vaccine 25:14-18, 2007.
39. Hofstadler G, et al: BCG lymphadenitis in an HIV-infected child 9.5 years after vaccination. AIDS Patient Care STDS 12:677-680, 1998.
40. Hesseling AC, et al: Bacille Calmette-Guerin vaccine-induced disease in HIV-infected and HIV-uninfected children. Clin Infect Dis 42:548-558, 2006.
41. Phongsamart W, et al: *Mycobacterium avium* complex in HIV-infected Thai children. J Med Assoc Thai 85(Suppl 2):S682-S689, 2002.
42. Horsburgh CR, Caldwell MB, Simonds RJ: Epidemiology of disseminated nontuberculous mycobacterial disease in children with acquired immune deficiency syndrome. Pediatr Infect Dis J 12:219-222, 1993.
43. Centers for Disease Control and Prevention: Recommendations on prophylaxis and therapy for disseminated *Mycobacterium avium* complex for adults and adolescents infected with human immunodeficiency virus. US Public Health service Task Force on prophylaxis and therapy for *Mycobacterium avium* complex. MMWR Recomm Rep 42(RR-9):14-20, 1993.
44. Abrams EJ: Opportunistic infections and other clinical manifestations of HIV disease in children. Pediatr Clin North Am 47:79-108, 2000.

45. Liebeschuetz S, et al: Diagnosis of tuberculosis in South African children with a T-cell-based assay: A prospective cohort study. Lancet 364:2196-2203, 2004.

46. Marais BJ, Pai M: Recent advances in the diagnosis of childhood tuberculosis. Arch Dis Child 92: 446-452, 2007.

47. Zar HJ, et al: Comparison of induced sputum with gastric lavage for microbiologic confirmation of pulmonary tuberculosis in infants and young children a prospective study. Lancet 365:130-134, 2005.

48. Abadco DL, Steiner P: Gastric lavage is better than bronchoalveolar lavage for isolation of *Mycobacterium tuberculosis* in childhood pulmonary tuberculosis. Pediatr Infect Dis J 11:735, 1992.

49. World Health Organization: Guidance for National Tuberculosis Programmes on the Management of Tuberculosis in Children. Accessed April 10, 2008. Available at: http//www.who.int.

50. Schaaf HS, et al: Recurrent culture-confirmed tuberculosis in human immunodeficiency virus-infected children. Pediatr Infect Dis J 24:685-691, 2005.

51. Puthanakit T, et al: Immune reconstitution syndrome after highly active antiretroviral therapy in human immunodeficiency virus-infected Thai children. Pediatr Infect Dis J 25:53-58, 2006.

52. Bonnet MM, et al: Tuberculosis after HAART initiation in HIV-positive patients from five countries with a high tuberculosis burden. AIDS 20: 1275-1279, 2006.

53. Lawn SD, et al: Immune reconstitution disease associated with mycobacterial infections in HIV-infected individuals receiving antiretrovirals. Lancet Infect Dis 5:361-373, 2005.

54. Zampoli M, et al: Tuberculosis during early antiretroviral-induced immune reconstitution in HIV-infected children. Int J Tuberc Lung Dis 11: 417-423, 2007.

55. Michailidis C, et al: Clinical characteristics of IRIS syndrome in patients with HIV and tuberculosis. Antivir Ther 10:417-422, 2005.

56. Hesseling AC, et al: Resistant *Mycobacterium bovis* bacillus Calmette-Guerin disease: Implications for management of bacillus Calmette-Guerin disease in human immunodeficiency virus-infected children. Pediatr Infect Dis J 23:476-479, 2004.

57. LoBue PA, Moser KS: Treatment of *Mycobacterium bovis* infected tuberculosis patients: San Diego County, California, United States, 1994-2003. Int J Tuberc Lung Dis 9:333-338, 2005.

58. Zar HJ, et al: The effect of isoniazid prophylaxis on mortality and TB incidence in HIV-infected children from a high tuberculosis prevalence area a randomised controlled trial. BMJ 334:136-139, 2007.

59. Madhi SA, et al: Increased burden of respiratory viral associated severe lower respiratory tract infections in children with human immunodeficiency virus type-1 J Pediatr 137:78-84, 2000.

60. Madhi SA, et al: Human metapneumovirus-associated lower respiratory tract infections among hospitalized human immunodeficiency virus type 1 (HIV-1)-infected and HIV-1-uninfected African infants. Clin Infect Dis 37:1705-1710, 2003.

61. Madhi SA, Klugman KP; Vaccine Trialist Group: A role for *Streptococcus pneumoniae* in virus-associated pneumonia. Nat Med 10:811-813, 2004.

62. Kovacs A, et al: Cytomegalovirus infection and HIV-1 disease progression in infants born to HIV-1-infected women. N Engl J Med 341:77-84, 1999.

63. Williams AJ, et al: *Pneumocystis carinii* pneumonia and cytomegalovirus infection in children with vertically acquired HIV infection. AIDS 15: 335-339, 2001.

64. Frenkel LM, et al: Oral ganciclovir in children: Pharmacokinetics, safety, tolerance, and antiviral effects. The Pediatric AIDS Clinical Trials Group. J Infect Dis 182:1616-1624, 2000.

65. Hatherill M, et al: Severe upper airway obstruction caused by ulcerative laryngitis. Arch Dis Child 85:326-329, 2001.

66. Derryck A, et al: Varicella and zoster in children with human immunodeficiency virus infection. Pediatr Infect Dis J 17:931-933, 1998.

67. De Carvalho V, et al: Measles in children with HIV infection: Report of five cases. Braz J Infect Dis 7:346-352, 2003.

68. Hussey GD, Klein M: A randomized, controlled trial of vitamin A in children with severe measles. N Engl J Med 323:160-164, 1990.

69. Zawadzka-Glos L, et al: Lower airway papillomatosis in children. Int J Pediatr Otorhinolaryngol 67:1117-1121, 2003.

70. Reeves WC, et al: National Registry for Juvenile-Onset Recurrent Respiratory Papillomatosis. Arch Otolaryngol Head Neck Surg 129:976-982, 2003.

71. Vernon SD, et al: A longitudinal study of human papillomavirus DNA detection in human immunodeficiency virus type 1-seropositive and -seronegative women. J Infect Dis 169:1108-1112, 1994.

72. St Louis ME, et al: Genital types of papillomavirus in children of women with HIV-1 infection in Kinshasa, Zaire. Int J Cancer 54:181-184, 1993.

73. Shehab N, Sweet BV, Hogikyan ND: Cidofovir for the treatment of recurrent respiratory papillomatosis: A review of the literature. Pharmacotherapy 25:977-989, 2005.

74. Simonds RJ, et al: Prophylaxis against *Pneumocystis carinii* pneumonia among children with perinatally-acquired human immunodeficiency virus infection in the United States. N Engl J Med 332:786-790, 1995.

75. Graham SM, et al: Clinical presentation and outcome of *Pneumocystis carinii* pneumonia in Malawian children. Lancet 355:369-373, 2000.

76. Zar HJ, et al: *Pneumocystis carinii* in HIV-infected children in South Africa. Pediatr Infect Dis J 19:603-607, 2000.

77. Ruffini DD, Madhi SA: The high burden of *Pneumocystis carinii* pneumonia in African HIV-1-infected children hospitalized for severe pneumonia. AIDS 16:105-112, 2002.

78. Hughes WT: *Pneumocystis carinii* pneumonia: New approaches to diagnosis, treatment and prevention. Pediatr Infect Dis J 10:391-399, 1991.

79. Fatti GL, Zar HJ, Swingler G: Clinical indicators of *P. jiroveci* pneumonia in South African children infected with HIV. Int J Infect Dis 10:282-286, 2006.

80. Madhi SA, et al: Ineffectiveness of trimethoprim-sulphamethoxazole prophylaxis and the importance of bacterial and viral coinfections in African children with *Pneumocystis carinii* pneumonia. Clin Infect Dis 35:1120-1126, 2002.

81. Kagawa FT, et al: Serum lactate dehydrogenase activity in patients with AIDS and *Pneumocystis carinii* pneumonia. Chest 94:1031-1033, 1988.

82. Garay SM, Greene J: Prognostic indicators in the initial presentation of *Pneumocystis carinii* pneumonia. Chest 95:769-772, 1989.

83. Sivit CJ, et al: Spectrum of chest radiographic abnormalities in children with AIDS and *Pneumocystis carinii* pneumonia. Pediatr Radiol 25:389-392, 1995.
84. Solomon KS, et al: Pneumothorax as the presenting sign of *Pneumocystis carinii* infection in an HIV-positive child with prior lymphocytic interstitial pneumonitis. Pediatr Radiol 26:559-562, 1996.
85. Holland, ET Saulsbury FT: Chronic *Pneumocystis carinii* pneumonia associated with extensive pneumatocele formation in a child with human immunodeficiency virus infection. Pediatr Pulmonol 35:144-146, 2003.
86. Bye MR, et al: *Pneumocystis carinii* pneumonia in young children with AIDS. Pediatr Pulmonol 9:251-253, 1990.
87. Vernon DD, et al: Respiratory failure in children with acquired immunodeficiency syndrome and acquired immunodeficiency syndrome-related complex. Pediatrics 82:223-228, 1988.
88. Thomas CF, Limper AH: *Pneumocystis* pneumonia. N Engl J Med 350:2487-2498, 2004.
89. Bye MR, Cairns-Bazarian AM, Ewig JM: Markedly reduced mortality associated with corticosteroid therapy of *Pneumocystis carinii* pneumonia in children with acquired immunodeficiency syndrome. Arch Pediatr Adolesc Med 148:638-641, 1994.
90. Briel M, et al: Adjunctive corticosteroids for *Pneumocystis jiroveci* pneumonia in patients with HIV-infection. Cochrane Database Syst Rev 3:CD006150, 2006.
91. Miller RF, et al: Probable mother-to-infant transmission of *Pneumocystis carinii* f. sp. *hominis* infection. J Clin Microbiol 40:1555-1557, 2002.
92. Heresi GP, et al: *Pneumocystis carinii* pneumonia in infants who were exposed to human immunodeficiency virus but were not infected: An exception to the AIDS surveillance case definition. Clin Infect Dis 25:739-740, 1997.
93. McNally LM, et al: Probable mother to infant transmission of *Pneumocystis jiroveci* from an HIV-infected woman to her HIV-uninfected infant. AIDS 19:1548-1549, 2005.
94. Rieder MJ, King SM, Read S: Adverse reactions to trimethoprim sulfamethoxazole among children with human immunodeficiency virus infection. Pediatr Infect Dis J 16:1028-1031, 1997.
95. Goodwin SD: *Pneumocystis carinii* pneumonia in human immunodeficiency virus-infected infants and children. Pharmacotherapy 13:640-646, 1993.
96. McLaughlin GE, et al: Effect of corticosteroids on survival of children with acquired immune deficiency syndrome an *Pneumocystis carinii*-related respiratory failure. J Pediatr 126:821-824, 1995.
97. Creery WD, et al: Surfactant therapy improves pulmonary function in infants with *Pneumocystis carinii* pneumonia and acquired immunodeficiency syndrome. Pediatr Pulmonol 24:370-373, 1997.
98. Marriage SC, Underhill H, Nadel S: Use of natural surfactant in an HIV-infected infant with *Pneumocystis carinii* pneumonia. Intensive Care Med 22:611-612, 1995.
99. Zar HJ: Prevention of HIV-associated respiratory illness in children in developing countries potential benefits. Int J Tuberc Lung Dis 7:820-827, 2003.
100. Chintu PC, et al: Co-trimoxazole as prophylaxis against opportunistic infections in HIV-infected Zambian children (CHAP): A double-blind randomised placebo-controlled trial. Lancet 364:1865-1871, 2004.
101. World Health Organization: Guidelines for cotrimoxazole prophylaxis for HIV-related infections among children, adolescents and adults in resource-limited settings. Recommendations for a public health approach. Accessed May 15, 2008. Available at: http/www.who.int/hiv/pub/guidelines/ctx.
102. Nachman S, et al: The rate of serious bacterial infections among HIV-infected children with immune reconstitution who have discontinued opportunistic infection prophylaxis. Pediatrics 115:e488-e494, 2005.
103. Barnett ED: Dapsone for prevention of *Pneumocystis* pneumonia in children with acquired immunodeficiency syndrome. Pediatr Infect Dis J 13:72-74, 1994.
104. Cruciani M, et al: Dapsone prophylaxis against *Pneumocystis carinii* pneumonia in human immunodeficiency virus-infected children. Pediatr Infect Dis J 13:80-81, 1994.
105. Orcutt TA, et al: Aerosolized pentamidine: A well-tolerated mode of prophylaxis against *Pneumocystis carinii* pneumonia in older children with human immunodeficiency virus infection. Pediatr Infect Dis J 11:290-294, 1992.
106. Hand IL, et al: Aerosolized pentamidine for prophylaxis of *Pneumocystis carinii* pneumonia in infants with human immunodeficiency virus infection. Pediatr Infect Dis J 13:100-104, 1994.
107. Chiou CC, et al: Esophageal candidiasis in pediatric acquired immunodeficiency syndrome: Clinical manifestations and risk factors. Pediatr Infect Dis J 19:729-734, 2000.
108. Bye MR, et al: Clinical *Candida* supraglottitis in an infant with AIDS-related complex. Pediatr Pulmonol 3:280-281, 1987.
109. Balsam D, Sorrano D, Barax C: *Candida* epiglottitis presenting as stridor in a child with HIV infection. Pediatr Radiol 22:235-236, 1992.
110. Rex JH, et al: Practice guidelines for the treatment of candidiasis. Clin Infect Dis 30:662-678, 2000.
111. Pons V, et al: Oropharyngeal candidiasis in patients with AIDS: Randomized comparison of fluconazole versus nystatin oral suspensions. Clin Infect Dis 24:1204-1207, 1997.
112. Galgiani JN, et al: Practice guidelines for treatment of coccidioidomycosis. Clin Infect Dis 30:658-661, 2000.
113. Norton KI, et al: Chronic radiographic lung changes in children with vertically transmitted HIV-1 infection. AJR Am J Roentgenol 176:1553-1558, 2001.
114. Berdon WE, et al: Pediatric HIV infection in its second decade—the changing pattern of lung involvement: Clinical, plain film, and computed tomographic findings. Radiol Clin North Am 31:453-463, 1993.
115. Katz BZ, Berkman AB, Shapiro ED: Serologic evidence of active Epstein-Barr virus infection in Epstein-Barr virus-associated lymphoproliferative disorders of children with acquired immunodeficiency syndrome. J Pediatr 120(2 Pt 1):228-232, 1992.
116. Simmank K, et al: Clinical features and T-cell subsets in HIV-infected children with and without lymphocytic interstitial pneumonitis. Ann Trop Paediatr 21:195-201, 2001.
117. Oldham SA, et al: HIV-associated lymphocytic interstitial pneumonia: Radiologic manifestations and pathologic correlation. Radiology 170(1 Pt 1):83-87, 1989.

118. Jeena PM, et al: Persistent and chronic lung disease in HIV-1 infected and uninfected African children. AIDS 12:1185-1193, 1998.
119. Sharland M, Gibb DM, Holland F: Respiratory morbidity from lymphocytic interstitial pneumonitis (LIP) in vertically acquired HIV infection. Arch Dis Child 76:334-336, 1997.
120. Amorosa JK, et al: Bronchiectasis in children with lymphocytic interstitial pneumonia and acquired immune deficiency syndrome: Plain film and CT observations. Pediatr Radiol 22:603-606, 1992.
121. Prosper M, et al: Clinical significance of resolution of chest x-ray findings in HIV-infected children with lymphocytic interstitial pneumonitis (LIP). Pediatr Radiol 25(suppl):S243-S246, 1995.
122. Gonzalez CE, et al: Lymphoid interstitial pneumonitis in pediatric AIDS: Natural history of the disease. Ann N Y Acad Sci 918:358-361, 2000.
123. Dufour V, et al: Improvement of symptomatic human immunodeficiency virus-related lymphoid interstitial pneumonia in patients receiving highly active antiretroviral therapy. Clin Infect Dis 36:e127-e130, 2003.
124. Becciolini V, et al: Lymphocytic interstitial pneumonia in children with AIDS: High-resolution CT findings. Eur Radiol 11:1015-1020, 2001.
125. Zuckier LS, Ongseng F, Goldfarb CR: Lymphocytic interstitial pneumonitis: A cause of pulmonary gallium-67 uptake in a child with acquired immunodeficiency syndrome. J Nucl Med 29:707-711, 1988.
126. Kornstein MJ, et al: The pathology and treatment of interstitial pneumonitis in two infants with AIDS. Am Rev Respir Dis 133:1196-1198, 1986.
127. Griffiths MH, Miller RF, Semple SJ: Interstitial pneumonitis in patients infected with the human immunodeficiency virus. Thorax 50:1141-1146, 1995.
128. Rubinstein A, et al: Corticosteroid treatment for pulmonary lymphoid hyperplasia in children with the acquired immune deficiency syndrome. Pediatr Pulmonol 4:13-17, 1988.
129. World Health Organization: WHO case definitions of HIV for surveillance and revised clinical staging and immunological classification of HIV-related disease in adults and children. Accessed May 20, 2008. Available at: http/www.who.int/hiv/.
130. Evlogias NE, et al: Severe cystic pulmonary disease associated with chronic *Pneumocystis carinii* infection in a child with AIDS. Pediatr Radiol 24:606-608, 1994.
131. French MA, Price P, Stone SF: Immune restoration disease after antiretroviral therapy. AIDS 18:1615-1627, 2004.
132. Siberry GK, Tessema S: Immune reconstitution syndrome precipitated by bacille Calmette Guerin after initiation of antiretroviral therapy. Pediatr Infect Dis J 25:648-649, 2006.
133. Puthanakit T, et al: Immune reconstitution syndrome due to bacillus Calmette-Guerin after initiation of antiretroviral therapy in children with HIV infection. Clin Infect Dis 41:1049-1052, 2005.
134. Sheikh S, et al: Bronchiectasis in pediatric AIDS. Chest 112:1202-1207, 1997.
135. Biggar RJ, Frisch M, Goedert JJ: Risk of cancer in children with AIDS. AIDS-Cancer Match Registry Study Group. JAMA 284:205-209, 2000.
136. Knowles DM: Etiology and pathogenesis of AIDS-related non-Hodgkin's lymphoma. Hematol Oncol Clin N Am 17:785-820, 2003.
137. Amir H, et al: Kaposi's sarcoma before and during a human immunodeficiency virus epidemic in Tanzanian children. Pediatr Infect Dis J 20:518-521, 2001.
138. Sinfield RL, et al: Spectrum and presentation of pediatric malignancies in the HIV era: Experience from Blantyre, Malawi, 1998-2003. Pediatr Blood Cancer 48:515-520, 2007.
139. Mbulaiteye S, et al: Molecular evidence for mother-to-child transmission of Kaposi sarcoma-associated herpesvirus in Uganda and K1 gene evolution within the host. J Infect Dis 193:1250-1257, 2006.
140. Von Roenn JH: Clinical presentations and standard therapy of AIDS-associated Kaposi's sarcoma. Hematol Oncol Clin N Am 17:747-762, 2003.
141. Naidich DP, et al: Kaposi sarcoma: CT-radiographic correlation. Chest 96:723-728, 1989.
142. Starc TJ, et al: Incidence of cardiac abnormalities in children with human immunodeficiency virus infection: The prospective P2C2 HIV Study. J Pediatr 141:327-334, 2002.
143. Lipshultz SE, et al: Left ventricular structure and function in children infected with human immunodeficiency virus. The prospective P2C2 HIV Multicenter Study. Pediatric Pulmonary and Cardiac Complications of Vertically Transmitted HIV Infection. Circulation 97:1246-1256, 1998.

CHAPTER **3**

Pulmonary Manifestations of Immunosuppressive Diseases Other than Human Immunodeficiency Virus Infection

JAMES M. STARK

Primary Immunodeficiencies 50
  Deficiencies in Immunoglobulin
    Production 50
  Deficiencies in Cellular Immunity 53
  Deficiencies in Phagocyte Numbers, Function,
    and Opsonization 59
Secondary Immunodeficiencies 62
  Overview 62
  Factors Contributing to the Secondary
    Immunodeficient State 63
  Pulmonary Complications of Cancer
    Therapy 64
  Transplant-Related Pulmonary
    Complications 67

**Diagnosis and Treatment of
  Respiratory Abnormalities in a Child
  with Secondary Immunocompromise
  Owing to Cancer or
  Transplantation** 74
  Radiography 74
  Sputum and Nasopharyngeal Washes, and
    Other Indirect Methods for Pathogen
    Detection 74
  Flexible Bronchoscopy 75
  Transthoracic Needle Aspiration Biopsy 75
  Open Lung Biopsy 75
Summary 76
  References 76

Infection in an immunocompromised child presents many diagnostic challenges. In patients with primary immunodeficiencies, the clinician is often faced with the difficulty of not only diagnosing the infectious agent in the lung but also determining whether this child with "too many" respiratory infections actually has an underlying immune problem predisposing to repeat or atypical infections. Many of the basic defects in patients with the primary immunodeficiencies come into play in those who are immunosuppressed by cancer chemotherapy or by specific antirejection therapies after organ transplantation: decreased number or function of B lymphocytes, T lymphocytes, and phagocytic cells as well. The conducting airways branch 20 to 25 times between the trachea and the alveoli. The large surface area of the conducting airways and alveolar surfaces ($>70m^2$ in an adult) poses a great challenge for the lung

defenses for even an immunocompetent host. The anatomy of the lung, lung products, cell receptors, and host cellular responses all contribute to the normal lung defense and disease prevention. A defect in any of these defenses can result in an increased susceptibility to infection.

This chapter first focuses on the primary immunodeficiencies and the associated cellular defects that predispose to pulmonary infections. In this section the discussion of roles of specific cell types in lung defenses provides background for the discussion of immune defects arising from cancer chemotherapy or use of immunosuppressive drugs after organ transplantation. Although this portion of the chapter cannot provide an exhaustive review of all pulmonary abnormalities in primary immunodeficiency states, we will also focus on the major immunodeficiencies as examples of alterations in the cellular immune system and their pulmonary manifestations. Readers are referred to several more recent reviews for more details on primary immunodeficiency states.[1-6]

The focus of the chapter changes to the general principles underlying the immune and nonimmune pulmonary complications of cancer chemotherapy and immunosuppressive therapy after organ transplantation. Many of the cellular defects described in the section on primary immunodeficiencies come into play in those patients with secondary immunocompromise. The chapter concludes with a discussion of diagnostic tools available for defining the underlying causes of pulmonary abnormalities in patients with immunodeficiency or immunosuppression.

Primary Immunodeficiencies

This section focuses on the pulmonary manifestations of primary immunodeficiency diseases. More than 100 primary immunodeficiency diseases are well-characterized clinically or at the molecular level, or both.[1,4] Antibody deficiencies are the most common primary immunodeficiency diseases, accounting for about 70% of cases.[7] Patients with deficiencies in antibody production typically acquire infections from encapsulated (*Streptococcus pneumoniae, Haemophilus influenzae*, and *Staphylococcus* species) and gram-negative (*Pseudomonas* species) organisms. Chronic fungal and opportunistic infections are rare. Viral infections are handled normally, with the exception of enteroviruses, which can cause persistent meningoencephalitis.[3,7]

In contrast, defects in T cell function lead to infections by viruses and opportunistic organisms. Affected infants can present early in life with chronic diarrhea and failure to thrive. Persistent infections with opportunistic organisms (*Candida albicans, Pneumocystis jiroveci* [formerly *P. carinii*]) and viral infections often can be fatal.[3,7] Patients with T cell defects cannot reject allografts, placing them at risk for fatal graft-versus-host disease (GVHD) if they receive nonirradiated blood or blood product transfusions. Infants with severe combined immunodeficiency (SCID) have absent T cell and B cell function, placing them at risk for infections manifested by immunoglobulin and T cell defects. The knowledge of the genetic defects underlying these immunodeficiency states continues to grow; there are now more than 10 known gene alterations associated with the phenotype of SCID.[4] As the molecular genetics of these diseases becomes better understood, the ability to treat the severe forms of primary immunodeficiency disease with stem cell transplant (SCT) or gene therapy has improved in recent years.

Deficiencies in Immunoglobulin Production

Overview

IgG and IgA are found in the epithelial airway–lining fluid and play important roles in lung defense against bacteria. Deficiencies in these antibodies occur in many primary immunodeficiencies and usually result in chronic sinopulmonary infections.

Secretory IgA is the predominant immunoglobulin isotype present in airway secretions.[2] Secretory IgA serves several functions, including neutralization of viruses and exotoxin, enhancement of lactoferrin and lactoperoxidase activities, and inhibition of microbial growth. Because dimeric IgA is able to bind two antigens simultaneously, it is capable of forming large antigen-antibody complexes. In this manner, IgA neutralizes microbes, facilitates their removal by mucociliary clearance, inhibits microbial binding to epithelial cells, and inhibits uptake of potential allergens. Although concentrations of IgG in the upper airway are less than the concentrations of IgA, all IgG subclasses are detectable in respiratory secretions, and it is the primary antibody found in lower respiratory secretions. As opposed to IgA, which is actively transported into the airway, IgG reaches the airway largely by transudation through the mucosa. IgG functions by opsonizing microbes for phagocytosis and killing, activating the complement cascade, and neutralizing many bacterial endotoxins and viruses.

Deficiencies in IgA and IgG result in loss of mucosal protection against numerous pathogens. Selective IgA deficiency (defined by a serum IgA concentration <0.05mg/mL) may be asymptomatic; it is often detected in healthy individuals during routine blood donor screening. Symptomatic individuals present with various manifestations, including recurrent sinusitis, otitis media, pharyngitis, bronchitis, pneumonia, chronic diarrhea, and autoimmune syndromes. Individuals with associated IgE deficiency tend to have less serious pulmonary disease, in contrast to individuals with normal or high IgE, who in addition to the aforementioned disorders may have allergic respiratory problems and pulmonary hemosiderosis. IgA deficiency is associated with increased frequency of neoplastic and autoimmune disorders.[2] IgG deficiency is associated with recurrent otitis media, sinusitis, bronchitis, and pneumonia. In addition, recurrence of airway infections may result in chronic airway injury with bronchiectasis more frequently in patients with IgG deficiency than in patients with isolated IgA deficiency. The combination of altered opsonic activity and bronchiectasis can result in chronic colonization with respiratory pathogens, such as *Pseudomonas aeruginosa*.

Compared with IgG and IgA, IgM seems to play little role in lung defense. Most IgM remains in the vascular space owing to its high molecular weight. IgM does gain access to the airway, however, by exudation or by active secretion via secretory components. IgM is capable of agglutinating bacteria and activating the complement cascade.

IgE seems to participate in immunity to parasites. It binds to the parasites, and eosinophils bind to the opsonized organisms via the IgE Fc receptors. Eosinophils are stimulated to release granular contents, resulting in lysis of the parasite. The major manifestation of the presence of IgE in the respiratory tract is related to its role in allergic disease.

Specific Diseases

Antibody production is altered in many primary immunodeficiency states (Table 3-1). Severe recurrent infections associated with bronchiectasis occur with combined deficiencies in IgA and IgG production. X-linked agammaglobulinemia, the first primary immunodeficiency disease to be recognized, by Bruton in 1952,[8] has been found to result from mutations in Bruton tyrosine kinase.[9,10]

Patients with X-linked agammaglobulinemia have a block in differentiation at all stages of B cell development, whereas T cell numbers and function are preserved. Initially, infants with X-linked agammaglobulinemia are protected by circulating maternal antibodies, but later develop recurrent sinopulmonary infections and may progress to bronchiectasis.[9,11,12]

Similar to X-linked agammaglobulinemia, common variable immunodeficiency is characterized by impaired antibody production of all major classes. In contrast to X-linked agammaglobulinemia, patients with common variable immunodeficiency have normal numbers of circulating B cells; however, these B cells do not differentiate into antibody-secreting plasma cells. Common variable immunodeficiency affects males and females, and in some cases seems to be inherited in an autosomal dominant pattern with incomplete penetrance. Patients can present in infancy but may present in late childhood to adulthood. Common variable immunodeficiency likely represents several different genetic disorders.[13-16]

Isolated IgA deficiency is the most common primary immunodeficiency disease, with an incidence of 1 in 333 to 1 in 700 in whites. The clinical manifestations of isolated IgA deficiency vary. Some affected patients are asymptomatic, whereas others can have recurrent respiratory and gastrointestinal infections, allergy, and increased incidence of autoimmune disease and malignancies.[2,3] Because these patients can make IgG, however, bronchiectasis is uncommon compared with X-linked agammaglobulinemia or common variable immunodeficiency.

Isolated IgM deficiency is not associated with recurrent respiratory infections. Individuals with IgM deficiency seem to have a specific defect in B lymphocyte maturation, but the B lymphocytes are capable of secreting other antibody isotypes. The autosomal recessive form of hyper-IgM syndrome is caused by deficiency in nucleotide-modifying enzymes, UNG (uracil nucleoside glycosylase) and AID (activation-induced cytidine deaminase), expressed only in B cells that operate on sequential steps in antibody class switching.[17] This form of hyper-IgM syndrome is accompanied by decreased

Table 3-1 Primary Immunodeficiencies with Antibody Underproduction

DEFICIENCY	INHERITANCE	GENE LOCUS	GENETIC DEFECT	CELLULAR DEFECTS	CLINICAL FINDINGS
X-linked agammaglobulinemia (Bruton agammaglobulinemia)	X-linked	Xq21.3-Xq22	Deficiency in Bruton tyrosine kinase	<1% circulating B cells; Block in B cell differentiation	Recurrent sinopulmonary infections; Most manifest in infancy, ~20% manifest in 3-5 yr old; Bronchiectasis in right middle lobe and bases
IgA deficiency	Variable (1/333-1/700 births)	17p11	TACI	Deficiency in immunoglobulins of all types and isotypes	Bacterial pneumonias, sinus disease
		Possibly 6p21.3	Others	Deficient isotype switch to IgA	Associated gastrointestinal infections; Increased atopy and neoplastic and autoimmune disorders
Common variable immunodeficiency (likely several diseases)	AD with incomplete penetrance	17p11.2	TACI	Impaired production of all major antibody classes	Onset from early childhood to adulthood
		2q33	ICOS	Absent immunoglobulins	Increased susceptibility to recurrent sinopulmonary infections
		16p11.2 22q13.1-22q12.21	Others	Normal number of B cells; Failure to differentiate into antibody-secreting cells; Abnormal T cells in 60%	Leads to bronchiectasis; Associated with autoimmunity in 20%
Autosomal recessive agammaglobulinemia	AR		Mutations in μ, α, $\lambda5$, *BLNK*, or *LRRCE* genes	All isotypes, decreased B cells	Severe bacterial infections
Immunoglobulin heavy chain deletions	AR	Δ14q32	Δ immunoglobulin heavy chains	Decreased IgG1, IgG2, IgG4, IgE, IgA1, IgA2	Recurrent bacterial infections
ICOS deficiency	AR	2q33	Mutation in ICOS gene	Decreased all isotypes	Recurrent bacterial infections
Hyper-IgM syndrome	AR	12p13 12q23-2q24.1	Mutation in AID and UNG	Decreased IgG and IgA; Deficient B cell switching; Normal T cells	Recurrent bacterial infections

AD, autosomal dominant; AID, activation-induced cytidine deaminase; AR, autosomal recessive; ICOS, inducible T cell costimulator; TACI, transmembrane activator and calcium modulator and cyclophilin ligand interactor; UNG, uracil nucleoside glycosylase.

levels of IgG and IgA, resulting in an increased propensity to bacterial infection (see Table 3-1).[17]

Isolated IgE deficiency has not been reported. IgE deficiency in combination with IgG4 deficiency has been described in a patient who had recurrent otitis media and sinusitis. Hyper-IgE syndrome is discussed in the section focusing on phagocytic disorders.

Diagnosis

In patients with suspected immunoglobulin deficiency, quantitation of total serum IgA and IgG, and IgG subclasses should be performed along with measurement of the antibody response to protein (diphtheria and tetanus toxoids) and polysaccharide (*S. pneumoniae, H. influenzae, Neisseria meningitidis*) vaccines. In addition, flow cytometry to quantify B and T cell numbers and B and T cell stimulation studies should be done if immunoglobulin levels are low. Specific genetic studies can be done to identify patients with several of the immunoglobulin primary immunodeficiency diseases (see Table 3-1).

Treatment

IgG-deficient patients with recurrent respiratory tract infections often benefit from prophylactic antibiotics, intravenous gamma globulin therapy, and the use of airway clearance techniques. Patients with selective IgA deficiency are treated symptomatically for respiratory, gastrointestinal, and allergic problems. Because most preparations of gamma globulin contain IgA, the use of gamma globulin increases the risk of anaphylaxis if the recipient has anti-IgA antibodies. Transfusion of blood products presents a similar problem for these individuals. In patients with a combined IgA and IgG deficiency who need immunoglobulin therapy or the transfusion of blood products, it is crucial to ensure that the recipient does not have IgA antibodies or use a preparation that does not contain IgA.

Deficiencies in Cellular Immunity

Overview

Bronchial-associated lymphoid tissue functions in the development of adaptive lung defense. Bronchial-associated lymphoid tissue comprises intraepithelial lymphocytes, macrophages, dendritic cells, and natural killer (NK) and NK-T cells that recognize foreign substances, invading organisms or their exoproducts, and products of cell injury using innate receptor systems. The dendritic cells or macrophages interact with them and interact with lymphocytes to create the cellular immune responses, or to signal antibody production. These cells migrate to local lymph nodes, tonsils, or adenoids; process antigens; generate cytokines; and generate the adaptive immune responses. Extensive reviews of humoral (B cell mediated) and cellular (T cell mediated) immunity, antigen presentation, and cellular activation are well beyond the scope of this chapter; however, we briefly discuss the roles of T lymphocytes and cellular immunity with respect to lung defense.

Several types of T lymphocytes contribute to lung immunity and tissue pathology.[18-23] Two major types of antigen receptors are used by T lymphocytes—the $\gamma\delta$ T cell receptor (discussed later) and the $\alpha\beta$ receptor (used by the $CD4^+$ and $CD8^+$ T cell populations). The $\alpha\beta$ T cell mounts cytolytic responses to infected cells, makes cytokines, and stimulates B cell responses (see later). $\alpha\beta$ T cells expressing the receptor protein, CD4, are termed T helper cells. $CD4^+$ T cells recognize antigens presented via the MHC class II antigen and provide effector function primarily by the release of cytokines. T helper cells can be differentiated further phenotypically into Th1 and Th2 populations based on their profiles of cytokine production. Th1 cells differentiate in the presence of interleukin (IL)-12 and IL-18, and produce interferon-γ, IL-2, and tumor necrosis factor-α in response to antigen. These cells have been regarded as responsible for the delayed hypersensitivity response to viral or bacterial infection, stimulating local macrophage activation and neutrophil recruitment, and altering specific T cell responses. Th2 cells are driven to differentiate by the presence of IL-4, and in the presence of antigen they respond by making IL-4, IL-5, IL-10, and IL-13. These cytokines are responsible for driving B lymphocytes to make antibodies and lead to the recruitment and activation of basophils and eosinophils. The Th2 phenotype has been associated with an allergic/asthmatic phenotype in mouse models and human studies.[24]

αβ T cells expressing CD8 are cytotoxic cells. In response to peptides presented by the MHC class I molecules, CD8[+] T cells function in target cell toxicity. CD8[+] T cell toxicity is mediated by the release of cellular granules containing perforin (perturbs the cell membrane) and granzymes (disrupt target cells by altering intracellular targets). In addition, CD8[+] T cells can initiate apoptosis in target cells by Fas-FasL interactions. CD8[+] cells reinforce viral defenses by rendering adjacent cells resistant to infection, presumably by release of interferons.

Three additional subsets of T cells contribute to innate lung responses, including recognition and elimination of tumor cells and certain pathogens using limited sets of conserved recognition receptors. NK cells are bone marrow–derived lymphocytes that are distinct from either B or T cells. NK-T cells are T cells that express the NK cell marker, NK1, a highly restricted/limited repertoire of the CD3/T cell receptor complex with specificity for antigens presented in association with CD1. These cells most closely resemble CD4[+] T cells in terms of cytokine production. Finally, γδ T cells have a limited diversity of T cell receptors that recognize self and bacterial/protozoan antigens. These innate lymphocytes are considered to be a first line of defense against tumors and infection, and in modulating inflammation in the lung.[25,26]

T cell responses are tightly regulated. T cell responses are necessary to eliminate pathogens and for immune memory; lack of T cell function can lead to serious life-threatening infections.[1,3,4,6,7,27] Uncontrolled responses can cause autoimmune inflammatory diseases, however.[28-33] In this section, we discuss primary immunodeficiency disease associated with T lymphocyte dysfunctions.

Specific Diseases

Mutations in the function of B cells or T cells result in immunodeficiencies of antibody production, cellular immunity, or both. The incidence of these deficiencies is unknown, but has been estimated to be 1 in 10,000 live births.[7] Children with defects in T cell function can present with abnormal ability to limit "usual" childhood respiratory viral infections, which can be persistent or life-threatening (e.g., respiratory syncytial virus [RSV], parainfluenza virus, influenza virus, and adenovirus). Common childhood viral infections, such as varicella-zoster virus and measles, can cause serious lung infections in immunodeficient or immunosuppressed children. Children with T cell immunodeficiencies are more susceptible to opportunistic pathogens—agents that typically do not cause infections except in the context of immunodeficiency or immunosuppression, such as cytomegalovirus (CMV) and *P. jiroveci* (Fig. 3-1). Children with T cell deficiencies can present in the first months of life with diarrhea and failure to thrive, or with persistent infections with *Candida albicans, P. jiroveci,* varicella-zoster virus, adenovirus, RSV, or CMV.[7,34] Patients with T cell primary immunodeficiency disease may show abnormalities in antibody production because B cell function in antibody production is T cell–dependent. T cell primary immunodeficiency disease can manifest with bacterial infections as in patients with primary antibody deficiencies as described earlier.[3]

Severe combined immunodeficiency (SCID) is an immunodeficiency characterized by a severe reduction in the number or function of T cells, which results in the absence of adaptive responses (Table 3-2).

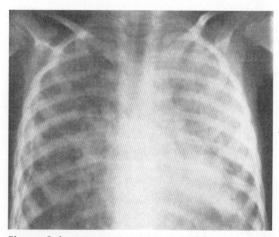

Figure 3-1. Chest radiograph shows bilateral interstitial and alveolar infiltrates in a child with acute lymphocytic leukemia and *Pneumocystis jiroveci* (formerly *P. carinii*) pneumonia. (*From Long S, et al: Principles and Practice of Pediatric Infectious Disease, 2nd ed. Philadelphia, Churchill Livingstone, 2003. page 578*)

Table 3-2 Primary Immunodeficiencies with T Cell Defects (Examples)

DEFICIENCY	INHERITANCE	GENE LOCUS	GENETIC DEFECT	CELLULAR DEFECTS	CLINICAL FINDINGS
T⁻B⁺NK⁻ SCID					
γc deficiency	XL	Xq13.1	Mutations in common γ chain of IL-2, IL-4, IL-7, IL-9, IL-15, and IL-21	Markedly decreased natural killer cells	Severe infections with opportunistic organisms soon after neonatal period
				Markedly decreased T cells	Manifest with failure to thrive, chronic diarrhea, persistent thrush, pneumonia, sepsis
				Decreased serum immunoglobulin	
CD45 deficiency	AR	1q31-1q32	Mutation in CD45 gene	As per γc SCID	As above
Jak3 deficiency	AR	19p13.1	Janus kinase-3 deficiency (Jak3)	As per γc SCID	As above
T⁻B⁺NK⁺ SCID					
IL7Rα deficiency	AR	5p13	Mutation in IL7RA gene	Marked decrease in T cells	As above
				Decreased serum immunoglobulin	
CD3δ deficiency	AR	11q23	Mutation in CD3D gene	As per IL7Rα	As above
CD3ε deficiency	AR	11q23	Mutation in CD3E gene	As per IL7Rα	As above
T⁻B⁻NK⁻ SCID					
ADA deficiency	AR	20q13.11	Mutation in ADA gene	As per γc SCID	As above
					Axial skeletal abnormalities

(Continued)

Table 3-2 Primary Immunodeficiencies with T Cell Defects (Examples)—Cont'd

DEFICIENCY	INHERITANCE	GENE LOCUS	GENETIC DEFECT	CELLULAR DEFECTS	CLINICAL FINDINGS
T⁻ B⁻ NK⁺ SCID					
RAG1/2 deficiency	AR	11p13	Mutation in *RAG-1* or *RAG-2*	Markedly decreased T and B cell numbers Decreased serum immunoglobulin Defective VDJ recombination	As above
Artemis deficiency	AR	10p13	Mutation in *artemis* gene	As above for RAG1/2	As above
Other T Cell Defects					
X-linked hyper-IgM syndrome	XL	Xq26-Xq27	Mutations in CD40 ligand (CD154)	Normal T cells Only IgM and IgD bearing B cells Neutropenia	Neutropenia, thrombocytopenia, opportunistic infections
CD8 deficiency	AR	2q12	Mutation in *CD8A* gene	Absent CD8, normal CD4 numbers	As for Artemis
TAP-1 and TAP-2 deficiency	AR	6p21.3	Mutation in *TAP-1* or *TAP-2*	As for CD8 deficiency	As for CD8, vasculitis occurs
DiGeorge syndrome	AD	22q11.2	*TBX1*	Decreased or absent CD3⁺ cells	Cardiac and thymic defects, variable TCID

AD, autosomal dominant; AR, autosomal recessive; SCID, severe combined immunodeficiency; TCID, T cell immunodeficiency; XL, X-linked.

This disease phenotype is the consequence of mutations in at least 10 different genes located on six different chromosomes (see Table 3-2).[4,5] Four lymphocyte phenotypes have been identified associated with SCID, based on the effects of the mutation on T cell, B cell, and NK cell maturation (T⁻B⁺NK⁺, T⁻B⁺NK⁻, T⁻B⁻NK⁺, T⁻B⁻NK⁻) (see Table 3-2). SCID causes severe infections with opportunistic infections in the neonatal period.

Because of lack of graft rejection capability, these infants are at risk for GVHD if transfused with nonirradiated blood products. They are also at risk for severe systemic infection when immunized with live viruses (e.g., polio, measles, or varicella) or with bacille Calmette-Guérin. Diagnosis is possible at birth, with most affected infants having lymphopenia (<2000 lymphocytes/μL blood) and decreased *in vitro* proliferation studies.[5] Even in the absence of a normal thymus, T cell development can be achieved after SCT, and this is the standard of care for these infants. Survival is improved if SCT occurs within the first 4 weeks of life.[5] The improved survival of early transplants is attributed to the acquisition of opportunistic infections and their complications.

The X-linked form of hyper-IgM syndrome is caused by a defect in the CD40 ligand (CD40L) expressed by activated CD4⁺ T cells (see Table 3-2). The CD40-CD40L interaction is crucial in B cell–T cell signaling. A defect in this interaction results in normal to elevated IgM; reduced serum IgG, IgA, and IgE; and reduced memory B cells.[17,35] In addition to the immunoglobulin defects, patients with X-linked hyper-IgM syndrome have opportunistic infections, neutropenia, thrombocytopenia, seronegative arthritis, inflammatory bowel disease, and greater likelihood of malignancies. The increased risk of opportunistic infections, autoimmune diseases, and malignancies is attributed to defective T cell–antigen-presenting cell interactions owing to the CD40L defect. *P. jiroveci* pneumonia has been reported in 40% of patients with mutations in CD40L.

The cellular immunodeficiency in DiGeorge syndrome results from primary T cell deficiency. DiGeorge syndrome is usually due to gene defects on chromosome 22, leading to abnormal development of the third and fourth pharyngeal pouches during embryogenesis. This leads to aberrant development of several organs, including the thymus, parathyroid glands, and heart. The degree of thymic hypoplasia varies, resulting in a variable severity in the T cell deficiency.[3,36] In 80% of patients, the immunodeficiency is mild. Severe T cell deficiency and secondary deficient antibody responses can result from the thymic hypoplasia, however, leading to a severe disease phenotype (approaching SCID in severity). It is important to evaluate the presence of a thymus in patients with conotruncal cardiac defects and hypocalcemia because the T cell deficiency in DiGeorge syndrome places these patients at risk of GVHD after transfusion with nonirradiated blood products.[3,36]

Not all T cell immunodeficiencies manifest with a severe propensity for infections. Isolated CD8⁺ T cell developmental and signaling defects can have a milder form of immunodeficiency. Mutations in the CD8α molecule prevent the final assembly of the CD8⁺ T cell receptor signaling complex. Mutations in the MHC-1 molecule (binds to the T cell receptor) caused by TAP1/TAP2 mutations or a mutation in the TAP-binding protein prevent normal antigen presentation to the T cell receptor. These mutations cause a deficiency in CD8⁺ T cell function but no deficiency in the CD4⁺ T cells, and lead to a milder disease phenotype (see Table 3-2).[1,5-7]

The dysregulation of cellular immunity can lead to immunodeficiency, autoimmunity, and malignancy, as described previously for X-linked hyper-IgM syndrome (Table 3-3). Wiskott-Aldrich syndrome is an X-linked disorder characterized by eczema, thrombocytopenia with small defective platelets, and recurrent infections. Patients with Wiskott-Aldrich syndrome have impaired response to polysaccharides and protein antigens and aberrant T cell function.[37] Systemic and chronic sinopulmonary infections develop in the first year of life. Pulmonary infections can be caused by encapsulated bacteria (*S. pneumoniae*), viruses (herpes simplex virus),

Table 3-3   Other Defined Immunodeficiency Syndromes with Autoimmunity or Malignancies

DEFICIENCY	INHERITANCE	GENE LOCUS	GENETIC DEFECT	CELLULAR DEFECTS	CLINICAL FINDINGS
Wiskott-Aldrich syndrome	XL	Xp11.22-11.23	Mutation in WASP gene	Cytoskeletal defect affecting hematopoietic stem cell derivatives	Thrombocytopenia Immunodeficiency Autoimmune disease Malignancy Progressive decrease in T cells
Ataxia-telangiectasia	AR	11q22-q23	ATM	Disorder of cell cycle checkpoint leading to chromosomal instability	Thymic hypoplasia Increased α-fetoprotein Telangiectasia Sensitivity to Ionizing Radiation Increased risk of malignancies, particularly lymphoid
X-linked lymphoproliferative disease	XL	Xq25	SH2D1A	Altered adapter protein regulating intracellular signaling	Uncontrolled T cell proliferation in Epstein-Barr virus infection, fatal mononucleosis, ineffective viral elimination, lymphoma, hypogammaglobulinemia
ALPS1a	AR	10q24.1	CD95	Excessive CD4$^-$CD8$^-$ $\alpha\beta$ TCR$^+$ T cells Defective lymphocyte apoptosis	Autoimmunity Hypergammaglobulinemia Lymphoproliferation Increased risk of lymphoma
ALPS1b	AR	1q23	CD95L	As above	As above, plus lupus syndrome
ALPS2b	AR	2q33-2q34	CASP8	Defective lymphocyte apoptosis and activation	Recurrent bacterial and viral infections Autoimmunity, hypergammaglobulinemia, lymphoproliferation

ALPS, autoimmune lymphoproliferative syndrome; AR, autosomal recessive; CASP, caspase; SH2D1A, gene encoding SAP (signaling lymphocytic activation molecule [SLAM]-associated protein); XL, X-linked.

or opportunistic organisms (*P. jiroveci*).[3,37] Patients rarely survive beyond teenage years without SCT. Death usually results from infection, vasculitis, autoimmune cell cytopenias, or lymphoreticular malignancy.[37]

Ataxia telangiectasia is another complex disease resulting from a disorder of cell cycle regulation that leads to chromosomal instability. Ataxia telangiectasia represents a combined immunodeficiency associated with neurologic, cutaneous, and immune abnormalities.[7] These patients have recurrent sinopulmonary infection. Their cells have defective DNA repair and are sensitive to ionizing radiation. A concern is that repeated exposure to x-rays used in usual diagnostic studies places them at risk for lymphoreticular cancers and adenocarcinoma.[38]

Several cellular defects can result in unchecked cell proliferation and susceptibility to infections and to tumors. X-linked lymphoproliferative disease is another example of immunodeficiency from aberrant cellular control (see Table 3-3). In X-linked lymphoproliferative disease, there is failure to control proliferation of cytotoxic T cells after infection with Epstein-Barr virus (EBV).[39] The most common presentation is severe infectious mononucleosis, which is fatal in 80% of patients. The defect is in the gene encoding an adapter protein, *SH2D1A,* a protein that helps regulate the proliferation of T cells and NK cells. Autoimmune lymphoproliferative syndrome results from defects in cellular apoptosis (regulated cell death) mediated by CD95 (FAS). These patients have autoimmunity, hypergammaglobulinemia, lymphoproliferation, and excessive numbers of CD3$^+$, CD4$^-$, and CD8$^-$ T lymphocytes (see Table 3-3).[5]

Diagnosis

In an infant with possible T cell deficiency, total blood lymphocyte counts are a reasonable place to begin for diagnosis. Functional studies (immunoglobulin responses to protein and polysaccharide antigen immunizations), activation studies, and B, T, and NK cell markers can define the nature of the deficiency further. Finally, specific genetic studies can be conducted to identify several of the defined mutant genes.

Treatment

Treatment depends on the specific immunodeficiency. Prophylactic antibiotics, antiviral agents, or intravenous immunoglobulin can be used to prevent or ameliorate serious infections.[40] For severe T cell deficiency, SCT early in life can be lifesaving. Thymic transplants have been performed to reconstitute the T cell defects in DiGeorge syndrome.[36] Gene therapy has been investigated for specific primary immunodeficiency disease, but success has been tempered by the occurrence of leukemia in subjects resulting from the insertion of the retrovirus vectors near oncogenes.[41] Newer vectors may improve the safety of this mode of therapy.

Deficiencies in Phagocyte Numbers, Function, and Opsonization

Overview

Neutrophils constitute about half the circulating white blood cell population, and their primary function is phagocytosis and killing of invading pathogens. For the neutrophil to accomplish this, it must respond to signals in the area of injury; adhere and transmigrate through the vascular endothelium; migrate to the area of infection; and recognize the pathogen, phagocytose, and kill it. Interruption of any of these steps would leave the host susceptible to infections. When the neutrophil has migrated into the tissue, its primary purpose is to recognize, ingest, and destroy pathogens. Phagocytosis comprises two steps: recognition and internalization of the foreign material into the phagosome. Killing or neutralization involves a secretory response. Materials may bind directly to the neutrophil, resulting in ingestion, or opsonization by serum proteins occurs. Neutrophils exhibit specific Fc-mediated binding and nonspecific binding using complement receptors CR1 and CR3. Intracellular killing generally is associated with the initiation of the respiratory burst. The importance of this process is shown by patients with chronic granulomatous disease (discussed later), whose neutrophils cannot undergo the oxidative burst.[42] Deficiencies in neutrophil numbers, ability to migrate, opsonization, phagocytosis, or function can render the host susceptible to infection (Table 3-4).

Table 3-4 Examples of Immunodeficiency Syndromes with Abnormal Neutrophils, Chemotaxis, or Opsonization

DEFICIENCY	INHERITANCE	GENE LOCUS	GENETIC DEFECT	CELLULAR DEFECTS	CLINICAL FINDINGS
Neutrophil Numbers					
Kostmann syndrome	AD	19p13.3 or 1p22	Defects in *ELA2* or *Gfi1*	Mistrafficking or repression of neutrophil elastase	Neutropenia; Susceptibility to bacterial and fungal infections
Congenital neutropenia	AD	19p13.3	*ELA2* defect	As per Kostmann syndrome	As above
Cyclic neutropenia	AD	19p13.3	*ELA2* defect	As per Kostmann syndrome	Susceptibility to infection at nadir of neutrophil counts
X-linked neutropenia	XL	Xp11.22-11.23	*WASP*	Defective regulator of actin cytoskeleton	Neutropenia, infections as per Kostmann syndrome
Chemotaxis					
LAD1	AR	21q22.3	*INTG2 (CD18)*	Defective neutrophil and lymphocyte migration from blood; Lack CD18	Delayed umbilical stump separation, recurrent gingivitis; Absent tissue neutrophils, blood neutrophilia
Function					
Hyper-IgE syndrome	ADv	4q21	Unknown	Unknown	High IgE and eosinophilia; Skin abscesses, pneumonia with pneumatocele formation
CGD	AD	Xp23	$CYBB{:}gp91^{phox}$	Absent cytochrome b ~70% of cases	Granulomatous lesions of lung, skin, lymph nodes, and liver: *Staphylococcus aureus*, *Burkholderia cepacia*, *Serratia marcescens*, *Nocardia* and *Aspergillus* species
	XL	16q24	$CYBA{:}p22^{phox}$	Absent cytochrome b <5% of cases	
	AR	7q11.23 1q225	$NCF1{:}p67^{phox}$ $NCF2{:}p67^{phox}$	Cytochrome positive	
IFNγR1 deficiency	AR, AD	6q23	*IfnγR1*	Loss of IFN-γ binding	Severe infections: *Salmonella*, HSV, CMV, parainfluenza, RSV, mycobacteria
IFNγR2 deficiency	AR, AD	21q22	*IfnγR2*	Loss of IFN-γ binding	As above
Opsonization					
Complement C2	AR	6p21.3	C2 defect	Absent complement activity	Pyogenic infection, vasculitis, SLE-like
Complement C3	AR	19p13.3-p13.2	C3 defect	As above	Recurrent pyogenic infections
MBL deficiency	AR	10q11.2-q21	*MBL2*	Deficiency in *MBL2*	Increased pyogenic infections and sepsis

AR, autosomal recessive; AD, autosomal dominant; ADv, autosomal dominant with variable penetrance; CGD, chronic granulomatous disease; CMV, cytomegalovirus; HSV, herpes simplex virus; IFN-γ, interferon-γ; LAD, leukocyte adhesion defect; MBL, mannose binding lectin; RSV, respiratory syncytial virus; SLE, systemic lupus erythematosus; XL, X-linked.

Specific Diseases

Defects in neutrophil numbers, such as Kostmann syndrome and cyclic neutropenia, can result from a deficiency in elastase 2 (see Table 3-4). In cyclic neutropenia, peripheral blood counts oscillate in about a 21-day cycle with a nadir approaching an absolute neutrophil count (ANC) of 0 and a peak near normal. Life-threatening infections occur during days around the nadir of neutrophil counts. In Kostmann syndrome, the neutropenia is static. One variant of Kostmann syndrome is caused by a deficiency in ELA2 (coding for neutrophil elastase 2). Mutations causing a deficiency of *Gfi1* (a zinc finger transcriptional repressor oncoprotein) result in ELA2 deficiency and neutropenia.[43,44]

Deficiencies in neutrophil migration from the circulation can result in recurrent infections. Patients with leukocyte adhesion deficiency are unable to recruit neutrophils into sites of inflammation, and, as a result, they sustain recurrent, life-threatening infections.[45] Patients with leukocyte adhesion deficiency lack the normal β_2 integrins to allow neutrophil recruitment from the circulation. These patients have peripheral neutrophilia, but do not form pus and have difficulty localizing infections because of their defect in neutrophil migration. Recurrent infections of the skin, upper and lower airways, bowel, and perirectal area are common and are usually caused by *Staphyloccocus aureus* or gram-negative bacilli.[46]

When neutrophils arrive at the site of infection, defective function can limit their ability to clear infection. Job syndrome (hyper-IgE syndrome) is caused by an unclear defect in phagocyte function and is characterized by recurrent skin and lower respiratory tract infections, eczema, elevated IgE levels, and eosinophilia. Symptoms occur within the first month of life with severe eczema, mucocutaneous infections, sinusitis, and lower respiratory tract infections with *S. aureus* or *H. influenzae*. Development of empyema, lung abscesses, and persistent pneumatoceles is common.

Chronic granulomatous disease is the most common phagocyte disorder, with the X-linked form accounting for two thirds of the reported cases (see Table 3-4). Chronic granulomatous disease is caused by defects in the reduced nicotinamide adenine dinucleotide phosphate (NADPH) oxidase complex responsible for production of superoxide.[3,46] Onset of the disease occurs early in life, with pulmonary infection the most frequent presentation, with fungal organisms predominating.[3,46] Five organisms cause most infections in chronic granulomatous disease: *S. aureus, Burkholderia cepacia, Serratia marcescens, Nocardia* species, and *Aspergillus* species. Bacteremia is rare. Patients with mutations leading to the complete loss of the interferon-γ receptors (IFNγR1 and IFNγR2) are less capable of killing mycobacteria and intracellular organisms. These patients have been identified because of extreme susceptibility to nontuberculous mycobacteria.[46] Viral agents, including herpes simplex virus, CMV, and RSV, also present severe problems. Mortality is high because of recurrent severe infection.

Opsonization is necessary for neutrophil killing of several organisms. Serum proteins reach the lung through transudation in response to inflammation, including the complement family and mannose-binding lectin (MBL) (see Table 3-4). The complement protein cascade is activated by three independent pathways: (1) the classic pathway, which is activated by antigen-antibody complexes (involving IgG or IgM); (2) the alternative pathway, which is activated by foreign carbohydrates, such as bacterial and fungal components; and (3) the lectin pathway (involving MBL[44]). The complement system functions to coat foreign particles in opsonin via the alternative pathway, making the particles more likely to be phagocytosed, to activate phagocytic cells by the local release of chemotactic agents such as C5a, and to lyse cells through the activation of the late complement components C5, C6, C7, C8, and C9 (the membrane attack complex). Other important aspects of the complement pathway are the generation of anaphylatoxins, such as C3a and C5a, which cause the release of vasoactive mediators from mast cells, and the generation of C3b and C4 on the cell surface, where they interact with specific receptors on phagocytic cells.[47]

Complement deficiency is associated with recurrent infections, glomerulonephritis, or collagen vascular diseases such as systemic lupus erythematosus. Early complement deficiencies are associated with systemic lupus erythematosus, glomerulonephritis, or other rheumatologic diseases. Pneumonia has been described in association with C1 deficiency, although bacterial meningitis is a more common manifestation. Pneumonia complicated by empyema, pneumatoceles, and liver abscesses has been described as a consequence of C1r deficiency. Autoimmune disorders are associated with C2 and C4 deficiency, although bacterial infections also occur in children with C2 deficiency (the most common complement deficiency). C3 deficiency (clinically the most severe and least common of the complement deficiencies) is associated with autoimmune disorders and recurrent infections. C3 acts as an opsonizing agent and plays roles in the classic and alternative pathways. C3 deficiency results in otitis media, pneumonia, sepsis, meningitis, and osteomyelitis, most commonly caused by *S. pneumoniae, N. meningitidis, Klebsiella* species, *Escherichia coli,* and *Streptococcus pyogenes.* C5 deficiency produces a complex defect owing to the loss of chemotactic and anaphylatoxin activities; it leads to decreased lung clearance of *S. pneumoniae,* but not *S. aureus,* in C5-deficient mice. The late complement deficiencies (C5 through C9) impair serum bactericidal and cytolytic activities. Susceptibility to systemic infection with encapsulated organisms, such as *N. meningitidis* and *S. pneumoniae,* is increased; however, pulmonary infections are uncommon. C3 deficiency manifests with the most severe disease phenotype.[44]

MBL also participates in opsonization through activation of the complement pathway.[44] MBL deficiency is common, occurring in 10% of the general population.[48] Although infections are uncommon in healthy individuals, MBL deficiency in patients receiving chemotherapy or SCT or with specific leukemias can result in suppression of phagocytic activity. MBL deficiency is associated with autoimmune and inflammatory diseases.[48]

Diagnosis

Assessment of neutrophil deficiency begins with performing cell counts and assessing the ANC. Specialized laboratories can perform specific measures of neutrophil chemotaxis and oxidative burst. Receptor levels (CD18,

IFNγR1, and IFNγR2) can be measured using flow cytometry. Oxidative burst can be measured using assays for superoxide production or by measuring NADPH oxidoreductase function in specialized laboratories. Measuring the CH50 or AH50 can perform functional screening for complement deficiency. Specific complement components and MBL can be measured using immunoassays.

Treatment

Cyclic neutropenia and congenital neutropenias can be treated with granulocyte colony-stimulating factor.[43] Prophylactic antibiotics and antifungal agents, and aggressive therapy during acute infections are keys for long-term survival. Patients with chronic granulomatous disease also are treated with prophylactic trimethoprim-sulfamethoxazole, antifungal therapy, and recombinant human interferon-γ. In addition, SCT has been performed with success in patients with chronic granulomatous disease.[43,46] Treatment of opsonic defects (complement and MBL) also involves prophylactic antibiotics and immunization against encapsulated organisms. Replacement therapy is usually ineffective.

Secondary Immunodeficiencies

Overview

Predisposition to infection occurs when there is an imbalance between the invading organism and the host's ability to prevent the infection. This imbalance can occur because of the organism itself (portal of entry, type of organism, antibiotic resistance, virulence factors) or host factors that prevent the ability of the host to prevent or limit invasion. Host defenses consist of innate and adaptive processes. Innate immunity provides the initial defense against infection, whereas adaptive immunity develops slowly and provides specific defense against specific invading organisms and memory to protect from reinfection.

Earlier in this chapter, we discussed primary defects in the immune system and how they predispose to infections. In this section, the focus is on secondary immunodeficiencies that arise after childhood cancers and chemotherapy, and related to transplantation (heart, liver, kidney, and lung transplantation, and SCT). Many of the concepts presented earlier apply to the secondary immunodeficient states. Deficient numbers of lymphocytes or phagocytic cells or defective functions that can occur in the primary immunodeficiency disease also can occur secondary to the underlying malignancy, chemotherapeutic agents used for the cancer, or immunosuppression after transplantation. The common themes and several disease-related processes that occur and predispose the host to lung complications are reviewed. We first consider the broad issues that apply in the secondary immunodeficiency states in general, then focus on problems specific to cancer chemotherapy, solid organ transplantation, SCT, and lung transplantation.

Factors Contributing to the Secondary Immunodeficient State

The airway epithelium is more than a passive barrier to airway water loss or a passive fortification against bacterial and viral infection. Published data support the active participation of the airway epithelium in the regulation of airway smooth muscle tone, the physical removal of inhaled substances through ciliary clearance, and secreting or transporting broad-spectrum antimicrobial substances. Finally, the respiratory epithelium is a functional interface between the pathogen and innate or adaptive immune response. The airway epithelium is a pivotal structure in respiratory physiology and pathology.

The respiratory epithelium participates in passive lung immunity in many different ways. The epithelium presents a physical barrier to viral and bacterial invasion, lining the respiratory tract from the nose to the alveoli with a wide range of cell phenotypes.[49,50] Ciliated epithelial cells are important in moving mucus up the airway, removing particulate material, and injury to these cells by agents such as oxidants can alter ability to remove mucus from the airway. Tracheobronchial glands and goblet cells are important sources of airway mucus, which nonspecifically traps particulates and potential pathogens. The

respiratory epithelium also serves functions in the regulation of water and ion movement into the airway mucus,[51] and serves as its own reservoir for injury repair.[50]

The respiratory epithelium also performs more specific interactions with the innate and adaptive immune systems. Alveolar type II cells manufacture surfactant proteins A and D (described later).[52,53] The respiratory epithelium can be induced to produce numerous bioactive cytokines,[54] and express numerous adhesion molecules that support interactions between the epithelial cell and inflammatory cells recruited to the lung. The other epithelial layers throughout the body serve similar functions. Disruption of the epithelial layer by injury caused by chemotherapeutic agents, irradiation, or GVHD can allow invasion by potentially pathogenic organisms, such as *S. aureus*, gram-negative bacilli, and *Candida* species, which normally colonize the various epithelial surfaces. Bypassing the epithelial barrier by transcutaneous catheters provides potential routes of entry for infection. Treatment with broad-spectrum antibiotics reduces the normal flora at the epithelial surfaces, allowing overgrowth of potentially more invasive organisms and potentially selecting for antibiotic-resistant organisms (Table 3-5).

The underlying disease state or chemotherapy (cytotoxic or immunosuppressive) can alter the numbers or function of lymphocytes and phagocytic cells, resulting in immunodeficient states similar to those discussed earlier in the sections on primary immunodeficiency disease. Organ failure resulting from the underlying disease state or secondary to chemotherapy can reduce further the host defenses to infection (e.g., renal failure with uremia, liver failure with loss of complement or MBL production, splenectomy secondary to malignancy). Thrombocytopenia may reduce healing, extending the duration of breakdown of the epithelial barriers. The underlying disease or its treatment can alter the nutritional state of the patient, further limiting healing and epithelial barrier functions (see Table 3-5).

Moreover, the patient's previous "immune experience" can alter his or her ability to fight infection. Preexisting antibody or immune memory can help protect the patient when subsequently exposed to the potentially infectious

Table 3-5	Factors Predisposing to Infection and Pulmonary Complications after Cancer Therapy or Organ Transplantation

Underlying Disease

Alteration in neutrophil, lymphocyte, or platelet function secondary to underlying disease, malignancy, or autoimmune state

Organ dysfunction secondary to underlying malignancy or autoimmune state

Change in Physical Barriers

Breakdown in physical barriers owing to mucositis, defective healing, chemotherapy, graft-versus-host disease

Changes in colonizing bacteria and fungi

New routes of entry (intravenous catheters, shunts)

Use of Broad-Spectrum Antibiotic Therapy for Acute Infections or Prophylaxis ("Rule Out" Infection)

Eliminate normal flora and allow secondary bacterial or fungal overgrowth

Select resistant organisms

Quantitative Defects in Normal Circulating Blood Cells

Neutropenia

Lymphopenia

Thrombocytopenia

Qualitative Differences in Function of Lymphocytes and Phagocytic Cells

Lymphocytes: antibody production and cytotoxic cells

Neutrophil and macrophage functional defects

Defective wound healing

Organ Dysfunction

Liver, heart, or renal failure; asplenia or splenic hypofunction

Epithelial defects allowing bacterial invasion

Diabetes mellitus

Nutritional Defects

Iron deficiency

Vitamin deficiency

Catabolic state

Previous Infections

Colonization (respiratory, gut, renal system)

Previous viral infections with persistent virus (EBV, CMV, HSV, herpesvirus 6)

Preexisting immunity owing to immunization or infection

Concurrent Infection

Infections acquired from donor organs or blood products

Naturally occurring infection that causes further immunosuppression

CMV, cytomegalovirus; EBV, Epstein-Barr virus; HSV, herpes simplex virus.

agent. CMV is a good example of an opportunistic infection that can be ameliorated if the patient had previous immune experience or exposure. Alternatively, CMV infection can be life-threatening in a patient on chemotherapy or immunosuppressants after organ transplantation with no previous immune experience.

Pulmonary Complications of Cancer Therapy

Pulmonary complications of cancer therapy can arise from the primary malignancy, from infections resulting from immunosuppression, or as complications to the cancer therapy (Table 3-6). Superior vena cava syndrome and tracheal compression can complicate the initial presentation of tumors or tumor therapy (see Chapter 7). Space-occupying tumors (non-Hodgkin lymphoma, Hodgkin disease, acute lymphoblastic leukemia, neuroblastoma, Ewing sarcoma, thyroid tumors, thymoma, rhabdomyosarcoma) can cause obstruction or compression of the superior vena cava and trachea, resulting in respiratory distress. Superior vena cava syndrome also can be a complication of thrombosis secondary to central lines in cancer patients. Patients may complain of

Table 3-6	Pulmonary Complications of Malignancies, Transplantation, and Related Medications	
COMPLICATIONS OF UNDERLYING MALIGNANCY	**INFECTIOUS COMPLICATIONS**	**NONINFECTIOUS COMPLICATIONS**
Immunosuppression (related to primary neoplasm or secondary to chemotherapy or radiation therapy)	Bacterial infection	Alveolar hemorrhage
Pulmonary invasion	Viruses (HSV, EBV, VZV, RSV, adenovirus)	Superior vena cava syndrome or superior mediastinal syndrome
Airway obstruction with secondary infection	Mycobacteria (*M. tuberculosis* and atypical mycobacteria)	Drug reactions
Leukemia and lymphomatous involvement with	Fungi (*Aspergillus, Nocardia, Pneumocystis*)	Secondary neoplasms
Leukostasis		Pulmonary embolism
Leukemic cell lysis		Pulmonary edema
Hyperleukocytic reaction		Airway obstruction owing to mucositis
		ARDS, acute lung injury
		Interstitial pneumonitis (drug or radiation induced)

ARDS, acute respiratory distress syndrome; EBV, Epstein-Barr virus; HSV, herpes simplex virus; RSV, respiratory syncytial virus; VZV, varicella-zoster virus.

dyspnea, orthopnea, hoarseness, chest pain, cough, or syncope. On examination, patients may present with signs of superior vena cava obstruction (cyanosis, swelling of face, neck, or upper arms), stridor or wheezing, and signs of pleural or pericardial effusions.[55] In these patients, presentation with signs and symptoms of airway obstruction can be a medical/surgical emergency. Surgical airway management can be lifesaving. Occasionally, airway decompression must be accomplished with radiation therapy, steroids, or other chemotherapeutic agents.[55]

The hyperleukocytosis syndrome (cells >100,000/μL) can occur in 50% of children with acute lymphoblastic leukemia and acute myeloblastic leukemia in the chronic phase (see Chapter 7). Pulmonary injury is the result of hyperviscosity leading to sluggish blood flow and aggregation of leukeuric cells; this can lead to oxygenation defects and pulmonary endothelial injury, leading to pulmonary hemorrhage. Chest radiographs show diffuse interstitial haziness. Therapy is aimed at decreasing the circulating cell numbers, and includes leukapheresis and exchange transfusion.[55]

Tumors can lead to pulmonary dysfunction by occupying space (see Chapter 7). Large

tumors within the thoracic or abdominal cavities can impair normal excursion of the diaphragm, impair normal chest wall motion, or decrease available volume for lung expansion. Benign tumors (ganglioneuroma, teratoma) can grow slowly and allow the child to adapt to the pulmonary function abnormality with minimal symptoms until critical restrictive deficits are present. Likewise, slow-growing tumors in the neck or mediastinum can cause upper airway or tracheal compression. Primary lung tumors are rare in children[56]; however, secondary invasion can occur. Lung tumors may manifest as hemoptysis or postobstructive pneumonias, and usually manifest in an advanced state. In addition, extrinsic compression of an airway can occur as a result of tumor or adenopathy, leading to stridor, wheezing, or postobstructive pneumonia. Secondary invasive solid tumors (Ewing sarcoma, neuroblastoma) on either side of the diaphragm can lead to pulmonary impairment—intrathoracic tumors by decreasing available space for lung expansion; extrathoracic tumors by impeding diaphragmatic excursion—leading to restrictive lung disease. Finally, intracranial tumors can lead to central apnea or central hypoventilation syndromes.[55]

Treatment of tumors with chemotherapeutic agents or radiation therapy can lead to secondary pulmonary complications (Table 3-7). Improved cancer survival has led to increasing awareness of short-term and long-term pulmonary complications of cancer therapies (chemotherapy and radiation therapy).[55,57-60] In addition to causing direct injury to the lung itself, disruption of the epithelial barriers or host primary defenses by cancer therapy (radiation therapy, cancer chemotherapy, immunosuppressive agents) or secondary organ dysfunction (kidney, liver, heart) can lead to pulmonary dysfunction or pneumonia (see Tables 3-5 and 3-6).

Acute and chronic side effects of chemotherapy have been recognized (see Table 3-7). Acute side effects include hypersensitivity reactions, bronchospasm, and urticaria (see Table 3-7). Chronic side effects include diffuse alveolar damage, interstitial fibrosis, interstitial pneumonitis, and bronchiolitis obliterans syndrome. In addition, radiation therapy to the lungs, mediastinal structures, and vertebrae can cause abnormal growth and lead to restrictive lung disease as the child continues to grow.

Pulmonary infections are common complications of cancer therapies.[55,61] Neutropenia and subsequent infection are major dose-limiting complications of these therapies. Neutropenia is defined as an ANC of less than 1500/μL, and the risk of infection increases with ANC values of less than 1000/μL. The magnitude and duration of the neutropenia determine the risk of infection by many agents (see Table 3-6).[55,61] Chemotherapy can result in altered neutrophil function, breakdown of mucosal barriers, and other

Table 3-7	Complications of Chemotherapeutic Agents

IMMEDIATE/SHORT-TERM COMPLICATIONS	
Agent	*Complication*
Carboplatin	Hypersensitivity
Etoposide	Hypersensitivity
Asparaginase	Hypersensitivity
Vindesine	Bronchospasm
Vinblastine	Bronchospasm
Cyclophosphamide	Urticaria, angioedema

LONG-TERM COMPLICATIONS	
Agent	*Complication*
Radiation therapy	Pneumonitis, fibrosis
Bleomycin	Diffuse alveolar damage, interstitial fibrosis/pneumonia, bronchiolitis obliterans syndrome
Alkylating Agents	
Busulfan	Diffuse alveolar damage, interstitial fibrosis
Cyclophosphamide	Diffuse alveolar damage, interstitial pneumonia, interstitial fibrosis, diffuse pulmonary hemorrhage
Melphalan	Diffuse alveolar damage, interstitial fibrosis
Nitrosoureas	
Carmustine	Diffuse alveolar damage, interstitial pneumonitis
Lomustine	Diffuse alveolar damage, interstitial pneumonitis
Semustine	Diffuse alveolar damage, interstitial pneumonitis
VM-26	Noncardiogenic pulmonary edema
Cyclophosphamide	Noncardiogenic pulmonary edema
Cytarabine	Noncardiogenic pulmonary edema, pulmonary hemorrhage
Methotrexate	Noncardiogenic pulmonary edema, hypersensitivity pneumonitis

dysfunctions (organ dysfunction, nutrition; summarized in Table 3-5) that allow microbial invasion, or prevent the child from fighting infection or healing mucosal surfaces appropriately.[55,61,62] Alkylating agents, purine analogues, and newer monoclonal antibody regimens can cause prolonged, severe, multilineage cytopenias.[62] These infections include common bacterial pathogens at the skin (*S. aureus,* other staphylococci, gram-negative bacilli) or mucosal surfaces (*Streptococcus viridans,* other streptococci, *Enterococcus,* gram-negative bacilli). Opportunistic infections can occur owing to impaired neutrophil and humoral immunity (members of the herpesvirus family, fungal infections including *P. jiroveci,* and *Toxoplasma*). In the immunocompromised state, common childhood infections may be life-threatening (e.g., RSV, varicella).[34,55,61,62] The febrile, neutropenic child is at great risk for sepsis or pneumonia. Diagnostic evaluation and treatment of this group of patients are discussed subsequently.

Transplant-Related Pulmonary Complications

Transplantation has become the curative treatment for many immunodeficiency diseases and for organ failure. Solid organ transplantation (liver, kidney, heart) is now so successful that more than 80% of children survive to become adolescents and adults,[63] largely owing to improvements in immunosuppression and antimicrobial prophylaxis regimens. Immunosuppression requires a balance: On the one hand, there is the need to prevent allograft rejection and to preserve organ function; on the other hand, this suppression leaves the host susceptible to infections, including pulmonary infection. The side effects of these agents can result in secondary organ failure and further pulmonary complications.[63,64]

Transplant rejection is mediated primarily by T cells, although B cell–mediated antibody production plays a role in hyperacute rejection (caused by preformed antibody to donor antigens, including HLA antigens). Acute and chronic cellular rejection involves T cell recognition of antigen on the surface of donor cells, or recipient antigen-presenting cell presentation of donor-derived peptides for solid organ transplants (Fig. 3-2). SCT is different because the donor T cells engraft, then respond to the recipient (GVHD). The ablative therapy before SCT removes host T cells. The immunosuppressive agents involve many classes of drugs often used in combination, which differ in their specificity for cell types or subtypes, or signaling pathway used by the effector cells (Table 3-8).[63,64]

In addition to their immunosuppressive effects, the use of these agents (see Table 3-8) can be accompanied by significant side effects with pulmonary implications. Cyclosporine and tacrolimus have significant renal side effects: nephrotoxicity occurring in 5% to 50%, and blood pressure abnormalities in 25% to 70% of treated patients.[63] Mycophenolate mofetil may have fewer renal complications, but causes bone marrow suppression and increases rates of sepsis. The use of monoclonal antibodies, such as basiliximab or daclizumab, may decrease renal toxicity by allowing lower doses of cyclosporine or tacrolimus. Post-transplant lymphoproliferative disorder (PTLD) and

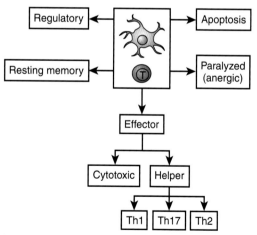

Figure 3-2. T cell responses can take many directions: Following an encounter with an antigen-presenting cell, naive T cells can respond in various ways, including apoptosis (programmed cell death), the induction of effector T cells, the induction of regulatory T cells, and a form of immunologic paralysis known as anergy. After initial T cell expansion, a few cells survive as long-lasting memory cells, ready to respond rapidly in the event of later exposure to the same antigen. (*From Taussig L, Landau L: Pediatric Respiratory Medicine, 2nd ed. St Louis, Mosby, 2008, p 43.*)

Table 3-8 Immunosuppressive Agents Used in Transplantation

AGENT	ACTIVITY
Corticosteroids	Potent, but least specific of immunosuppressive agents
	Negative regulation effect in lymphocytes by directly inhibiting transcription factors AP-1 and NF-κB
	Anti-AP-1 effect: blocks IL-2 production
	Anti-NF-κB effect: prevents upregulation of IL-1, IL-2, IL-3, IL-6, IFN-γ, CD40 ligand, TNF-α, GMCSF, MHC molecules
	Interfere with breakdown of cytokine mRNA and interfere with tyrosine phosphorylation
	Inhibit functions of many nonlymphoid cells, including APC, inhibiting MHC class II expression
Calcineurin inhibitors	Inhibit T cell activation by binding to intracellular immunophyllins
	Calcineurin, a calmodulin-activated serine-threonine phosphatase, dephosphorylates inactive NFAT, leading to nuclear translocation and subsequent activation of T cells
Cyclosporine	Binds to cyclophilin A, inhibiting action
	Inhibits production of IL-1β, IL-2, IL-6, IL-8, IFN-γ, and TNF-α
	Inhibits Jun N terminal kinase and p38 pathways
	Suppresses antigen presentation by APC
Tacrolimus	Binds to FK-binding protein 12, inhibiting action
	Activity as for cyclosporine
	Preferentially inhibits Th1 cells over Th2 cells
	Less anti-HLA antibody formation
	Inhibits glucocorticoid-induced apoptosis of antigen-stimulated T cells
Antimetabolites	
Azathioprine	Antimetabolite agent: inhibits DNA and RNA production
	Lymphocytes use de novo pathway for purine synthesis. Blocks de novo synthesis, preventing clonal expression of T cells and B cells
	Inhibits DNA synthesis, purine metabolism, nucleotide synthesis, and CD28 costimulation pathway
	Inhibits production of AMP and GMP
	Results in suppression of all hematopoietic cell lines
Mycophenolate mofetil	More potent and selective inhibitor of de novo purine pathway
	No significant effect on hematopoietic or neutrophil populations
	Inhibits proliferation of T cells and B cells, blocks antibody formation, and decreases generation of NK cells
Target of rapamycin inhibitors	
Sirolimus (rapamycin)	Bind to kinase named target of rapamycin, preventing translation of mRNA responsible for cell cycle regulation
	Inhibits FK binding proteins
	Prevents T cell proliferation by blocking progress from G_1 to S phase
	Inhibits growth factor–driven proliferation of smooth muscle, fibroblasts, and endothelial cells—leads to high incidence of anastomotic dehiscence when used in lung transplantation
Everolimus	Same activity as sirolimus

Agent	Description
Polyclonal antilymphocyte antibodies	Polyclonal antibody made in animals specific for target cell lines (lymphocytes, thymocytes, T cell lines) Lymphocyte depletion owing to complement-mediated opsonization or Fas-mediated apoptosis Cause profound, long-lasting lymphopenia Very nonspecific—contain antibodies to wide variety of lymphocytes and costimulatory molecules
Monoclonal antibodies	More specific, directed against specific T cell antigens or cytokine receptors
OKT3 (Muromonab-CD3)	Murine IgG2a monoclonal antibody directed against the epsilon subunit of CD3 CD3 facilitates translation expression of TcR-α and TcR-β chains on cell surface for intracellular killing—needed for $CD4^+$ cell activation Initially activates T cells, causing cytokine release, but within hours causes internalization of TcR-α and TcR-β chains, rendering T cell unresponsive to antigen Causes nonspecific T cell depletion M-CD3 also causes T cell opsonization and removal from circulation by liver and spleen Causes apoptosis of activated T cells and NK-T cells
Daclizumab	Humanized mouse monoclonal
Basiliximab	Human/mouse chimeric monoclonal antibody Directed against α-chains of CD25 molecule (IL-2 receptor) Inhibits IL-2 induced T cell proliferation Eliminates activated T cells through Fas-Fas ligand interactions (apoptosis) No depletion of other T cell populations
Efalizumab	Humanized mouse IgG1 against CD11α chain Non-lymphocyte depleting Blocks LFA-1:ICAM-1 interactions preventing T cell adhesion, activation, and trafficking
LEA29Y	Antibody against CD80 and CD86 (B7 molecules), a costimulatory signal necessary for T cell activation
Rituximab	Human-mouse chimeric anti-CD20 (B cell antibody): depletes B cells, eliminating hyperacute antibody-mediated rejection in cardiac, renal, and liver transplantation
Alemtuzumab	Anti-CD52/campath-1H Humanized IgG1 antibody: depletes T cells by complement-mediated cell lysis (T, B, NK, and dendritic cells, not hematopoietic stem cells)
FTY720	Sphingosine-1 phosphate receptor agonist Reduces recirculation of lymphocytes from lymph nodes back into the circulation, causes peripheral lymphopenia

AP-1, activating protein 1; NF-κB, nuclear factor kappa B; Anti-AP-1: anti-activating protein 1; IFN-γ, interferon gamma; TNF-α, tumor necrosis factor alpha; GMCSF, granulocyte-macrophage-colony stimulating factor; MHC, major histocompatibity complex; APC, adenomatous polyposiscoli; LFA-1, lymphocyte function associated antigen; ICAM-1, intercellular adhesion molecule; NK-T, natural killer T lymphocytes.

secondary malignancies can result from long-term immunosuppression in a small but significant number of patients. It is important to differentiate these noninfectious complications from infection in this group of patients.

The overall risk of infection or rejection in a transplant patient results from the balance of net state of immunosuppression, the type of transplant, and the degree of exposure to the particular pathogen (see Table 3-5).[63,64] Comorbid conditions (preexisting or secondary to the transplantation or immunosuppressive agents) can increase susceptibility to infectious or noninfectious complications further (see Table 3-6). Infectious complications of solid organ transplantation occur in a predictable pattern.[65] Based on the type of organism and the timing of occurrence, prophylactic regimens have developed over the years to prevent these infections,[63-68] including the use of prophylaxis for *P. jiroveci, Candida,* and CMV. Latent infections (either latent in the host or the donor organ) occur early after transplantation (CMV, herpes simplex virus, EBV), as can azole-resistant fungal infections. Duncan and Wilkes[64] review the common "time lines" for appearance of various infectious agents and the effects of prophylaxis on the appearance of these agents.

Heart Transplantation

The 10-year survival of cardiac transplant in children is 60% to 80%.[63] With this good prognosis, prevention of acute rejection while minimizing the side effects of immunosuppressive agents is important.[63,69] Freedom from acute rejection after 5 years was found to be 40% with cyclosporine, 56% with tacrolimus, and 62% with mycophenolate mofetil treatment for immunosuppression.[63,69] This suppression comes with a price of nephrotoxicity (4%), hypertension (35%), PTLD (17%), and secondary malignancies (1% to 4%). In addition, chronic rejection can lead to organ failure requiring retransplantation (5%).[70-72] Infectious and noninfectious events can cause pulmonary complications as listed in Table 3-6. Pneumonias in heart transplant patients are frequently multimicrobial in origin; CMV was the most common single pathogen and copathogen in this patient group.[70-73] Many of these infections likely resulted from reactivation of latent infection.

Renal Transplantation

Renal transplants were among the first successful transplants done in children. With current immunosuppressive protocols, the 1-year graft survival is expected to be greater than 90% with an acute rejection rate of 22%.[74] Ten-year graft survival approaches 70%. Complications of immunosuppressive therapy include hypertension (70%), PTLD (7%), malignancy (17%), and overall retransplantation rates of 25% (improved with newer immunosuppressive protocols). The incidence of immunosuppressive nephrotoxicity is uncertain because of difficulties in distinguishing drug toxicity from chronic rejection.[63] Use of mycophenolate mofetil or sirolimus for maintenance prevents significant renal dysfunction and can be steroid-sparing. CMV and EBV infections are common in immunosuppressed renal transplant patients because of the lack of effective immunization before transplant and the high incidence of infection by these viruses in adult donors. In one study, 12% of kidney recipients developed CMV disease—the incidence of developing CMV disease increased significantly if the donor was seropositive.[75]

Liver Transplantation

Significant progress has been made in pediatric liver transplantation, largely owing to improvements in immunosuppressive therapies. The current 10-year survival rate is 80% to 85% after liver transplantation.[63,64,76] Side effects of immunosuppression in this group include nephrotoxicity (5%), hypertension (28%), PTLD (5% to 7%), secondary malignancy (12%), and organ failure requiring retransplantation (5% to 10%). EBV and CMV infections pose major problems in the liver transplant patient.[63,76] Many protocols include prophylaxis for CMV with intravenous or oral ganciclovir for 3 months posttransplantation.

Hepatopulmonary syndrome and portopulmonary hypertension can present major problems in the patient before transplantation.[77,78] Hepatopulmonary syndrome is characterized by pulmonary vascular dilation and abnormal gas exchange (see Chapter 5). Structurally, the parenchyma of the lung is normal, but there is generalized vasodilation at the capillary level resulting in arteriovenous communication (shunt) and severe hypoxemia. Hepatopulmonary syndrome is recognized as an independent risk factor for death in patients with advanced liver disease. Portopulmonary hypertension is a process defined by pulmonary hypertension associated with portal hypertension. Histologically, it appears identical to primary pulmonary hypertension with smooth muscle hypertrophy, intimal fibrosis, and plexiform lesions in small lung injury. It is initially asymptomatic, but evolves to rapidly progressive impairment of right heart function. The prognosis is poor, with mean survival of 15 months after diagnosis. Hepatopulmonary syndrome frequently reverses after liver transplantation, whereas portopulmonary hypertension seems to resolve less frequently. Both of these entities must be considered in a patient with dyspnea before or just after liver transplantation.[77,78]

Lung Transplantation

Lung transplantation presents a unique set of problems for the balance of immunosuppression in the transplanted organ (prevention of rejection versus risk of infection) in part because the transplanted lung is an interface between the outside environment and the host defenses. The large epithelial surface area in the conducting airways and at the alveolar surfaces ($>70m^2$ in the adult) poses a great challenge for the lung defenses, particularly in the context of immunosuppression. The anatomy of the lung, lung products, cell receptors and subsequent signaling mechanisms activated, and host cellular responses all contribute to the normal lung defense and disease prevention. A defect in any of these defenses can result in an increased susceptibility to infection or increased propensity to inflammation, which can lead to rejection or development of obliterative bronchiolitis (see later) that can be life-threatening in the lung transplant patient.[76,79-81]

Immunosuppressive agents used to prevent transplant rejection alter the lung defenses. Local alteration of lung defenses contribute further to propensity to infection: denervation of the transplanted organ results in decreased cough reflex; ischemic injury to the mucosa causes impairment in mucociliary clearance; the anastomosis between host and transplanted organ

provides a point of possible narrowing of the airway. Infectious agents can be transferred passively from the donor to the recipient during transplantation. The additional complications related to lung transplantation likely account for the lower survival statistics compared with other solid organ transplants (1-year survival 77%, 3-year survival 63%, and 5-year survival 54%).[80] Graft failure accounts for most deaths in the first 60 days post-transplant (56%), whereas infection is an uncommon cause of early death. Late deaths primarily result from obliterative bronchiolitis (62%), infection (22%), and malignancies (14%).[80,81]

Immunosuppression after lung transplantation often consists of cyclosporine or tacrolimus, corticosteroids, and mycophenolate mofetil. The steroid dose is commonly tapered 2 to 3 months post-transplant.[80,81] Infection, allograft rejection, PTLD, and obliterative bronchiolitis are major pulmonary complications in the post-transplant period. The antibiotic regimen is tailored to the most likely pathogens. In a patient without cystic fibrosis, a first-generation cephalosporin is likely the first-line treatment, unless a center has a high incidence of methicillin-resistant *S. aureus*. In cystic fibrosis patients, antibiotics are directed to the pathogens present in the most recent respiratory culture; antifungal agents are initiated based on previous or current positive cultures.

Viruses can pose serious problems in a post–lung transplant patient; as in other solid organ transplants, CMV and EBV are important pathogens.[81] Most centers use ganciclovir or valganciclovir as prophylaxis for the first 5 to 6 months post-transplant. In the context of immunosuppression, however, infection by common respiratory viruses (particularly RSV, parainfluenza virus, adenovirus, or vaccinia) can be life-threatening. Prophylaxis with palivizumab (anti-RSV monoclonal antibody) can provide passive immunity for young infants at risk for RSV infection. It also is advantageous to keep these children out of the daycare setting. Aside from acute pneumonias, viral infections may be associated with early graft loss and rapid development of obliterative bronchiolitis.

PTLD occurs more commonly in pediatric lung transplant patients than in adults.

Because the first response to development of PTLD is reduction in immunosuppression, survival from PTLD often is complicated by episodes of rejection or obliterative bronchiolitis. Use of rituximab (anti-CD-20 antibody) has resulted in a significant reduction in morbidity and mortality from PTLD.

Allograft rejection is less common in children than in adults; however, surveillance and timely and accurate diagnosis of rejection may be more important and more difficult in children because of the frequency of respiratory viral infections. Spirometry is employed after lung transplantation to assess allograft function, and evidence for restrictive lung disease is concerning for the development of acute or chronic rejection. Computed tomography (CT) scans can be helpful in assessing for changes associated with rejection. Lung biopsy remains the only accurate method of diagnosing acute and chronic rejection; however, the utility of lung biopsy is limited by sampling error (small samples obtained with the pediatric biopsy forceps and skip areas). Rejection is diagnosed on the basis of standard histopathologic markers, and immunosuppressive therapy is adjusted accordingly.[80]

Obliterative bronchiolitis (formerly bronchiolitis obliterans) is rare in healthy children, but its incidence is markedly increased in the context of lung transplantation or SCT. Obliterative bronchiolitis is characterized by partial or complete occlusion of the lumens of terminal and respiratory bronchioles by inflammatory and fibrous tissue. The initiating event in the chain of events that leads to obliterative bronchiolitis is unclear. The primary trigger is thought to relate to epithelial injury in the small airways leading to transient derangements in epithelial cell function or local necrosis. This local necrosis leads to the generation of fibrinopurulent exudates that induce ingrowth of myofibroblasts, cellular proliferation, capillary immigration, and the development of an intraluminal polyp. Ongoing injury to the airway epithelium perpetuates this process, leading to narrowing or obliteration of the airway lumen.

Although injury and infection likely play a role in the changes that lead to obliterative bronchiolitis, the high incidence of obliterative bronchiolitis in lung transplant and SCT recipients provides strong evidence that immunopathologic response contributes to the development of obliterative bronchiolitis in the transplant setting. After lung transplantation, recurrent episodes of acute rejection are a risk factor for developing obliterative bronchiolitis. Early and accurate diagnosis of acute rejection and aggressive treatment are thought to be important in preventing the long-term development of obliterative bronchiolitis. Because of sampling limitations in transbronchial biopsies and risk associated with performing the biopsy itself, investigators have sought sensitive and noninvasive methods to detect early acute rejection and obliterative bronchiolitis.

In 1993, a consensus statement suggested using the term "bronchiolitis obliterans syndrome," defined by changes in pulmonary function as a possible surrogate marker for obliterative bronchiolitis.[82] These recommendations were later modified to use forced mid expiratory flow in addition to changes in forced expiratory volume in 1 second (focusing on early changes in small airways), and to use percent predicted values in addition to absolute values (to account for lung growth in small children).[83] Other surrogate clinical markers of obliterative bronchiolitis have been investigated, including cytokine measurements, measurement of cell surface receptors, and soluble cytokines and receptors in bronchoalveolar lavage (BAL).[79] BAL neutrophilia in the absence of detectable infectious agents has been shown to be a reproducible marker of obliterative bronchiolitis in adult and pediatric transplant patients.[79]

The optimal therapy for obliterative bronchiolitis in lung transplant and SCT patients is controversial. Alteration of immunosuppressive agents (see Table 3-8), inhaled cyclosporine, extracorporeal phosphophoresis, and the use of macrolide antibiotics have been studied in small groups of patients with variable results.[79] Despite these therapies, it is estimated that 35% to 60% of long-term survivors of lung transplantation develop obliterative bronchiolitis, which is the most common cause of death in this patient population.[79]

Stem Cell Transplantation

SCT presents an even greater challenge to the host defenses against pneumonia and lung injury because of the combined challenges of the initial conditioning regimen and the need for the recipient to develop a functional immune system from donor-derived stem cells. Serious infection occurs in the first 2 years after SCT in 50% of recipients with uncomplicated transplants from histocompatible sibling donors and in 80% to 90% of recipients from matched unrelated donors.

The immune deficits after SCT can be categorized into three phases. In the pre-engraftment phase (0 to 30 days post-transplant), infections arise primarily as a result of prolonged neutropenia and breaks in the mucosal barriers resulting from mucositis from the induction regimen before transplant. Myelosuppressive drugs can prolong this period. Repopulation of the lungs by donor-derived alveolar macrophages and recovery of circulating neutrophil counts occur during this period. Recovery of lymphocyte counts takes longer (the post-engraftment phase, 30 to 100 days post-transplant), and cellular immunity remains impaired. Response to alloantigens may not return for at least 6 months after SCT, and return of B cell function and humoral antibody production may take 1 year (late phase, >100 days post-transplant).[34,61,84]

The temporal sequence of the immunologic recovery and immunosuppressive therapy determines SCT recipients' susceptibility to pulmonary infection at any given time point. During the pre-engraftment phase, patients are most susceptible to bacterial infections and viral infections, including herpes simplex virus, CMV, and RSV. After neutrophil recovery (postengraftment phase), T cell and B cell immunity remains abnormal, predisposing the patient to infections with fungi, viruses, mycobacteria, and parasites. Patients can remain susceptible to encapsulated organisms because of inability to generate specific antibody responses. The development of GVHD further increases susceptibility to infection.[34,61,84-86]

Several noninfectious complications occur after SCT, including airway obstruction by mucositis, diffuse alveolar hemorrhage, pulmonary edema, and pulmonary embolism. Chronic obstructive pulmonary disease can be detected in 20% of long-term survivors of SCT; this is mainly associated with chronic GVHD, but other risk associations include the preparatory regimen (total body irradiation (TBI), methotrexate) and infection.[34,86] Mortality can be high, particularly if there is an early onset and rapid decline in forced expiratory volume in 1 second. Immunosuppressive therapies may be beneficial, but less than 50% of patients receiving such therapies show improvement in lung function or symptoms. Late-onset pulmonary disease includes obliterative bronchiolitis, cryptogenic organizing pneumonia (formerly bronchiolitis obliterans–organizing pneumonia[87,88]), diffuse alveolar damage, and interstitial pneumonia.[34,86]

PTLD is often associated with T cell dysfunction in the presence of EBV. The mean interval to development of PTLD was 5 to 6 months post-transplantation, with a cumulative incidence of 1% at 10 years. The use of quantitative polymerase chain reaction for EBV DNA has improved diagnosis dramatically. Using the EBV viral load, patients can be identified with low tumor burden. Use of rituximab (anti-CD20 monoclonal antibody) has shown promise in the treatment of PTLD in SCT patients.[86]

Obliterative bronchiolitis develops in 10% of SCT recipients who develop GVHD.[79] As with obliterative bronchiolitis in lung transplant recipients, immunologic and nonimmunologic factors are believed to play a role in the development of obliterative bronchiolitis in SCT recipients. These nonimmunologic factors include the pre-SCT conditioning regimen, intercurrent illness (particularly viral pneumonitis), the use of immunosuppressive medications, and the underlying disease that necessitated the SCT. Viral agents, such as CMV, adenovirus, influenza, parainfluenza, and RSV, have been implicated in the development of obliterative bronchiolitis. Several medications have been used in SCT recipients for the treatment of chronic GVHD and obliterative bronchiolitis; however, response was usually limited to skin, soft tissue, and oral mucosa.

Diagnosis and Treatment of Respiratory Abnormalities in a Child with Secondary Immunocompromise Owing to Cancer or Transplantation

In an immunocompromised child, aspects of the medical history, physical examination, and routine microbial surveillance (or previous antibody titers) are important first steps. Timing of the symptoms relative to drug therapies or changes in immunosuppressants could point to the infection or noninfectious complications. The presence of sinusitis, otitis media, and rhinitis would point to respiratory virus infections as an important consideration. The presence of severe mucositis or evidence of skin GVHD could point to anaerobic organisms, oral flora, or gut enterics as causes for the respiratory symptoms or infiltrates on chest x-ray. The history and physical examination can only suggest the causes of lung complications or lung symptoms and physical findings, however. Because there is a good probability of full recovery if the pathogen is uncovered, early and aggressive diagnostic studies are warranted to direct appropriate antimicrobial or antiviral therapy. This is particularly true in the context of fever in a neutropenic patient.

Radiography

Pulmonary changes on chest radiographs may be delayed or modified in an immunocompromised patient because of the inability to generate an inflammatory response. Still, the time course, evolution, and appearance of the pneumonias can provide important diagnostic clues. Radiographic changes in an immunocompromised child can be classified according to their appearance: (1) diffuse alveolar or interstitial pneumonias, (2) localized alveolar lobar or lobular consolidation, (3) nodular infiltrates or abscesses, or (4) hyperinflation.[34,65] Interstitial/alveolar infiltrates can arise from viral (CMV, RSV, varicella-zoster virus, adenovirus) and fungal (P. jiroveci pneumonia, Cryptococcus, Candida,

Histoplasma) infection, and pulmonary edema or early obliterative bronchiolitis, rejection, and GVHD. Consolidation can arise from bacterial infections (S. pneumoniae, H. influenzae, S. aureus, gram-negative organisms, M. tuberculosis, or atypical mycobacteria) and fungal infections (Cryptococcus, Nocardia, Aspergillus, Mucor), and pulmonary thromboembolic disease, pulmonary hemorrhage, and pulmonary edema. Nodular infiltrates arise from bacterial infections, fungal infections, P. jiroveci pneumonia, and M. tuberculosis. The early changes of obliterative bronchiolitis manifest as hyperinflation with clear lung fields. There is considerable overlap between these basic radiographic patterns and their causes, so more aggressive diagnostic studies are indicated to show the cause and direct appropriate therapy.[34,65]

CT scan of the chest is particularly useful when the chest radiograph is negative, or when findings on chest x-ray are nonspecific. CT is useful in defining areas of lung involvement for more invasive studies (e.g., biopsy, BAL). Spiral CT and ventilation/perfusion studies can be diagnostic if pulmonary thromboembolism is a consideration. A "mosaic" pattern of lung hyperinflation and infiltrate can suggest the development of obliterative bronchiolitis.

Sputum and Nasopharyngeal Washes, and Other Indirect Methods for Pathogen Detection

Spontaneous or induced sputum samples can be studied by culture and special stains for pulmonary pathogens: Gram stain, fungal stains, acid-fast bacillus stain, and silver stains can be performed to diagnose bacterial and fungal causes of pulmonary infiltrates. Blood cultures are rarely positive, but can be diagnostic for bacterial pneumonias. In addition, nasal aspirates can be studied by immunologic methods or culture to identify common viral pathogens (RSV, influenza, parainfluenza viruses, adenovirus) that can cause pulmonary infections in immunocompromised patients. Viral cultures can be useful in detecting the common viral pathogens in addition to members of the herpesvirus family (CMV, herpes simplex virus). Genetic probes are available to detect CMV and EBV in blood samples, and quantitative polymerase chain reaction can provide a measure of viral load. Probes also are available for detecting *P. jiroveci, Legionella, Mycobacterium,* and *Mycoplasma.* These studies also can be applied to samples obtained by more invasive methods (bronchoscopy and lung biopsy) as described subsequently.

Flexible Bronchoscopy

Flexible fiberoptic bronchoscopy can provide BAL or bronchial lavage samples and biopsy materials for diagnosis of pulmonary complications in immunocompromised patients. Bronchoscopy with lavage performed early in the course of evaluation of an immunocompromised patient can enhance the probability of identifying a pathogen in the lung. BAL can provide materials for culture (i.e., bacterial, viral, fungal, acid-fast bacillus), cytology, and immunohistochemistry, potentially identifying pathogens in the lung. In addition, bronchoscopy can identify endobronchial obstruction owing to infection or tumor. Protected brush specimens can decrease the potential for BAL samples to be contaminated by upper airway flora during passage through the nasopharynx. Although bronchoscopy with BAL can provide important diagnostic information, it has limitations. BAL cultures in patients already on broad-spectrum antibiotics are often negative. Pathogens present in small numbers (e.g., *P. jiroveci,* mycobacteria) may be missed on stains or cytology, although more sensitive polymerase chain reaction techniques may increase the yield. Invasive pathogens (*Aspergillus*) may be missed by lavage when obvious on biopsy samples.

Bronchoscopy also can be used to perform transbronchial lung biopsies.[34,80] Transbronchial biopsy can be difficult in young children because the size of available bronchoscopes and their small suction channel (1.2 mm) require obtaining several samples for adequate material for histology and culture. In older children, small adult bronchoscopes can be used with standard size biopsy forceps. These biopsy samples can help in identifying pathogens missed by standard BAL (e.g.,

invasive *Aspergillus*), in addition to helping to identify acute rejection (lung transplant), GVHD, and obliterative bronchiolitis (SCT and lung transplant).[34,80] Most centers have a protocol for surveillance post-transplantation to screen for rejection. Open biopsy is usually needed to make the diagnosis of obliterative bronchiolitis.

Lung lavage can be done in intubated patients by passing a catheter through an existing endotracheal tube and performing saline washes. This technique is "blind," but can provide important diagnostic material in a critically ill child too sick to tolerate standard BAL techniques.

Transthoracic Needle Aspiration Biopsy

Needle aspiration of the lung under CT or fluoroscopic guidance can have high yields in sampling peripheral lung lesions (particularly suspected fungal lesions) that cannot be reached by standard flexible fiberoptic bronchoscopy techniques. The major risks of transthoracic biopsy are pneumothorax and bleeding. In addition, because of the small needle size, sampling error can occur ("missing" nearby involved areas).

Open Lung Biopsy

Open lung biopsy remains the gold standard for diagnosis of pulmonary abnormalities in an immunocompromised patient. It allows the surgeon to obtain adequate quantities of lung tissue for analysis, provides the opportunity to sample multiple sites, and allows the surgeon to visualize and select optimal sites for biopsy. The use of a mini-thoracotomy or video-assisted thoracoscopic surgery allows for a smaller incision. Although open lung biopsy provides the most definitive information in an immunocompromised patient, timing of the biopsies and the potential need for repeated biopsies (particularly if rejection and obliterative bronchiolitis are considerations) limit the use of this technique. A patient who does not respond to therapy based on other diagnostic techniques (including bronchoscopy and needle biopsy) usually would benefit from open biopsy.

Summary

Pulmonary symptoms and pulmonary complications in an immunocompromised patient provide a diagnostic challenge for clinicians. The immunologic defects resulting from primary immunodeficiencies or immunosuppression in patients can allow lung infection by common pathogens or by opportunistic organisms (in patients with primary or secondary T cell defects or immunosuppressed patients after transplantation). Infection must be discriminated from potentially treatable noninfectious complications resulting from thrombosis, organ failure, and complications of chemotherapeutic agents or organ rejection. The clinician caring for these patients must maintain a high index of suspicion for infectious and noninfectious pulmonary complications and must be methodical in the evaluation of these complex patients.

References

1. Bonilla FA, Geha RS: 2. Update on primary immunodeficiency diseases. J Allergy Clin Immunol 117:S435-S441, 2006.
2. Pilette C, Ouadrhiri Y, Godding V, et al: Lung mucosal immunity: Immunoglobulin-A revisited. Eur Respir J 18:571-588, 2001.
3. Buckley RH: Pulmonary complications of primary immunodeficiencies. Paediatr Respir Rev 5(Suppl A): S225-S233, 2004.
4. Notarangelo L et al: Primary immunodeficiency diseases: An update. J Allergy Clin Immunol 114:677-687, 2004.
5. Cunningham-Rundles C, Ponda PP: Molecular defects in T- and B-cell primary immunodeficiency diseases. Nat Rev Immunol 5:880-892, 2005.
6. Chinen J, Shearer WT: Basic and clinical immunology. J Allergy Clin Immunol 116:411-418, 2005.
7. Buckley RH: Primary immunodeficiency diseases due to defects in lymphocytes. N Engl J Med 343:1313-1324, 2000.
8. Bruton OC: Agammaglobulinemia. Pediatrics 9:722-728, 1952.
9. Ochs HD, Notarangelo LD: X-linked immunodeficiencies. Curr Allergy Asthma Rep 4:339-348, 2004.
10. Maas A, Hendricks RW: Role of Bruton's tyrosine kinase in B cell development. Dev Immunol 8:171-181, 2001.
11. Chinen J, Shearer WT: Basic and clinical immunology. J Allergy Clin Immunol 111:S813-S818, 2003.
12. Stewart DM, Lian L, Nelson DL: The clinical spectrum of Bruton's agammaglobulinemia. Curr Allergy Asthma Rep 1:558-565, 2001.
13. Goldacker S, Warnatz K: Tackling the heterogeneity of CVID. Curr Opin Allergy Clin Immunol 5: 504-509, 2005.
14. Salzer U, Grimbacher B: TACItly changing tunes: Farewell to a yin and yang of BAFF receptor and TACI in humoral immunity? New genetic defects in common variable immunodeficiency. Curr Opin Allergy Clin Immunol 5:496-503, 2005.
15. Bayry J, et al: Common variable immunodeficiency: The immune system in chaos. Trends Mol Med 11:370-376, 2005.
16. Grimbacher B, Schaffer AA, Peter HH: The genetics of hypogammaglobulinemia. Curr Allergy Asthma Rep 4:349-358, 2004.
17. Durandy A, et al: Hyper-immunoglobulin M syndromes caused by intrinsic B-lymphocyte defects. Immune Rev 203:67-79, 2005.
18. Pulendran B, Ahmed R: Translating innate immunity into immunological memory: Implications for vaccine development. Cell 124:849-863, 2006.
19. Davey GM, et al: SOCS1: A potent and multifaceted regulator of cytokines and cell-mediated inflammation. Tissue Antigens 67:1-9, 2006.
20. Sigal LH: Basic science for the clinician 32: T-cells with regulatory function. J Clin Rheumatol 11:286-289, 2005.
21. Ochoa JB, Makarenkova V: T lymphocytes. Crit Care Med 33:S510-S513, 2005.
22. Bleackley RC: A molecular view of cytotoxic T lymphocyte induced killing. Biochem Cell Biol 83: 747-751, 2005.
23. Bacchetta R, Gregori S, Roncarolo MG: CD4+ regulatory T cells: Mechanisms of induction and effector function. Autoimmun Rev 4:491-496, 2005.
24. Boyton RJ, Openshaw PJ: Pulmonary defenses to acute respiratory infection. Br Med Bull 61:1-12, 2002.
25. Jameson J, Witherden D, Havran WL: T-cell effector mechanisms: γδ and CD1d-restricted subsets. Curr Opin Immunol 15:349-353, 2003.
26. Yokoyama WM, Kim S, French AR: The dynamic life of natural killer cells. Annu Rev Immunol 22:405-429, 2004.
27. Fischer A, de Saint BG, Le Deist F: CD3 deficiencies. Curr Opin Allergy Clin Immunol 5:491-495, 2005.
28. Cardell SL: The natural killer T lymphocyte: A player in the complex regulation of autoimmune diabetes in non-obese diabetic mice. Clin Exp Immunol 143:194-202, 2006.
29. Firestein GS: Immunologic mechanisms in the pathogenesis of rheumatoid arthritis. J Clin Rheumatol 11:S39-S44, 2005.
30. Kay AB: The role of T lymphocytes in asthma. Chem Immunol Allergy 91:59-75, 2006.
31. Krzych U, Schwenk J: The dissection of CD8 T cells during liver-stage infection. Curr Top Microbiol Immunol 297:1-24, 2005.
32. Walter U, Santamaria P: CD8+ T cells in autoimmunity. Curr Opin Immunol 17:624-631, 2005.
33. Ferrara JL, Yanik G: Acute graft versus host disease: Pathophysiology, risk factors, and prevention strategies. Clin Adv Hematol Oncol 3:415-419, 428, 2005.
34. Stokes DC: Pulmonary infections in the immunocompromised host. In Chernick V, et al, eds: Kendig's Disorders of the Respiratory Tract in Children, 7th ed. Philadelphia, Saunders, 2006, pp 453-462.
35. Etzioni A: Immune deficiency and autoimmunity. Autoimmun Rev 2:364-369, 2003.
36. Hong R: The DiGeorge anomaly. Clin Rev Allergy Immunol 20:43-60, 2001.
37. Ochs HD, Thrasher AJ: The Wiskott-Aldrich syndrome. J Allergy Clin Immunol 117:725-738, 2006.
38. Taylor AM, Groom A, Byrd PJ: Ataxia-telangiectasia-like disorder (ATLD)—its clinical presentation and molecular basis. DNA Repair (Amst) 3:1219-1225, 2004.

39. Nichols KE, et al: Molecular and cellular pathogenesis of X-linked lymphoproliferative disease. Immunol Rev 203:180-199, 2005.

40. Orange JS, et al: Use of intravenous immunoglobulin in human disease: A review of evidence by members of the Primary Immunodeficiency Committee of the American Academy of Allergy, Asthma and Immunology. J Allergy Clin Immunol 117:S525-S553, 2006.

41. Chinen J, Puck JM: Successes and risks of gene therapy in primary immunodeficiencies. J Allergy Clin Immunol 113:595-603, 2004.

42. Kobayashi SD, Voyich JM, DeLeo FR: Regulation of the neutrophil-mediated inflammatory response to infection. Microbes Infect 5:1337-1344, 2003.

43. Berliner N, Horwitz M, Loughran TP Jr: Congenital and acquired neutropenia. Hematology (Am Soc Hematol Educ Program) 2004:63-79, 2004.

44. Wen L, Atkinson JP, Giclas PC: Clinical and laboratory evaluation of complement deficiency. J Allergy Clin Immunol 113:585-593, 2004.

45. Anderson DC, Springer TA: Leukocyte adhesion deficiency: An inherited defect in the Mac-1, LFA-1, and p150, 95 glycoproteins. Annu Rev Med 38:175-194, 1987.

46. Rosenzweig SD, Holland SM: Phagocyte immuno-deficiencies and their infections. J Allergy Clin Immunol 113:620-626, 2004.

47. Watford WT, Ghio AJ, Wright JR: Complement-mediated host defense in the lung. Am J Physiol Lung Cell Mol Physiol 279:L790-L798, 2000.

48. Thiel S, Frederiksen PD, Jensenius JC: Clinical manifestations of mannan-binding lectin deficiency. Mol Immunol 43:86-96, 2006.

49. Breeze RG, Wheeldon EB: The cells of the pulmonary airways. Am Rev Respir Dis 116:705-777, 1977.

50. Evans MJ, et al: Cellular and molecular characteristics of basal cells in airway epithelium. Exp Lung Res 27:401-415, 2001.

51. Knowles MR, Boucher RC: Mucus clearance as a primary innate defense mechanism for mammalian airways. J Clin Invest 109:571-577, 2002.

52. Crouch E, Wright JR: Surfactant proteins A and D and pulmonary host defense. Annu Rev Physiol 63:521-554, 2001.

53. Shepherd VL: Distinct roles for lung collectins in pulmonary host defense. Am J Respir Cell Mol Biol 26:257-260, 2002.

54. Strieter RM, Belperio JA, Keane MP: Cytokines in innate host defense in the lung. J Clin Invest 109:699-705, 2002.

55. Meyer S, et al: Pulmonary dysfunction in pediatric oncology patients. Pediatr Hematol Oncol 21:175-195, 2004.

56. Lal DR, et al: Primary epithelial lung malignancies in the pediatric population. Pediatr Blood Cancer 45:683-686, 2005.

57. Nysom K, et al: Pulmonary function after treatment for acute lymphoblastic leukaemia in childhood. Br J Cancer 78:21-27, 1998.

58. Nysom K, et al: Relationship between cumulative anthracycline dose and late cardiotoxicity in childhood acute lymphoblastic leukemia. J Clin Oncol 16:545-550, 1998.

59. Kaplan E, et al: Pulmonary function in children treated for rhabdomyosarcoma. Med Pediatr Oncol 27:79-84, 1996.

60. Kaplan EB, et al: Late effects of bone marrow transplantation on pulmonary function in children. Bone Marrow Transplant 14:613-621, 1994.

61. Joos L, Tamm M: Breakdown of pulmonary host defense in the immunocompromised host: Cancer chemotherapy. Proc Am Thorax Soc 2:445-448, 2005.

62. Allen UD: Factors influencing predisposition to sepsis in children with cancers and acquired immunodeficiencies unrelated to human immunodeficiency virus infection. Pediatr Crypt Care Med 6:S80-S86, 2005.

63. Kelly DA: Long-term challenges of immunosuppression in pediatric patients. Transplant Proc 37:1657-1662, 2005.

64. Duncan MD, Wilkes DS: Transplant-related immunosuppression: A review of immunosuppression and pulmonary infections. Proc Am Thorac Soc 2:449-455, 2005.

65. Fishman JA, Rubin RH: Infection in organ-transplant recipients. N Engl J Med 338:1741-1751, 1998.

66. Turgeon N, et al: Safety and efficacy of granulocyte colony-stimulating factor in kidney and liver transplant recipients. Transpl Infect Dis 2:15-21, 2000.

67. Turgeon N, et al: Prevention of recurrent cytomegalovirus disease in renal and liver transplant recipients: Effect of oral ganciclovir. Transpl Infect Dis 2:2-10, 2000.

68. Fishman JA, et al: Dosing of intravenous ganciclovir for the prophylaxis and treatment of cytomegalovirus infection in solid organ transplant recipients. Transplantation 69:389-394, 2000.

69. Groetzner J, et al: Cardiac transplantation in pediatric patients: Fifteen-year experience of a single center. Ann Thorac Surg 79:53-60, 2005.

70. Ross M, et al: Ten- and 20-year survivors of pediatric orthotopic heart transplantation. J Heart Lung Transplant 25:261-270, 2006.

71. Minami K, et al: Long-term results of pediatric heart transplantation. Ann Thorac Cardiovasc Surg 11:386-390, 2005.

72. Azeka E, et al: Heart transplantation in children: Clinical outcome during the early postoperative period. Pediatr Transplant 9:491-497, 2005.

73. Cisneros JM, et al: Pneumonia after heart transplantation: A multi-institutional study. Spanish Transplantation Infection Study Group. Clin Infect Dis 27:324-331, 1998.

74. European best practice guidelines for renal transplantation: Section IV. Long-term management of the transplant recipient. IV.11. Pediatrics (specific problems). Nephrol Dial Transplant 17(Suppl 4):55-58, 2002.

75. Robinson LG, et al: Predictors of cytomegalovirus disease among pediatric transplant recipients within one year of renal transplantation. Pediatr Transplant 6:111-118, 2002.

76. McDiarmid SV: Management of the pediatric liver transplant patient. Liver Transpl 7:S77-S86, 2001.

77. Bottari G, Mazzeo AT, Santamaria LB: The importance of predicting the prognosis in patients with hepatopulmonary syndrome: A simple scoring system. Transplant Proc 38:795-797, 2006.

78. Martinez-Palli G, et al: Liver transplantation in high-risk patients: Hepatopulmonary syndrome and portopulmonary hypertension. Transplant Proc 37:3861-3864, 2005.

79. Kurland G, Michelson P: Bronchiolitis obliterans in children. Pediatr Palomino 39:193-208, 2005.

80. Mallory GB, Spray TL: Paediatric lung transplantation. Eur. Respir J 24:839-845, 2004.

81. Mallory GB, Elidemir O: Management of posttransplant lung disease. Clin Pulm Med 12:269-280, 2005.

82. Cooper JD, et al: A working formulation for the standardization of nomenclature and for clinical staging of chronic dysfunction in lung allografts. International Society for Heart and Lung Transplantation. J Heart Lung Transplant 12:713-716, 1993.

83. Estenne M, et al: Bronchiolitis obliterans syndrome 2001: An update of the diagnostic criteria. J Heart Lung Transplant 21:297-310, 2002.

84. Veys P, Owens C: Respiratory infections following haemopoietic stem cell transplantation in children. Br Med Bull 61:151-174, 2002.

85. Boeckh M, et al: Emerging viral infections after hematopoietic cell transplantation. Pediatr Transplant 9(Suppl 7):48-54, 2005.

86. Socie G, Tichelli A: Long-term care after stem-cell transplantation. Hematol J 5(Suppl 3):S39-S43, 2004.

87. Schlesinger C, Veeraraghavan S, Koss MN: Constructive (obliterative) bronchiolitis. Curr Opin Pulm Med 4:288-293, 1998.

88. Schlesinger C, Koss MN: The organizing pneumonias: An update and review. Curr Opin Pulm Med 11:422-430, 2005.

CHAPTER 4

Pulmonary Manifestations of Cardiac Diseases

MARLYN S. WOO AND JACQUELINE R. SZMUSZKOVICZ

Overview of the Cardiovascular
  Circulation 79
  Pulmonary Circulation 79
  Bronchial Circulation 80
  Lymphatic Circulation 80
Cardiovascular Lesions That Increase
  the Work of Breathing 80
  Large Volume Left-to-Right Shunts 81
  Outflow or Inflow Obstruction of the
    Systemic Ventricle 87

Vascular Anomalies That Cause Airway
  Obstruction 89
Lesions with Increased Venous Admixture 92
Idiopathic Pulmonary Arterial
  Hypertension 95
Other Pulmonary Conditions Associated with
  Cardiac Disease or Surgery 96
Summary 96
  References 97

Sharing the same body cavity, the heart and lungs are closely interconnected by the pulmonary vasculature. An increase or decrease in pulmonary vascular pressures leads to changes in the blood vessels, which directly affect the airways, lung interstitium, alveoli, and pleura. Heart disease often leads to respiratory failure as a result of its impact on gas exchange, water/solute exchange, and pulmonary mechanics. The appearance of lung disease secondary to cardiac disease depends on whether the changes in the pulmonary vascular pressures are acute or chronic. Clinical manifestations of cardiac disease include pulmonary edema, pleural effusion, hypoxemia, pulmonary hypertension, atelectasis, and plastic bronchitis.

Noninfectious pulmonary complications, such as bronchiectasis, prolonged postoperative mechanical ventilation, extubation failure, airway complications (e.g., tracheobronchomalacia, subglottic stenosis, bronchial stenosis), and obstructive sleep apnea, have been extensively described in pediatric patients after cardiac surgery.[1-4] Although many of the physiologic mechanisms are similar, this chapter concentrates on pediatric heart diseases and disorders that have an impact on the pulmonary system.

Overview of the Cardiovascular Circulation

The cardiopulmonary vascular system comprises two components: the pulmonary circulation and the bronchial circulation. The bronchial circulation constitutes a very small portion of the output of the left ventricle, and it supplies part of the tracheobronchial tree with systemic arterial blood. The pulmonary circulation constitutes the entire output of the right ventricle, and it supplies the lung with the mixed venous blood draining from all the tissues of the body. This blood undergoes gas exchange with alveolar air in the pulmonary capillaries. Under normal circumstances, these systems change with the maturational stage of the individual. It is important to understand the vascular changes that occur with normal growth over time. A brief review of the cardiovascular circulation follows.

Pulmonary Circulation

The normal mature pulmonary circulation is a low-resistance system compared with the general systemic circulation.[5] Despite receiving about the same amount of blood flow, the pulmonary arterial pressure is only about 20% of the systemic circulation pressure. The plasticity of the pulmonary circulation can be attributed to two related factors: (1) the pulmonary vessels are thin-walled and dilate with mild increases in pressure, and (2) this augmentation of the vessel radius passively recruits underperfused vessels, which leads to an increase in overall cross-sectional area.

In contrast to the mature pulmonary circulation, the fetal pulmonary resistance is higher than the systemic resistance. The high pulmonary system resistance in the fetus permits shunting of blood from the systemic venous to the systemic arterial circulation via the ductus arteriosus to the aorta and through the foramen ovale to the left atrium. The following three factors contribute to the high fetal pulmonary circulation resistance: (1) In the fetus, the pulmonary arteries are exposed to the full systemic blood pressure via the ductus arteriosus, and their walls are very muscular. (2) The fetal lung exists in an airless state. (3) There is hypoxic vasoconstriction within the intrauterine environment.

With the onset of air breathing and inflation of the lungs, the pulmonary circulatory resistance decreases with the loss of the placental circulation. The inflation of the lungs causes expansion of the pulmonary vessels, and the increase in oxygenation results in vasodilation. With subsequent involution of the arterial muscle, there is remodeling of the pulmonary arteries. This remodeling involves thinning of the arterial muscular wall and the normal branching and growth of the airways and alveoli. Although the pulmonary veins have thinner walls compared with the arteries, veins do have a muscular layer, which can become hypertrophied in response to elevated pulmonary pressure.[5,6]

Bronchial Circulation

In contrast to the pulmonary circulation, the bronchial circulation is small, carrying only 1% of the cardiac output. The bronchial arteries carry oxygenated blood to the lungs as part of the general systemic circulatory system. Bronchial arteries respond to stimuli, as do the other systemic arteries (dilation in response to hypoxia). Conversely, the pulmonary arteries constrict to hypoxia. The bronchial arteries arise from the aorta and the intercostal arteries, and then divide along with the bronchial divisions. Despite the differences between the pulmonary and bronchial circulations, there are intricate interconnections between them. Anastomotic vessels connect the bronchial arteries to the pulmonary arterioles and to the pulmonary veins. These anastomotic connections permit flexibility of flow to and from pulmonary and bronchial circulations. The drainage of the bronchial arteries to a vascular plexus permits great flexibility of bronchial venous drainage. The bronchial venous drainage can move to either the right or the left side of the heart. Extrapulmonary bronchial vessels supplying large airways drain to the right atrium through the azygos and hemiazygos veins. The intrapulmonary vessels drain to the pulmonary veins and to the left atrium. The venous drainage permits flexibility in drainage route, depending on changing hemodynamic pressures.

Lymphatic Circulation

The pulmonary lymphatic circulation lies in the connective tissue of the lung. There is continuous filtration of liquid and protein through the lung microcirculation. Passive flow of liquids proceeds along a pressure gradient to reach the lymphatic capillaries and is returned via active pumping to the systemic circulation. Disruption of the intravascular pulmonary pressures also alters the lymphatic circulation.[5,7]

Cardiovascular Lesions That Increase the Work of Breathing

Generally, three types of cardiovascular problems cause disturbances in mechanical function of the lungs and increase the work of breathing: (1) large volume left-to-right shunts, (2) outflow or inflow obstruction of the systemic ventricle, and (3) vascular anomalies that obstruct the airways.

Large Volume Left-to-Right Shunts

Lesions that allow communication between the systemic and pulmonary circulations and cause a large left-to-right shunt are the most frequent congenital cardiac anomalies. These include common problems such as ventricular septal defect (VSD), atrial septal defect (ASD), and patent ductus arteriosus (PDA), and defects with similar physiologic consequences, but more complex anatomy, such as single ventricle, aorticopulmonary window, and truncus arteriosus. These lesions are characterized by the recirculation of oxygenated blood through the lungs and pulmonary vascular congestion. The shunt produces excessive pulmonary blood flow and increased return of pulmonary venous blood to the left side of the heart. In addition, when the abnormal communication is large and occurs at the level of the ventricles or great vessels, the high pressure of the left side of the heart is transmitted to the pulmonary circulation, causing pulmonary artery hypertension.

The volume of blood traversing the pulmonary circulation in the presence of an anomalous intracardiac communication or between the great arteries depends on the size of the communication and the relative resistances of the pulmonary and systemic circulations. When the communication is small, it offers a high resistance to the passage of blood. As a result there is a large pressure decrease between the high-pressure chamber and vessel (usually, the left ventricle or aorta) and the low-pressure chamber or vessel (usually, the right ventricle or pulmonary artery), and the left-to-right shunt is limited. When the communication is large, there is virtually no resistance to the flow of blood from the systemic to the pulmonary side of the circulation. Consequently, the pressures become equal in both sides, and the size of the shunt is no longer governed by the size of the communication, but rather by the relative magnitudes of the systemic and pulmonary vascular resistances. Because the pulmonary vascular resistance of the term newborn is very high, it is not surprising that even large communications such as those caused by a large VSD or PDA produce little left-to-right shunt for days, or even weeks, after birth. As pulmonary vascular resistance declines postnatally, signs of pulmonary congestion develop quickly.

Numerous factors have been identified that influence the decrease in pulmonary vascular resistance associated with the transition to extrauterine life. In the immediate postnatal period, the expansion of the alveoli, the increase in alveolar PO_2, and the decrease in the alveolar PCO_2 cause recruitment of pulmonary capillaries and dilation of pulmonary arterioles, decreasing pulmonary vascular resistance. As the arterial musculature becomes thinner, and new vessels gradually grow in the lungs, pulmonary vascular resistance decreases even further. Finally, the postnatal decline in hematocrit—so-called physiologic anemia—also contributes significantly to the decrease in pulmonary vascular resistance by reducing blood viscosity.

Left-to-right shunts can cause increased symptoms after the decrease in the pulmonary arterial pressure and pulmonary vascular resistance that normally occurs after birth. As mentioned before, these shunts can be intracardiac (ASD, VSD, or atrioventricular septal defect) or extracardiac (PDA or aorticopulmonary window). Intracardiac shunts usually are associated with increased pulmonary blood flow without an increase in pressure in the early stage of the disease. Extracardiac shunts (depending on their size) may expose the pulmonary vascular circulation to systemic pressures that would cause earlier development of vascular changes. Shunt lesions, such as a VSD, ASD, or PDA, may not cause a significant murmur in a neonate because of the normally elevated pulmonary vascular resistance at birth causing the shunting to be low velocity. As the pulmonary vascular resistance decreases to normal levels over the first 1 to 2 months of life, the shunt becomes more prominent. The normal systemic vascular resistance is about 25 Wood units/m^2, and normal pulmonary vascular resistance is about 3 Wood units/m^2, so blood shunts from the left (systemic) circulation to the right (pulmonary) circulation.

Pathophysiology of Pulmonary Edema and Pleural Effusion

One of the main pathophysiologic effects of the left-to-right shunt is to redistribute part of the left ventricular output from the systemic to the pulmonary circulation (Fig. 4-1). When this occurs, pulmonary blood flow increases, increasing the right ventricular afterload, left ventricular preload, left atrial pressure, and the work performed by the heart muscle. In normal circumstances, the venous pressure in the lung is low and varies only a little during the cardiac cycle. An increase in left ventricular end-diastolic or left atrial pressure can cause increased pressure in the pulmonary veins, however, with subsequent pressure increases in the capillary vessels and then in the pulmonary arteries. As a result, fluid starts to accumulate in the interstitium and alveoli, causing pulmonary edema. Edema usually forms in response to increased pulmonary venous pressures. As the intravascular pressure increases, more extravascular fluid is filtered through the pulmonary interstitium to the lymphatic system. When this microvasculature filtration system becomes overwhelmed, there is accumulation of fluid in the interstitial lung tissue.[8] An early feature

of this fluid buildup, or edema, is the accumulation of fluid around the bronchovascular bundles. This accrual of bronchovascular bundle fluid can be seen on chest radiographs, particularly in the fissures.

When the pulmonary lymphatic system cannot clear the interstitial fluid, the fluid accumulation must leave by other means. One route is to form a transudate through the interlobular septa and then to the pleural space, which leads to pleural effusion. When in the pleural space, the liquid is absorbed into the parietal pleural lymphatic system. Transport of interstitial fluid to the pleural space reduces the possibility of alveolar edema, which is associated with altered gas exchange and pulmonary mechanics. In contrast, pleural effusion alone generally is not associated with severe derangements in pulmonary function. Alterations in blood flow and in pulmonary vascular pressures are associated with pathologic changes in the pulmonary arteries (Table 4-1).

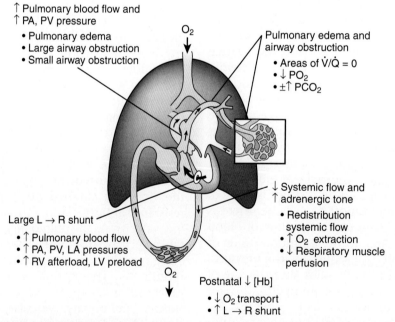

Figure 4-1. Pathophysiology of a large left-to-right shunt. Proceeding in a clockwise direction, this schema shows the factors that contribute to respiratory and circulatory compromise. With a large left-to-right (L → R) shunt, pulmonary blood flow and pulmonary arterial (PA), pulmonary venous (PV), and left atrial (LA) pressures increase, as does right ventricular (RV) afterload and left ventricular (LV) preload. These changes promote pulmonary edema formation, and cause large or small airway obstruction. The restrictive and obstructive lung disease creates areas of the lung with true intrapulmonary shunt ($\dot{V}/\dot{Q} = 0$), and can depress arterial PO_2 and increase arterial PCO_2. Because of the reduced systemic perfusion and increased adrenergic tone, systemic blood flow is redistributed, O_2 extraction increases, and respiratory muscle perfusion is diminished. The postnatal decline in hemoglobin concentration [Hb] further aggravates the circulatory imbalance by decreasing O_2 transport and increasing further the left-to-right shunt. (*From Lister, and G Perez Fontan JJ. Congenital Heart Disease and Respiratory Disease in Children. Loughlin G and Eigen H. Eds. Baltimore, Williams & Wilkins, 1994, p 603.*)

Table 4-1	Diagnoses Associated with Increased Pulmonary Arterial Pressure

Aorta

Patent ductus arteriosus

Aorticopulmonary window

Truncus arteriosus

Postsurgical shunts

 Blalock-Taussig (subclavian artery to ipsilateral pulmonary artery)

 Potts (descending aorta–left pulmonary artery)

 Waterston (ascending aorta–right pulmonary artery)

Atrium

Atrial septal defect

Common atrium

Total or partial anomalous pulmonary venous connection

Transposition of the great arteries with atrial septal defect

Ventricle

Ventricular septal defect

Single ventricle

Atrioventricular canal

Associated lesions with ventricular septal defect

Transposition of the great arteries

Double-outlet right ventricle

Tricuspid atresia without pulmonary stenosis

Mitral atresia

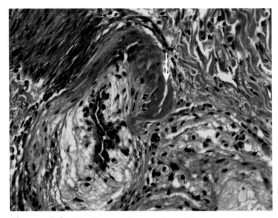

Figure 4-2. Plexiform lesion on lung biopsy specimen of a patient with severe pulmonary arterial hypertension.

The earliest change to increased pressure in the pulmonary arteries is medial thickening, which is the response to increased intramural vascular pressure. The medial thickening may come about from hypertrophy and hyperplasia of smooth muscle cells. The next change is an increase in intimal thickening. Intimal thickening can be due to an increase in the number of cells or an accumulation of dense fibrous tissue. The development of irreversible change is heralded by the formation of plexiform lesions (Fig. 4-2).

As the pulmonary vascular disease gradually worsens from the increased pressure, the pulmonary vascular resistance also increases and results in decreased pulmonary blood flow. When the pulmonary vascular resistance becomes higher than the systemic vascular resistance, the shunt flow (initially left-to-right shunt) reverses direction, leading to a right-to-left shunt. At this point, the elevated pulmonary vascular resistance with a right-to-left shunt is defined as Eisenmenger syndrome.

Clinical Findings of Acute Increased Pulmonary Venous Pressure

Patients with acute pulmonary edema may be asymptomatic in the early stages. On auscultation, the lung sounds can be normal, or there may be mild wheezing. As the condition progresses with alveolar edema, the patient may experience tachypnea and possible cough productive of foamy secretions. At this stage, coarse crackles (rales) are usually heard. Conditions associated with acute increase of pulmonary venous pressure are outlined in Table 4-2.

The chest radiograph is more sensitive than the history or physical examination in detecting acute elevation of pulmonary venous pressure (Fig. 4-3). The chest radiograph shows increased vascular markings and changes in the cardiac silhouette, depending on the underlying heart disease. Kerley B lines are seen in the periphery of the lungs, indicating accumulation of fluid

Table 4-2	Diagnoses Associated with Acute Increase of Pulmonary Venous Pressure

Aortic regurgitation

Left atrium

 Mitral regurgitation

 Mitral stenosis or obstruction

Left ventricular failure

 Myocarditis

 Pericardial tamponade

 Tachyarrhythmia

in the interlobular septa. Alveolar edema is represented radiologically as fluffy infiltrates. Pleural effusion may also appear, usually bilaterally beginning with blunting of the costophrenic angles (Fig. 4-3).

Even with interstitial edema and pleural effusion, pulmonary function changes little in patients with acute increased pulmonary venous pressure. Alveolar edema is associated with significant decreases in the PaO_2, however. With increased alveolar flooding, there is also a decrease in lung volume and compliance. Airway resistance increases because of the decrease in lung volume and liquid filling the airway lumen.

Pulmonary edema renders the alveoli unstable, and it makes the lung stiff, increasing the work that the respiratory muscle must perform to maintain adequate ventilation. Pulmonary edema is not the only mechanism, however, by which the work of breathing becomes greater in subjects with a left-to-right shunt. These patients can also develop extrinsic airway compression. Pulmonary "overcirculation" along with pulmonary hypertension may cause extrinsic compression of the main and lobar bronchi by enlarged pulmonary arteries (usually affecting the right main stem bronchus, the lingular and left upper lobe bronchi, or the left main stem bronchus) or by distention of the left atrium (affecting the left lower

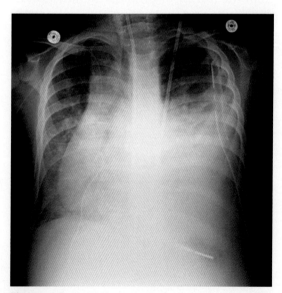

Figure 4-3. Pleural effusion in a child with severe congestive heart failure.

lobe bronchus).[9] In addition, there is usually compression of small intraparenchymal airways by engorged peribronchial vessels or by bronchial wall or peribronchial edema.

The term "cardiac asthma" is often applied to describe the wheezing caused by compression of large and small intrathoracic airways. Affected infants often may have respiratory symptoms so prominent that they overshadow or mask the underlying cardiac disease. The shunt may be recognized only when a clinician notes the coexistence of cardiomegaly and air trapping on a chest radiograph. Bronchial compression at these locations also can produce lobar emphysema or atelectasis. This complication is seen most frequently in 2 to 9-month-old infants. The age range predilection may be linked to the gradual decrease of pulmonary vascular resistance over the first few months of life that results in an increase in pulmonary blood flow and the small airway caliber and less cartilaginous airway support in infants.[6] Evaluation for underlying cardiac disease also should be part of the assessment of an infant or young child with atelectasis or lobar emphysema.

Pulmonary edema, and the mechanical disturbances that it produces, also impairs gas exchange within the lung. In the presence of a left-to-right shunt, overall ventilation to perfusion is low, and there are areas that are perfused but not ventilated (true right-to-left intrapulmonary shunt). However, the recirculation of arterial blood through the lung and the high saturation of pulmonary arterial blood (owing to the left-to-right shunt) minimize the effects, of intrapulmonary right-to-left shunting on arterial oxygen saturation. Arterial PO_2 and PCO_2 are usually near-normal, unless there is respiratory fatigue caused by increased respiratory rate and effort.

Patients with ASD are usually asymptomatic in early life, although they may have an increased incidence of respiratory tract infections. With the onset of pulmonary hypertension (usually in adulthood), dyspnea and fatigue may occur. Patients with left-to-right shunts at the aortic and ventricular levels may develop biventricular congestive heart failure in infancy. Symptoms include dyspnea, grunting, apnea, and poor feeding. The early congestive heart failure also predisposes these infants to respiratory infections and poor growth. When the disease has progressed to Eisenmenger syndrome, all patients have cyanosis (at rest and during exercise) and dyspnea. The clubbing that is apparent is due to chronic hypoxia; the peripheral tissue capillaries dilate to increase the oxygen supply, causing digital swelling. Other symptoms that occur after disease progression to Eisenmenger syndrome are chest pain, syncope, and hemoptysis. The hemoptysis can be caused by pulmonary infarction from low pulmonary blood flow or congestion, polycythemia, or bronchial arterial bleeding.

Patients with PDA characteristically have a continuous murmur. When the disease progresses to Eisenmenger syndrome, a patient with an uncorrected PDA has differential cyanosis (upper body is pink and lower body is blue owing to right-to-left shunt beyond the left subclavian artery). Isolated digital clubbing of the toes without clubbing of the fingers may occur because of the difference in upper versus lower body oxygenation.

Treatment of Large Volume Left-to-Right Shunts

Although corrective or palliative surgery is the ultimate therapy for each of the conditions described in this section, initial medical management is essential for stabilizing an infant with critical congestive heart failure. For an infant with large left-to-right shunt, treatment traditionally has focused on improving myocardial function, removing excess fluid accumulated in the lungs, and, in some patients, providing assisted respiration. These infants have increased caloric needs, and close assessment of growth is an essential part of their management and part of the decision-making process in determining the timing of corrective surgery. They have increased energy requirements and sometimes have difficulty feeding secondary to shortness of breath.

In an acutely decompensated infant, an intravenous inotropic agent, such as dopamine, dobutamine, or isoproterenol, is most useful. For long-term use, a medication that can be given enterally, such as digoxin, is more appropriate. Diuretics can improve respiratory function by controlling the

accumulation of pulmonary edema. In particular, the combination of diuretics and inotropic drugs can decrease filling pressure in the left atrium and reduce pulmonary microvascular pressure, attenuating edema formation. Depending on the specific lesion and the size of the patient, often interventional cardiac catheterization offers an alternative to cardiac surgery. These less invasive techniques are currently widely used for the closure of secundum ASDs and PDAs.

Clinical Manifestations of Chronic Increased Pulmonary Venous Pressure

Several conditions are associated with chronic increased pulmonary venous pressure (Table 4-3). The gradual onset of increased pulmonary venous pressure leads to an almost imperceptible onset of symptoms. These early symptoms may include dyspnea, fatigue, and decrease in endurance or exercise tolerance.

Table 4-3	Diagnoses Associated with Chronic Increase of Pulmonary Venous Pressure

Aortic Valve
Aortic regurgitation
Aortic stenosis
Left Atrium
Atrial myxoma
Ball-valve thrombus
Cor triatriatum
Left Ventricle
Chronic heart failure
Congenital subaortic stenosis
Constrictive pericarditis
Hypertrophic cardiomyopathy
Restrictive cardiomyopathy
Mitral Valve
Mitral regurgitation
Mitral stenosis
Pulmonary Veins
Congenital pulmonary vein stenosis
Mediastinal fibrosis
Mediastinal neoplasms
Mediastinitis
Veno-occlusive disease
Thoracic Aorta
Coarctation of aorta
Supravalvular aortic stenosis

When these patients are otherwise stable, symptoms may be minimal. Acute increases in cardiac output (e.g., fever or exercise) or decreases in filling time (e.g., tachyarrhythmias) can lead to sudden worsening of dyspnea (Fig. 4-4). Hemoptysis is a late complication and is caused by rupture of the dilated bronchial anastomotic vessels.

Pediatric patients can have a severe, rapidly progressive form of veno-occlusive disease.[10] This form of veno-occlusive disease can be sporadic or familial. The initial chest radiograph may show only cardiomegaly with mild lung changes, or may show pulmonary effusion or edema (Fig. 4-5). These patients present with progressive dyspnea and then syncope. As a postcapillary form of pulmonary hypertension, patients are often misdiagnosed as having arterial hypertension. Although cardiac catheterization and computed tomography (CT) of the chest can be diagnostic,[11] a lung biopsy may be needed to confirm the diagnosis. On pulmonary function tests, there is reduction of vital capacity, forced expiratory volume in one second, and arterial oxygen saturation or diffusing capacity for carbon monoxide.[12] There is no effective medical or surgical therapy for most of these cases. There have been some case reports that immunosuppressant therapy may ameliorate the disease progression.[13] Although gentle vasodilator therapy may be effective in some cases, use of vasodilator therapy also can lead to (sometimes acutely) increased

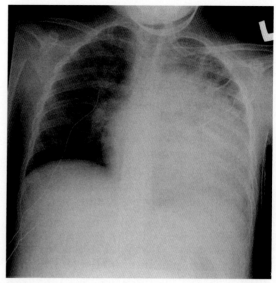

Figure 4-5. Chest radiograph of a child with pulmonary veno-occlusive disease.

vascular congestion, atelectasis, and pleural effusion.[14] Vasodilators should be used sparingly and extremely cautiously in pediatric patients with veno-occlusive disease. Consultation with a lung transplant team is recommended at the time of diagnosis.

As with acute increased pulmonary venous pressure, the chest radiograph may be the most sensitive noninvasive test to alert the clinician to the possibility of chronic venous hypertension. On the radiograph, the pulmonary arteries become attenuated initially at the bases and then toward the apex. Kerley B lines appear due to the presence of dilated lymphatics and interlobular fibrosis, rather than owing to interstitial edema, as in the patient with acute increased pulmonary venous pressure. Diffuse nodularity resulting from hemosiderin-laden macrophages may fill the lower lobe alveoli. Rarely, ossified nodules also may be found at the lung bases (Fig. 4-6).

The chest radiograph also is useful in determining the level of the venous obstruction. If the level of obstruction is preventricular (atrial myxoma or cor triatriatum), the left ventricular silhouette may be normal, although the left atrium may show an enlarged shadow. If the level of obstruction is at the ventricle due to myocardial disease or to valvular disease, the heart is likely to appear enlarged on the chest radiograph.

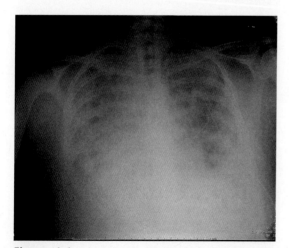

Figure 4-4. Acute decompensation of a patient with chronic pulmonary venous hypertension after spontaneous left pneumothorax.

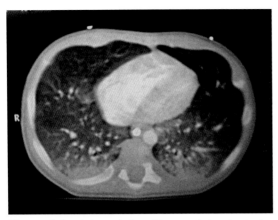

Figure 4-6. High-resolution CT scan of the chest of a patient with idiopathic/sporadic pulmonary veno-occlusive disease.

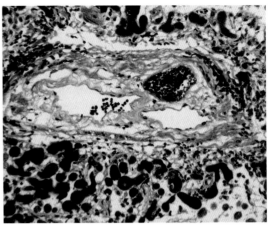

Figure 4-7. Photomicrograph of lung biopsy specimen taken from a child with pulmonary venous obstruction. Note the thickened walls of the pulmonary vein with narrowing of the lumen. Also note the dilated capillaries in the interstitium.

Initial changes in pulmonary function are due to congestion of the lungs and interstitial edema. Pulmonary congestion and interstitial edema may lead to decreases in airway caliber with a decrease in forced expiratory volume in one second. With increasing years, chronic changes, including interlobular fibrosis develop and lead to a decrease in lung recoil and volume. In time, the chronic hemodynamic and pulmonary functional limitation may lead to changes in respiratory muscle function as shown by decreases in maximal strength.

With the chronic interstitial edema, lymphatic distention, and possible intermittent extravasation of blood into the interstitium, interstitial fibrosis develops around septa and blood vessels. The pulmonary veins show characteristic changes of medial hypertrophy. Later venous changes include intimal thickening and fibrosis (Fig. 4-7). An external elastic membrane characteristic of arteries may form—the so-called arterialization of the pulmonary veins. These venous changes are pathognomonic of pulmonary venous hypertension but nonspecific as to the underlying causes. Calcium deposition and ossification are the most extreme changes, however, which are seen only in long-standing mitral stenosis.

Outflow or Inflow Obstruction of the Systemic Ventricle

Anomalies that commonly cause left-sided (systemic ventricular) obstruction include aortic stenosis or atresia, coarctation of the aorta, interruption of the aortic arch, and obstruction to pulmonary venous return. These anomalies generally are characterized by decreased systemic perfusion and pulmonary venous congestion. Infants with obstruction of the left heart usually develop clinical manifestations at an earlier postnatal age and have more severe respiratory compromise because closure of the ductus arteriosus, which usually occurs within the first few days after birth, may substantially reduce blood flow through the aorta and decrease systemic perfusion. When the pulmonary artery pressure is suprasystemic, as in total anomalous pulmonary venous return and obstruction, ductus closure eliminates a mechanism for amelioration of the pulmonary hypertension via right-to-left shunting. The pulmonary and systemic venous congestion can occur precipitously.

Pathophysiology of Obstruction of the Systemic Ventricle

The problems occurring with left heart obstruction arise from its effects on systemic blood flow, ventricular loading, and pulmonary function. For a better understanding of the pathophysiology of left ventricular obstruction, it is helpful to separate the lesions into outflow and inflow obstruction.

Left Ventricular Outflow Obstruction. These lesions cause an increased afterload of the left ventricle, which is tolerated very poorly if the obstruction is severe or if it occurs abruptly. The hemodynamic consequences of outflow obstruction are increased ventricular end-diastolic, left atrial, and pulmonary venous and pulmonary arterial pressures, which cause variable degrees of pulmonary venous congestion and pulmonary edema (interstitial and alveolar) and obstruction of large and small airways, just as with the large left-to-right shunt. In the most severe forms of obstruction, usually found in neonates, there are always signs of poor systemic perfusion (increased capillary refill time, decreased or absent peripheral pulses, cool extremities) accompanied by lactic acidosis.

Left Ventricular Inflow Obstruction. These anomalies (i.e., mitral atresia or stenosis) impede left ventricular filling and increase the afterload on the right ventricle. The preload on the right ventricle also becomes increased by the excess blood flow entering the right ventricle from the portion of the pulmonary venous return, which is shunted from the left to the right atrium through the foramen ovale. The impairment of systemic perfusion depends on the amount if any, of anterograde (aortic) flow from the systemic ventricle and the right-to-left shunt, through the ductus arteriosus. When there is atresia of the mitral or aortic valve, the left-to-right atrial shunt represents the only means for blood to reach the systemic circulation (via the right ventricle and through the ductus arteriosus to the descending aorta).

Aortic Stenosis
Aortic stenosis causes a spectrum of disease in children, based on the severity of the valvular narrowing. The valvular pathology involves thickening of the tissue and varying degrees of separation of the commissures. Clinical findings vary widely with the severity of the valvular obstruction. Most children with mild aortic stenosis have normal growth and development and come to a cardiologist's attention when a heart murmur is heard. On the other end of the spectrum, infants with critical aortic stenosis can be hemodynamically unstable and exhibit severe endocardial fibroelastosis at birth, requiring immediate relief of the obstruction through interventional cardiac catheterization or a surgical approach.

The findings on chest radiograph also vary with the severity of the obstruction. Severe obstruction may show edema on the chest film, along with left ventricular enlargement. In most patients with mild or moderate aortic stenosis, the heart size is normal or only mildly enlarged. Intervention for aortic stenosis, when indicated, can be accomplished by percutaneous balloon valvuloplasty in the cardiac catheterization laboratory or by surgical valvulotomy or valve replacement.

Coarctation of the Aorta
Coarctation of the aorta often manifests as a discrete stenosis in the proximal thoracic aorta, just opposite the PDA insertion. There is a wide spectrum of this disease, however, including long segment coarctation and abdominal coarctation. Associated lesions, such as PDA, VSD, aortic stenosis, or mitral stenosis, also affect the pathophysiology and clinical presentation.

The clinical presentation of isolated coarctation of the aorta varies. Newborns with severe coarctation and PDA closure present with congestive heart failure and cardiogenic shock or low cardiac output. If a right-to-left ductal shunt is present, differential cyanosis of the lower extremities is seen. On the other end of the spectrum, coarctation can manifest later in childhood when systolic hypertension or a heart murmur is being evaluated. The systolic blood pressure in the upper extremity is elevated proximal to the coarctation, and there is a gradient noted between the arm and leg systolic blood pressures. The arterial pulse in the leg is diminished and delayed when palpated at the same time as the arm pulse. The blood pressure and pulse should be evaluated in all four limbs.

The chest radiograph of an infant with severe coarctation of the aorta usually shows cardiomegaly and pulmonary vascular congestion. In older children being evaluated for a murmur or hypertension, the heart size usually is not prominent, and in isolated coarctation, the pulmonary markings are normal. The contour of the aortic arch is often abnormal, with an indentation seen at the site of coarctation (the "3" sign). Rib notching also can occur in older patients; this is caused by erosion of the inferior rib by the collateral circulation or dilated intercostals arteries.

Treatment for many children consists of surgical repair of the coarctation. This is usually performed via a left thoracotomy. Sometimes, when an associated lesion also is being repaired, a sternotomy is performed.[15] Percutaneous balloon angioplasty, stent placement, or both, for a discrete coarctation or recoarctation are other treatment options.[16-18]

Vascular Anomalies That Cause Airway Obstruction

Compression of the trachea and bronchi can be caused by developmental abnormalities of both of the major arterial branches of the aorta or the pulmonary vessels (Table 4-4). These lesions, which generally arise from failure of normal regression of one or more segments of the early fetal paired branchial arches, can produce substantial distortion of the trachea and large bronchi.[19] The most common types involve either complete encirclement of the tracheoesophageal complex by vascular structures (vascular rings) or compression of the trachea or bronchi by vessels that follow an anomalous trajectory.

An example of the latter is the pulmonary artery sling. The left pulmonary artery arises from an elongated main pulmonary artery or distally from the right pulmonary artery. It crosses the midline between the trachea and the esophagus, sometimes with a crossover segment of the left pulmonary artery supplying the right upper lobe. This condition also is strongly associated with long segment congenital tracheal stenosis.

The most likely types of vascular rings include double aortic arch and right aortic arch with aberrant left subclavian artery, which arises from the descending aorta and passes behind the esophagus. The vascular ring is completed by the left ligamentum arteriosum, which courses from the origin of the left subclavian artery to the left pulmonary artery (Fig. 4-8). The left subclavian

Table 4-4	Causes of Vascular Compression of the Airway in Children

- Anomalies of the aorta
  - Double aortic arch
  - Interrupted aortic arch (after surgical repair)
  - Right-sided aortic arch
    - With aberrant left subclavian artery
    - With mirror-image branching and right ligamentum arteriosum
  - Left-sided aortic arch
    - With aberrant right subclavian artery and right ligamentum arteriosum
    - Right-sided descending aorta with right ligamentum arteriosum
  - Cervical aortic arch
- Absent pulmonary valve syndrome
- Aberrant left pulmonary artery ('pulmonary artery sling')
- Acquired cardiovascular disease
  - Dilated cardiomyopathy
  - Aneurysm
    - Ascending aorta
      - Ductus arteriosus

Adapted from McLaren CA, Elliott MJ, Roebuck DJ: Vascular compression of the airway in children. Paediatr Respir Rev 9:85-94, 2008.

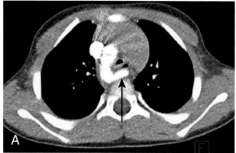
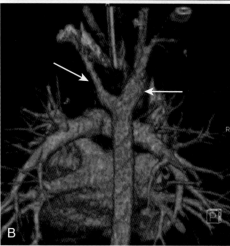

Figure 4-8. A 5-year-old boy with a right-sided aortic arch and aberrant left subclavian artery. **A,** Axial CT scan of the thorax shows compression of the trachea by the aberrant artery (*arrow*). **B,** Three-dimensional volume rendered image (posterior view) shows the right-sided aortic arch (*white arrow on right*) and the aberrant left subclavian artery (*white arrow*) arising from the descending aorta. (*Adapted from McLaren CA, Elliott MJ, Roebuck DJ: Vascular compression of the airway in children. Paediatr Respir Rev 9:85-94, 2008.*) (See Color Plate)

artery often originates from an outpouching of the descending aorta, called Kommerell diverticulum. Other patterns of right aortic arch include mirror-image branching and right ligamentum arteriosum, anomalous innominate arising farther to the left than usual and passing anterior to the trachea, anomalous left carotid artery arising further to the right than usual and passing anterior to the trachea, and aberrant right subclavian artery.

As a group, vascular anomalies obstruct the intrathoracic airways exclusively. Consequently, their manifestations are predominantly expiratory and include wheezing and lung hyperinflation. When the compression is severe, inspiratory stridor also is heard indicating the relatively fixed nature of the obstruction. Infants are often brought to medical attention when an intercurrent infection causes increased respiratory distress. Some patients are labeled as having "recurrent bronchitis" or "steroid-resistant asthma" before the diagnosis of a vascular ring is made. In older children, a (often more "loose") vascular ring can manifest with dysphagia or choking. Other patients remain asymptomatic and are diagnosed incidentally.

Barium esophagogram is an important tool for the initial evaluation of infants and children suspected to have airway compression by an anomalous vessel. A large posterior esophageal indentation in association with an anterior notch in the tracheal air column is usually caused by complete vascular rings (double aortic arch or a right aortic arch with an aberrant left subclavian artery or ligamentum arteriosum or both) encircling the trachea and esophagus (Fig. 4-9).

A complete vascular ring can be associated with intracardiac defects, such as VSD, which can divert attention from the extracardiac anomalies. Another radiographic finding is the presence of an isolated anterior tracheal indentation. This pattern occurs when there is an anomalous innominate artery that arises too far from its normal origin and has to cross the midline in front of the trachea. In contrast to the complete vascular rings, anterior tracheal compression may be an incidental observation and produce few to no symptoms. Finally,

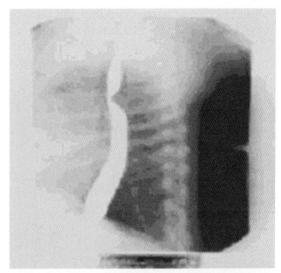

Figure 4-9. Lateral projection of a barium esophagogram in a 3-month-old infant with a double aortic arch causing posterior compression of the esophagus.

an uncommon radiographic finding is an anterior esophageal indentation with a posterior impression on the tracheal air column. This combination is seen when the left pulmonary artery originates from the right pulmonary artery (pulmonary artery sling). The anomalous left pulmonary artery must find its way to the left lung anterior to the esophagus and posterior to the trachea. In the process, it passes over the right main stem bronchus, behind the trachea, and down over the left main stem bronchus, and may compress any of these structures, frequently causing air trapping or atelectasis in either lung.

The diagnosis of vascular rings and slings is confirmed by magnetic resonance imaging (MRI)[20] and computed tomography (CT). These are the most useful imaging techniques because they provide information about the tracheobronchial tree, the cardiovascular structures, and their relationship to each other. CT data are generally useful to diagnose the type and severity of airway compression, but multiplanar reconstruction and three-dimensional volume rendered images provide further useful information. Virtual bronchoscopy images also can be generated from CT data but rarely add diagnostic information and cannot yet be used as a substitute for flexible bronchoscopy. MRI has excellent contrast resolution and multiplanar imaging capabilities.[20] Evaluation of cardiac anatomy and physiology with MRI is usually superior to CT. Most MRI studies for vascular compression are quite prolonged (>30 minutes), however, requiring sedation or general anesthesia in young children. Sedation risks for children with a compromised airway are significant.

In practice, the increased speed and quality of multiplanar reconstruction provided by CT technology means that CT is used more often than MRI in most centers. A limitation of MRI and CT is that obliterated vascular segments (e.g., the ligamentum arteriosum or an atretic aortic arch) cannot be directly visualized. Echocardiography is essential for the evaluation of associated congenital heart disease and usually clearly shows abnormal vascular structures. Echocardiography is useful to the surgeon for understanding complex three-dimensional relationships. Cross-sectional imaging is probably much better than bronchoscopy at determining the nature of the vascular compression of the airway. Yet, current CT and MRI techniques do not reliably distinguish, between dynamic and static airway narrowing. This is an important practical issue because many children with prolonged airway compression develop secondary malacia. Flexible bronchoscopy is currently the best technique for this purpose. Airway malacia should be assessed only when the patient is breathing spontaneously. Diagnostic catheter angiography has largely been replaced by cross-sectional imaging.

Surgery is advised for symptomatic patients with diagnostic imaging evidence of tracheal compression. The left arch is generally small, nondominant (hypoplastic), and often transected in patients with double aortic arch. Compression produced by a right aortic arch and aberrant left subclavian artery with a ligamentum arteriosum is relieved by transection of the latter. Anomalous innominate or carotid arteries cannot be divided; attaching the adventitia of these vessels to the sternum usually relieves the tracheal compression. An anomalous left pulmonary artery is corrected during cardiopulmonary bypass by division at its origin and reimplantation to the main pulmonary artery with the simultaneous repair of a long segment congenital tracheal

stenosis, if present. Surgery does not usually eliminate all the respiratory manifestations immediately, if ever, because the residual tracheal obstruction tends to persist for months. In some cases, it is unclear whether the airway ever becomes normal.[21]

Congenital Absence of the Pulmonary Valve

Congenital absence of the pulmonary valve is characterized by the presence of enlarged pulmonary arteries and hypoplastic pulmonary valve cusps. This lesion often occurs in association with tetralogy of Fallot, VSD, and right ventricular outflow tract obstruction. There is also a strong association with DiGeorge syndrome.

Regurgitation of blood through the pulmonary outflow tract results in extremely enlarged pulmonary arteries (Fig. 4-10). These arteries compress the trachea and main stem bronchi, causing lobar collapse or lobar emphysema and severe respiratory distress. Airway compression can be unilateral or bilateral. Respiratory difficulty occurs as the pulmonary artery becomes gradually dilated when the postnatal decrease in pulmonary vascular resistance increases left-to-right shunting and pulmonary regurgitation. Surgical repair of the cardiac anomaly and placement of an artificial pulmonary valve are invariably necessary. As a result of the residual tracheomalacia, there is, in many patients, a need for mechanical ventilation for weeks or months after surgical repair even if the hemodynamic function is near-normal, and there is no regurgitation.

Pathophysiology of Respiratory Manifestations

From a clinical point of view, all the cardiovascular anomalies we have described until now are characterized by the severity of their respiratory manifestations. Regardless of the exact nature of the anomaly, these manifestations always include an increase in the work that the respiratory system must perform to maintain adequate ventilation. The increased work takes a further toll on the already limited energy reserves of most patients and often leads to respiratory failure as the first indication of the presence of the anomaly.

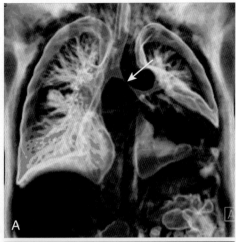

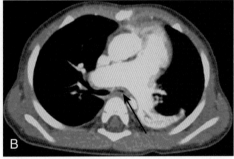

Figure 4-10. Tetralogy of Fallot and absent pulmonary valve syndrome with airway compression in a 15-month-old boy. **A,** CT volume-rendered image shows compression of the left main bronchus (*arrow*). **B,** Axial CT scan of the thorax shows severe compression of the airway between the vertebral body and the grossly enlarged pulmonary arteries. (*From McLaren CA, Elliott MJ, Roebuck DJ: Vascular compression of the airway in children. Paediatr Respir Rev 9:85-94, 2008.*) (See Color Plate)

The mechanisms responsible for the increase in work of breathing vary depending on the mechanical alterations produced by each cardiovascular anomaly. Most patients with a large left-to-right shunt or a left ventricular obstruction develop pulmonary edema. As a result, their alveoli become unstable and collapse, causing an increase in the force that the respiratory muscles have to generate to overcome the elastic recoil of the lungs. Under these circumstances, intercostal and subcostal retractions develop, and the respiratory pattern becomes rapid and shallow. The patient frequently tries to preserve lung volume by closing the glottis at the end of expiration, producing a grunt.

A group of children with similar heart disease can develop airway obstruction as their predominant respiratory abnormality. Whether it is caused by direct compression of the trachea and large bronchi by enlarged vessels or heart chambers or by narrowing of the small intraparenchymal airways by edema, the obstruction is almost always intrathoracic, and as such is exacerbated during expiration. In these patients, respiration tends to be slower and deeper, and the physical examination reveals wheezing and prolonged expiration. The chest x-ray shows hyperinflation.

The increase in the work of breathing represents a challenge for patients who are usually in a poor nutritional state and whose respiratory muscles may have a reduced ability to increase their blood flow because of reduced systemic perfusion. In addition, the mechanical abnormalities produced by the disease itself tend to decrease the efficiency with which the respiratory system uses its limited resources (Fig. 4-11).

The development of severe retractions creates an extra burden on the diaphragm, which for the same amount of work performed by the lungs has to use more energy to deform the rib cage. Likewise, flattening of the diaphragm in the presence of airway obstruction causes the muscle to generate less volume displacement for the same degree of fiber shortening and diminishes its area of apposition to the rib cage. Under such conditions, it is not unsurprising that the energy cost of breathing becomes extraordinary. Such demands cannot always be fully met, particularly under stressful conditions. Respiratory failure then develops.

Lesions with Increased Venous Admixture

Cyanotic children have defects that allow venous blood to mix with arterial oxygenated blood. Children may have an isolated right-to-left shunt or obstruction to pulmonary blood flow in addition to the right-to-left shunt. Another example of cyanotic heart disease is when the great arteries are transposed, causing the systemic venous blood to return directly to the aorta. Examples of each of these types of cyanotic heart lesions are discussed subsequently.

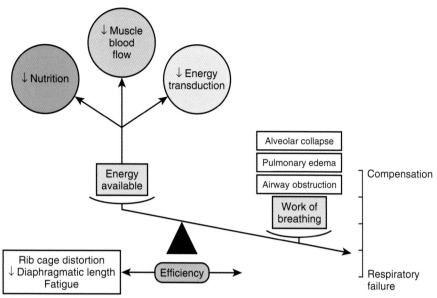

Figure 4-11. Schematic representation of the balance between the energy available to the respiratory muscles and the work that these muscles do during breathing in the presence of mechanical alteration. Whether the balance tips toward compensation or respiratory failure depends not only on the relative magnitudes of the energy available to the muscles and the increased workload (represented by the weights on both sides of the balance) but also on the efficiency with which the energy is transformed into work (represented by the position of the fulcrum). The presence of heart disease, alveolar collapse, pulmonary edema, and airway obstruction can increase the workload; poor nutrition, decreased blood flow, and, in general, the inability of the muscle's contractile machinery to transduce energy into work can decrease the energy available. Under such circumstances, decreased efficiency caused by rib cage distortion (retractions), a flattened diaphragm, or muscle fatigue can easily displace the fulcrum to the left, precipitating respiratory failure. (*From Lister, G and Perez Fontan JJ. Congenital Heart Disease and Respiratory Disease in Children. Loughlin G and Eigen H. Eds. Baltimore, Williams & Wilkins, 1994, p 603.*)

Tricuspid Atresia

Infants with tricuspid atresia do not have a normal pathway for blood to flow from the right atrium to the right ventricle because the tricuspid valve is not patent. The blood in the right atrium instead takes a path across an ASD to mix with the oxygenated blood in the left atrium. Patients with tricuspid atresia can have normally related great arteries, D-transposed great arteries, or L-transposition of the great arteries. Some have pulmonary stenosis or atresia, and some have VSDs of varying sizes. Associated cardiac anomalies may produce decreased, increased, or normal pulmonary blood flow. Patients with decreased pulmonary blood flow appear cyanotic, while patients with excessive pulmonary blood flow develop congestive heart failure. Patients with tricuspid atresia who present in the first days of life are typically cyanotic, have a leftward superior axis and left ventricular hypertrophy on electrocardiogram, and have decreased pulmonary vascular markings on chest radiograph. Surgical palliation is directed at

the main underlying physiologic issue, whether it is the need to increase pulmonary blood flow, decrease pulmonary overcirculation, or eliminate interatrial obstruction.

Tetralogy of Fallot

When there is an obstruction to pulmonary outflow and a right-to-left shunt, the pulmonary blood flow can decrease to less than systemic flow (Table 4-5). The most common cardiac anomaly associated with decreased pulmonary arterial pressure is tetralogy of Fallot.

With low pulmonary blood flow, the bronchial circulation may assume a more prominent role in supplying blood to the lungs

Table 4-5	Diagnoses Associated with Decreased Pulmonary Arterial Pressure
Ebstein anomaly	
Pulmonary valvular stenosis with patent foramen ovale	
Tetralogy of Fallot	

for gas exchange. With severe pulmonary outflow obstruction, cyanosis appears early, occurring when the patient is crying or straining. The mechanism is presumed to be an increase in pulmonary vascular resistance by a Valsalva-like maneuver. The cyanosis becomes severe, and the children are usually dyspneic. Their characteristic pose, squatting to relieve their shortness of breath, is believed to help increase systemic resistance, which increases the pulmonary blood flow and improves their oxygenation. On physical examination, these children have cyanosis, digital clubbing, and growth failure. Electrocardiograms and echocardiograms show right ventricular and atrial hypertrophy. On chest radiograph, there is a prominent right ventricle and a small pulmonary artery, which appears as the characteristic "boot-shaped" cardiac silhouette (Fig. 4-12).

Except for significant hypoxemia, there are minimal alterations in pulmonary function. One study found reduced lung volumes in young adults with congenital pulmonic stenosis compared with normal controls. It has been proposed that low pulmonary blood pressures can cause pulmonary hypoplasia.[22] Patients with tetralogy of Fallot undergo complete surgical repair; sometimes severely ill cyanotic infants require a palliative Blalock-Taussig shunt before definitive repair.

D-Transposition of the Great Arteries

D-transposition of the great arteries is a cyanotic heart lesion that occurs when the aorta arises from the right ventricle, and the pulmonary artery arises from the left ventricle (ventriculoarterial discordance). A parallel circulation is set up, and a mixing lesion (VSD, ASD, or PDA) is essential for survival.

Clinically, an infant who does not have adequate mixing appears severely cyanotic. A hyperoxia test can be performed to distinguish cyanotic heart disease from severe pulmonary disease by placing the patient on 100% FiO_2 for 10 minutes. If the PO_2 increases greater than 150mmHg, pulmonary disease should be suspected. The classic chest radiograph is described as an "egg on a string" because the great vessels are in an anteroposterior relationship (Fig. 4-13). The chest radiograph also can appear normal in these patients, or may exhibit increased pulmonary vascular markings and enlarged cardiac silhouette if a large VSD is present.[23] If mixing of the pulmonary and systemic circulations is inadequate at birth, an atrial septostomy can be performed in the cardiac catheterization laboratory to create an ASD. This palliative procedure is followed by the arterial switch surgery, with reimplantation of the coronary arteries to restore normal circulatory flow.

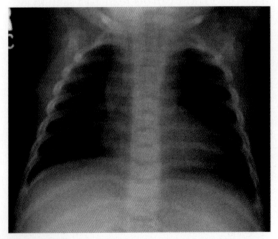

Figure 4-12. Chest radiograph of a child with tetralogy of Fallot.

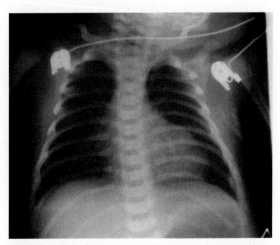

Figure 4-13. Chest radiograph of a child with D-transposition of the great arteries.

Idiopathic Pulmonary Arterial Hypertension

Although idiopathic pulmonary arterial hypertension (IPAH) is not a primary cardiac disease, children with IPAH are usually referred to pediatric cardiologists for evaluation of their symptoms or cardiomegaly or both (Fig. 4-14). Children with IPAH (previously known as primary pulmonary hypertension) have a worse prognosis than adults.[24] The definition of pulmonary arterial hypertension is the same for children and adults: mean pulmonary arterial pressure greater than 25mmHg at rest or greater than 30mmHg during exercise, with normal pulmonary artery wedge pressure (i.e., <15 mmHg), and an increased pulmonary vascular resistance index (>3 Wood units/m^2). The diagnosis of IPAH is made only when all other causes of pulmonary hypertension have been ruled out (Table 4-6).[24,25] A careful family history also must be obtained to rule out familial pulmonary arterial hypertension. Children with IPAH often have insidious onset of vague symptoms, including fatigue, decreased endurance, or abdominal pain (older children and adolescents may have chest pain). They also may present with recurrent exertional or nocturnal syncope. If the child with IPAH fails to respond to vasodilator therapy or is not treated in this manner, the prognosis is poor. The pulmonary arteries become greatly dilated throughout the lung parenchyma (Fig. 4-15), and patients develop progressive right heart failure accompanied by hemoptysis.

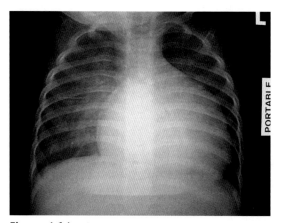

Figure 4-14. Chest radiograph of a child with idiopathic pulmonary arterial hypertension.

Table 4-6	Pulmonary Hypertension Diagnostic Classification

Pulmonary Arterial Hypertension
Familial
Sporadic
Related to:
  Connective tissue disease
  Congenital heart disease
  Portal hypertension
  Human immunodeficiency virus infection
  Drugs and toxins
  Other—type 1 glycogen storage disease, Gaucher disease, hemoglobinopathies, myeloproliferative disorders, hereditary hemorrhagic telangiectasia (Rendu-Osler-Weber disease)
Pulmonary Arterial Hypertension with Significant Venule or Capillary Involvement
Pulmonary veno-occlusive disease
  Familial
  Sporadic
Pulmonary capillary hemangiomatosis
Persistent Fetal Circulation (Persistent Pulmonary Hypertension of the Newborn)
Pulmonary Venous Hypertension
  Pulmonary venous obstruction (discrete)
  Left-sided heart disease
Pulmonary Hypertension Associated with Disorders of Respiratory System or Hypoxemia
Hyaline membrane disease
Bronchopulmonary dysplasia
Congenital diaphragmatic hernia
Pulmonary hypoplasia
Alveolar capillary dysplasia
Cystic fibrosis
Chronic obstructive pulmonary disease
Interstitial lung disease
Sleep-disordered breathing
Alveolar hypoventilation disorders
Chronic exposure to high altitude
Pulmonary Hypertension due to Chronic Thrombotic or Embolic Disease
Thromboembolic obstruction of proximal pulmonary arteries
Thromboembolic obstruction of distal pulmonary arteries
Pulmonary embolism (tumor, parasites, foreign material)
Miscellaneous
Sarcoidosis
Histiocytosis X
Fibrosing mediastinitis
Adenopathy and tumors
Lymphangiomatosis

From Rosenzweig EB, Widlitz AC, Barst RJ: Pulmonary arterial hypertension in children. Pediatr Pulmonol 38:2-22, 2004.

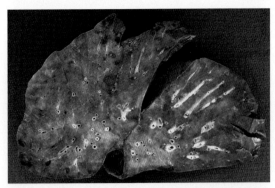

Figure 4-15. Explanted lung from a young adolescent girl with idiopathic pulmonary arterial hypertension. Note the markedly dilated pulmonary arteries extending to the peripheral portions of the lung.

Diagnosis generally starts with an echocardiogram with Doppler, to evaluate the cardiac anatomy, and if a shunt is present, to determine shunt flow direction and to quantify the shunt velocity (Fig. 4-16). Patients proceed to cardiac catheterization for measurement of pressures and evaluation of response to acute therapy (e.g., nitric oxide, prostacyclin). If the child fails to respond to vasodilator therapy, the prognosis is poor.

Few pulmonary function changes other than cyanosis occur with disease progression. Until congestive heart failure occurs, the lung parenchyma is relatively spared. Increase in airway resistance with mild nonreversible airway obstruction has been reported, in these patients, however.

Other Pulmonary Conditions Associated with Cardiac Disease or Surgery

Plastic Bronchitis

Plastic bronchitis can occur in children and adults.[26,27] The disease is characterized by severe obstruction of the large airways by bronchial casts (Fig. 4-17). Affected patients are usually classified by the type of airway cast.[26] Type I or inflammatory casts have fibrin, eosinophils, and Charcot-Leiden crystals. Type II or noninflammatory/acellular casts consist primarily of mucin with a paucity of cells. Type II casts usually occur in children with cyanotic congenital heart disease and after cardiac surgery. A new classification scheme has been proposed that is based on the associated disease and the histology of the cast.[27] Treatment usually consists of urgent/emergency removal of the casts from the large airways by means of flexible or rigid bronchoscopy. Aerosolized medications (rhDNase, heparin, tissue plasminogen activator) and other medications (corticosteroids, low-dose azithromycin) also have been used in published case reports.[28-31] Thoracic duct ligation has been performed in two patients with Fontan circuits who had recurrent episodes of plastic bronchitis that failed to respond adequately to medical management.[32]

Summary

Because of the close proximity and interconnected circulatory systems of the cardiac and respiratory system, alteration in cardiac function has profound effects on

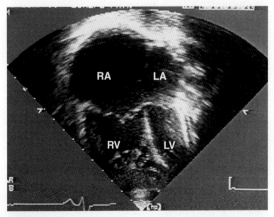

Figure 4-16. Echocardiogram of a patient with severe pulmonary arterial hypertension. There is severe right ventricular and right atrial dilation.

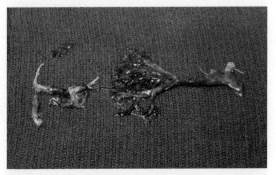

Figure 4-17. Bronchial casts ("plastic bronchitis") removed by flexible fiberoptic bronchoscopy from a patient with congenital heart disease with acute airway obstruction and respiratory failure.

the entire respiratory system. Understanding the physiologic mechanisms of this interrelationship and the early signs and symptoms of dysfunction of the cardiopulmonary circulatory systems can aid in the early detection and initiation of best available treatment for children with cardiac disease.

References

1. Ip P, Chiu CS, Cheung YF: Risk factors prolonging ventilation in young children after cardiac surgery: Impact of noninfectious pulmonary complications. Pediatr Crit Care Med 3:269-274, 2002.
2. Thomas B, et al: Chronic respiratory complications in pediatric heart transplant recipients. J Heart Lung Transplant 26:236-240B, 2007.
3. Bandla HP, et al: Pulmonary risk factors compromising postoperative recovery after surgical repair for congenital heart disease. Chest 116:740-747, 1999.
4. Weissman C: Pulmonary complications after cardiac surgery. Semin Cardiothorac Vasc Anesth 8:185-211, 2004.
5. Broaddus VC: Cardiac disease. In Murray JF, ed: Pulmonary Complications of Systemic Disease. New York, Marcel Dekker, 1992, pp 149-190.
6. Lister G, Pitt BR: Cardiopulmonary interactions in the infant with congenital cardiac disease. Clin Chest Med 4(2):219-232, 1983.
7. Bates DV: Inter-relationships between cardiac and pulmonary function. In: Respiratory Function in Disease, 3rd ed. Philadelphia, WB Saunders, 1989, pp 250-264.
8. Remetz MS, Cleman MW, Cabin HS: Pulmonary and pleural complications of cardiac disease. Clin Chest Med 10(4):545-592, 1989.
9. Stanger P, Lucas R, Edwards J: Anatomic factors causing respiratory distress in acyanotic congenital heart disease: Special reference to bronchial obstruction. Pediatrics 47:760-769, 1969.
10. Wagenvoort CA, Wagenvoort TN, Takahashi T: Pulmonary veno-occlusive disease: Involvement of pulmonary arteries and review of the literature. Hum Pathol 16:1033-1041, 1985.
11. Resten A, et al: Pulmonary hypertension: CT of the chest in pulmonary venoocclusive disease. AJR Am J Roentgenol 183:65-70, 2004.
12. Thadani U, et al: Pulmonary veno-occlusive disease. QJM 44:133-159, 1975.
13. Sanderson JE, et al: A case of pulmonary veno-occlusive disease responding to treatment with azathioprine. Thorax 32:140-148, 1977.
14. Davis LL, et al: Effect of prostacyclin on microvascular pressures in a patient with pulmonary veno-occlusive disease. Chest 108:1754-1756, 1995.
15. Dittrich S, et al: Comparison of sodium nitroprusside versus esmolol for the treatment of hypertension following repair of coarctation of the aorta. Interact Cardiovasc Thorac Surg 2:111-115, 2003.
16. Weber HS, Cyran SE: Endovascular stenting for native coarctation of the aorta is an effective alternative to surgical intervention in older children. Congen Heart Dis 3:54-59, 2008.
17. Lee CL, et al: Balloon angioplasty of native coarctation and comparison of patients younger and older than three months. Circ J 71:1781-1784, 2007.
18. Mendelsohn AM, Lloyd TR, Crowley DC, et al: Late follow-up of balloon angioplasty in children with a native coarctation of the aorta. Am J Cardiol 74:696-700, 1994.
19. McLaren CA, Elliott MJ, Roebuck DJ: Vascular compression of the airway in children. Paediatr Respir Rev 9:85-94ss, 2008.
20. Malik TH, et al: The role of magnetic resonance imaging in the assessment of suspected extrinsic tracheobronchial compression due to vascular anomalies. Arch Dis Child 91:52-55, 2006.
21. Murphy TM, et al: Pulmonary function sequelae in children with operated vascular rings. Chest 86(2):295, 1984.
22. De Troyer A, Yernault J-C, Englert M: Lung hypoplasia in congenital pulmonary valve stenosis. Circulation 56:647-651, 1977.
23. Levin DL, et al: D-Transposition of the great vessels in the neonate: A clinical diagnosis. Arch Intern Med 137:1421-1425, 1977.
24. Rosenzweig EB, Widlitz AC, Barst RJ: Pulmonary arterial hypertension in children. Pediatr Pulmonol 38:2-22, 2004.
25. Simonneau G, et al: Clinical classification of pulmonary hypertension. J Am Coll Cardiol 43:5S-12S, 2004.
26. Brogan TV, et al: Plastic bronchitis in children: A case series and review of the medical literature. Pediatr Pulmonol 34:482-487, 2002.
27. Madsen P, Shah SA, Rubin BK: Plastic bronchitis: New insights and a classification scheme. Paediatr Respir Rev 6:292-300, 2005.
28. Wang G, et al: Effective use of corticosteroids in treatment of plastic bronchitis with hemoptysis in Chinese adults. Acta Pharmacol Sin 27:1206-1212, 2006.
29. Wakeman MK, et al: Long-term treatment of plastic bronchitis with aerosolized tissue plasminogen activator in a Fontan patient. Pediatr Crit Care Med 6:76-78, 2005.
30. Kamin W, Klar-Hlawatsch B, Truebel H: Easy removal of a large mucus plug with flexible paediatric bronchoscope after administration of rhDNase (Pulmozyme). Klin Padiatr 218:88-91, 2006.
31. Schultz KD, Oermann CM: Treatment of cast bronchitis with low-dose oral azithromycin. Pediatr Pulmonol 35:139, 2003.
32. Shah SS, Drinkwater DC, Christian KG: Plastic bronchitis: Is thoracic duct ligation a real surgical option? Ann Thorac Surg 81:2281-2283, 2006.

CHAPTER 5

Pulmonary Manifestations of Gastrointestinal Diseases

JOSEPH LEVY

Gastroesophageal Reflux Disease   99
    Pathophysiology   99
    Developmental Aspects   100
    Congenital Anomalies   100
    Diagnosis   102
    Diagnostic Approach   103
    Reflux as Etiology of Pulmonary
        Pathology   104
    Gastroesophageal Reflux Disease and
        Asthma   105
    Apparent Life-Threatening Events   105
Heiner Syndrome   106
    Diagnostic Approach   107
Inflammatory Bowel Disease   108
    Pulmonary Manifestations   108
    Clinical Manifestations   110

    Diagnostic Approach   110
    Clinical Management   110
Hepatopulmonary Syndrome   111
    Clinical Manifestations   111
    Pathophysiology   111
    Diagnostic Approach   112
    Clinical Management   113
Pancreatitis   114
    Etiology   114
    Pulmonary Manifestations   114
    Pathophysiology   115
    Diagnostic Approach   116
    Clinical Management   116
Acknowledgments   117
    References   117

This chapter addresses the pulmonary involvement observed in gastrointestinal diseases, particularly gastroesophageal reflux (GER), Heiner syndrome, inflammatory bowel disease (IBD), the hepatopulmonary syndrome (HPS), and pancreatitis. Although the purported mechanisms currently invoked to explain their concurrent associations vary, several general modes of involvement include (1) the direct effect of spillage of food or gastric contents into the airway, resulting in aspiration pneumonia; (2) a secondary, immune-mediated process, inflaming specific elements of the lung; and (3) injury to the lung from medications used to treat specific gastrointestinal disorders, such as sulfa derivatives or immunosuppressive agents integral to the management of IBD. The true etiology of the observed involvement is still unclear, and much work is being done to unravel the molecular mechanisms at play. This is a fruitful field for translational research and wide open for the development of novel pharmacologic agents with precise targets.

The pulmonary involvement concurrent with gastrointestinal diseases is often clinically subtle and requires a high index of suspicion. The radiologic manifestations might lag behind the establishment of respiratory compromise, and only specialized testing such as high-resolution computed tomography (CT), permeability studies with labeled proteins, or comprehensive pulmonary function tests (PFTs) may be sensitive enough to detect the evolving pathophysiology. Increased use of these techniques, in addition to bronchoalveolar lavage and validation of various biomarkers, would allow better definition of the prevalence of these disorders and their natural history. As in many fields of pediatrics, the data on pulmonary manifestations of gastrointestinal diseases are limited by sample size and general research investment. Much of the data is extrapolated from adult studies or animal models.

For the most part, management is supportive and conservative. Increasing recognition of specific entities such as immune-mediated alveolitis or granulomatous involvement of the airway would result in the implementation of therapies that can be lifesaving or significantly improve the patient's prognosis.

Gastroesophageal Reflux Disease

GER, defined as the passage of gastric contents into the esophagus, is a common physiologic event of little consequence in most infants. It occurs throughout the day, and is most frequent in the immediate postprandial period. In the first 3 months of life, more than 50% of full-term infants regurgitate more than once a day, and 15% regurgitate more than four times a day. These numbers increase from 4 to 6 months of age, when greater than 80% regurgitate. By the time the child is 18 months old, the prevalence of reflux decreases to 5%.[1]

In contrast to GER, gastroesophageal reflux disease (GERD) refers to the significant clinical manifestations of excessive reflux, which manifest in a wide spectrum of settings, including failure to thrive, irritability, feeding difficulties (especially feeding aversion), bleeding, and anemia. Extraesophageal manifestations include chronic hoarseness, upper airway obstruction owing to vocal cord edema, recurrent bronchitis or pneumonia, and exacerbation of reactive airway disease.[2]

The pulmonary manifestations of GERD are controversial. Pathophysiologically, it is often impossible to ascribe a causal relationship to these two phenomena, presenting a which-came-first conundrum: Are the pulmonary complications observed in children with reflux a direct result of the exposure of the airway to acid or gastric contents, or are the cough, bronchospasm, and deranged diaphragmatic mechanics the primary causes of the suspected reflux? Acid spillage into the distal esophagus may trigger increased vagal tone resulting in bronchospasm and worsening reflux as the infant mobilizes abdominal muscles to aid in exhalation against the bronchospasur constricted airways.

The clinical manifestations of airway disease in which reflux is suspected as an etiologic factor include recurrent pneumonia, chronic bronchitis/bronchiolitis, chronic cough, asthma, and apparent life-threatening events (ALTEs).[3,4] Neonatal conditions that are associated with a heightened risk of GER include prematurity, postrepair esophageal atresia with or without associated tracheoesophageal fistula, congenital diaphragmatic hernia, and chronic lung disease of infancy.

Pathophysiology

It is now believed that the primary mechanism responsible for reflux in children is an inappropriate relaxation of the lower esophageal sphincter.[5] In contrast to in adults, the resting pressure of the sphincter is rarely abnormally low in children. Other factors contributing to reflux in this patient population include reduced esophageal capacitance and increased intra-abdominal pressure. Important developmental factors also play a role, including decreased fundic compliance, discoordination of gastric emptying, and the shorter length of the intra-abdominal esophagus. Esophageal peristalsis and mucosal protective factors are less efficient in infants, especially when born prematurely, and this helps explain the increased occurrence of pathologic reflux in this vulnerable population.[5]

Experimental work in animals and some studies in humans suggest that pulmonary involvement in the presence of acid reflux can be the result of at least two very different, but potentially complementary or synergistic mechanisms. Exposure of the lower esophagus of kittens to hydrochloric acid has been associated with a mild increase in measured bronchial smooth muscle tone.[6-9] Similar results have not been consistently documented in adults or in children, although evidence suggests that there is a loss of protective lower esophageal sphincter tone in the presence of established esophagitis. A second mechanism considered pertinent to the pathophysiology of reactive airways in the presence of reflux is the stimulation, through vagal mediators, of receptors in the upper airway by microaspiration of acid or other irritants.[10,11]

Loss of the protective reflexes, which normally prevent aspiration from above, would aggravate pulmonary manifestations in any patient with concomitant risk factors. The most vulnerable children presenting with pulmonary signs and symptoms suggestive of GERD are children with associated neuro-muscular handicaps that place them at risk for aspiration.[12,13]

Developmental Aspects

The mechanisms that coordinate breathing and swallowing are not fully developed until 34 weeks gestation.[14] Premature infants are often treated for apnea suspected to be caused by reflux; however, acidic and non-acidic events occur frequently in this popula-tion, and they are not always causally related to the respiratory irregularities or apnea that occurs regularly in this setting of central ner-vous system immaturity.[15-17] The technique of intraluminal electrical impedance, which is limited to institutions with a research inter-est, allows identification not only of the direction and volume of the bolus (antegrade or retrograde), but also the effectiveness of the esophageal clearance mechanisms.[18] When paired with a pH sensor, this tech-nique can shed light on important factors not otherwise detected with the more com-monly used gold standard,—prolonged pH intraesophageal monitoring.[19]

As infants mature, the larynx descends and moves more effectively to provide a tight seal during sucking and to close the trachea with a well-developed epiglottis; the risk of aspiration decreases significantly.[20] For many former premature infants, however, the vulnerabilities can persist for years and become a major challenge in their day-to-day management; this is especially the case with infants who have sustained intracranial bleeds or injuries, infants with hydrocepha-lus, infants with anoxic encephalopathy, and infants who have required prolonged respiratory support and artificial orogastric or gavage feedings.[3] In children who are fed by gastrostomy tube, GER is common even when studies before gastrostomy tube place-ment are negative for GER.

In children with spastic cerebral palsy and other syndromes that may include men-tal retardation, constipation is common.

A particularly dangerous form of aspiration occurs when stool softeners and laxatives containing mineral oil are administered orally for management of chronic constipa-tion. Medium-chain triglycerides (MCT) oil used to increase the caloric density of formu-las also may cause a lipoid pneumonia when aspirated. Lipoid pneumonia can manifest insidiously from continued microaspiration, but also can have a sudden onset when a large aspiration of lipid occurs. Oropharyn-geal discoordination, loss of protective cough reflexes, and airway penetration all contrib-ute to the development of lipoid pneumonia. The pulmonary injury can manifest insidi-ously over months or years with tachypnea and unexplained fever, but little cough or congestion.[21] The findings on radiologic studies can be impressive (Fig. 5-1).

Congenital Anomalies

Infants born with congenital anomalies affecting the oropharynx and other midline structures (e.g., cleft palate, laryngotracheal cleft) and infants with disproportionately large tongues or small mandibles (macroglos-sia, as seen in various syndromes or in the Pierre Robin sequence) are at a major disad-vantage with respect to their capacity to prevent aspiration from above and in the presence of reflux (Fig. 5-2).[22,23] The presence of abnormal communication between the esophagus and the airway (tracheoesophageal

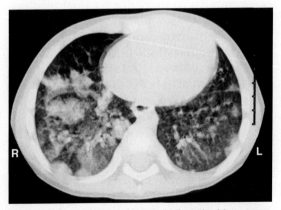

Figure 5-1. Aspiration of mineral oil resulted from treat-ment of constipation in a 14-year-old child with profound mental retardation and seizure disorder. Extensive, severe, bilateral basilar chronic pneumonia is documented in this chest CT scan.

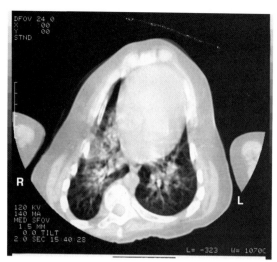

Figure 5-2. CT scan of a patient with nemaline myopathy and compromised chest motion secondary to his paralytic thorax shows extensive basilar atelectasis and pneumonia resulting from recurrent aspiration. Bronchiectasis also is present bilaterally.

fistulas) results in spillage of saliva and particulate food into the airway. Even after repair of the fistula, most children with these anomalies have a dysmotility of their foregut, with more severe GER, and increased likelihood of associated tracheomalacia or laryngomalacia.[24]

Serious respiratory and gastrointestinal complications, such as recurrent pneumonia, obstructive airway disease, airway hyperreactivity, GERD, and esophageal stenosis, are frequent in patients with a history of esophageal atresia/tracheoesophageal fistula, although the frequency of such events seems to decrease significantly with age. Because chronic aspiration can lead to recurrent pneumonia and impaired pulmonary function, it is essential in patients with a history of esophageal atresia/tracheoesophageal fistula that these recognized respiratory complications be excluded before respiratory symptoms are simply attributed to "asthma." Common etiologies of respiratory symptoms in patients with a history of esophageal atresia/tracheoesophageal fistula include retained secretions owing to impaired mucociliary clearance secondary to tracheomalacia, and aspiration related to impaired esophageal peristalsis or esophageal stricture or both, recurrence of the tracheoesophageal fistula, or GERD.

Children with neuromuscular disorders, including children with certain forms of spastic cerebral palsy, spinal muscular atrophy, or bulbar involvement, can have recurrent aspiration because of their inability to coordinate the five muscle groups that form the intrinsic muscles of the larynx. These groups are innervated by the trigeminal, facial, hypoglossal, and vagus nerves, along with the important branches, the superior and recurrent laryngeal nerves. Sensory abnormalities and autonomic dysfunction (such as encountered in children with familial and nonfamilial dysautonomic syndromes) can result in prominent and life-threatening lung disease (Fig. 5-3; see Fig. 5-2).[25]

Another at-risk group for chronic reflux and pulmonary disease are children with congenital diaphragmatic hernia.[26,27] The presence of the herniated viscus during the development of the lung often becomes the most life-threatening component of the defect because it profoundly affects lung development and results in pulmonary hypertension.[28] The pulmonary compromise poses the most serious prognostic implications for the child. The effects on esophageal motility can be serious; often there is an associated delayed gastric emptying and severe feeding intolerance.[26] Infants born with congenital diaphragmatic hernia

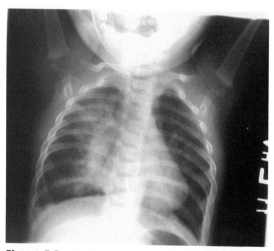

Figure 5-3. Chest x-ray in a patient with familial dysautonomia (Riley-Day syndrome) shows hyperinflation, extensive right upper lobe and parahilar areas of atelectasis, and pneumonia. Oropharyngeal and gastroesophageal reflux also were documented. The patient's x-rays improved after a Nissen fundoplication was performed.

often also have various degrees of pulmonary hypertension, which is usually proportional to the extent of lung hypoplasia. GER is a major problem after surgical repair of the diaphragm because with the stomach in the chest during fetal development, these infants fail to develop a cardiac sphincter, and their esophagus tends to be short and intrinsically dysmotile, as is the rest of the foregut. After surgery (even if an antireflux procedure is performed at the initial surgery), recurrence of GER is common when there is a paraesophageal hernia or slippage of the antireflux wrap. This is a common event when the diaphragm is repaired with a Gore-Tex patch owing to stretch of the patch with growth of the infant allowing slippage of the stomach through the wrap.

There is also an increased risk of reflux in esophageal atresia because even after esophageal anastomosis, these infants are at very high risk for esophageal stricture at the site of the anastomosis and poor distal esophageal motility. Similar to infants with congenital diaphragmatic hernia, these infants rarely have a competent gastroesophageal sphincter.

Penetration of gastric contents, acid, or nasal or oral secretions into the airway has deleterious effects on the surface epithelium, triggering the production of mucus, the recruitment of inflammatory cells, and the activation of inflammatory pathways. Surfactant damage, alveolar obliteration, atelectasis, and progressive parenchymal damage result. As a result, interstitial fibrosis can develop with secondary changes in the pulmonary circulation.[29]

Table 5-1	Differential Diagnosis of Vomiting in Pediatric Patients
Structural/Anatomic	
Pyloric stenosis	
Malrotation	
Intestinal stenosis/atresia	
Intussusception	
Hirschsprung disease	
Infections	
Pyelonephritis/cystitis	
Pneumonia	
Central nervous system infections	
Gastroenteritis	
Otitis	
Sepsis	
Metabolic Disorders	
Organic acidurias	
Galactosemia	
Hereditary fructose intolerance	
Urea cycle defects	
Fatty acid oxidation defects	
Central Nervous System Disorders	
Hydrocephalus	
Ventricular or intracerebral hemorrhage	
Chronic subdural hematoma	
Tumors	
Gastrointestinal Etiologies	
Acute appendicitis	
Gastritis	
Pancreatitis	
Allergic enteropathies	
GERD	
Cholelithiasis/cholecystitis	
Hepatitis (infectious, autoimmune, metabolic, drugs)	
Miscellaneous	
Medication side effects	
Lead toxicity	
Dysautonomic crisis	

Diagnosis

The differential diagnosis of vomiting in a child is multifactorial (Table 5-1), and a diagnosis of "reflux" should not be considered seriously until other important reasons for vomiting are ruled out by a thorough history and physical examination. When necessary, ancillary tests help define potentially serious etiologies of vomiting.

Vomiting in an infant is often the presenting symptom for an underlying structural problem or obstruction. In pyloric stenosis, the vomiting is typically projectile and nonbilious. The presence of bilious vomiting is always an emergency because it can result from malrotation or intussusception. Delay in diagnosis of volvulus can have catastrophic consequences, with ischemic damage to the midgut. Vomiting also is a common clinical manifestation of an underlying infection in infants and children, including central nervous system infection, urinary tract infection, otitis media, and pneumonia. Inborn errors of metabolism often manifest with vomiting and failure to thrive. In specific disorders, intolerance to certain carbohydrates (galactose, fructose) or to proteins (urea cycle disorders) can confuse the clinical picture and result in inappropriate management for presumed reflux. Because the child is vomiting, tests designed to identify reflux of gastric contents into the esophagus would invariably be positive, reinforcing the false assumption of reflux as the underlying primary pathology.

Diagnostic Approach

Given the numerous tests available to identify reflux (Table 5-2), it behooves the practitioner to choose the most appropriate test to answer a specific clinical question. A guiding principle in the choice of test to identify reflux is to consider how the results would help guide or change management.[30] Radiologic visualization of the esophagus and stomach is neither particularly sensitive nor specific to identify reflux, but radiography is an excellent and widely available screening test for detecting anatomic defects, such as the critical conditions of obstruction or malrotation.

The modified barium swallow, performed under videofluoroscopic control with the guidance of a feeding or speech therapist who works closely with the radiologist, can provide extremely useful information regarding the mechanics of suck and

Table 5-2	Diagnostic Tests Used in the Investigation of Gastroesophageal Reflux–Associated Pulmonary Involvement	
TEST	**ADVANTAGES**	**LIMITATIONS**
Barium swallow/upper GI series	Commonly available; inexpensive; best suited to identify anatomic abnormalities	Poor specificity; procedure performed supine; easy to elicit reflux in frightened, crying infant
Modified barium swallow	Allows accurate definition of phases of swallow and abnormal structural positions of involved structures; physiologic posture; helps in the management of infants and children with dysphagia and other feeding difficulties	Requires collaboration between experienced speech/feeding and radiology services; not widely available
Prolonged pH probe monitoring	Accurate capture of acid reflux events; allows correlation with symptoms; reflects esophageal acid clearance; presents physiologic events over time (18-24 hr), and their timing during the day and night; helps in titration of antacid therapy	Does not identify nonacidic reflux events; difficult to perform in children receiving nasogastric or continuous feedings; not useful in the identification of GER-related ALTEs (see text)
Milk scan	Affords a more physiologic setting to determine gastric emptying compared with inert barium	Insensitive to detect aspiration, unless it occurs while isotope is still in the stomach; requires child to be completely immobile for >1 hr under the gamma camera
Salivagram	High concentration of isotope allows better demonstration of aspiration from above; helps in visualizing retropharyngeal pooling and esophageal clearance	Not commonly performed; no standards available
Intraluminal impedance	Best test available to show bidirectional fluid movement in the esophagus; acid and nonacid events can be identified	Available only in a very limited number of centers at present; analysis is time-consuming and dependent on experience of reader
Polysomnography	Provides a wealth of physiologic data reflective of most systems potentially involved in ALTE episodes—EEG, air flow, end-tidal CO_2, EMG, abdominal and chest wall motion, saturation, ECG video recording, and pH probe; allows temporal correlation between variables	Only performed in a few pediatric centers in the U.S.; requires overnight hospitalization (home monitoring sometimes available through commercial services)

ALTE, apparent life-threatening event; ECG, electrocardiogram; EEG, electroencephalogram; EMG, electromyogram; GER, gastroesophageal reflux; GI, gastrointestinal.

swallow and the safety of oral feedings (Fig. 5-4).[31,32] This study is performed with the infant in a more physiologic position (sitting up, as opposed to lying down, as is the case for a routine upper gastrointestinal series) while various textures and barium consistencies are offered via a nipple or cup. In addition to delineating the appropriateness of lip and tongue coordination, bolus propulsion, and traverse through the retropharynx and into the upper esophagus, the test allows an appreciation of the esophageal sweeping peristaltic waves and the effective relaxation of the lower esophageal sphincter during swallows.

Monitoring of the changes in acidity occurring in the esophagus is still considered one of the most valuable diagnostic tests to quantify acid reflux and to determine its correlation to symptoms such as irritability, neck posturing and arching, feeding refusal, or nocturnal cough.[33] The pH probe monitoring test can now be performed with slender probes that have proximal and distal sensors; this allows determination of the level reached by the acid refluxate in the esophagus. It also is useful in determining the adequacy of acid-suppressive therapy, a recurrent and very relevant clinical issue that arises when symptoms persist despite what is believed to be an appropriate dose of H_2-blocker or proton pump inhibitor.

A gastric scintiscan using a Tc 99m–labeled meal also can be performed. This study allows detection of reflux and quantifies gastric emptying over 2 hours. In some cases, markedly delayed gastric emptying appears to contribute to the reflux.

Reflux as Etiology of Pulmonary Pathology

Determining the possible contribution of reflux to pulmonary disease remains a formidable challenge. As already noted, no single test can help make the distinction between aspiration or reflux of food and saliva from above, or of acid and gastric contents from below. Correlation with respiratory events, including apnea, bronchospasm, and cough, requires the simultaneous recording of multiple variables, usually best performed in a sleep laboratory or similarly specialized testing facility. Polysomnography allows measurement of airflow and chest movements and cardiovascular parameters and oxygen saturation, while also capturing REM sleep and, if indicated, swallowing movements. Correlating events that are separated by milliseconds and trying to determine cause-and-effect relationships can be a daunting task and can help explain the dearth of "definitive" studies pertaining to this topic.

Theoretically, labeling of saliva with nuclear isotopes should provide a sensitive way to detect aspiration of secretions from above.[34,35] The "salivagram" has never been validated as a useful tool for this indication, however.[36] It sometimes provides information on esophageal clearance and even gastric emptying, similar to a formal gastric emptying test performed with labeled formula or solids.[37] Identifying aspiration of gastric contents during a gastric emptying test depends on the

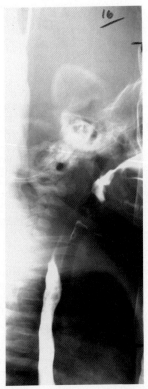

Figure 5-4. Direct tracheal aspiration documented during a modified barium swallow in a patient with bulbar dysfunction. Retention of the contrast material at the level of the vallecula also can be appreciated.

aspiration event occurring while there is still sufficient isotope left in the stomach. It does not easily or reliably duplicate the clinical setting of nocturnal aspiration.

Gastroesophageal Reflux Disease and Asthma

The etiologic role of GERD in some patients with the more refractory forms of asthma has not been firmly established, although there is evidence (albeit controversial) to suggest that aggressive management of GERD can change the natural history of unremitting steroid dependency and severe bronchial inflammation in some patients.[38] For most patients with uncomplicated asthma, however, it is unclear to what degree stimulation of esophageal vagal mediators plays a role in triggering or aggravating bronchospasm, or even whether reflux exerts its deleterious effects in this population through (micro) aspiration and airway penetration.[39]

Clinical Management
Typical acid reflux symptoms are often absent in patients with asthma referred to a pediatric gastroenterologist for evaluation. Severe bronchospasm and cough can result in chest pain, epigastric discomfort, and nausea indistinguishable from GERD. Increased secretions promote triggering of the gag reflex and nausea, adding to the diagnostic difficulties. In practical terms, the possibility of GERD-aggravated asthma is considered when response to appropriate therapy is inadequate, and when asthma symptoms seem to worsen at night or recur without obvious explanation. Steroid dependence and difficulties in maintaining airway quiescence while receiving anti-inflammatory and bronchodilator therapy should be a "red flag" pointing to GERD as a possible contributor to the refractory nature of asthma. A positive pH probe is more likely in patients with severe asthma than in patients without severe asthma.[40]

In 2001, the North American Society for Pediatric Gastroenterology and Nutrition published clinical practice guidelines for evaluation and treatment of GER in infants and children.[30] In this evidence-based review, a meta-analysis of 13 case series involving 668 patients documented the presence of abnormal pH monitoring studies in more than 60% of infants and children with asthma. Nevertheless, only half of the patients with chronic asthma and abnormal pH studies ever reported gastrointestinal symptoms (including vomiting, regurgitation, and heartburn) suggestive of underlying reflux disease. No clinical features of asthma predicted which children had abnormal pH scores.

There is no pediatric experience that helps predict which children with asthma but without GER symptoms might benefit from empiric antireflux therapy, or how to approach patients with severe asthma who have negative prolonged esophageal pH probe studies. Regarding surgery, a review of six case series involving 258 patients with steroid-dependent asthma showed that 85% of patients who underwent an antireflux operation (fundoplication) were reported to have a decrease in the frequency and intensity of their asthma attacks and were able to reduce their bronchodilator and anti-inflammatory medication dose. The American Thoracic Society and the National Institutes of Health Expert Panel on the Diagnosis and Management of Asthma have issued recommendations to investigate reflux as a possible cause of poorly controlled asthma (in adults), including documenting reflux with pH probe studies, if indicated.[41,42]

There is some evidence that GER is a possible trigger or aggravating factor in a subgroup of patients with severe asthma. In patients who have frequent exacerbations, nocturnal attacks or cough, frequent need for steroids, or steroid dependence, a trial of aggressive acid suppression (preferably with a proton pump inhibitor) and lifestyle modifications for at least 3 months can be beneficial and should be recommended. For patients without any GER symptoms, but with a positive pH study or a clinical profile that includes recurrent pneumonia, nighttime wheezing, and steroid dependence, the same recommendations apply.

Apparent Life-Threatening Events

In the spectrum of pulmonary complications related to reflux disease, ALTEs hold a special place, given the high anxiety generated by the episodes and the costly evaluation to which many of these infants are subjected when they are admitted to the hospital for investigation of the episode.[43] ALTEs are defined as frightening events affecting infants who, during the episode, appear to require resuscitation (usually mouth-to-mouth breathing for perceived apnea) and look cyanotic (or pale) and lifeless, and who were sometimes observed to have had a preceding gasping, choking, or gagging trigger.[44] In the typical case, an otherwise healthy infant has an ALTE episode when placed supine on a changing table soon after a feed or a bottle. It is not unusual to elicit a history of finding formula in the infant's mouth, or noticing the infant cough just as the airway clears and the long episode (15 to 40 seconds) subsides. Characteristically, by the time emergency personnel arrive at the home and bring the infant to the emergency department, there is little to support the parents' concerns about a life-threatening event.

In addition to certain infections (e.g., respiratory syncytial virus in premature infants), the differential diagnosis of ALTEs includes cardiac arrhythmias, central nervous system disorders (including seizures), and metabolic derangements. It is important to consider defects of fatty acid oxidation and other, less common entities because they can be difficult to diagnose unless there is a high index of suspicion and specific tests are obtained shortly after the event.[45,131,132]

GER plays a role in a large proportion of children with ALTEs (80% can have abnormal pH monitoring studies, although they seldom are found to correlate with ALTE episodes). Frequent regurgitation is elicited in the history of 60% to 70% of infants presenting with ALTEs.[43]

The understanding of the sequence of events leading to apnea in this setting is that the activation of protective reflexes in the upper airway leads to airway obstruction when refluxate reaches the upper larynx or is about to penetrate the airway. Vagally mediated reflexes can explain the vasomotor and cardiorespiratory changes after the obstructive episode. The likelihood of GER being responsible for the ALTE episode increases if the event occurred within the first hour postprandially, and if the infant was awake (or semiawake) and supine.[44] Changes in position are known to promote relaxation of the lower esophageal sphincter, and the presence of a full stomach in the recumbent position favors regurgitation.

Clinical Management

Management of ALTEs associated with reflux focuses on measures geared to decrease the likelihood of reflux; avoidance of the supine position within 1 hour of feedings and thickened feedings have been recommended. If there is a history of symptomatic reflux, acid suppression and improvement in the degree of esophagitis would optimize sphincter function. Diagnostically, a pH monitoring study rarely is helpful because the ALTEs are so random that capturing a whole GER-obstruction-apnea sequence is seldom successful or worth the effort. Conservative treatment is recommended for most infants with ALTEs. This recommendation represents a significant change in the indication for surgery (fundoplication), which used to be the standard of care in some centers for management of GERD-related ALTEs.[46]

All parents, and especially parents whose infants have had an ALTE, should be instructed on *back to sleep,* the recommendation to encourage sleeping in the supine position. This recommendation has been associated with a major reduction in the incidence of sudden infant death syndrome. Severe GERD has been considered a special circumstance, however, in which a semiprone position can be allowed, provided that the infant is carefully observed and monitored, and the infant's face rests against a firm mattress. In addition, bottle propping or bottle in bed is recognized as a risk factor for ALTE and aspiration and chronic bronchitis from aspiration as the infant falls asleep with the bottle in the mouth.

Heiner Syndrome

Heiner syndrome is a very rare form of pulmonary hemosiderosis, believed to be due to cow's milk allergy because in the initial report all infants had precipitins to cow's milk proteins in their serum.[47] The symptoms in these children were not the symptoms normally expected in idiopathic pulmonary hemosiderosis[48] (recurrent hemoptysis or intermittent blood-streaked sputum, varying degrees of anemia, and radiographic findings of symmetric diffuse alveolar infiltrates predominant in perihilar regions and lower zones), and all had nonspecific complaints of chronic lung disease and upper respiratory tract disease. These patients apparently improved on a milk-free diet.

In more recent decades, enthusiasm for cow's milk allergy as the cause of idiopathic pulmonary hemosiderosis has waned. In a very large series of patients with idiopathic pulmonary hemosiderosis, no such association was present. Some patients with pulmonary hemosiderosis did not have milk precipitins, whereas many children with milk precipitins did not have pulmonary hemosiderosis. Because of the reported association between cow's milk allergy and pulmonary hemosiderosis, many children with idiopathic pulmonary hemosiderosis are placed on milk-free diets, but unless there is unequivocal evidence of true milk allergy, this approach is unjustified.[49,50] The possible role played by exposure to foreign food proteins should be actively elicited during the history. The onset of symptoms depends on the time of introduction of milk and solid foods and varies in different geographic areas and cultural backgrounds. As mentioned, cow's milk seems to be the major offender, but individual experiences suggest soy, eggs, and pork also can play a role.[47]

The reported clinical improvement that results from withdrawal of the offending protein seems to be marked. It also is followed by radiologic improvement, which can lag behind symptomatic relief. Demonstration of the causal relationship with cow's milk protein exposure is not always feasible because parents might be reluctant to allow re-exposure after they have witnessed the dramatic resolution of chronic symptoms and the resumption of normal weight gain and growth.

Heiner syndrome may be considered in any atopic infant or young child who presents with recurrent or chronic respiratory symptoms. A history of chronic cough, pneumonia, bronchitis, and bronchiolitis is often elicited, and a history of frequent visits to the emergency department for wheezing and a suspected diagnosis of asthma. Hemoptysis can occur when the inflammation and alveolar damage progress to intrapulmonary bleeding.[48,51] Some children can have transient hives and other urticarial rashes, periorbital edema, and allergic shiners. As a result of the chronic nature of the pulmonary involvement, many children are debilitated and have poor weight gain and failure to thrive.[52] Gastrointestinal manifestations are nonspecific and include vomiting and abdominal pain. Diarrhea is more common than constipation, although in some cases, both may be present.

Diagnostic Approach

The chest x-ray findings are nonspecific and reflect the underlying interstitial changes and air trapping caused by small and large airway obstruction. Diffuse and variable infiltrates, patchy pneumonia, interstitial lung disease, and fibrosis can be documented at various times during the course and progression of the condition. Chronic intrapulmonary bleeding results in a microcytic, hypochromic anemia and iron deficiency that can be severe and debilitating.

The precipitins against cow's milk protein fractions can be identified by the micro-Ouchterlony technique; their appearance and concentration can vary depending on the state of sensitization and the temporal proximity of the exposure to the offending protein.[50] These circulating IgG antibodies are not pathognomonic, however, because, as mentioned previously, they have been reported in children who do not manifest pulmonary hemosiderosis. Identification of iron-laden alveolar macrophages in bronchoalveolar lavage is good evidence that bleeding has occurred recently, and that the disease process is still active. The finding of hemosiderin in macrophages from gastric aspirates also is suggestive of the diagnosis, but is less direct than bronchoalveolar lavage. Nevertheless, their presence—

notwithstanding the suspected specific protein exposure trigger—should raise the possibility of other entities responsible for pulmonary hemorrhage/hemoptysis in children (Fig. 5-5).[49,53,54]

Heiner syndrome remains a controversial entity because circulating precipitins, although necessary, are insufficient to predict clinical symptoms. The role of genetic and environmental factors has not been elucidated in most reported cases of pulmonary hemosiderosis, but it is important to consider alternative, or concurrent, triggers resulting in iron deposition in the lungs.[55,56]

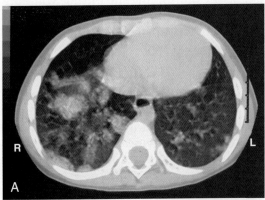

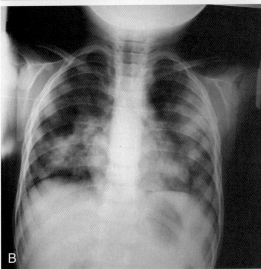

Figure 5-5. A, Chest CT scan of a 2-year-old patient with hemosiderin-laden macrophages in bronchoalveolar lavage shows multiple nodular masses involving the upper and lower lobe fields. **B,** Chest x-ray shows bilateral nodular masses of varying sizes. The appearance of the chest radiographs improved between attacks of febrile respiratory distress. Although this patient was initially diagnosed with idiopathic pulmonary hemosiderosis, her subsequent benign course suggests that she might have had Heiner syndrome.

Inflammatory Bowel Disease

Inflammatory bowel disease (IBD) refers to the two most common forms of chronic, idiopathic inflammation affecting the intestinal tract: Crohn disease and ulcerative colitis. These conditions presently are believed to be due to the intersection of predisposing genetic factors, environmental triggers, and a dysregulation of immune control resulting in varying degrees of damage.[57] In the case of Crohn disease, the inflammation is transmural and segmental, involving any portion of the small or large bowel, and often progressing to cicatricial stricture. In contrast, the involvement in ulcerative colitis is limited to the large bowel. The inflammation is mucosal, begins at the rectum, and is contiguous, without skip lesions. At worst, ulcerative colitis affects the whole colon (universal colitis), but sometimes only the rectum (proctitis) or left colon is affected.

The clinical manifestations depend on the severity and location of the inflammation and range from mild, intermittent abdominal pain to severe bloody diarrhea with or without extraintestinal involvement. In a quarter of children, the gastrointestinal manifestations can be subtle; delayed growth and pubertal development is more prominent.[58] Fatigue, low-grade fever, and night sweats sometimes can be confused for hematologic or oncologic etiologies; rheumatologic manifestations also are common.[59]

Pulmonary Manifestations

The multisystemic involvement in IBD has long been recognized, and the extraintestinal manifestations are believed to reflect the effects of deranged immunologic regulation.[60] Changes in intestinal permeability that allow translocation of bacteria, fungal, or viral products (including endotoxin) can stimulate the formation of antibodies targeting similar epitopes. Also, a common embryologic origin (as is the case with the gut and the lung or with elements of the eye or the joints) can result in distant inflammation in conjunction with or independent of the bowel disease.[61]

The involvement of the lung is perhaps the least recognized of the extraintestinal manifestations of IBD, and there are no reliable figures to describe true incidence and prevalence rates.[133] It is possible that a systematic study would bring to light many cases that are mild and subclinical, or that would be identifiable only by abnormalities in PFTs, including the diffusing capacity for carbon monoxide, or by increased lung permeability as identified by Tc 99m DTPA clearance.[62] It is believed that as a whole, extraintestinal manifestations are more common in Crohn disease than in ulcerative colitis, although pulmonary complications in particular seem to be more common in ulcerative colitis.[63] Also, when a patient has one extraintestinal complication, generally there is a higher likelihood of involvement in another organ.

Parenchymal and Pleural Disease

Ascribing an etiologic role to the immune mechanisms that underlie IBD may be difficult because reactions to drugs used in its management can confound the picture. Hypersensitivity pneumonitis with eosinophilia is a known complication of exposure to certain drugs, including sulfa and some of its derivatives—a class of drugs that is commonly used in the long-term treatment of IBD patients.[64,65] Clinical manifestations of drug-related pneumonitis are nonspecific and include fever, dyspnea, chest pain, and productive cough. A mixed obstructive-restrictive lung disease pattern is often shown on PFTs.

Confirming the presence of eosinophilic pleural effusions or alveolar fibrosis and resolution of clinical symptoms and signs or radiologic findings is sometimes the only way that a presumptive diagnosis of a drug-induced complication can be considered. Response to drug withdrawal and steroids can be lifesaving, particularly in cases in which the inflammation potentially could progress to pulmonary fibrosis.[65] For the most part, the offending agent is believed to be the sulfapyridine moiety of sulfasalazine, although there have been isolated reports of eosinophilic pneumonia in patients receiving only mesalamine.[66-68]

Airway Disease

Airway damage in IBD has been documented at all levels of the tracheobronchial tree, most commonly as the development of bronchiectasis and suppurative bronchitis.[63,67] The spectrum of involvement includes bronchial and bronchiolar inflammation, bronchiolitis obliterans organizing pneumonia,[67] and severe upper airway stenosis.[69,70] In Crohn disease, metastatic granulomatous involvement of the larynx, trachea, and bronchi has been reported.[69] Most of the published series involve adults, although single case reports have shown that children also can develop these complications.[71] In the spectrum of extraintestinal manifestations, pulmonary disease is much less common than joint, skin, or eye involvement.

The presence of lymphocytes in the bronchoalveolar lavage of some patients with Crohn disease suggests an immune-mediated damage. Along these same lines, the changes observed histologically in instances of small airway disease have been similar to those found in patients with a graft-versus-host disease after bone marrow or lung transplantation. In patients with ulcerative colitis, pulmonary complications can occur 1 to 2 years after colectomy (Fig. 5-6). One study suggests that colectomy might represent an independent risk factor for the onset of the lung disease.[72] In some patients, there is no correlation between the degree of inflammatory activity in the bowel and the timing of appearance of the respiratory disease.[63]

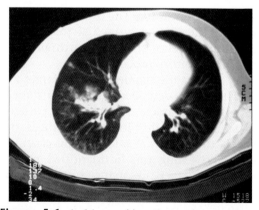

Figure 5-6. A 16-year-old patient, who underwent colectomy for ulcerative colitis, developed bronchiectasis in the right mid-lung field 1 year later. Clinical manifestations included recurrent fever, productive cough, and dyspnea on exertion. Management included antibiotics for acute exacerbations and prophylactically, postural drainage, and inhaled bronchodilator.

Clinical Manifestations

The most common manifestations of pulmonary disease in IBD are cough and dyspnea. In bronchiectasis, the cough is productive, and the secretions are copious and thick—although there are reports of well-documented bronchiectasis with neither cough nor sputum production. In patients with few (if any) symptoms, pulmonary disease can only be surmised on the basis of abnormal radiologic findings or abnormal PFTs. In more severe cases of suppurative disease, dyspnea and hypoxemia can be significant.[73]

Diagnostic Approach

The airway and interstitial changes that occur as a result of the immune-mediated damage are not always accompanied by identifiable radiologic changes in plain chest films, even when the clinical situation has progressed, and the patient is clearly symptomatic.[63] A more representative picture is obtained through the use of high-resolution CT, particularly if care is exercised in obtaining full inspiration and expiration views.[74] The presence of bronchiectasis is identified by the discrepant caliber of the bronchus in relation to its corresponding artery. The bronchus appears of a homogeneous diameter even in images that extend to the periphery, where the size would be expected to diminish. The presence of secretions in the dilated bronchial tree reflects the stasis and suppuration occurring during the inflammatory process.

Changes in the diameter of the larger airways have been described in isolated instances of glottis and tracheal stenosis in patients with ulcerative colitis. In these instances, the trachea can appear as a long, rigid channel. Mucosal swelling can be identified prominently in magnetic resonance imaging scans with gadolinium enhancement.[71]

Parenchymal characteristics on high-resolution CT reflect the inflammatory exudates present in various portions of the lung and appear in a ground-glass pattern. Centrilobular nodules and branching linear opacities can give what has been described as a "tree

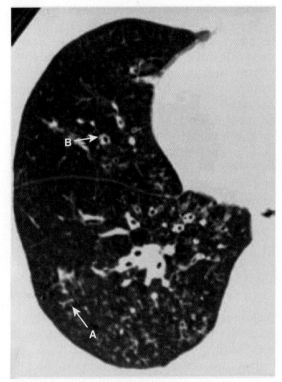

Figure 5-7. "Tree in bud" pattern on high-resolution CT. (*From Mahadeva R, et al: Clinical and radiological characteristics of lung disease in inflammatory bowel disease. Eur Resp J 15:41-48, 2000.*)

in bud" pattern (Fig. 5-7).[75] Air trapping can be prominent and can be reversible with steroid treatment. Pathophysiologically, this pattern often seems to be associated with more severe coughing, much as bronchiectasis is often accompanied by productive cough.

Clinical Management

Systemic steroids are the mainstay of treatment for inflammatory lung disease when it occurs in the context of IBD. The inflammatory changes in the lungs do not always parallel the degree of activity of the underlying intestinal disease and need to be managed in their own right, regardless of whether the intestine is quiescent or not. In some instances of suppurative bronchial or bronchiolar disease, the response to steroids can be dramatic and has been the indication for recurrent courses of treatment during the course of the illness. Similarly, patients with stenosing airway presentations, in which airway wall edema is prominent, have benefited greatly from steroids. In some instances of interstitial pneumonia, methylprednisolone has been administered directly in the form of bronchial lavages.[76] In this respect, the therapeutic response is similar to what is seen in immune-mediated lung disorders, including autoimmune and vasculitic syndromes, or in graft-versus-host disease.

Hepatopulmonary Syndrome

HPS is a recognized complication of cirrhotic and noncirrhotic liver disease that is accompanied by portal hypertension. HPS is characterized by the clinical triad of (1) chronic liver disease, (2) arterial hypoxemia, and (3) formation of abnormal intrapulmonary vascular dilations.[77] The initial description of HPS dates to the turn of the 19th century, but the pathophysiologic processes underscoring the intrapulmonary shunting, and the molecular mechanisms responsible for those changes, have begun to be appreciated only in the past 2 decades.[78]

HPS has a profound impact on the survival of patients who develop it. It raises the Model End-Stage Liver Disease score for patients awaiting liver transplantation because orthotopic liver transplantation remains the only proven therapy at this time.[79] Liver transplantation brings about a resolution of the pulmonary findings in greater than 80% of patients. The reversibility of the syndrome reinforces the notion that HPS is secondary to functional abnormalities occurring in the endothelium of the pulmonary vasculature.[80] These abnormalities seem to be mediated by various key circulating molecular species released into the venous circulation, particularly nitric oxide and carbon monoxide, which contribute to the vasodilation and subsequent microvascular changes.[81]

It is important to distinguish between HPS and portopulmonary hypertension (PPHTN) because these two entities are pathophysiologically distinct. Their underlying mechanisms are diametrically opposed. In PPHTN,

pulmonary vasoconstriction leads to compromised oxygenation in the presence of portal hypertension.[82]

HPS is found in 30% to 40% of patients with chronic liver disease (range 13% to 47%).[83] PPHTN is much less common, diagnosed in about 5% of patients with chronic liver disease. The symptoms of PPHTN are those of hemodynamic compromise, with right ventricular dysfunction and cor pulmonale. PPHTN is associated with mortality rates of 40% within 15 months of diagnosis.[80] In contrast to HPS, PPHTN is much less likely to reverse after successful liver transplantation.

Clinical Manifestations

Initially, patients with HPS can be asymptomatic, although as the alveolar-arterial gradient increases, dyspnea and cyanosis inevitably ensue. In addition, digital clubbing can be prominent. In some patients, orthodeoxia—the decrease in arterial oxygenation caused by pooling of blood in the dilated capillary vasculature when a patient stands up (as blood moves with gravity to the lower lobes of the lungs)—develops.[84] Patients also have clinical signs of the underlying chronic liver disease, most commonly hyperbilirubinemia, spider angiomas, splenomegaly, and other signs of portal hypertension.

Pathophysiology

New insights into the possible mechanisms of development of HPS have been gained from detailed studies in a mouse model of common bile duct ligation. After ligation of the common bile duct, progressive changes in the pulmonary vasculature are consistent with the changes shown in the concentrations of nitric oxide in the lung: hypoxia results.[81] The postulated mechanism is a chain reaction triggered by production of the mediator endothelin-1 (ET-1) by cholangiocytes, which become hypertrophic after the ligation. Overexpression of endothelial endothelin B (ET_B) receptor promoted by the shear stress in the pulmonary circulation increases the production of nitric oxide in the lung. This cascade possibly is initiated by absorption of bacterial endotoxin in the gut, triggering tumor necrosis factor-α release, which upregulates cyclic adenosine monophosphate and the intrinsic nitric oxide synthesis pathway.[85]

Factors playing a role in the formation of pulmonary arteriovenous shunts and dilated microcapillaries differ from the factors that are involved in the hyperdynamic circulation most characteristic of patients with cirrhotic liver disease. In all patients with cirrhosis, systemic vasodilation occurs uniformly as a function of time, whereas HPS is seen in only about one third of this population, pointing to other mechanisms involved in the pathogenesis.[86] It also has become clear that, in rare instances, HPS can develop even when cirrhosis is not firmly established, suggesting that activation of nitric oxide–mediated pathways can occur in the presence of preserved hepatic synthetic function[84] or transiently, in the setting of acute or chronic hepatitis.[87,88]

In the above-described experimental model of common bile duct ligation, ET-1 plays an important role in producing an overexpression of the ET_B receptor, which brings about vascular dilation.[85] It is paradoxical that ET-1, a well-recognized vasoconstrictor, would result in vasodilation in the pulmonary circulation. The explanation seems to lie in selective activation of ET_B receptors on the luminal surface of the vascular endothelial cells in the lung by ET-1, which is the final mediator of vasodilation. ET_B receptor expression was found to be significantly increased in the presence of portal hypertension secondary to biliary or nonbiliary cirrhosis. The increase in ET_B receptor concentration mediates the sensitization of the pulmonary vasculature to the vasodilating effects of ET-1, with activation of the endothelial nitric oxide synthase pathway.[81]

One consequence of this vasodilation is the development of a perfusion/ventilation mismatch, owing in part to increased perfusion in under ventilated areas where the abnormal dilation has developed. In addition, there are direct shunts between the arterial and venous plexuses creating a bypass physiology (Fig. 5-8).[86] The dilation

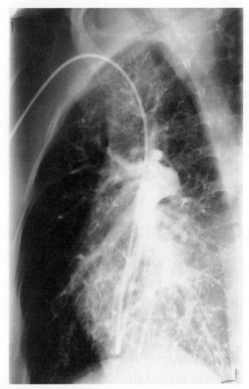

Figure 5-8. Patient with cystic fibrosis, established biliary cirrhosis, and portal hypertension shows arteriovenous shunting by right and left selective pulmonary arteriograms. Findings are characteristic of the hepatopulmonary syndrome and resulted in hypoxemia and orthodeoxia (see text).

of the capillary bed interrupts the normal physiologic steady state characterized by the movement of single red blood cells through the capillary bed with highly efficient oxygen transfer to hemoglobin. This transfer cannot occur when four or five red blood cells are traversing the capillary bed simultaneously, as has been shown in pathologic preparations.[82] Depending on the extent of the phenomenon, a pressure difference between the oxygen in the alveoli and the arteries can result in either no symptoms or in severe dyspnea, with consequent hypoxemia.

Diagnostic Approach

The diagnosis of HPS depends on identification of dilated capillary channels in the periphery of the lung. Four common methods of identifying this process are (1) contrast-enhanced echocardiography, (2) Tc 99m–labeled macroaggregated albumin (MAA) scan, (3) pulmonary angiography, and (4) high-resolution CT.

In contrast-enhanced echocardiography, indocyanine green or normal saline is injected intravenously while a transthoracic echocardiogram is performed. In the presence of a dilated capillary bed in the lungs, the 8 to 15μm bubbles are noted to appear in the heart after five or six cardiac cycles owing to the "escape" of the microbubbles through the dilated channels, which may be 500 μm in diameter.[89] The delayed opacification seen after three to six cardiac cycles is a reflection of the time it takes for the microbubbles to permeate through the pulmonary capillaries, and is a specific sign of the intrapulmonary shunting that is taking place. The presence of a positive contrast-enhanced echocardiography study is not enough, however, to ensure a diagnosis of HPS. In some instances, some patients have been found to have a positive contrast-enhanced echocardiography study, but normal alveolar-arterial gradient. These patients would not technically qualify for a diagnosis of HPS.

A similar principle applies to the passage of Tc 99m MAA molecules through the dilated channels in a Tc 99m MAA study. The sensitivity of these tests is not high, but they are specific in the absence of intracardiac shunting.[90] The oxygenation in the pulmonary artery when 100% oxygen is inspired has been shown to be significantly worse in HPS when pulmonary nonvascular comorbidities are present. This finding is of clinical significance because mortality is increased when decreased oxygenation is present while breathing room air and when there is an increase in the shift of Tc 99m MAA to the brain.

Echocardiography, especially if the transesophageal approach is used, has better sensitivity for distinguishing between intrapulmonary and intracardiac shunting than the regular transthoracic echocardiogram. Because it requires anesthesia, however, transesophageal echocardiography poses practical risks in the setting of compromised liver function and the possible presence of esophageal varices.[91]

From a structural point of view, high-resolution CT may facilitate determining the ratio of the pulmonary artery (main pulmonary trunk, right and left main pulmonary arteries) and the diameter of pulmonary vasculature. These changes can be shown best on the "parenchymal" windows on the CT scan, in contrast to the "mediastinal" windows, which seem better suited for the vascular measurements. The ratio of the diameter of the right lower lobe basal segmental pulmonary artery to the diameter of the lumen of the accompanying bronchus, known as the pulmonary artery/bronchus ratio, can be calculated. In high-resolution chest CT, there is a correlation between the diameter of the right lower lobe basal segmental artery and the partial pressure of oxygen in HPS. An increased pulmonary artery/bronchus ratio may be helpful in diagnosing HPS in patients with liver disease and hypoxemia. High-resolution CT also can identify the presence of pleural or direct arteriovenous communications in dilated channels, and provide information on the lung parenchyma.[92] More experience with this technique is needed because these findings have been inconsistent.[93]

The appearance of the chest x-ray in HPS is usually nonspecific. Some chest radiographs might show "mottled" shadows bilaterally, which have been suspicious enough to warrant treatment for suspected tuberculosis. Increased bilateral interstitial markings also have been described. It is believed that these markings are a result of the intrapulmonary vascular dilations.

Clinical Management

The presence of HPS is associated with increased mortality in patients with liver disease. It is important to evaluate periodically the presence and progression of the gradient and the presence of hypoxemia in any patient with chronic liver disease. Because HPS is reversible only by transplantation, it constitutes at present an indication for early liver transplantation. Transplantation results have been positive; greater than 80% of transplant recipients have near-complete resolution of pathologic changes.[94] The return to normal occurs over months in patients surviving the transplant. As mentioned, it is important to ensure beforehand that no pulmonary comorbidities are present, particularly the presence of PPHTN.

Pancreatitis

Acute pancreatitis is often a self-limited condition characterized by abdominal pain and elevation in the serum concentrations of amylase and lipase. Inflammation of the pancreas is the result of activation of the digestive enzymes normally maintained in an inactive proform in the exocrine portion (the acini) of the gland. Autodigestion is potentially a serious consequence, although self-limited mild inflammation is more common than fulminant, necrotizing pancreatitis.[95]

The hallmarks of pancreatitis include abdominal pain and abnormalities in the measured circulating pancreatic enzymes, principally amylase and lipase.[96] The abdominal pain—typically referring to pain in the back and epigastrium—can be excruciating, requiring narcotics for management. Nausea, vomiting, and the sensation of bloating often accompany the pain. In many cases, pancreatitis can be asymptomatic, however, and can be suspected only from the presence of biochemical abnormalities.

Etiology

The most common triggers for pancreatitis in adults are gallstones and alcohol ingestion. In children, the etiology often remains elusive or idiopathic; Table 5-3 lists the broad categories to be considered in the differential diagnosis. In addition to infections and medications, some metabolic disorders and hereditary forms of recurrent pancreatitis are now being increasingly recognized as possible causes, with mutations in genes involved in the stability of trypsinogen and other protective mechanisms.[97,98] An important cause of pancreatitis in children is blunt abdominal trauma; bicycle

Table 5-3	Etiology of Pancreatitis in Children

Idiopathic (20%-30% of cases)
Trauma (including child abuse)
Drugs*
  Thiazides
  Azathioprine
  Asparaginase
  Antiretrovirals
  Valproic acid
Infections (congenital and acquired)
  Viral/bacterial—mumps, rubella, coxsackievirus, influenza, hepatitis A and B, *Mycoplasma pneumoniae*
  Parasitic—*Ascaris, Echinococcus, Clonorchis sinensis*
Metabolic disorders
  Hyperparathyroidism
  Hyperlipidemia types I, IV, V
  Hypercalcemia
  Vitamin D deficiency
Hereditary conditions
  Cystic fibrosis
  Shwachman-Diamond syndrome
  Familial recurrent pancreatitis
Collagen vascular disorders
  Systemic lupus erythematosus
  Periarteritis nodosa
Congenital anatomic abnormalities
  Choledochal cyst
  Enteric duplications
  Cholelithiasis

*List is not comprehensive.

handlebar injuries are notorious in this regard,[99] but the possibility of child abuse needs to be considered.[100]

Pulmonary Manifestations

Lung involvement in the course of acute pancreatitis has long been recognized as a potentially extremely serious complication, manifesting in 5% of cases as acute respiratory distress syndrome (ARDS) with high mortality rates of 50% to 75%. In adults, the incidence of lung complications has been reported to be 15% to 55%.[101] Data for pediatric patients are unavailable, and only anecdotal case reports have been published.[102,103]

The changes leading to pleural effusions and to alveolar damage are not fully understood, but intensive work in several animal models of pancreatitis has helped expand understanding of the pathophysiologic steps involved in the process. Cystic fibrosis also can manifest as recurrent pancreatitis. These patients often have similar *CFTR* gene mutations, class IV (abnormal conductance) and class V (reduced synthesis or trafficking). In these two classes, lung dysfunction is often recognized only after complete genetic evaluation.[134]

Early in the course of the attack of acute pancreatitis, changes can occur in the lung ranging from asymptomatic hypoxemia to fulminant respiratory failure. The degree of hypoxemia is not correlated to the severity of the underlying pancreatic involvement. Tachypnea, dyspnea, and shallow breathing can be present, with the last-mentioned reflecting the presence of diaphragmatic irritation secondary to accumulated pleural effusions. Effusions have been shown in more than 15% of patients and are preferentially left-sided, for unclear reasons, but perhaps related to direct irritation of the diaphragm.[101] The effusion fluid is usually rich in amylase, and the enzyme concentrations can remain elevated even after the circulating pancreatic enzymes have normalized.[104]

Pathophysiology

Experimental pancreatitis, induced in rats either by intraperitoneal injections of cerulein (an analogue of cholecystokinin) or by intrabiliary ductal injection of the bile acid taurocholate, has allowed identification of several important mechanisms participating in the observed multiorgan dysfunction.[105,106] As autodigestion of the gland occurs, chemokines and cytokines are released into the circulation, resulting in recruitment of activated cellular mediators capable of producing intense changes in the alveolar endothelium and the pulmonary vasculature.[105] Among the cellular mediators, mast cells and macrophages are believed to play central roles, whereas activated trypsinogen generates trypsin, a potent protease.[107-109]

Damaged acini release the powerful membrane and cellular digestive enzymes normally kept in their proenzyme granular storage form. Elastase and phospholipase A are considered key players in this process.[110] When the inflammatory cascade is triggered, upregulation of the genes encoding for nuclear factor κB and tumor necrosis factor-α has been shown.[111]

Important changes occur in the pulmonary capillary bed, resulting from recruitment of neutrophils and translocation of serum proteins into the lung interstitium (this can be shown with the use of chromium-labeled albumin or transferrin). Pulmonary infiltrates are seen radiologically. Thickening of basement membranes and lysis of the surfactant proteins and phospholipids results in the clinical picture of ARDS and profound hypoxemia.[112]

Various adhesion molecules, such as intracellular adhesion molecule-1, are synthesized in higher quantities in the presence of inflammation.[111] They play a role in the activation of lymphocytes, macrophages, and neutrophils; they further contribute to the endothelial damage and the leaking of proteins into the lung parenchyma. The role of endotoxemia is strongly suspected as another important promoter of progressive damage and multiorgan failure because severe pancreatitis is frequently associated with infection of the necrotic gland; the most common organisms are enteropathogens believed to have translocated as a result of the above-described diffuse capillary permeability changes.[113]

Structural changes in the alveolar integrity parallel severe impairment in oxygen diffusing capacity and bronchial reactivity. Vital capacity piratory volume in 1 second are diminished, although the functional residual capacity does not seem as affected.[114] On the basis of results provided by labeled transferrin studies, it has been established that the main drive for the pathophysiologic changes in the lung results from the changes in vascular permeability and protein exudation into the peribronchiolar and parenchymal space.[115] After this process takes place, mortality increases significantly.[116]

The most dreaded complication of pancreatitis is the progression to fulminant necrotizing destruction of the gland. As noted, this occurs via autodigestion and activation of inflammatory pathways by virtue of a wide variety of mediators capable of affecting the circulation in profound ways, with rapid progression to systemic inflammatory syndrome, capillary leak, and irreversible shock. The pulmonary changes are manifested by subclinical hypoxia or by frank ARDS, with serious implications for the patient's prognosis.[117]

Diagnostic Approach

In addition to the biochemical abnormalities, pancreatitis is characterized by radiologically identifiable changes in the gland, best documented by abdominal CT with oral and intravenous contrast enhancement. The presence of glandular edema and peripancreatic fluid accumulation are common in the acute phase of the process, whereas calcifications, fat necrosis, and scarring are sequelae of chronic pancreatitis.[118]

Ultrasonography is useful in identifying concomitant gallbladder pathology, bile duct dilation, and cholelithiasis, but the presence of intraluminal gas makes it an unreliable examination to visualize the pancreas.[119] Newer techniques using magnetic resonance (magnetic resonance cholangiopancreatography [MRCP]) can accurately visualize the pancreatic and biliary tree, often obviating the need for the more invasive endoscopic retrograde cholangiopancreatography (ERCP).[120,121] ERCP is more commonly used in adults, but advances in equipment design and miniaturization of video processors have made ERCP applicable in infants and children.[122,123] Concurrent improvements in the magnetic signal acquisition and processing have reduced the resolution of MRCP and expanded its usefulness for pediatric patients.[120,121,124]

Radiologically, the lung changes during acute pancreatitis are nonspecific and are often mild or unappreciated, even when pulmonary function abnormalities are present. The presence of effusions already has been alluded to, and increased markings, infiltrates, and atelectasis all can be present during the evolution of the pulmonary deterioration. High-resolution CT can help demarcate the alveolar damage and the exudative process that ultimately result in the picture of ARDS.[125] The pulmonary picture is similar to the one observed in shock, or in what is now termed "systemic inflammatory response syndrome."

Clinical Management

Management of pancreatitis is conservative, addressing the following factors: (1) support of cardiovascular homeostasis, (2) judicious use of antibiotics when infected collections or peritonitis is believed to be imminent or established, and (3) nutritional support. More recent evidence suggests improved survival with early introduction of enteral feedings (intragastric or transpyloric) and avoiding reliance on intravenous alimentation, which carries a high risk for serious bacteremia and fungemia.[126-128] Patients benefit from the expertise of tertiary centers with excellent intensive care units and access to important ancillary services such as intervention radiology, gastroenterology, and surgery.

Experimental approaches aimed at inhibiting the inflammatory cascade triggered by noxious cytokines have not changed the natural course of the disease, and much work continues in this field of clinical research. The interruption of systemic absorption and widespread distribution of toxic vasoactive and proteolytic substances by ligation or external draining of the thoracic duct has been promising, but has not been confirmed by additional studies.[101] In an attempt to decrease pancreatic secretion, the somatostatin analogue octreotide and the platelet-activating factor antagonist lexipafant have been tried with mixed results, although the exact mechanism of the purported beneficial effect could not be determined with certainty. In addition to its effects on exocrine and endocrine pancreatic secretion, it is believed that somatostatin has a direct immunomodulator effect, which could play a part in the observed decreased progression to ARDS.[129,130]

The complexity of the processes at play, the variety of cellular and chemical mediators, and the individual genetic predispositions to pancreatic damage under certain stressors all are responsible for the current state of uncertainty regarding best practices beyond supportive medical therapy. Future application of the expanding knowledge in this area would allow effective blockade of the destructive proinflammatory processes, while buttressing the counter-regulatory forces at play triggered by the activation and extravasation of digestive enzymes.

Acknowledgments

The author is deeply grateful to Dr. Walter Berdon for selecting informative cases from his teaching files, for his thoughtful comments regarding the radiologic manifestations of the entities discussed, and for his valuable insights.

References

1. Nelson SP, et al: Prevalence of symptoms of gastroesophageal reflux during childhood: A pediatric practice-based survey. Pediatric Practice Research Group. Arch Pediatr Adolesc Med 154:150-154, 2000.
2. Rudolph CD: Supraesophageal complications of gastroesophageal reflux in children: Challenges in diagnosis and treatment. Am J Med 115(Suppl 3A):150S-156S, 2003.
3. Sivarao DV, Goyal RK: Functional anatomy and physiology of the upper esophageal sphincter. Am J Med 108(Suppl 4a):27S-37S, 2000.
4. Euler AR: Upper respiratory tract complications of gastroesophageal reflux in adult and pediatric-age patients. Dig Dis 16:111-117, 1998.
5. Vandenplas Y, Hassall E: Mechanisms of gastroesophageal reflux and gastroesophageal reflux disease. J Pediatr Gastroenterol Nutr 35:119-136, 2002.
6. Harding SM, Guzzo MR, Richter JE: 24-h esophageal pH testing in asthmatics: Respiratory symptom correlation with esophageal acid events. Chest 115:654-659, 1999.
7. Schan CA., et al: Gastroesophageal reflux-induced bronchoconstriction: An intraesophageal acid infusion study using state-of-the-art technology. Chest 106:731-737, 1994.
8. Gustafsson PM, Kjellman NI, Tibbling L: Bronchial asthma and acid reflux into the distal and proximal oesophagus. Arch Dis Child 65:1255-1258, 1990.
9. Tuchman DN, et al: Comparison of airway responses following tracheal or esophageal acidification in the cat. Gastroenterology 87:872-881, 1984.
10. Herve P, et al: Intraesophageal perfusion of acid increases the bronchomotor response to methacholine and to isocapnic hyperventilation in asthmatic subjects. Am Rev Resp Dis 134:986-989, 1986.
11. Boyle JT, et al: Mechanisms for the association of gastroesophageal reflux and bronchospasm. Am Rev Respir Dis 131:S16-S20, 1985.
12. Gustafsson PM, Tibbling L: Gastro-oesophageal reflux and oesophageal dysfunction in children and adolescents with brain damage. Acta Paediatr 83:1081-1085, 1994.
13. Heine RG, Reddihough DS, Catto-Smith AG: Gastro-oesophageal reflux and feeding problems after gastrostomy in children with severe neurological impairment. Dev Med Child Neurol 37:320-329, 1995.
14. Berseth CL: Gastrointestinal motility in the neonate. Clin Perinatol 23:179-190, 1996.
15. Wenzl TG: Evaluation of gastroesophageal reflux events in children using multichannel intraluminal electrical impedance. Am J Med 115(Suppl 3A):161S-165S, 2003.
16. Wenzl TG, et al: Esophageal pH monitoring and impedance measurement: A comparison of two diagnostic tests for gastroesophageal reflux. J Pediatr Gastroenterol Nutr 34:519-523, 2002.
17. Wenzl TG, Skopnik H: Intraluminal impedance: An ideal technique for evaluation of pediatric gastroesophageal reflux disease. Curr Gastroenterol Rep 2:259-264, 2000.
18. Castell DO, Mainie I, Tutuian R: Non-acid gastroesophageal reflux: Documenting its relationship to symptoms using multichannel intraluminal impedance (MII). Trans Am Clin Climatol Assoc 116:321-333; discussion 333-334, 2005.
19. Gustafsson PM, Tibbling T: 24-hour oesophageal two-level pH monitoring in healthy children and adolescents. Scand J Gastroenterol 23:91-94, 1988.
20. Sasaki CT, Isaacson G: Functional anatomy of the larynx. Otolaryngol Clin North Am 21:595-612, 1988.
21. Bandla HP, Davis SH, Hopkins NE: Lipoid pneumonia: A silent complication of mineral oil aspiration. Pediatrics 103:E19, 1999.
22. Monasterio FO, et al: Swallowing disorders in Pierre Robin sequence: Its correction by distraction. J Craniofac Surg 15:934-941, 2004.
23. Hoffman W: Outcome of tongue-lip plication in patients with severe Pierre Robin sequence. J Craniofac Surg 14:602-608, 2003.
24. Nasr A, Ein SH, Gerstle JT: Infants with repaired esophageal atresia and distal tracheoesophageal fistula with severe respiratory distress: Is it tracheomalacia, reflux, or both? J Pediatr Surg 40:901-903, 2005.
25. Axelrod FB, et al: Fundoplication and gastrostomy in familial dysautonomia. J Pediatr 118:388-394, 1991.
26. Stolar CJ: What do survivors of congenital diaphragmatic hernia look like when they grow up? Semin Pediatr Surg 5:275-279, 1996.
27. Stolar CJ, et al: Anatomic and functional abnormalities of the esophagus in infants surviving congenital diaphragmatic hernia. Am J Surg 159:204-207, 1990.
28. Ijsselstijn H, Tibboel D: The lungs in congenital diaphragmatic hernia: Do we understand? Pediatr Pulmonol 26:204-218, 1998.
29. Kovesi T, Rubin S: Long-term complications of congenital esophageal atresia and/or tracheoesophageal fistula. Chest 126:915-925, 2004.

30. Rudolph CD, et al: Guidelines for evaluation and treatment of gastroesophageal reflux in infants and children: Recommendations of the North American Society for Pediatric Gastroenterology and Nutrition. J Pediatr Gastroenterol Nutr 32 (Suppl 2):S1-S31, 2001.
31. Bastian RW: Videoendoscopic evaluation of patients with dysphagia: An adjunct to the modified barium swallow. Otolaryngol Head Neck Surg 104:339-350, 1991.
32. Kendall KA, Leonard RJ, McKenzie S: Airway protection: Evaluation with videofluoroscopy. Dysphagia 19:65-70, 2004.
33. Vandenplas Y, Hegar B: Diagnosis and treatment of gastro-oesophageal reflux disease in infants and children. J Gastroenterol Hepatol 15:593-603, 2000.
34. Akbunar AT, et al: Diagnosis of orotracheal aspiration using radionuclide salivagram. Ann Nucl Med 17:415-416, 2003.
35. Bar-Sever Z, Connolly LP, Treves ST: The radionuclide salivagram in children with pulmonary disease and a high risk of aspiration. Pediatr Radiol 25(Suppl 1):S180-S183, 1995.
36. Baikie G, et al: Agreement of aspiration tests using barium videofluoroscopy, salivagram, and milk scan in children with cerebral palsy. Dev Med Child Neurol 47:86-93, 2005.
37. Van Den Driessche M, Veereman-Wauters G: Gastric emptying in infants and children. Acta Gastroenterol Belg 66:274-282, 2003.
38. Harding SM, Guzzo MR, Richter JE: The prevalence of gastroesophageal reflux in asthma patients without reflux symptoms. Am J Respir Crit Care Med 162:34-39, 2000.
39. Field SK: Gastroesophageal reflux and asthma: Can the paradox be explained? Can Respir J 7:167-176, 2000.
40. Andze GO, et al: Diagnosis and treatment of gastroesophageal reflux in 500 children with respiratory symptoms: The value of pH monitoring. J Pediatr Surg 26:295-299; discussion 299-300, 1991.
41. Wenzel SE: Proceedings of the ATS Workshop on Refractory Asthma. Am J Respir Crit Care Med 162:2341-2351, 2000.
42. National Institutes of Health National Heart, Lung, and Blood Institute, Expert Panel Report 2: Guidelines for the Diagnosis and Management of Asthma. NIH Publication 97-4051. 1997.
43. Mousa H, et al: Testing the association between gastroesophageal reflux and apnea in infants. J Pediatr Gastroenterol Nutr 41:169-177, 2005.
44. Dewolfe CC: Apparent life-threatening event: A review. Pediatr Clin North Am 52:1127-1146, 2005.
45. McGovern MC, Smith MBH: Yield of diagnostic testing in infants who have had an apparent life-threatening event. Pediatrics 116:1599-1600; author reply 1600, 2005.
46. Fonkalsrud EW, Ament ME: Gastroesophageal reflux in childhood. Curr Probl Surg 33:1-70, 1996.
47. Moissidis I, et al: Milk-induced pulmonary disease in infants (Heiner syndrome). Pediatr Allergy Immunol 16:545-552, 2005.
48. Gonzalez-Crussi F, Hull MT, Grosfeld JL: Idiopathic pulmonary hemosiderosis: Evidence of capillary basement membrane abnormality. Am Rev Respir Dis 114:689-698, 1976.
49. Godfrey S: Pulmonary hemorrhage/hemoptysis in children. Pediatr Pulmonol 37:476-484, 2004.
50. Heine RG, et al: Cow's milk allergy in infancy. Curr Opin Allergy Clin Immunol 2:217-225, 2002.
51. Gorbunov NV, et al: Inflammatory leukocytes and iron turnover in experimental hemorrhagic lung trauma. Exp Mol Pathol 80:11-25, 2006.
52. Le Clainche L, et al: Long-term outcome of idiopathic pulmonary hemosiderosis in children. Medicine 79:318-326, 2000.
53. von Vigier RO, et al: Pulmonary renal syndrome in childhood: A report of twenty-one cases and a review of the literature. Pediatr Pulmonol 29:382-388, 2000.
54. Bass TL, et al: Traumatic adult respiratory distress syndrome. Chest Surg Clin North Am 7:429-442, 1997.
55. Dearborn DG, et al: Clinical profile of 30 infants with acute pulmonary hemorrhage in Cleveland. Pediatrics 110:627-637, 2002.
56. Saeed MM, et al: Prognosis in pediatric idiopathic pulmonary hemosiderosis. Chest 116:721-725, 1999.
57. Plevy S: The immunology of inflammatory bowel disease. Gastroenterol Clin North Am 31:77-92, 2002.
58. Heyman MB, et al: Children with early-onset inflammatory bowel disease (IBD): Analysis of a pediatric IBD consortium registry. J Pediatr 146:35-40, 2005.
59. Urlep D, Mamula P, Baldassano R: Extraintestinal manifestations of inflammatory bowel disease. Min Gastroenterol Dietol 51:147-163, 2005.
60. Danese S, et al: Extraintestinal manifestations in inflammatory bowel disease. World J Gastroenterol 11:7227-7236, 2005.
61. Bhagat S, Das KM: A shared and unique peptide in the human colon, eye, and joint detected by a monoclonal antibody. Gastroenterology 107:103-108, 1994.
62. Diot P, et al: Characterization of 99mTc-DTPA aerosols for lung permeability studies. Respiration 68:313-317, 2001.
63. Storch I, Sachar D, Katz S: Pulmonary manifestations of inflammatory bowel disease. Inflamm Bowel Dis 9:104-115, 2003.
64. Shepherd GM: Hypersensitivity reactions to drugs: Evaluation and management. Mt Sinai J Med 70:113-125, 2003.
65. Parry SD, et al: Sulphasalazine and lung toxicity. Eur Respir J 19:756-764, 2002.
66. Pascual-Lledo JF, et al: Interstitial pneumonitis due to mesalamine. Ann Pharmacother 31:499, 1997.
67. Haralambou G, et al: Bronchiolitis obliterans in a patient with ulcerative colitis receiving mesalamine. Mt Sinai J Med 68:384-388, 2001.
68. Bitton A, et al: Mesalamine-induced lung toxicity. Am J Gastroenterol 91:1039-1040, 1996.
69. Vandenplas O, et al: Granulomatous bronchiolitis associated with Crohn's disease. Am J Respir Crit Care Med 158(5 Pt 1):1676-1679, 1998.
70. Spira A, Grossman R, Balter M: Large airway disease associated with inflammatory bowel disease. Chest 113:1723-1726, 1998.
71. Rickli H, et al: Severe inflammatory upper airway stenosis in ulcerative colitis. Eur Respir J 7:1899-1902, 1994.
72. Mahadeva R, et al: Clinical and radiological characteristics of lung disease in inflammatory bowel disease. Eur Respir J 15:41-48, 2000.
73. Rosen MJ: Chronic cough due to bronchiectasis: ACCP evidence-based clinical practice guidelines. Chest 129(1 Suppl):122S-131S, 2006.

74. Garg K, Lynch DA, Newell JD: Inflammatory airways disease in ulcerative colitis: CT and high-resolution CT features. J Thorac Imaging 8:159-163, 1993.
75. Chooi WK, Morcos SK: High resolution volume imaging of airways and lung parenchyma with multislice CT. Br J Radiol 77(Spec No 1):S98-S105, 2004.
76. Camus P, et al: The lung in inflammatory bowel disease. Medicine 72:151-183, 1993.
77. Rodriquez-Roisin R, et al: Highlights of the ERS Task Force on pulmonary-hepatic vascular disorders (PHD). J Hepatol 42:924-927, 2005.
78. Chongsrisawat V, et al: Relationship between vasoactive intestinal peptide and intrapulmonary vascular dilatation in children with various liver diseases. Acta Paediatr 92:1411-1444, 2003.
79. Krowka MJ, Plevak D: The distinct concepts and implications of hepatopulmonary syndrome and portopulmonary hypertension. Crit Care Med 33:470, 2005.
80. Meyer CA, White CS, Sherman KE: Diseases of the hepatopulmonary axis. RadioGraphics 20:687-698, 2000.
81. Fallon MB: Mechanisms of pulmonary vascular complications of liver disease: Hepatopulmonary syndrome. J Clin Gastroenterol 39(4 Suppl 2):S138-S142, 2005.
82. Ratti L, Pozzi M: The pulmonary involvement in portal hypertension: Portopulmonary hypertension and hepatopulmonary syndrome. Gastroenterol Hepatol 29:40-50, 2006.
83. Moller S, Henriksen JH: Cardiopulmonary complications in chronic liver disease. World J Gastroenterol 12:526-538, 2006.
84. Gupta D, et al: Prevalence of hepatopulmonary syndrome in cirrhosis and extrahepatic portal venous obstruction. Am J Gastroenterol 96:3395-3399, 2001.
85. Luo B, et al: Cholangiocyte endothelin 1 and transforming growth factor beta1 production in rat experimental hepatopulmonary syndrome. Gastroenterology 129:682-695, 2005.
86. Hira HS, et al: A study of hepatopulmonary syndrome among patients of cirrhosis of liver and portal hypertension. Ind J Chest Dis Allied Sci 45:165-171, 2003.
87. Regev A, et al: Transient hepatopulmonary syndrome in a patient with acute hepatitis A. J Viral Hepat 8:83-86, 2001.
88. Tzovaras N, et al: Reversion of severe hepatopulmonary syndrome in a non cirrhotic patient after corticosteroid treatment for granulomatous hepatitis: A case report and review of the literature. World J Gastroenterol 12:336-339, 2006.
89. Santamaria F, et al: Noninvasive investigation of hepatopulmonary syndrome in children and adolescents with chronic cholestasis. Pediatr Pulmonol 33:374-379, 2002.
90. Abrams GA, et al: Use of macroaggregated albumin lung perfusion scan to diagnose hepatopulmonary syndrome: A new approach. Gastroenterology 114:305-310, 1998.
91. Aller R, et al: Diagnosis of hepatopulmonary syndrome with contrast transesophageal echocardiography: Advantages over contrast transthoracic echocardiography. Dig Dis Sci 44:1243-1248, 1999.
92. Lee KN, et al: Hypoxemia and liver cirrhosis (hepatopulmonary syndrome) in eight patients: Comparison of the central and peripheral pulmonary vasculature. Radiology 211:549-553, 1999.
93. McAdams HP, et al: The hepatopulmonary syndrome: Radiologic findings in 10 patients. AJR Am J Roentgenol 166:1379-1385, 1996.
94. Kim HY, et al: Outcomes in patients with hepatopulmonary syndrome undergoing liver transplantation. Transplant Proc 36:2762-2763, 2004.
95. Werlin SL, Kugathasan S, Frautschy BC: Pancreatitis in children. J Pediatr Gastroenterol Nutr 37:591-595, 2003.
96. Jackson WD: Pancreatitis: Etiology, diagnosis, and management. Curr Opin Pediatr 13:447-451, 2001.
97. Teich N, Mossner J: Genetic aspects of chronic pancreatitis. Med Sci Monit 10:RA325-RA328, 2004.
98. Cavestro GM, et al: Genetics of chronic pancreatitis. J Pancreas 6(1 Suppl):53-59, 2005.
99. Stringer MD: Pancreatitis and pancreatic trauma. Semin Pediatr Surg 14:239-246, 2005.
100. Iuchtman M, et al: Post-traumatic intramural duodenal hematoma in children. Isr Med Assoc J 8:95-97, 2006.
101. Pastor CM, Matthay MA, Frossard J-L: Pancreatitis-associated acute lung injury: New insights. Chest 124:2341-1251, 2003.
102. Yoshikawa H, Yamazaki S, Abe T: Acute respiratory distress syndrome in children with severe motor and intellectual disabilities. Brain Dev 27:395-399, 2005.
103. Pezzilli R, et al: Acute pancreatitis in children: An Italian multicentre study. Dig Liver Dis 34:343-348, 2002.
104. Segura RM: Useful clinical biological markers in diagnosis of pleural effusions in children. Paediatr Respir Rev 5(Suppl A):S205-S212, 2004.
105. Zhao X, et al: Influence of mast cells on the expression of adhesion molecules on circulating and migrating leukocytes in acute pancreatitis-associated lung injury. Lung 183:253-264, 2005.
106. Zaninovic V, et al: Cerulein upregulates ICAM-1 in pancreatic acinar cells, which mediates neutrophil adhesion to these cells. Am J Physiol Gastrointest Liver Physiol 279:G666-G676, 2000.
107. Pastor CM, et al: Role of macrophage inflammatory peptide-2 in cerulein-induced acute pancreatitis and pancreatitis-associated lung injury. Lab Invest 83:471-478, 2003.
108. Leindler L, et al: Importance of cytokines, nitric oxide, and apoptosis in the pathological process of necrotizing pancreatitis in rats. Pancreas 29:157-161, 2004.
109. Hartwig W, et al: Trypsin and activation of circulating trypsinogen contribute to pancreatitis-associated lung injury. Am J Physiol Gastrointest Liver Physiol 277(5 Pt 1):G1008-G1016, 1999.
110. Lungarella G, et al: Pulmonary vascular injury in pancreatitis: Evidence for a major role played by pancreatic elastase. Exp Mol Pathol 42:44-59, 1985.
111. Hartwig W, et al: Membrane-bound ICAM-1 is upregulated by trypsin and contributes to leukocyte migration in acute pancreatitis. Am J Physiol Gastrointest Liver Physiol 287:G1194-G1199, 2004.
112. Frossard J-L: Pathophysiology of acute pancreatitis: A multistep disease. Acta Gastroenterol Belg 66:166-173, 2003.
113. Pastor CM, et al: Role of Toll-like receptor 4 on pancreatic and pulmonary injury in a mice model of acute pancreatitis associated with endotoxemia. Crit Care Med 32:1759-1763, 2004.

114. Ates F, Hacievliyagil SS, Karincaoglu M: Clinical significance of pulmonary function tests in patients with acute pancreatitis. Dig Dis Sci 51:7-10, 2006.

115. Foitzik T, et al: Persistent multiple organ microcirculatory disorders in severe acute pancreatitis: Experimental findings and clinical implications. Dig Dis Sci 47:130-138, 2002.

116. Steer ML: Relationship between pancreatitis and lung diseases. Resp Physiol 128:13-16, 2001.

117. Bhatia M, et al: Pathophysiology of acute pancreatitis. Pancreatology 5(2-3):132-144, 2005.

118. Graziani R, et al: The various imaging aspects of chronic pancreatitis. J Pancreas 6(1 Suppl):73-88, 2005.

119. Gupta V, Toskes PP: Diagnosis and management of chronic pancreatitis. Postgrad Med J 81:491-497, 2005.

120. Pamuklar E, Semelka RC: MR imaging of the pancreas. Magn Reson Imaging Clin N Am 13:313-330, 2005.

121. Arcement CM, et al: MRCP in the evaluation of pancreaticobiliary disease in children. Pediatr Radiol 31:92-97, 2001.

122. Cheng C-L, et al: Diagnostic and therapeutic endoscopic retrograde cholangiopancreatography in children: A large series report. J Pediatr Gastroenterol Nutr 41:445-453, 2005.

123. Rocca R, et al: Therapeutic ERCP in paediatric patients. Dig Liver Dis 37:357-362, 2005.

124. Hamada Y, et al: Magnetic resonance cholangiopancreatography on postoperative work-up in children with choledochal cysts. Pediatr Surg Int 20:43-46, 2004.

125. Puneet P, Moochhala S, Bhatia M: Chemokines in acute respiratory distress syndrome. Am J Physiol Lung Cell Mol Physiol 288:L3-L15, 2005.

126. Kaushik N, et al: Enteral feeding without pancreatic stimulation. Pancreas 31:353-359, 2005.

127. O'Keefe SJD, McClave SA: Feeding the injured pancreas. Gastroenterology 129:1129-1130, 2005.

128. Eatock FC, et al: A randomized study of early nasogastric versus nasojejunal feeding in severe acute pancreatitis. Am J Gastroenterol 100:432-439, 2005.

129. Heinrich S, et al: Evidence-based treatment of acute pancreatitis: A look at established paradigms. Ann Surg 243:154-168, 2006.

130. Hoogerwerf WA: Pharmacological management of pancreatitis. Curr Opin Pharmacol 5:578-582, 2005.

131. McGovern MC, Smith MBH: Causes of apparent life threatening events in infants: A systematic review. Arch Dis Child 89:1043-1048, 2004.

132. Kozzi DA, et al: Pathogenesis of ALTE in infants with esophageal atresia. Pediatr Pulmonol 41:488-493, 2001.

133. Black H, Mendoza M, Murin S: Thoracic manifestations of inflammatory bowel disease. Chest 131:524-532, 2007.

134. DeBoeck K, et al: Pancreatitis among patients with cystic fibrosis: Correlation with pancreatic status and genotype. Pediatrics 115:463-469, 2005.

CHAPTER 6

Pulmonary Manifestations of Renal Diseases

Nelson L. Turcios

Role of the Kidney in Fetal Lung
  Growth   121
Physiologic Connections Between the
  Lungs and the Kidneys   121
Diseases That Affect Lungs and
  Kidneys   123
  Wegener Granulomatosis   123
  Systemic Lupus Erythematosus   124
  Goodpasture Syndrome   124
Respiratory Effects of Chronic Renal
  Failure   124
  Pulmonary Edema   125
  Fibrinous Pleuritis   125
  Tuberculosis   125

Pulmonary Calcifications   126
  Urinothorax   126
  Sleep Apnea   127
  Anemia   127
  Pulmonary Embolism   128
  Hemodialysis-Related Hypoxemia   129
Respiratory Effects of Acute Renal
  Failure   130
How Critical Illness and Mechanical
  Ventilation Can Damage the
  Kidneys   131
Summary   132
  References   132

The relationships between the kidneys and the lungs are clinically important ones in health and disease. This chapter first reviews the role of the kidney in fetal lung development and the interactions between respiratory and renal function under normal conditions. Then a brief overview is provided of the large group of diseases that affect the lungs and the kidneys. Most of these conditions are uncommon in pediatric patients, although three of them—Wegener granulomatosis, systemic lupus erythematosus, and Goodpasture syndrome—may be encountered frequently by clinicians. They are discussed in detail elsewhere in this book. This chapter describes how chronic renal failure may affect respiratory function and the intrathoracic structures, and provides a brief review of the corresponding manifestations of acute renal failure and the ways in which they affect respiratory care in children. The phenomenon of dialysis-related hypoxemia is described and explained. Finally, the ways in which critical illness and its management may adversely affect kidney function are summarized.

Role of the Kidney in Fetal Lung Growth

Lung development continues during the middle trimester with branching morphogenesis and is completed postnatally with the development of alveoli. Fetal urine is an important component of the amniotic fluid during late gestation and contributes to lung growth. During fetal development, the kidney also is a major source of proline. Proline aids in the formation of collagen and mesenchyme in the lung, explaining the severe pulmonary hypoplasia secondary to prolonged or severe oligohydramnios (amniotic fluid index <4 for >2 weeks) seen in fetal renal agenesis, urinary tract obstruction, bilateral renal dysplasia, and bilateral cystic kidneys.

Physiologic Connections Between the Lungs and the Kidneys

Lung and kidney function are intimately related in health and disease.[1] Respiratory changes help modulate the systemic effects of renal acid-base disturbances, and the reverse is also true, although renal compensation occurs more slowly than its respiratory counterpart. Under normal circumstances, the lungs and kidneys work together to maintain acid-base balance in the body, according to the relationship described by the Henderson-Hasselbalch equation[1,2]:

$$pH = pK + \log \text{(base concentration/ acid concentration)}$$

According to this equation, the overall acidity or alkalinity of the blood, which is quantified by the negative logarithm of the hydrogen ion concentration (or pH), is determined by the relationship between the amount of base and the amount of acid present, also expressed logarithmically, as modified by a mathematical constant (pK) for the particular acid involved. The bicarbonate-carbonic acid system is the major buffering system of the extracellular fluid. Bicarbonate (HCO_3^-) dissociates into CO_2 and water in the presence of the enzyme carbonic anhydrase, so that the acid-base quotient in the previous equation can be thought of as the HCO_3^- concentration divided by the CO_2 concentration. The CO_2 concentration is related to the partial pressure of CO_2 ($PaCO_2$) in the arterial blood by the solubility constant 0.03, so the Henderson-Hasselbalch equation can be rewritten in terms of what clinicians typically measure:

$$pH = 6.1 + \log [HCO_3^- \text{concentration/} (Paco_2 \times 0.03)]$$

Because the kidneys normally determine the concentration of the HCO_3^-, and the alveolar ventilation regulates the $PaCO_2$, the relationship also can be rewritten conceptually as:

$$pH = pK + \text{(kidneys/lungs)}$$

A decrease in HCO_3^- concentration (metabolic acidosis),[3] whether from an increase in acids in the blood or an overall loss of HCO_3^-, provokes an increase in alveolar ventilation (respiratory alkalosis),[4] which tends to restore the balance between the two and bring the low arterial pH (acidemia) back toward normal. This process may be thought of as respiratory compensation for metabolic acidosis. The stimulus to increase the ventilation is chiefly the action of H^+ ions on the peripheral chemoreceptors.

An increase in HCO_3^- concentration (metabolic alkalosis)[5] causes an increase in arterial pH (alkalemia), which tends to decrease alveolar ventilation (respiratory acidosis).[6] In this instance, respiratory compensation is usually less vigorous, however, because the respiratory stimulant effect of hypercapnia is much stronger than the respiratory depressant effect of alkalemia. The familiar clinical presentation of diabetic ketoacidosis is an example of respiratory compensation for severe metabolic acidosis. Patients with this disorder may hyperventilate to $PaCO_2$ levels of 10 mm Hg or less, which diminishes (but does not completely correct) their severe acidemia. In both instances, the respiratory changes are immediate (within a few minutes) because of the rapidity of equilibration between alveolar gas and pulmonary capillary blood.

In the less frequent situation of primary metabolic alkalosis, as is seen with protracted vomiting or the ingestion of excess alkali, patients typically present with only modest hypercapnia (e.g., $PaCO_2$ 48 to 50 mm Hg) despite pH greater than 7.60. An increase in $PaCO_2$ stimulates the kidneys to retain HCO_3^-, producing metabolic alkalosis, which tends to normalize arterial pH. Conversely, hypocapnia prompts an increased loss of HCO_3^-, causing a compensatory metabolic acidosis that decreases arterial pH. The renal responses to respiratory acid-base disturbances occur much more slowly, however—over a few days—than do respiratory adjustments to metabolic disturbances. As a result, because carbonic acid/HCO_3^- buffering acts immediately, but is relatively weak, sudden alterations in respiratory acid-base status cause more sudden and severe changes in arterial pH than do their primary metabolic counterparts. An example of the more gradual adjustment of metabolic status with changes in ventilatory status is respiratory acidosis in patients with cystic fibrosis. When such patients present with a severe exacerbation, they may be severely acidemic if hypercapnia has developed rapidly, whereas the same

Table 6-1	Renal Compensation for Respiratory Acidosis		
	Normal	Acute Respiratory Acidosis*	Chronic Respiratory Acidosis[†]
pH	7.40	7.24	7.38
$PaCO_2$ (mm Hg)	40	56	56
HCO_3^- (mEq/L)	24	25	33

*Minutes to hours; no renal compensation.
[†]Days to weeks; renal compensation present.
Adapted from Pierson DJ: Respiratory considerations in the patient with renal failure. Respir Care 51:413-422, 2006.

$PaCO_2$ in a clinically stable patient tends to be associated with a much more normal pH (Table 6-1).

A more comprehensive discussion of the different types of acid-base disturbance, their effects on respiratory and renal function, and their management is beyond the scope of this brief review. More recent reviews of these topics are available, however.[3-8] The kidneys also regulate fluid balance in the body,[1] and derangements in overall volume status can affect pulmonary function, as discussed subsequently.

Diseases That Affect Lungs and Kidneys

There are many "pulmonary-renal syndromes" that affect the lungs and the kidneys.[1,9-11] These disorders most commonly manifest with hemoptysis from diffuse alveolar hemorrhage, along with renal failure associated with either acute glomerulonephritis or other vasculitis. Patients may develop pulmonary hemorrhage without evidence of renal involvement, however, with the latter appearing only later in the clinical course. The reverse sequence may also occur. Many of these diseases have overlapping and variable features, prompting investigators to classify them in various ways. Schwarz and colleagues[12,13] have used the presence or absence of pulmonary capillaritis as a means of categorizing these diseases (Table 6-2).

Another classification of patients with pulmonary hemorrhage and nephritis uses the presence or absence of anti–glomerular basement membrane antibody; antineutrophil cytoplasmic antibody; or small, medium, or large vessel vasculitis, although overlapping features in different cases often make clear

Table 6-2	Diseases That Affect Lungs and Kidneys
Diseases that cause alveolar hemorrhage in the presence of pulmonary capillaritis	
Wegener granulomatosis	
Henoch-Schönlein purpura	
Microscopic polyangiitis	
Immune complex–associated glomerulonephritis	
Pauci-immune glomerulonephritis	
Mixed cryoglobulinemia	
Diseases that cause alveolar hemorrhage with pulmonary capillaritis variably present	
Systemic lupus erythematosus	
Other connective tissue diseases	
Goodpasture syndrome	
Diseases that cause alveolar hemorrhage without pulmonary capillaritis	
Thrombotic thrombocytopenic purpura	
Drug-induced (e.g., penicillamine)	
Diseases in which alveolar hemorrhage is not a typical feature	
Churg-Strauss syndrome	

Adapted from Pierson DJ: Respiratory considerations in the patient with renal failure. Respir Care 51:413-422, 2006.

distinction difficult.[14] Three of the most familiar diseases with pulmonary and renal manifestations are Wegener granulomatosis, systemic lupus erythematosus, and Goodpasture syndrome (see Chapter 11).

Wegener Granulomatosis

Wegener granulomatosis is a clinical syndrome consisting mainly of necrotizing granulomatous vasculitis of the upper and lower respiratory tract, along with glomerulonephritis.[9,15] The eyes, ears, heart, skin, joints, and central nervous system also may be involved. It is the most common vasculitis involving the lungs and most frequently affects school-age children and adolescents. Sinusitis is the most common clinical manifestation, followed by fever, arthralgias, cough, rhinitis, hemoptysis, otitis media, epistaxis, and ocular inflammation.[9,15] Although Wegener granulomatosis may be confined to the kidneys, the lungs are involved in more than 80% of all patients with the disease. Likewise, some patients have pulmonary but not renal involvement. The pulmonary involvement varies, but localized infiltrates or nodules or both, either bilateral or unilateral, are most common.

Cavitations may occur in 10% to 20% of cases. The cause of the disease is unknown, but it is characterized by the presence of positive tests for antineutrophil cytoplasmic antibody in at least 90% of affected patients. Wegener granulomatosis was almost always fatal within a few months before the advent of combination therapy with corticosteroids and cytotoxic agents, but today more than three quarters of all patients achieve complete remission, with long-term survival.[11,15]

Systemic Lupus Erythematosus

Systemic lupus erythematosus is a multisystem inflammatory disorder of unknown cause, which is most common in young women.[16] It is characterized by the presence of antinuclear antibodies. Its many manifestations include a characteristic but highly variable malar rash, photosensitivity, arthritis, various neuropsychiatric problems, and hematologic and immune defects. Pulmonary and renal involvements are very common. Thoracic manifestations include pleuritis, acute lupus pneumonitis, interstitial pulmonary fibrosis, pulmonary vasculitis, diffuse alveolar hemorrhage, pulmonary hypertension, organizing pneumonia, and the "shrinking lung syndrome."[17] Pleuritis, with pleuritic pain and effusions, is common, as is acute pneumonitis. Although these usually occur in patients with an established diagnosis of lupus, either of them, and any of the other intrathoracic processes listed, may be the initial manifestation of the disease. Systemic lupus erythematosus has a highly variable course, and the response to treatment and the overall prognosis may be difficult to predict.

Goodpasture Syndrome

Goodpasture syndrome is a disorder of unknown etiology, manifested by diffuse alveolar hemorrhage and glomerulonephritis. It is also known as anti–glomerular basement membrane antibody disease because the presence of such antibodies is characteristic and believed to account for at least some of its manifestations. It is most common in young men, particularly in the fourth decade of life, and manifests with cough, hemoptysis, and fatigue. Alveolar hemorrhage seems to be more common among patients who smoke. Although either pulmonary or renal involvement may be present in isolation, at least at the time of presentation, most patients with Goodpasture syndrome have both. The diagnosis is typically made with renal biopsy. The disease is treated with plasmapheresis, corticosteroids, and cytotoxic drugs, but the prognosis is guarded at best, and dialysis or renal transplantation is often necessary.

Respiratory Effects of Chronic Renal Failure

Numerous complications related to the respiratory system occur in patients with chronic renal disease (Table 6-3).[1,18-20] Some of these are related to alterations in volume status, plasma oncotic pressure, bone and mineral metabolism, concomitant heart failure, and altered immune function in such patients, although in other instances the precise mechanisms are not well understood.

Table 6-3	Respiratory Complications of Chronic Renal Failure
Pulmonary edema	
Fibrinous pleuritis	
Tuberculosis	
Pulmonary calcification	
Urinothorax	
Sleep apnea	
Anemia	
Pulmonary embolism	
Dialysis-associated hypoxemia	

Adapted from Pierson DJ: Respiratory considerations in the patient with renal failure. Respir Care 51:413-422, 2006.

Pulmonary Edema

Pulmonary edema (Fig. 6-1) is a common complication in acute and chronic renal failure.[1] Its pathogenesis is not fully understood. Uremia may be associated with pulmonary edema as the result of overhydration, expansion of the blood volume, and elevation of the pulmonary microvascular pressures, compounded by anemia and reduced colloid osmotic pressures. Hypoalbuminemia, characteristic of chronic renal failure, decreases plasma oncotic pressure and promotes movement of fluid out of the pulmonary capillaries. The increased hydrostatic pressure that occurs may result from the altered vascular permeability caused by the increased metabolic products of uremia, which also fosters such movement. One would assume that the edema fluid resulting from these processes would be low in protein, as is characteristic of cardiogenic or hydrostatic pulmonary edema. The finding of increased protein concentrations in the edema fluid of patients with renal failure[21] suggests, however, that capillary permeability also is altered. Such a suggestion is supported by the occurrence of pulmonary edema in patients who are clinically normovolemic and do not have other features of heart failure. Other studies of the edema fluid in patients with chronic renal failure[22] have found low protein levels, however, more consistent with those found in heart failure than

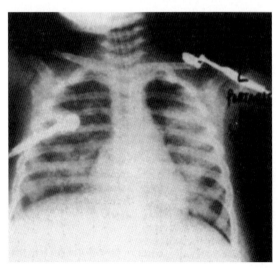

Figure 6-1. Pulmonary edema as seen in a chest x-ray of a 4-year-old child with nephrotic syndrome.

in inflammatory conditions such as acute respiratory distress syndrome (ARDS).

Left ventricular failure is common in chronic renal failure, further complicating attempts to clarify the nature of pulmonary edema in patients with this condition. Pulmonary congestion in patients with chronic renal failure is associated with a restrictive pattern on pulmonary function testing, and reduced airflow rates can be observed on spirometry. These abnormalities have been shown to improve or resolve with hemodialysis.[23-25] This observation would seem to strengthen the argument that increased lung water results primarily from overall hypervolemia in the presence of low serum albumin levels in this condition, and accounts for the symptoms and signs traditionally associated with "uremic lung."[19]

Fibrinous Pleuritis

Pleural disease is common in patients with chronic renal failure, being present in as many as 20% to 40% of autopsies on adult patients with this condition.[1,26,27] The most common manifestation encountered clinically is pleural effusion, which was present in 3% of all patients with end-stage renal disease in one series.[28] The effusion is typically an exudate and may be hemorrhagic.[27,29] Effusions are typically unilateral and can be quite large. Most patients with fibrinous pleuritis are asymptomatic. Dyspnea is the most common symptom, but this condition also can be associated with fever and pleuritic chest pain, sometimes with an audible friction rub on auscultation. Fibrothorax also can occur.

Tuberculosis

The incidence of tuberculosis is increasing worldwide. Compared with the general population, patients with chronic renal failure and patients on long-term dialysis have at least a several-fold greater risk of developing tuberculosis.[30] Patients with chronic renal failure are immunocompromised. Because of an impairment of cellular immunity, patients with chronic renal failure are susceptible to reactivation of tuberculosis. Seventy patients were treated by continuous ambulatory peritoneal dialysis in a pediatric nephrology department during an 8-year period.[31] Tuberculosis was diagnosed in four patients, representing 5.7% of all continuous ambulatory peritoneal dialysis patients in that study. One patient had extrapulmonary tuberculosis (tuberculosis osteomyelitis), and the others had pulmonary tuberculosis. All patients were treated with antituberculous drugs. Two patients with pulmonary tuberculosis were cured. Symptoms improved in the other two patients, but they died at home of unknown causes.

An 8-year-old boy receiving maintenance hemodialysis for chronic renal failure developed mediastinal lymph node tuberculosis. He showed only intermittent fever, recurring every 2 weeks, with no other symptoms suggesting tuberculosis. Although tuberculosis skin test was negative, and staining and culture of gastric aspirate specimens failed to provide evidence of tuberculosis, a lymph node biopsy specimen showed caseating granulomas. Antituberculous therapy with isoniazid, rifampin, pyrazinamide, and ethambutol was given for 12 months, resulting in complete resolution of the tuberculosis, with no subsequent recurrence.[32] It is recommended that all children with chronic renal failure in regions of high prevalence of tuberculosis should be investigated for tuberculosis, especially if they have a cough or fever of unknown etiology.

Renal insufficiency complicates the management of tuberculosis because the kidneys clear some antituberculosis medications. Management may be complicated further by the removal of some antituberculosis agents via hemodialysis. Some adjustment in dosing is commonly necessary in patients with renal insufficiency and end-stage renal disease receiving hemodialysis. Increasing the dosing interval, instead of decreasing the dose of the antituberculosis agent, is recommended and either estimating or measuring creatinine clearance.[30]

Pulmonary Calcifications

Calcifications occur as a complication of chronic renal failure in adult patients and may be found in various visceral organs and soft tissues. Calcifications have been implicated as causes of ischemic necrosis, cardiac arrhythmias, and respiratory failure. Soft tissue calcification has been regarded as rare, however, in pediatric renal patients. In a retrospective review of clinical, biochemical, and autopsy data of 120 patients with uremia, on dialysis, or after renal transplantation,[33] soft tissue calcification was found in 72 patients (60%). Forty-three patients (36%) had systemic calcinosis; the lung was the most frequent site of mineral deposition. By multiple logistic regression analysis, the use of vitamin D or its analogues, the form of vitamin D medication prescribed, the peak calcium × phosphorus product, the age at onset of renal failure, and male sex were together associated with calcinosis. Vitamin D therapy showed the strongest independent association with calcinosis, and the probability of calcinosis was greater in patients receiving calcitriol compared with dihydrotachysterol and vitamin D_2 or D_3. The duration of renal failure, peak serum calcium, serum calcium and phosphorus at death, and primary renal diagnosis were not statistically associated with calcinosis.

The rapid administration of sodium bicarbonate to correct severe metabolic acidosis has been associated with soft tissue calcification. Acidosis increases while alkalosis decreases the proportion of ionized calcium, and calcium deposition in soft tissues may occur during the rapid correction or overcorrection of acidosis or with alkalosis. Alkalinization or overcorrection of an acidosis may facilitate the development of ectopic calcification.[34]

When calcification occurs in the lungs, it is frequently asymptomatic. Although sometimes not apparent on chest radiography, pulmonary calcification usually can be detected on computed tomography (CT), or, more specifically, on Tc 99m diphosphonate scanning.[35] When visible on the standard chest radiograph, pulmonary calcification most often produces small nodular opacities, which occasionally may coalesce into larger infiltrates (Fig. 6-2).[36,37]

Urinothorax

Urinothorax, or collection of urine in the pleural space, is a very rare complication of obstructive uropathy.[38] Most patients who

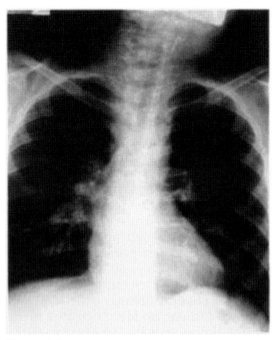

Figure 6-2. Pulmonary calcifications on a chest x-ray of a 4-year-old child with chronic renal failure.

are found to have urinothorax also have a urine collection (urinoma) in the abdominal cavity or retroperitoneal space.[39] Leakage from the urinary tract may cause urinoma, which can lead to urinothorax. The urinothorax usually disappears within a few days after adequate urinary drainage has been established. Reported underlying causes include posterior urethral valves, nephrolithiasis, blunt renal trauma, ureteral instrumentation, or ureteral surgery.[39] The pleural fluid in urinothorax is a transudate, although the lactate dehydrogenase level can be high, causing misclassification as an exudate.[38] The pH and glucose levels tend to be low. An elevated pleural fluid-to-serum creatinine ratio (which should be about 1, but may be ≥10 in urinothorax) confirms the diagnosis.

Sleep Apnea

Sleep apnea is common in adults with chronic renal failure.[1,40-42] Its prevalence is said to be 10-fold higher in adults with end-stage renal disease than in the general population,[43] and studies have found that at least 60% of patients on long-term hemodialysis have the disorder.[18,44] Other sleep disturbances, such

as restless legs syndrome and periodic limb movement disorder, also are common in this population.[44] Several potential explanations have been proposed, but the mechanism remains unknown. There seems to be a strong link between sleep apnea and nocturnal hypoxemia and cardiovascular complications in patients with chronic renal failure.[45,46] Hemodialysis during the night is said to have an ameliorating effect on sleep apnea,[43,47,48] although the reason for this also remains unclear. As in obstructive sleep apnea unassociated with renal disease, treatment with continuous positive airway pressure is effective. Breathing disorders during sleep complicating chronic renal failure in children is an area that warrants investigation.

Anemia

Normochromic normocytic anemia is a common and important manifestation in children with chronic renal failure when their glomerular filtration rate is less than 35 mL/min/1.73 m² body surface area, but it may develop earlier in some forms of renal disease. An inadequate erythropoiesis due to insufficient erythropoietin synthesis in the kidneys is the main cause of renal anemia. Other reasons include reduced red blood cell life span, chronic blood loss, iron deficiency, inhibitors of erythropoiesis, and malnutrition. The presence of anemia contributes to many of the symptoms of uremia, including decreased appetite, decreased energy, poor cardiac function, and poor school performance.[49,50]

If the anemia is untreated, hemoglobin concentrations typically decrease to less than 10 g/dL, and frequently to half or less of the normal value. With blood oxygen carrying capacity markedly diminished, cardiac output must increase to maintain normal tissue oxygen delivery, and even in the absence of pulmonary disease, patients are vulnerable to tissue hypoxia during exertion and at times of acute illness. Correction of anemia dramatically improves the quality of life of a child with chronic renal failure. Presently, the goal of anemia management is to maintain hematocrit concentrations at 33% to 36% and a hemoglobin concentration of at least 11 g/L. This objective can be accomplished by weekly intravenous or subcutaneous administration of recombinant erythropoietin and iron preparations. If adequate iron stores cannot be maintained with oral therapy, intravenous iron should be considered. Treatment with recombinant human erythropoietin corrects anemia, avoids the requirement for blood transfusions, and improves quality of life and exercise tolerance.[51] To optimize anemia management in children with chronic renal failure, future research should concentrate on the normalization of hemoglobin early in the course of chronic renal failure, and the long-term effects on the child's development.

Pulmonary Embolism

Pulmonary embolism is an uncommon complication in children with renal diseases, but a potentially serious and fatal disease. Children with nephrotic syndrome are at increased risk of thromboembolic events. The incidence of this complication in children is 2% to 5%, which represents a much lower risk than that of adults with nephrotic syndrome.[72] Nephrotic syndrome is primarily a pediatric disease. The characteristic features of nephrotic syndrome are heavy proteinuria (>40 mg/m^2/hr), hypoalbuminemia (<2.5 g/dL), edema, and hypercholesterolemia.[73] Most children (90%) with nephrotic syndrome have a form of idiopathic nephrotic syndrome.[74] The risk of thrombosis is related to increased prothrombotic factors (fibrinogen, thrombocytosis, hemoconcentration, relative immobilization) and decreased fibrinolytic factors (urinary losses of antithrombin III, proteins C and S).[75]

The effects of pulmonary embolism depend on the extent to which it obstructs the pulmonary circulation, coexistent cardiopulmonary disease, and vasoactive mediators. Acute pulmonary embolism, obstructing more than 50% of the pulmonary circulation, increases right ventricular afterload. Because the thin-walled right ventricle is not accustomed to working against a sudden obstruction, right ventricular dilatation occurs, and the right ventricular and pulmonary artery pressures

increase. Right ventricular dilatation leads to tricuspid regurgitation and may eventually compromise the filling of the left ventricle. In addition, right ventricular enlargement causes leftward shift of the interventricular septum, resulting in an impaired left ventricular filling during diastole. Cardiac output decreases, and the patient becomes hypotensive. The increased right ventricular pressure compresses the right coronary artery, decreasing subendocardial perfusion, and as a consequence, cardiac ischemia may develop.

The clinical manifestations of pulmonary embolism vary, and no group of physical findings yields a high positive predictive value. Pleuritic chest pain, dyspnea, apprehension, and cough are the most common complaints, and tachypnea is the most common physical finding. Other potential findings include crackles, increased intensity of the pulmonary component of the second heart sound, tachycardia, diaphoresis, wheezing, and hemoptysis. Patients with severe pulmonary embolism can even present with hemodynamic instability, cor pulmonale, and shock. Fever, chest pain, and respiratory manifestations may suggest heart disease, or masquerade as pneumonia; however, significant hypoalbuminemia may raise the index of suspicion.

Because the clinical diagnosis lacks sensitivity and specificity, objective diagnostic imaging is necessary to establish or rule out the presence of pulmonary embolism. An electrocardiogram and arterial blood gases are useful in ruling out other diseases. The measurement of the breakdown product of cross-linked fibrin (D-dimer) in plasma is a sensitive but nonspecific test for suspected venous thrombosis. In adults, studies showed that it is safe to exclude pulmonary embolism in patients with a normal D-dimer level. Chest radiographs are often normal in patients with pulmonary embolism. Ventilation/perfusion imaging displays regional blood flow and ventilation defects by noninvasive means and is safe and inexpensive. A normal ventilation/perfusion scan does not exclude a pulmonary embolism, however. Helical (spiral) CT is becoming the first-choice diagnostic test for pulmonary embolism in many centers. An iodinated contrast agent that is injected in a peripheral vessel visualizes the pulmonary vessels. Pulmonary embolism is seen as partial or complete filling defects in pulmonary arteries. This scan is particularly useful in patients with concomitant lung disease. Pulmonary angiography is the gold standard diagnostic test for pulmonary embolism.[76]

The optimal treatment of hypercoagulability in nephrotic syndrome has not been prospectively investigated, and randomized trials to guide the therapy are lacking. Prophylactic anticoagulation is not recommended in children unless they have had a previous thromboembolic event. Overaggressive diuresis should be avoided, and use of indwelling catheters should be limited because these factors may increase the likelihood of clotting complications. Unfractionated heparin should be used in the initial phase of anticoagulation.[76,77] It functions as an antithrombotic agent by binding to and potentiating the activity of antithrombin. Careful monitoring of the activated partial thromboplastin time and platelets is important. Low-molecular-weight heparin is an equally effective alternative to unfractionated heparin.[76,77] Similar to unfractionated heparin, the anticoagulant activity of low-molecular-weight heparin results from catalyzing the ability of antithrombin to inactivate coagulation factors. Monitoring of the anti–factor Xa assay should be done. Warfarin (Coumadin), which suppresses vitamin K–dependent clotting factors, should be started 24 to 48 hours after heparin therapy is begun. Generally, anticoagulation therapy for a minimum of 6 to 12 months is recommended.[77] Some authors have suggested continuing anticoagulation for as long as the patient is nephrotic.[77]

Thrombolytic agents such as plasminogen activators, including urokinase, streptokinase, and tissue plasminogen activator, also are useful. In most centers, tissue plasminogen activator is favored over the other thrombolytic agents because of fibrin specificity and affinity and low immunogenicity.[76] Thrombolytic therapy causes faster resolution of the embolus than heparin therapy.

Open surgical embolectomy can be beneficial in hemodynamically unstable patients for whom thrombolysis is contraindicated.[76]

There are several techniques. Effective fragmentation of central emboli and dislocation of the fragments to the periphery has been reported in children.

Hemodialysis-Related Hypoxemia

Shortly after it was introduced in the treatment of renal failure, most patients undergoing hemodialysis were discovered to develop hypoxemia while connected to the dialysis apparatus.[1] This phenomenon has generated much interest among renal and respiratory clinicians as to its possible mechanisms. Proposed explanations included a shift in the oxyhemoglobin dissociation curve because of the increased pH during dialysis, depression of central ventilatory drive, impairment of oxygen diffusion, leukostasis in small pulmonary vessels leading to mismatching of ventilation and perfusion, and alveolar hypoventilation because of diffusion of CO_2 into the dialysate.[18]

Studies in animals and humans showed that leukocytes did accumulate in the lungs during hemodialysis, with activation of complement and other events associated with inflammation.[54,55] For several years, "dialysis lung" was a subject of intense interest at the bedside and in the laboratory. It was shown that PaO_2 decreases within a few minutes of the initiation of hemodialysis, usually by 10 to 15 mm Hg, but sometimes considerably more, reaching a nadir after 30 to 60 minutes and then returning to predialysis levels on termination of the procedure.[18,56] The magnitude of the decrease in PaO_2 varies according to the chemical composition of the dialysate and the type of membrane used.[57] Current understanding of dialysis-related hypoxemia is based on the fundamentals of alveolar ventilation, as taught in physiology class. Leukostasis and complement activation do occur during dialysis, but they are almost certainly unrelated to the observed changes in PaO_2. The hypoxemia is explained by decreased alveolar ventilation in response to diffusion of CO_2 into the dialysate (Fig. 6-3).

As CO_2 diffuses into the dialysate, the CO_2 content in venous blood decreases. Because ventilation is tightly controlled by the peripheral and central chemoreceptors in response

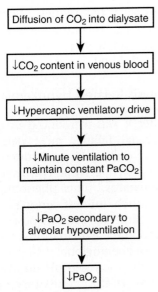

Figure 6-3. Pathogenesis of dialysis-associated hypoxemia.

to changes in $PaCO_2$, this decrease in blood CO_2 content diminishes central ventilatory drive and decreases minute ventilation. Because some of the body's CO_2 production is being eliminated through dialysis, to maintain a normal $PaCO_2$, less CO_2 must be eliminated via the lungs. As alveolar ventilation falls and oxygen extraction remains the same, alveolar Po_2 (Pao_2) decreases, and Pao_2 decreases.

That this basic physiologic sequence is responsible for dialysis-associated hypoxemia was finally shown by a series of studies of ventilation and perfusion in several laboratories.[56,58,59] This mechanism is an example of alveolar hypoventilation without hypercapnia,[60] something that is possible only if CO_2 is being removed from the body by some route other than the lungs.

Respiratory Effects of Acute Renal Failure

Acute renal failure is common in the intensive care unit (ICU).[1] An observational study of nearly 30,000 adults admitted to the ICUs of 54 hospitals in 23 countries found that 5.7% of all patients had acute respiratory failure during their stay, and that nearly 75% of these required some form of renal replacement therapy.[52] Development of acute renal failure predisposes patients to overall fluid overload, and

decreased plasma oncotic pressure from hypoalbuminemia and hemodilution promotes leakage of fluid from pulmonary capillaries. The restrictive effects of pulmonary interstitial and alveolar edema, pleural effusion, and chest wall edema increase the work of spontaneous breathing and may contribute to the development of acute ventilatory failure. In addition, the metabolic acidosis present in most instances of acute renal failure increases the demand for ventilation through compensatory respiratory alkalosis, further disrupting the relationship between the patient's ventilatory needs and capabilities. Pulmonary edema and ventilation at low lung volumes can cause or worsen hypoxemia.

Acute renal failure may necessitate numerous adjustments to the management of mechanical ventilation (Table 6-4). Higher airway pressure is required to maintain the same level of ventilation in the presence of

Table 6-4	Ways in Which Acute Renal Failure Affects Ventilator Management
Decreased Respiratory System Compliance	
Intrapulmonary causes	
Pulmonary edema	
Airway edema	
Extrapulmonary causes	
Pleural effusion	
Pericardial effusion	
Chest wall edema	
Clinical implication	
Requirement for higher airway pressure	
Increased Airway Resistance	
Causes	
Airway edema	
Decreased lung volumes	
Clinical implication	
Increased likelihood of hyperinflation and auto-PEEP	
Metabolic Acidosis	
Cause	
Impaired excretion of acid and metabolic products	
Clinical implications	
Need for compensatory hyperventilation	
Worse acidemia with lung protective ventilation	
Increased minute ventilation requirement may interfere with weaning	

Adapted from Pierson DJ: Respiratory considerations in the patient with renal failure. Respir Care 51:413-422, 2006.

pulmonary edema, pleural effusion, or total body fluid overload. Airway mucosal edema can reduce effective airway diameter, predisposing to air trapping and endogenous positive end-expiratory pressure, which can reduce venous return, compromising cardiac function further and increasing the risk of alveolar rupture.[53]

The management of acute lung injury (ALI) and ARDS using lung protective ventilation is made more difficult in the presence of metabolic acidosis, which increases ventilatory drive and worsens acidemia related to permissive hypercapnia. Because low tidal volume, lung protective ventilation substantially improves survival in ALI and ARDS, its use should not be abandoned because of acidemia in the face of acute renal failure. Using a dialysate solution with a higher concentration of bicarbonate can facilitate "compensation" for hypercapnia and permit renal replacement therapy and lung protective ventilation to be maintained. Weaning in the face of a metabolic acidosis is challenging because of the requirement that the patient be able to maintain higher than usual minute ventilation. Otherwise healthy patients may have no trouble with this requirement, but in patients with severe obstructive lung disease or ARDS, weaning may have to be deferred until either ventilatory function improves or the required hyperpnea diminishes.

How Critical Illness and Mechanical Ventilation Can Damage the Kidneys

Patients may be admitted to the ICU because of illness or injury causing acute renal failure. There are several ways, however, in which critical illness not initially involving the kidneys, and the management of that illness in the ICU, can precipitate iatrogenic renal damage (Table 6-5).[1] Just as acute processes that precipitate the systemic inflammatory response syndrome predispose patients to ALI and ARDS, these same processes are associated with the development of acute renal failure in the ICU.[61] Urinary tract infection, the most common hospital-acquired infection, can lead to

Table 6-5	Mechanisms by Which Critical Illness and Its Management Can Damage the Kidneys

Systemic effects of sepsis

Intensive care unit–acquired urinary tract infection

Drug toxicity

Abdominal compartment syndrome

Ventilator-induced renal injury

Adverse effects of permissive hypercapnia and hypoxia on renal blood flow

Renal hypoperfusion owing to decreased cardiac output (increased intrathoracic pressure)

Effects of systemic inflammatory mediators released in response to mechanical ventilation

Adapted from Pierson DJ: Respiratory considerations in the patient with renal failure. Respir Care 51:413-422, 2006.

renal failure, particularly in patients with underlying renal disease. A host of drugs used in the ICU can cause or aggravate renal failure. Shock from any cause is a known precipitant of acute renal failure, as are conditions that predispose to diminished renal perfusion.

One of the latter conditions that has received increasing attention in recent years is abdominal compartment syndrome.[62-64] In this syndrome, increased intra-abdominal pressure impairs venous return to the heart, diminishes cardiac output, and causes venous congestion of the abdominal organs, including the kidneys. Clinically, the abdominal compartment syndrome is characterized by hypotension, increased airway pressure, and oliguria. In this clinical setting, its presence is confirmed by measurement of pressure in the urinary bladder. Although some authors consider intravesical pressures greater than 12 mm Hg to be associated with adverse effects,[64] others use a pressure of 30 cm H_2O or greater to diagnose the syndrome.[65]

Although ventilator-induced lung injury is now a widely accepted entity and a much-investigated subject,[66-68] until more recently, much less attention was focused on the potential association between mechanical ventilation and renal injury. An increasing body of experimental evidence supports the concept that ventilatory support, particularly with high airway pressure and distending volume, can damage the kidneys and the lungs.[69-71] In addition, permissive hypercapnia and permissive hypoxemia, although potentially protecting the lungs from mechanical and biochemical damage, may be associated with adverse effects on renal perfusion and excretory function.[69] The emerging concept of biotrauma,[68] through which mechanical events in the lungs and airways initiate systemic processes that adversely affect other tissues and organs, may apply to the kidneys and to the lungs.[69]

Summary

Awareness of the relationship of respiratory and renal function is important in managing patients with diseases of the lungs and the kidneys. Among the disease processes with pulmonary and renal manifestations, Wegener granulomatosis, systemic lupus erythematosus, and Goodpasture syndrome may be commonly encountered in respiratory care. Patients with chronic renal failure are subject to several important respiratory complications, including pulmonary edema, pleural effusions, and other manifestations of fibrinous pleuritis. In managing acute renal failure, the clinician often must contend with respiratory manifestations of volume overload and metabolic acidosis. Mechanical ventilation in patients with renal failure can be especially challenging, particularly with respect to lung protective ventilation and weaning. Although it was previously believed to be caused by pulmonary leukostasis and complement activation triggered by the dialysis membranes, hypoxemia during dialysis is now understood to be a predictable effect of the loss of CO_2 into the dialysate. Critical illness of any primary cause predisposes patients not only to ALI and ARDS, but also to development of acute renal failure. Finally, there is currently an increasing appreciation of the potential for ventilator-induced renal injury, and this subject of investigation is sure to see more activity in the future.

References

1. Pierson DJ: Respiratory considerations in the patient with renal failure. Respir Care 51:413-422, 2006.
2. Adrogue HE, Adrogue HJ: Acid-base physiology. Respir Care 46:328-341, 2001.
3. Swenson ER: Metabolic acidosis. Respir Care 46:342-353, 2001.
4. Foster GT, Vaziri ND, Sassoon CS: Respiratory alkalosis. Respir Care 46:384-391, 2001.
5. Khanna A, Kurtzman NA: Metabolic alkalosis. Respir Care 46:354-365, 2001.
6. Epstein SK, Singh N: Respiratory acidosis. Respir Care 46:366-383, 2001.
7. Kraut JA, Madias NE: Approach to patients with acid-base disorders. Respir Care 46:392-403, 2001.
8. Madias NE, Adrogue HJ: Cross-talk between two organs: How the kidney responds to disruption of acid-base balance by the lung. Nephron Physiol 93:61-66, 2003.
9. Akikusa JD, et al: Clinical features and outcomes of pediatric Wegener's syndrome. Arthritis Rheum 57:837-844, 2007.
10. Godfrey S: Pulmonary hemorrhage and hemoptysis in children. Pediatr Pulmonol 37:476-484, 2004.
11. von Vigier RO, et al: Pulmonary renal syndrome in childhood: A report of twenty-one cases and a review of the literature. Pediatr Pulmonol 29:382-388, 2000.
12. Schwarz MI, Collard HR, King TE Jr: Diffuse alveolar hemorrhage and other rare infiltrative disorders. In Mason RJ, et al, eds: Murray and Nadel's Textbook of Respiratory Medicine. Philadelphia, WB Saunders, 2005, pp 1656-1678.
13. Collard HR, Schwarz MI: Diffuse alveolar hemorrhage. Clin Chest Med 25:583-592, 2004.
14. Niles JL, et al: The syndrome of lung hemorrhage and nephritis is usually an ANCA-associated condition. Arch Intern Med 156:440-445, 1996.
15. Fauci AS, et al: Wegener's granulomatosis: Prospective clinical and therapeutic experience with patients for 21 years. Ann Intern Med 98:76-85, 1983.
16. Gutiérrez-Suárez R, et al: A proposal for a pediatric version of the Systemic Lupus International Collaborating Clinics/American College of Rheumatology Damage Index based on the analysis of 1,015 patients with juvenile-onset systemic lupus erythematosus. Arthritis Rheum 54:2989-2996, 2006.
17. Eid NS, Buchino JJ, Schikler KN: Pulmonary manifestations of rheumatic diseases. Pediatr Pulmonol Suppl 18:91-92, 1999.
18. Rodriguez-Roisin R, Barbera JA: Pulmonary complications of abdominal disease. In Mason RJ, et al, eds: Murray and Nadel's Textbook of Respiratory Medicine. Philadelphia, WB Saunders, 2005, pp 2223-2241.
19. Grassi V, et al: Uremic lung. Contrib Nephrol 106:36-42, 1994.
20. Gavelli G, Zompatori M: Thoracic complications in uremic patients and in patients undergoing dialytic treatment: State-of-the-Art. Eur Radiol 7:708-717, 1997.
21. Rackow EC, et al: Uremic pulmonary edema. Am J Med 64:1084-1088, 1978.
22. Rocker GM, et al: Pulmonary vascular permeability to transferrin in the pulmonary oedema of renal failure. Thorax 42:620-623, 1987.
23. Zidulka A, et al: Pulmonary function with acute loss of excess lung water by hemodialysis in patients with chronic uremia. Am J Med 55:134-141, 1973.
24. Stanescu DC, et al: Lung function in chronic uraemia before and after removal of excess fluid by hemodialysis. Clin Sci Mol Med 47:143-151, 1974.
25. Prezant DJ: Effect of uremia and its treatment on pulmonary function. Lung 168:1-14, 1990.
26. Fairshter RD, Vaziri ND, Mirahmadi MK: Lung pathology in chronic hemodialysis patients. Int J Artif Organs 5:97-100, 1982.

27. Nidus BD, et al: Uremic pleuritis—a clinicopathological entity. N Engl J Med 281:255-256, 1969.
28. Berger HW, et al: Uremic pleural effusion: A study in 14 patients on chronic dialysis. Ann Intern Med 82:362-364, 1975.
29. Maher JF: Uremic pleuritis. Am J Kidney Dis 10:19-22, 1987.
30. Hussein MM, Mooij JM, Roujouleh H: Tuberculosis and chronic renal disease. Semin Dial 16:38-44, 2003.
31. Ekim M, et al: Tuberculosis in children undergoing continuous ambulatory peritoneal dialysis. Pediatr Nephrol 13:577-579, 1999
32. Okada M, et al: A boy undergoing maintenance hemodialysis who developed mediastinal lymph node tuberculosis. Clin Exp Nephrol 10:152-155, 2006.
33. Milliner DS, et al: Soft tissue calcification in pediatric patients with end-stage renal disease. Kidney Int 38:931-936, 1990.
34. Nakagawa M, et al: Serious cardiac and pulmonary calcification in a young peritoneal dialysis patient: Potential role of continuous correction of acidosis. Clin Nephrol 63:313-316, 2005.
35. Faubert PF, et al: Pulmonary calcification in hemodialyzed patients detected by technetium-99 m diphosphonate scanning. Kidney Int 18:95-102, 1980.
36. Justrabo E, Genin R, Rifle G: Pulmonary metastatic calcification with respiratory insufficiency in patients on maintenance hemodialysis. Thorax 34:384-388, 1979.
37. Conger JD, et al: Pulmonary calcification in chronic dialysis patients. Ann Intern Med 83:330-336, 1975.
38. Garcia-Pachon E, Padilla-Navas I: Urinothorax: Case report and review of the literature with emphasis on biochemical diagnosis. Respiration 71:533-536, 2004.
39. Buyukcelik M, et al: An unusual cause of pleura effusion, urinothorax in a child with urinary stone disease. Pediatr Nephrol 20:1487-1489, 2005.
40. Fletcher EC: Obstructive sleep apnea and the kidney. J Am Soc Nephrol 4:1111-1121, 1993.
41. Zoccali C, Mallamaci F, Tripepi G: Sleep apnea in renal patients. J Am Soc Nephrol 12:2854-2859, 2001.
42. Kraus MA, Hamburger RJ: Sleep apnea in renal failure. Adv Perit Dial 13:88-92, 1997.
43. Hanly P: Sleep apnea and daytime sleepiness in end-stage renal disease. Semin Dial 17:109-114, 2004.
44. Parker KP: Sleep disturbances in dialysis patients. Sleep Med Rev 7:131-143, 2003.
45. Zoccali C, et al: Left ventricular hypertrophy and nocturnal hypoxemia in hemodialysis patients. J Hypertension 19:287-293, 2001.
46. Zoccali C, Mallamaci F, Tripepi G: Nocturnal hypoxemia predicts incident cardiovascular complications in dialysis patients. J Am Soc Nephrol 13:729-733, 2002.
47. Mendelson WB, et al: Effects of hemodialysis on sleep apnea in end stage renal disease. Clin Nephrol 33:247-251, 1990.
48. Fein AM, et al: Reversal of sleep apnea in uremia by dialysis. Arch Intern Med 147:1355-1356, 1987.
49. Pendse S, Singh AK: Complications of chronic kidney disease: Anemia, mineral metabolism, and cardiovascular disease. Med Clin North Am 89:549-561, 2005.
50. Peco-Antic A: Management of renal anemia Turk J Pediatr 47(Suppl):19-27, 2005.
51. Cody J, et al: Recombinant human erythropoietin for chronic renal failure anemia in pre-dialysis patients. Cochrane Database Syst Rev 3:CD003266, 2005.
52. Uchino S, et al: Acute renal failure in critically ill patients: A multinational, multicenter study. JAMA 294:813-818, 2005.
53. Blanch L, Bernabe F, Lucangelo U: Measurement of air trapping, intrinsic positive end-expiratory pressure, and dynamic hyperinflation in mechanically ventilated patients. Respir Care 50:110-123, 2005.
54. Craddock PR, et al: Complement and leukocyte-mediated pulmonary dysfunction in hemodialysis. N Engl J Med 296:769-774, 1977.
55. Carlon GC, et al: Hypoxemia during hemodialysis. Crit Care Med 7:497-499, 1979.
56. Patterson RW, et al: Hypoxemia and pulmonary gas exchange during hemodialysis. J Appl Physiol 50:259-264, 1981.
57. Munger MA, et al: Cardiopulmonary events during hemodialysis: Effects of dialysis membranes and dialysate buffers. Am J Kidney Dis 36:130-139, 2000.
58. Romaldini H, et al: The mechanisms of arterial hypoxemia during hemodialysis. Am Rev Respir Dis 129:780-784, 1984.
59. Ralph DD, et al: Inert gas analysis of ventilation-perfusion matching during hemodialysis. J Clin Invest 73:1385-1391, 1984.
60. Martin L: Hypoventilation without elevated carbon dioxide tension. Chest 77:720-721, 1980.
61. Wan L, et al: The pathogenesis of septic acute renal failure. Curr Opin Crit Care 9:496-502, 2003.
62. Burch JM, et al: The abdominal compartment syndrome. Surg Clin North Am 76:833-842, 1996.
63. Walker J, Criddle LM: Pathophysiology and management of abdominal compartment syndrome. Am J Crit Care 12:367-371, 2003.
64. Sugrue M: Abdominal compartment syndrome. Curr Opin Crit Care 11:333-338, 2005.
65. Benditt JO: Esophageal and gastric pressure measurements. Respir Care 50:68-75, 2005.
66. Ranieri VM, et al: Mechanical ventilation as a mediator of multisystem organ failure in acute respiratory distress syndrome. JAMA 284:43-44, 2000.
67. Plotz FB, et al: Ventilator-induced lung injury and multiple system organ failure: A critical review of facts and hypotheses. Intensive Care Med 30:1865-1872, 2004.
68. Slutsky AS: Ventilator-induced lung injury: From barotrauma to biotrauma. Respir Care 50:646-659, 2005.
69. Kuiper JW, et al: Mechanical ventilation and acute renal failure. Crit Care Med 33:1408-1415, 2005.
70. Chien CC, King LS, Rabb H: Mechanisms underlying combined acute renal failure and acute lung injury in the intensive care unit. Contrib Nephrol 144:53-62, 2004.
71. Pannu N, Mehta RL: Effect of mechanical ventilation on the kidney. Best Pract Res Clin Anaesthesiol 18:189-203, 2004.
72. Hoyer PF, et al: Thromboembolic complications in children with nephrotic syndrome: Risk and incidence. Acta Paediatr Scand 75:804-810, 1986.
73. Nephrotic syndrome in children: Prediction of histopathology from clinical and laboratory characteristics at time of diagnosis. A report of the International

Study of Kidney Disease in Children. Kidney Int 13:159-165, 1978.

74. The primary nephrotic syndrome in children: Identification of patients with minimal change nephrotic syndrome from initial responses to prednisone. A report of the International Study of Kidney Disease in Children. J. Pediatr 98:561-564, 1981.

75. Singhal R, Brimble KS: Thromboembolic complications in the nephrotic syndrome: Pathophysiology and clinical management. Thromb Res 118:397-407, 2006.

76. Van Ommen CH, Peters M: Acute pulmonary embolism in childhood. Thromb Res 118:13-25, 2006.

77. Jones CL, Hebert D: Pulmonary thrombo-embolism in the nephrotic syndrome. Pediatr Nephrol 5: 56-58, 1991.

CHAPTER 7

Pulmonary Manifestations of Hematologic and Oncologic Diseases

RAUL C. RIBEIRO*, CARLOS RODRIGUEZ-GALINDO, AND GUILLERMO CHANTADA

Oncologic Diseases   135
  Complications Related to Disease and Acute
    Treatment   135
  Solid Tumors   141
  Primary Lung Neoplasms   146
  Inflammatory Pseudotumor   147
Hematologic Disorders   147
  Sickle Cell Disease   147
  Histiocytic Disorders of the Lung   152

**Complications of Treatment of
  Hematologic and Oncologic
  Disorders**   154
  Hematopoietic Stem Cell
    Transplantation   154
  Transfusion-Related Acute Lung Injury   156
  Chemotherapy-Induced Lung Toxicity   158
  Radiation Therapy   162
Acknowledgments   163
  References   163

Pulmonary complications are a common side effect of pediatric hematologic and oncologic disorders and their treatment. Respiratory signs and symptoms can be the presenting manifestations of several types of pediatric malignancies. The anatomic structures typically affected by this group of disorders are the mediastinum, airways (trachea and bronchus), alveolocapillary units, lung parenchyma, pleura, diaphragm, and chest wall. Many of these thoracic structures, as exemplified by the thymus, continue to develop intensively after birth and are common targets of malignant transformation. This chapter describes the pulmonary symptoms and management of pediatric hematologic and oncologic disorders that directly or indirectly affect the respiratory system.

Oncologic Diseases

Complications Related to Disease and Acute Treatment

Pediatric acute leukemias and lymphomas are clonal disorders of the blood-forming cells

(erythroid, myeloid, lymphoid, and megakaryocytic) that result from the transformation of immature progenitor cells of these hematopoietic lineages. These disorders are grouped in four broad categories: acute lymphoblastic leukemia (ALL), acute myeloid leukemia (AML), non-Hodgkin lymphoma (NHL), and Hodgkin disease (HD). They are classified further by the type of specific progenitor cells involved in the process.[1] Because the hematopoietic system is functionally diverse and has a wide anatomic distribution, the clinical and biologic characteristics of leukemias and lymphomas in young patients vary substantially.

In the United States, of the approximately 13,000 new cases of cancer diagnosed per year in children, adolescents, and adults younger than 20 years old, 18.7% are ALL, 8.8% are HD, 6.5% are NHL, and 3.5% are AML.[2,3] Of the neoplasias in children and adolescents, 50% are hematologic malignancies. The incidence of leukemias and lymphomas varies with age. ALL represents 17% of all cases of pediatric cancer in neonates and infants, 46% of cases of cancer

*This work was supported in part by Cancer Center Support (CORE) grant P30 CA-21765 from the National Institutes of Health, by a Center of Excellence Grant from the State of Tennessee, and by the American Lebanese Syrian Associated Charities (ALSAC)

135

in children 2 to 3 years old, and 9% of cases of cancer in individuals 15 to 20 years old. Although the incidence of AML also varies with age, the rates are highest in the first 2 years of life, after which they decrease to a nadir at the end of the first decade, and then gradually increase during the second decade of life. Conversely, the rates of NHL and HD increase with age. The incidence of HD increases with age, with 43.2 cases per 1 million for individuals 19 years old.

The pattern of age distribution among leukemia and lymphomas suggests that etiologic factors differ in these diseases. Generally, the process of malignant transformation of a specific hematopoietic progenitor cell is believed to occur during fetal development in acute leukemias[4] and postnatally in lymphomas[5]—hence, the incidence of lymphomas is greatly affected by environmental factors. In some areas of Africa, Burkitt lymphoma and Kaposi sarcoma are two common types of pediatric malignancy.[6]

The intrathoracic cavity harbors primary (thymus) and secondary (lymph nodes and mucosa-associated lymphatic aggregates) lymphoid organs; thoracic lymphoid structures are commonly affected in lymphoid leukemias and lymphomas. Enlargement of the thymus or its associated lymph nodes is very common in T cell ALL, lymphoblastic NHL, and HD.[7-9] Mediastinal involvement is extremely rare in AML. Chest radiography is an effective screening tool to identify children with mediastinal mass and should be obtained in any patient newly diagnosed with leukemia or lymphoma. A large mediastinal mass in a child should be considered a medical emergency and managed in a tertiary care hospital by a multidisciplinary team. Depending on the size, location, organ compression, and progression time, a particular constellation of clinical signs and symptoms indicates whether the airways, great vessels, or both are predominantly affected.[10,11] A detailed assessment of the patient's medical history and results of the physical examination can provide clues regarding whether the compression is affecting the airways, great vessels, heart, or more than one of these structures.

Tracheal Compression and Superior Vena Cava Syndrome

Large tumors in the anterior mediastinum can cause tracheal compression, superior vena cava (SVC) syndrome, or both. The most common tumors in this area are HD and NHL. Tracheal compression may cause cough, stridor, dyspnea, or orthopnea. In these cases, chest radiograph may reveal an anterior mediastinal mass, prominent hilar lymph nodes, posterior tracheal deviation, atelectasis, and pleural effusion. Tracheal compression is not always obvious, however, from the physical examination or chest radiograph. It may become apparent when a patient is unable to lie supine because of increased dyspnea; the patient should be considered at high risk for complete tracheal obstruction.[11,12] The SVC is particularly susceptible to compression because it is surrounded by lymph nodes and is in direct contact with rigid anatomic structures. It has a delicate vessel wall and low intraluminal pressure.

Symptoms resulting from moderate to severe SVC compression include headache, dizziness, syncope, and cardiovascular collapse secondary to decreased venous return (Fig. 7-1).[13] Physical examination may be unremarkable or may show facial and periorbital edema, cyanosis, plethora, neck and chest vein distention, papilledema, and edema of the upper extremities. The severity of the clinical manifestations of SVC syndrome depends on how rapidly the obstruction arises, and whether sufficient time has elapsed for new collateral blood vessels to develop.

Children with tracheal compression or SVC syndrome are often anxious and diaphoretic. They resist efforts to be placed in the supine position and should not be forced into this position. Assessment of airway patency with computed tomography (CT) scan or flexible bronchoscopy is ill-advised because patients do not tolerate these procedures well and may be very difficult to resuscitate if they experience cardiorespiratory collapse. Total airway occlusion has been reported during the induction of general anesthesia, tracheal intubation or extubation, movement of a patient to a supine or flexed position (for lumbar puncture), and conscious sedation.[14] Flow-volume loops have been used to indicate the degree of central airway obstruction and may be helpful in distinguishing fixed from variable intrathoracic airway lesions.[15]

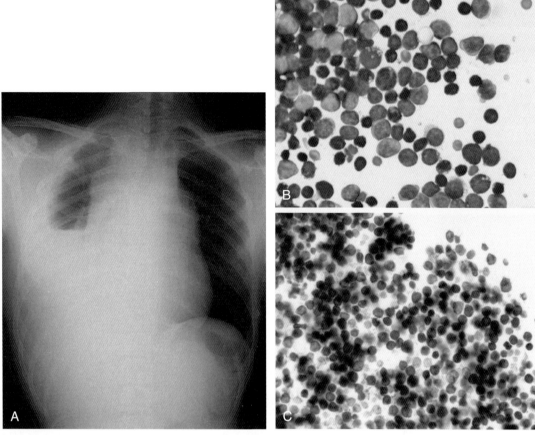

Figure 7-1. An 11-year-old boy with lymphoblastic lymphoma. **A**, Posteroanterior chest radiograph shows large anterior mediastinal mass and pleural effusion. **B** and **C**, Cytocentrifuge examination of the pleural effusion shows FAB L1 lymphoblasts (**B**) (Wright-Giemsa) of T cell origin (**C**) (anti-CD3 staining). (See Color Plate)

Whole-body positron emission tomography (PET) has been increasingly used to determine the extent of disease and response to therapy. NHL and HD are metabolically active, and so they can be detected with this method. Although PET/CT (Fig. 7-2) is still considered a research tool in disease staging and prognosis, some studies have shown the superiority of PET/CT to PET or CT alone in the management of NHL and HD.[15] The least invasive technique is used to obtain tissue for diagnosis. The diagnosis often can be made from bone marrow aspirate or peripheral lymph node biopsy, which can be obtained with topical anesthesia. Similarly, if pleural effusion is present, thoracentesis can be used in making a diagnosis (Fig. 7-3).

A proper regimen of chemotherapy should be started as soon as a diagnosis is established. Intravenous access should be started in the lower extremities because most of the venous return proceeds through the inferior vena cava. Although SVC syndrome per se does not represent a medical emergency, most children with SVC syndrome experience some degree of airway compression. Therapy with radiation to the mid-plane or corticosteroids (hydrocortisone, 2 mg/kg every 6 hours) or both usually alleviates symptoms. Most mediastinal masses in children and adolescents are highly sensitive to chemotherapy. These patients are at high risk of uric acid nephropathy and consequently kidney dysfunction.[17,18] Hyperhydration and alkalinization used for patients at high risk of tumor lysis syndrome (hyperuricemia)[17] should be avoided in patients with SVC syndrome, however, because of the risk of respiratory insufficiency and worsening of existent pleural effusion. Rasburicase is very

Figure 7-2. A, A 14-year-old boy with lymphoblastic lymphoma complicated by vena cava compression syndrome. The compression was predominantly vascular; the patient had no signs of respiratory distress. **B**, A 10-year-old boy with lymphoblastic lymphoma, superior vena cava syndrome, and tracheal compression. In addition to having increased collateral circulation in the frontal and cervical regions, the patient was plethoric and was experiencing respiratory distress. (See Color Plate)

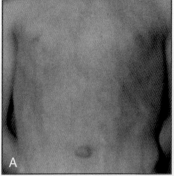
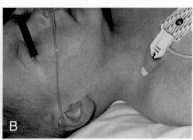

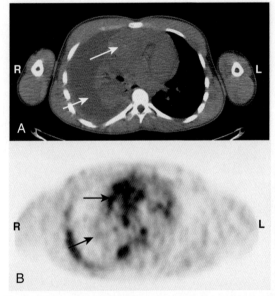
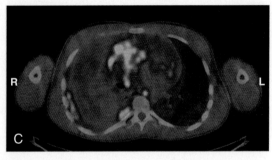

Figure 7-3. PET/CT images of a 15-year-old boy with non-Hodgkin lymphoma. **A**, CT image, transverse plane, shows large mediastinal mass (*top arrow*) and large pleural effusion (*bottom arrow*). Collapse of the right lung and mediastinal shift to the right are evident. **B**, PET image at same anatomic level as **A** shows irregularly increased uptake of fludeoxyglucose F 18 (FDG) in mediastinal mass (*top arrow*). The pleural effusion (*bottom arrow*) shows no uptake of FDG. Increased uptake of FDG, which represents pleural involvement, is evident along the periphery of the effusion, however. **C**, Fused image of **A** and **B** overlies the anatomic image in **A** and the functional image in **B**. (See Color Plate)

effective in rapidly decreasing plasma urate, avoiding the need for hyperhydration and alkalinization.[19]

Doppler ultrasonography and echocardiography may be indicated for evaluating flow through the great vessels and myocardial function. If thrombosis is detected, use of unfractionated or low-molecular-weight heparin should be considered to prevent propagation of the thrombus. In rare cases, catheter-directed thrombolysis has been performed to relieve obstruction.[20] Most importantly, prompt specific chemotherapy for primary malignancy should be instituted as soon as the diagnosis is established.

Pulmonary Leukostasis Syndrome
Approximately 50% of children with ALL and AML present with an abnormally elevated blood leukocyte count. Severe leukocytosis (defined as peripheral leukocytes $\geq100,000/mm^3$) occurs in approximately 20% of children with ALL and 15% of children with AML.[21,22] Most of these patients have no pulmonary signs or symptoms associated with this abnormality. Depending on

the number of leukocytes and the type of leukemia, however, a constellation of signs and symptoms, known as pulmonary leukostasis syndrome, may occur.[23] Leukostasis can affect any organ, but it most commonly involves brain and lungs. Clinically, pulmonary involvement is characterized by shortness of breath, tachypnea, dyspnea on exertion, and pleuritic chest pain. Mortality in patients with leukostasis is approximately 20%, usually secondary to pulmonary or intracranial hemorrhage.[24]

Patients with AML tend to develop symptomatic leukostasis at much lower leukocyte counts than do patients with ALL.[25] Postmortem evidence of leukostasis in AML, including extensive leukemic infiltration of the alveoli and parenchyma, and occlusion of small pulmonary vessels, has been found in patients presenting with a wide range of leukocyte counts.[26,27] Symptomatic pulmonary leukostasis occurs almost exclusively in children with AML.[28]

Respiratory distress and early death resulting from hyperleukocytosis (defined as leukocyte counts $\geq 200,000/mm^3$) is more common in children with AML, occurring in 6% of patients. A high initial white blood cell count seems to be the only marker associated with the development of respiratory complications.[29] In addition, because myeloblasts express adhesion molecules that attach to the pulmonary vascular endothelium, they are more tissue-invasive than lymphoblasts. These factors apparently are more relevant to the severity of pulmonary leukostasis syndrome than the number of leukemia cells. The adverse interactions between leukemic cells and organs such as lungs, brain, and kidneys seem to be worsened further in M5 AML and M4 AML because these subtypes of AML[31-34] release many proinflammatory cytokines and lysozymes.[30,35]

Chest radiographs can be normal, or they may reveal variable degrees of diffuse alveolar-interstitial infiltrates and pulmonary vessel enlargement. Findings of chest CT scans include bilateral thickening of the interlobular septa with patchy areas of ground-glass opacity that resemble that of interstitial edema. A ventilation/perfusion lung scan can show mismatched defects,[36] but is not specific for leukostasis, and reliance on it

can lead to the misdiagnosis of pulmonary embolism. Imaging studies are nonspecific for pulmonary leukostasis.[37]

Hypoxemia in patients with hyperleukocytosis can be a true or false finding. Causes of true hypoxemia in these patients include infection, hemorrhage, pulmonary embolism, pulmonary alveolar proteinosis (PAP), and occlusion of the pulmonary vasculature by leukocyte thrombi. False hypoxemia can result from technical inaccuracies in the measurement of PaO_2, and often may reflect that leukemic cells are metabolically active *in vitro*.[38-41] In this situation, low levels of PaO_2 reflect consumption of dissolved oxygen by leukocytes or platelets after the arterial blood specimen is obtained, a phenomenon called "oxygen steal."[42] Consistent with this concept is the observation that PaO_2 values are negatively correlated with the number of circulating leukocytes. Because pulse oximetry measures capillary oxygen instead of whole-blood oxygen saturation, this method is considered the most accurate way to assess oxygenation in patients with hyperleukocytosis.[43]

Acute leukemia complicated by severe hyperleukocytosis should be considered a medical emergency. Admission of the patient to an intensive care unit and proper management of aggravating factors, such as dehydration, electrolyte or metabolic imbalances, infection, thrombocytopenia, and coagulopathy, should be initiated immediately. Fluid balance is required to avoid excessive fluid retention. Transfusion of platelet concentrate or fresh frozen plasma is used to reduce the risk of bleeding. Prophylaxis of thromboembolic phenomena with heparin is not indicated. Transfusion of packed red blood cells should be withheld or be given with caution to prevent an increase in blood viscosity before the reduction of the leukocyte count.[44] Anemia in patients with hyperleukocytosis can be seen as an adaptive mechanism. Inhaled nitric oxide to produce pulmonary vasodilation and ventilation/perfusion mismatch reduction has been used by some investigators.[45-47] Leukapheresis or exchange transfusion (for young children) is commonly considered as a temporary measure until specific antileukemia treatment is initiated.[48-53] The efficacy of leukapheresis in reducing mortality or life-threatening complications has not been evaluated in controlled clinical trials.

Pulmonary Alveolar Proteinosis

PAP can rarely be a cause of respiratory failure in patients with acute leukemia, particularly AML.[54] PAP is characterized by the intra-alveolar accumulation of surfactant proteinaceous material, resulting in impaired alveolocapillary gas exchange (Fig. 7-4).[55-57] Three types of PAP have been recognized: congenital,[58-62] associated with or secondary to systemic disease,[63-65] and idiopathic. The last-mentioned is the most common form of PAP and believed to have an autoimmune basis.[66-68]

The mechanism of PAP has not been firmly established, although surfactant homeostasis apparently is impaired in this disease.[69] Although only 10% of surfactant comprises proteins, denominated A, B, C, and D, they are crucial to surfactant metabolism, opsonization of microorganisms, and stimulation of alveolar macrophage.[70-72] Alveolar type II epithelial cells and alveolar macrophage control surfactant synthesis, storage, and catabolism. Alveolar macrophages, which are produced by bone marrow hematopoietic cells, internalize and catabolize surfactant by a process believed to depend on granulocyte-macrophage colony-stimulating factor (GM-CSF) signaling.[73-75] Several lines of evidence suggest that abnormality of the GM-CSF signaling in the lung is associated with PAP pathogenesis. First, histologically similar PAP lung changes occur in mice genetically deficient in GM-CSF or its receptor.[76,77] Abnormal clearance of surfactant lipids is impaired in GM-CSF–deficient mice, providing an explanation for the intra-alveolar accumulation of PAS-positive material. PAP in GM-CSF–deficient mice can be corrected by the local expression of GM-CSF in the lungs,[78,79,84] or by bone marrow transplantation from a wild-type mouse.[80] Second, PAP occurs in individuals harboring constitutional mutations in the genes encoding surfactant proteins B or C or the β_c chain of the GM-CSF receptor.[58-62] Finally, autoantibodies that bind and neutralize GM-CSF are found in bronchoalveolar lavage (BAL) of patients with the idiopathic form of PAP.[66]

Imaging studies of the lungs suggest PAP.[85] The chest radiograph usually shows bilateral airspace disease characterized as ground-glass opacities suggestive of pulmonary edema, but without other signs of left-sided heart dysfunction. There is no relationship between clinical and radiographic findings, with the latter being disproportionately more severe.[85] High-resolution CT scans reveal a pattern referred to as "crazy-paving," which is characterized by ground-glass opacifications with superimposed interlobular septal and intralobular thickening.[86]

BAL specimens can be used to establish the diagnosis.[87] Lung biopsy is the gold standard for the diagnosis of PAP, but it sometimes can yield false-negative results.

The incidence of PAP associated with leukemia is unknown, but a study by Cordonnier and colleagues[63] suggested that it can be 10% in patients with leukemia and respiratory failure. Treatment of PAP consists of overall supportive care because many of these patients have severe neutropenia from previous chemotherapy, and whole-lung lavage for patients with severe respiratory distress.[88-93] Most cases of chemotherapy-induced PAP usually improve with the resolution of neutropenia.

Because the mechanism of PAP has been associated with GM-CSF deficiency, administration of GM-CSF has been proposed as a

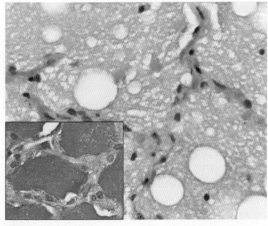

Figure 7-4. Pulmonary alveolar proteinosis (accumulation of amorphous, eosinophilic, periodic acid-Schiff-positive material) in pulmonary alveolar lumens. (Hematoxylin and eosin, 40× original magnification.) *Inset* shows PAS stain counterstained with hematoxylin. (See Color Plate)

treatment of PAP. In a study of 25 patients with idiopathic PAP, subcutaneous administration of GM-CSF improved oxygenation and decreased alveolar-arterial oxygen gradient in approximately 50% of the patients.[94] Whether GM-CSF has a therapeutic value in children with leukemia and respiratory distress associated with clinical and laboratory features of PAP remains to be determined. Defective expression of GM-CSF/interleukin-3/interleukin-5 receptor common β chain has been shown to occur in children with AML associated with respiratory failure.[95]

Solid Tumors

Solid malignancies in children differ markedly from such tumors in adults; biology and histology define a very distinct group of neoplasms, most of them of dysontogenetic origin, with unique clinical manifestations and natural history. Epithelial malignancies are extremely rare in children; sarcomas and dysontogenetic tumors constitute most solid cancers. Generally, these groups of malignancies are aggressive, and systemic dissemination (microscopic or macroscopic) is present at the time of diagnosis. For this reason, an extensive metastatic work-up is necessary, and most malignancies require systemic therapy regardless of the local stage.

Osteosarcoma

Osteosarcoma, a malignant neoplasm derived from primitive mesenchymal cells and characterized by the presence of osteoid-producing spindle cell stroma, is the most common malignant bone tumor in pediatric patients.[92] Osteosarcoma accounts for 2.6% of all neoplasms in children, with an estimated annual incidence of 3.9 per 1 million in white children and 4.5 per 1 million in African-American children.[93] Most osteosarcomas occur during the first 2 decades of life, a period characterized by rapid skeletal growth. Overt macroscopic metastatic disease is seen in a significant proportion of patients, and has a grave prognosis when present.[94] The most common site for metastatic spread is the lung; 14% to 24% of patients have macroscopic pulmonary disease at the time

of diagnosis.[95-98] Approximately 5% of all osteosarcomas are multifocal (i.e., involving two or more bones at the time of diagnosis). Multifocal osteosarcoma has a more aggressive clinical behavior, a higher incidence of pulmonary metastases, and a very poor prognosis.[99]

When osteosarcoma is diagnosed, even the most accurate staging procedures detect metastases in only a few patients. Without adequate treatment, however, most patients with seemingly localized disease develop secondary metastases within 1 year.[100] This finding implies that micrometastases are already present at diagnosis in most patients.

With appropriate treatment, 60% to 70% of patients with localized disease are expected to be cured. The outcome of patients with clinically detectable metastatic disease at diagnosis is usually very poor; less than 30% of patients are expected to survive.[94,101-103] Care of these patients needs to combine a multimodal approach, with intensive preoperative and postoperative chemotherapy and resection of the primary tumor and all the metastatic lesions.[102-105] Using these guidelines, more recent research reports 2- to 5-year, progression-free survival rates of 25% to 45%.[102,106-108] Factors that affect outcome include number of metastases, laterality, and the ability to perform a complete resection.[102,105]

The lungs also are the most common sites of treatment failure in patients with osteosarcoma. For patients with recurrent disease, a surgical approach is recommended; the 5-year postrelapse survival of patients in whom a complete resection of all macroscopic disease can be achieved is almost 40%, whereas it is 0% for patients with unresectable disease.[104,109] Prognostic factors for survival after recurrence include isolated lung metastases, late (>24 months) recurrences, and small number of pulmonary nodules.[105,109,110]

Plain chest radiographs detect lung metastases in most cases. High-resolution CT of the chest is the procedure of choice, however. False-positive results occur, particularly with smaller lesions, and biopsy confirmation of the lung disease is usually required. Osteoid matrix produced by osteosarcoma cells forms bone and causes calcification in pulmonary nodules. Seventy-five percent of metastatic osteosarcoma nodules lack calcification, however. Conversely, only 50% of calcified nodules in newly diagnosed patients with osteosarcoma are malignant, whereas 65% of noncalcified lesions are found to be metastatic osteosarcoma.[111] Mediastinal adenopathies are very rare in patients newly diagnosed with osteosarcoma, and their presence in the context of lung nodules favors the diagnosis of a nonmalignant condition; 60% of patients with benign nodules have mediastinal disease compared with less than 20% of patients with metastases.[111]

CT is often unable to distinguish benign from malignant pulmonary disease, and a surgical procedure is often required for confirmation. CT can miss 40% to 50% of the lesions that are found later during the surgical procedure.[112] This finding highlights the importance of manual palpation during open thoracotomy; minimal access procedures such as thoracoscopy should not be the approach if the goal is resection.

In patients who have undergone thoracotomy for metastatic disease, new nodules are likely to be metastatic, and surgical intervention is warranted. Surgical scarring often makes the diagnosis of recurrent disease difficult, however. McCarville and associates[111] evaluated the imaging patterns of recurrent nodules after thoracotomy in patients with osteosarcoma. Pulmonary nodules recurred in 90% of patients who underwent thoracotomy, and metastatic disease was found in 90% of patients who underwent another surgical procedure. Only one third of the nodules appeared to be calcified on CT scans. A consistent pattern suggestive of malignancy was the presence of progressive pleural thickening. In contrast to newly diagnosed patients, in most patients who had undergone thoracotomy, recurrent pulmonary disease was associated with the presence of mediastinal adenopathies. With subsequent recurrence, the proportion of malignant lesions and the incidence of malignant mediastinal disease increased.[111] Also, half of the new lesions occurred in previous scars, and the estimated probability that a recurrent nodule in the site of a scar was malignant was 82%.[111]

The ability to control the pulmonary micrometastatic disease after completion of therapy would result in a significant improvement in outcome. Muramyl tripeptide phosphatidylethanolamine (MTP-PE), a synthetic lipophilic analogue of muramyl dipeptide (a component of the cell wall of bacille Calmette-Guérin), has been encapsulated in liposomes to deliver the agent selectively to monocytes and macrophages to activate their tumoricidal properties. In an animal model, the administration of liposome-encapsulated muramyl tripeptide (L-MTP-PE) resulted in activation of pulmonary macrophages and eradication of pulmonary micrometastases.[113] In the cooperative Children's Cancer Group and Pediatric Oncology Group intergroup INT0133 clinical trial, patients with localized osteosarcoma received standard treatment with methotrexate-cisplatin-doxorubicin regimen. Patients were first randomly assigned to receive ifosfamide, L-MTP-E, or a combination of both. Adding a combination therapy with ifosfamide and L-MTP-PE to the standard regimen resulted in a significantly better outcome than the other three regimens.[114] This improved outcome could be due to the synergistic effect of L-MTP-PE and ifosfamide.[115]

It also is possible to induce activation of alveolar macrophages by nebulization of GM-CSF. Based on encouraging preliminary data, the Children's Oncology Group is currently evaluating this approach in patients with metastatic osteosarcoma. Another similar approach is the interleukin-12 gene transfer by aerosol using a nonviral vector, such as polyethylenimine, a polycationic DNA carrier. Interleukin-12 has a well-known activity against various tumors. The systemic administration of interleukin-12 is limited by its toxicity. In animal models, aerosol therapy resulted in a significant decrease in the size and number of metastatic nodules.[116,117] Interleukin-12 also has been shown to enhance the sensitivity of osteosarcoma cells in vitro to 4-hydroxy-cyclophosphamide by a mechanism involving the Fas pathway, which suggests that this approach may act synergistically with ifosfamide.[115] The same polyethylenimine transfer technology has been shown to provide an antitumor effect using *p53* transfection.[117]

Aerosolized technology also has been developed to deliver chemotherapeutic agents directly to the lungs. In an animal model, aerosolized 9-nitrocamptothecin liposome was administered to mice that had subcutaneous xenografts of various human cancers and to mice with lung metastases of osteosarcoma. The results were encouraging; a significant antitumor effect was noted in the xenografts and in the pulmonary disease, suggesting not only a local, but also a systemic effect.[118] Clinical trials to assess this form of therapy are under way.[119]

Ewing Sarcoma Family of Tumors

The term "Ewing sarcoma family of tumors" (ESFT) refers to a group of small round cell neoplasms of neuroectodermal origin. Ewing sarcoma of the bone is the least differentiated form, and primitive neuroectodermal tumor and peripheral neuroepithelioma are the most differentiated forms. Of all types of pediatric malignancy, 3% are ESFT; these tumors are rare in nonwhites.[120] Approximately 40% of all bone cancers in children are ESFT of the bone, the second most common type of bone malignancy in children after osteosarcoma.[120] Patients with ESFT commonly present with symptoms during the second decade of life; 80% of patients with EFST are younger than 18 years, and the median age at diagnosis is 14 years.[120-122] ESFT has a tendency to involve the shaft of long tubular bones, the pelvis, and the ribs, but almost every bone can be affected. More than 50% of the tumors arise from axial bones, with the pelvis being the most commonly involved (23% to 27%). Primary ESFT of the chest wall, previously known as Askin tumor, occurs in 12% of patients with ESFT.[120-123]

ESFT are aggressive neoplasms; systemic manifestations including fever and anemia are present in 10% to 15% of patients,[124] and approximately 20% to 25% of cases have clinically apparent metastatic disease at the time of diagnosis.[125-127] Metastatic disease seems to be associated with older age[128] and large tumors[128-130] or with pelvic primary tumors.[125,126,129] Isolated lung disease, usually bilateral, occurs in 25% to 45% of patients with

metastases; most (50% to 60%) have extrapulmonary disease (usually of the bone and bone marrow).[122,125-127,131] Overall, approximately 10% of patients have lung metastases at the time of diagnosis (Fig. 7-5).[129]

The most important prognostic factor is the presence of metastatic disease at diagnosis.[122] Advances in the treatment of ESFT have resulted in only a very modest improvement in the survival of patients with metastases.[122,126,132] Even among patients with metastatic disease, however, there is some heterogeneity. Patients with isolated lung metastases may have a better prognosis than patients with extrapulmonary metastases, with long-term survival rates approaching 40% to 45%.[125,130,131] Among patients with lung metastases, patients with unilateral disease[130] and patients with good histologic response to induction chemotherapy[129] seem to have a survival advantage.

In approximately 50% of patients with isolated lung metastases, treatment failures occur as isolated pulmonary disease again,[129,130] suggesting that further response consolidation might improve the outcome of these patients. In contrast to osteosarcoma cells, ESFT cells are very sensitive to radiation therapy, and lung radiation is an alternative to lung surgery. In the first American Intergroup Ewing Sarcoma Study, lung radiation was associated with a lower incidence of lung (and distant) recurrences.[133] With the development of more intensive chemotherapeutic regimens, lung radiation of localized disease was abandoned. It remains a therapeutic option, however, for

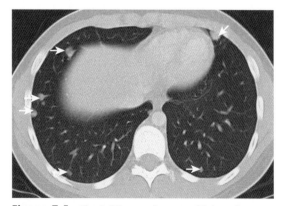

Figure 7-5. Chest CT scan shows multiple pulmonary metastases (*arrows*) in a patient with Ewing sarcoma.

patients with metastatic disease. In this regard, whole-lung radiation seems to provide a modest survival advantage in patients with metastatic disease.[129] Preliminary data of the European Bone Marrow Transplant Registry[134] suggest that an alternative approach to the treatment of patients with isolated lung metastases may be high-dose chemotherapy using a busulfan-based regimen and autologous stem cell rescue.

Patients with primary ESFT of the chest wall represent a distinct group. Many of these patients have infiltration of the pleura, have pleural effusion, or may develop intraoperative contamination of the pleural space. They may be at high risk of disease relapse within the pleural compartment, and many groups have used hemothorax radiation covering the entire pleural space. The use of hemithorax radiation seems to reduce systemic relapse rates (mainly in lung metastases) and to provide a survival advantage.[135]

Soft Tissue Sarcomas

Pediatric soft tissue sarcomas (STS) are broadly divided into rhabdomyosarcoma (RMS) (40% to 45%) and non-RMS soft tissue sarcomas (NRSTS) (55% to 60%), which include several histologic subtypes, each one of which constitutes less than 5% to 10% of STS. Altogether, STS represent approximately 6% to 7% of the cases of malignancy in individuals younger than 20 years. The incidence of RMS is highest in infancy and during the first years of life, and it decreases and levels out at later ages, whereas NRSTS have their highest incidence in adolescence, although a peak is observed in infants.[136]

RMS recapitulates the phenotypic and biologic features of developing skeletal muscle. Two broad categories are identified: Embryonal RMS with its botryoid and spindle cell variants accounts for two thirds of the cases, and alveolar RMS and undifferentiated RMS account for the remaining cases. RMS is clinically heterogeneous; it can arise anywhere in the body where mesenchymal tissue is found. One third of the cases arise in the head and neck region (orbit, parameningeal, and nonparameningeal sites); 25% arise in the genitourinary tracts, primarily bladder and prostate; and 18% arise in the extremities. RMS occur much less frequently in the trunk and pelvis.

Approximately 10% to 15% of patients with RMS have metastatic disease at the time of diagnosis. The incidence of metastatic disease is higher in patients with alveolar RMS (25% to 30%) than in patients with embryonal RMS (5% to 10%).[137-139] Most cases of alveolar RMS are characterized by the presence of the t(2;13)(q35;q14) or, less frequently, t(1;13)(p36;q14) translocations, which result in the *PAX3-FKHR* or *PAX7-FKHR* chimeric genes. Patients with the *PAX3* translocation have more widespread metastatic disease and a worse outcome. The *PAX7* translocation seems to be associated with a lower incidence of lung metastases.[140]

Approximately 5% of patients with RMS have lung metastases at the time of diagnosis.[138] Only 15% to 25% of patients with metastatic disease have isolated lung metastases; in most cases, the presence of lung disease is a sign of more widespread metastatic RMS.[141,142] The presence of isolated lung metastases is associated with favorable features, such as embryonal histology and negative nodal involvement. Patients with metastatic disease have a generally poor prognosis, with long-term survival estimates of less than 30%. Patients with isolated lung metastases seem to benefit from lung radiation, however, and have a slightly better outcome, with 4-year overall survival rates of 40%.[142]

NRSTS comprise a very heterogeneous group of neoplasms of mesenchymal origin. The most common subtypes in children are dermatofibrosarcoma protuberans, synovial sarcoma, malignant fibrous histiocytoma, fibrosarcoma, and malignant peripheral nerve sheath tumor. Because each tumor is individually rare in pediatric patients, little is known about their biology and natural history in children. Most have clinical behavior similar to tumors in adults; however, there are notable exceptions, such as infantile fibrosarcoma and infantile hemangiopericytoma, neoplasms that are associated with characteristically good prognosis despite aggressive histologic features.

Lung metastases are present in 5% to 10% of the cases at diagnosis.[143,144] Only 12% of children who have undergone gross tumor resection experience metastatic tumor recurrence.

Patients with large (≥5 cm), invasive, or high-grade tumors have a significantly higher (25% to 35%) risk of distant disease recurrence, however, usually in the lungs.[145-147] If patients are at high risk of distant metastases after local control or have unresectable or metastatic tumors at presentation, chemotherapy must be considered.

Among all the histologic subtypes of NRSTS, alveolar STS warrants special mention. This rare tumor accounts for only 1% of all STS. Of patients with this form of sarcoma, 65% have lung metastases at the time of diagnosis, however. This sarcoma has a very indolent course, and even in the presence of metastases, 5-year overall survival rates exceed 70% to 80%.[148]

Wilms Tumor

Wilms tumor is the most common childhood renal tumor, accounting for approximately 6% of all pediatric malignant disease. The most common presentation is an asymptomatic abdominal mass in a young child (typically <5 years old), although approximately one third of such patients present with abdominal pain, anorexia, and malaise. Hypertension is present in 25% of the cases, and congenital anomalies, such as aniridia, genitourinary malformations, or hemihypertrophy, are present in 10% to 20% of children.[149] Histologic characteristics are the most important prognostic indicators; anaplasia (which occurs in 10% of cases) is associated with an adverse outcome. Lung metastases are present in approximately 10% of patients with favorable histology and in 20% of patients with anaplasia.[150,151] In contrast to most other types of pediatric malignancy, Wilms tumor with lung metastases has a good outcome, with 5-year overall survival estimates exceeding 80% for patients with favorable histology.[152] Lung radiation is an integral component in the management of these patients with lung metastases.

Plain chest radiographs have been used to define the presence of metastatic disease in patients with Wilms tumor. In approximately 10% of patients with lung nodules, plain chest x-rays are normal, however, and the lesions are visible only on CT scan.[153] Nonmalignant nodular lesions are frequently identified on chest CT scans, but not on plain radiographs in children.[154,155] In adults, 50% to 60% of

lesions identified on CT only are not malignant.[156] For these reasons, the role of lung radiation in this group of patients with CT-only lung nodules is unclear. In such patients treated on the National Wilms Tumor Studies 3 and 4, the 4-year event-free survival estimates were 89% for patients receiving radiation and 80% for patients treated with chemotherapy only.[157] Similarly, results of a study by the International Society of Pediatric Oncology showed that patients with lung nodules identified only on CT and who achieved a complete response to chemotherapy had a 5-year overall survival estimate of 83%.[158] These results contrast with the findings of the United Kingdom Children's Cancer Study Group, which indicated much lower (65%) survival rates if no radiation was used.[159]

Because this issue remains unresolved, future trials by investigators in the Children's Oncology Group are expected to assess the necessity of lung radiation for patients whose tumors have favorable biologic and histologic features and show rapid response to chemotherapy. It is possible that some children with stage IV favorable histology Wilms tumor may be treated successfully without lung radiation.[152] Finally, an important consideration is the frequent extension of Wilms tumor into the renal vein and proximal inferior vena cava, which is sometimes associated with pulmonary embolism.[160] In most cases, tumor thrombus can be removed en bloc with the kidney. If the tumor extends to the hepatic level or into the atrium, however, the risk of operative morbidity is very high, and preoperative chemotherapy is recommended.

Neuroblastoma

Neuroblastoma is the most common extracranial solid tumor in children, accounting for 10% of all childhood cancers. Approximately two thirds of patients with neuroblastoma have metastatic disease at diagnosis, typically of the bone or bone marrow, and their prognosis is very poor, although it varies according to many clinical and biologic risk factors.[161] Pulmonary involvement at diagnosis is extremely rare, occurring in less than 1% of patients.[162] In patients with metastatic disease, lung metastases may be present in

4% of patients, are never isolated, and are always found in the context of a very aggressive clinical and biologic behavior. On radiographs, these lesions appear as multiple, small, bilateral, noncalcified nodules.[163]

Hepatoblastoma

Hepatoblastoma is a very rare malignancy in the overall population, but it accounts for 75% of all liver cancers in children. Lung metastases are very common; 20% of pediatric patients have pulmonary disease at diagnosis, and the lungs are the most common site of recurrence.[164-166] Metastatic hepatoblastoma is curable if the tumor responds to chemotherapy and the lung metastases are resected. With this aggressive approach, the 5-year overall survival estimates are approximately 50%.[164,166]

Imaging Considerations

Multiple studies have shown that even in children with tumors known to metastasize to the lungs, a significant proportion of lesions found on chest CT scans are benign.[167,168] Although granulomas develop less frequently in children than in adults, several other benign conditions may develop in the lungs of children, including the growth of normal intrapulmonary lymph nodes, hamartoma, round pneumonia, atelectasis (particularly in children requiring sedation or anesthesia), and inflammatory pseudotumor. Distinguishing benign from malignant pulmonary nodules may be difficult (Fig. 7-6).

The availability of helical CT has improved the quality of the chest images by diminishing the effect of breathing and cardiac motion on the readability of the scan. McCarville and associates[169] investigated the imaging features of 81 pulmonary nodules in 41 patients with solid tumors who had undergone a thoracotomy. The new chest CT scans were able to detect 75% of the nodules found at surgery; 44% of the patients had benign lesions only. Sharply defined nodules were more likely to be malignant in children than in adults.[169] Although node size was not always a predictor of malignancy, small (<5 mm) nodules were less likely to be malignant, particularly small solitary nodules.[169,170] New technologies such

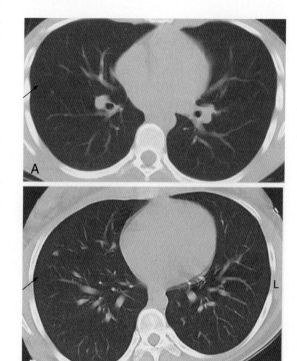

Figure 7-6. A and **B**, Chest CT scans show single pulmonary nodules (*arrows*) of similar characteristics in two patients with osteosarcoma. Both patients underwent a thoracotomy. Examination of a tissue specimen helped establish a diagnosis of histoplasmosis in the patient shown in **A** and metastatic osteosarcoma in the patient shown in **B**.

as PET/CT may allow us to assess more accurately and noninvasively the metabolic activity of pulmonary nodules.

Primary Lung Neoplasms

Pleuropulmonary blastoma (PPB) is a unique dysontogenetic neoplasm of childhood that appears as a pulmonary or pleural-based mass, with a primitive, histologically variable mixed blastomatous and sarcomatous appearance. It usually manifests in the first 3 to 4 years of life with respiratory distress, fever, cough, or chest pain. Cystic changes and pneumothorax are common on CT scans. The lower lobes are more commonly involved, and pleural invasion and effusion are typical. PPB can be divided into three morphologic types or subtypes based on the cystic, cystic and solid, or solid appearance of the tumor, as determined by the gross and microscopic examination. The exclusively cystic or type I PPB is the least complex, manifests at an earlier age than the other two forms, and is more readily resectable. The rhabdomyosarcomatous component is a prominent feature of type II and type III PPB, and it is the exclusive malignant element in type I. PPB is an aggressive malignancy, and metastases to the brain are common.

Type I PPB usually has a good prognosis if complete resection is achieved. The outcome associated with type II and type III PPB is much worse, with 5-year survival rates of less than 50%. These patients need a very aggressive treatment approach, with wide resection and systemic chemotherapy.[171] Other, less common primary malignancies of the lungs include carcinoid and primary sarcomas such as malignant peripheral nerve sheath tumor and fibrosarcoma.

Inflammatory Pseudotumor

Inflammatory pseudotumor (plasma cell granuloma, inflammatory myofibroblastic tumor) is a rare benign neoplasm consisting of histiocytes, myofibroblasts, plasma cells, and spindle-shaped mesenchymal cells. Inflammatory pseudotumor most often affects children and young adults, and it can be found in pulmonary and extrapulmonary locations, most commonly the abdomen. Despite its benign nature, it may be difficult to differentiate from a malignancy because of its local invasiveness and its tendency to recur. Pulmonary pseudotumor is often encountered as an incidental finding in a chest radiograph.

When a pseudotumor is symptomatic, patients may present with nonspecific respiratory symptoms, such as cough, shortness of breath, chest pain, hemoptysis, and clubbing. Laboratory findings consistent with inflammation are common. The etiologic factors are not clearly established, although an infectious cause is suspected. Although there are some anecdotal cases of spontaneous regression, the treatment of pulmonary inflammatory pseudotumor is surgical. Local recurrences are well described; for this reason, an aggressive surgical resection at diagnosis is always recommended.[172,173]

Hematologic Disorders

Sickle Cell Disease

Sickle cell disease (SCD) comprises a group of inherited hemoglobinopathies characterized by a predominance of hemoglobin (Hb) S. Included in SCD are sickle cell anemia (Hb SS, the homozygous state for the β S globin gene), Hb SC (Hb S and Hb C), sickle β-thalassemia syndrome (either Hb $β^0$ thalassemia or Hb $β^+$ thalassemia in combination with Hb S), and other combinations of Hb S and abnormal hemoglobins. These hemoglobinopathies result from the substitution of valine for glutamic acid at position 6 of the β globin chain, which alters the quaternary structure of hemoglobin and reduces the solubility of deoxyhemoglobin S to approximately 10% of that of the normal deoxyhemoglobin A. After deoxygenation of the erythrocyte, Hb S undergoes intracellular polymerization. As the concentration of Hb S increases, the erythrocytes collapse into a sickle shape, either reversibly or irreversibly. Repeated cycles of polymerization induce a series of erythrocyte abnormalities, including cytoplasmic and membrane rigidity and cellular dehydration. Elevated blood viscosity and microvascular occlusion then develop. The clinical features of the sickle cell syndromes include chronic hemolytic anemia, frequent infections owing to loss of splenic function, and microvascular obstruction producing acute and chronic anemia and organ damage from infarction and fibrosis.[174]

Patients with sickle cell anemia frequently experience acute pulmonary complications, such as asthma, thromboembolism, and acute chest syndrome (ACS). Results of several studies suggest that asthma is a significant contributing factor for acute pulmonary complications, and 35% of children with SCD have obstructive lung disease.[175] Individuals with SCD seem to be at risk of thromboembolism because of a hypercoagulable state. The term "acute chest syndrome" reflects the difficulty of establishing a definitive cause for these acute pulmonary episodes, particularly in distinguishing infection from pulmonary infarction by microvascular occlusion (Fig. 7-7).

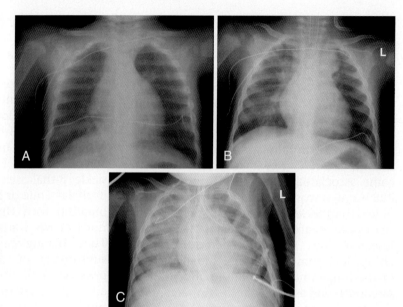

Figure 7-7. An 18-month-old girl with hemoglobin SS disease and respiratory distress. **A-C**, Radiographs reflect the rapid progression typical of acute chest syndrome at the time of admission (**A**), 24 hours later (**B**), and 72 hours later (**C**).

Acute Chest Syndrome

Definition. ACS is a clinical pulmonary exacerbation of SCD manifested by fever; a new infiltrate on chest radiograph; and one or more pulmonary signs or symptoms, such as cough, dyspnea, and chest pain.[177] As with pneumonias in children without SCD, the initial radiograph may not show a new infiltrate. The most common presenting signs are fever, cough, tachypnea, crackles, and hypoxemia. Fever is more common in children with ACS, and pain is more common in adults. ACS is the second leading reason for hospitalization (after vaso-occlusive painful crisis) and the leading cause of death in patients with SCD.[176] Sudden death in the setting of ACS may be associated with acute exacerbations of pulmonary hypertension.

Epidemiology. Vaso-occlusive painful crisis and ACS are the most common sickle cell–related events during the first decade of life. The risk of vaso-occlusive painful crisis and ACS begins in the first year and increases steadily; ACS is experienced by half of all patients with Hb SS disease by 6 years of age. Of patients with sickle cell anemia (Hb SS) experiencing a first ACS, 25% have a recurrent event in 6 months. The risk is decreased with greater levels of fetal hemoglobin (Hb F) and is increased with the magnitude of the anemia and with ele-vated steady-state white blood cell counts. Patients with Hb SC disease also are at risk, although the incidence and frequency of vaso-occlusive episodes, including ACS, is lower.[178]

Etiology. The etiology of ACS is complex and heterogeneous. In addition to the expected intravascular pulmonary thrombosis, ACS is marked by the co-occurrence of infection, fat embolism (presumably from bone infarcts), hypoventilation, edema, and reactive airway disease, and by secondary problems of mucus hypersecretion and atelectasis. Pulmonary infarction is the presumed cause in 16% of cases, and fat embolism is the presumed cause in 9%. Because multiple etiologic factors are usually involved, the diagnostic label of ACS is strongly preferred to pneumonia. A specific cause of ACS can be identified in 50% of the cases.

In children with SCD, infections are more commonly documented, as are associated bacteremias. An infectious etiology can be identified in one third of the patients; the most common agents are viruses, such as respiratory syncytial virus, parvovirus, and rhinovirus, particularly during winter months. These can be diagnosed through the immunofluorescent assessment of nasal secretions or by serial measurements of specific antibody titers. Atypical bacteria, such as *Mycoplasma pneumoniae* and *Chlamydia pneumoniae*, mostly cause bacterial infections. Pneumonia from these agents is more severe in SCD than in normal children. In the era of long-term antibiotic prophylaxis and immunizations for *Streptococcus pneumoniae* and *Haemophilus influenzae*, these bacteria are less commonly responsible for ACS than previously, and other causes such as community-acquired pneumonia have arisen.[178] In 45% of the cases, an etiology cannot be identified.[177]

The vasculopathy of SCD progresses in the first years of life to render the spleen incapable of performing its immune functions, including the generation of antibodies to encapsulated organisms. In addition to this "functional asplenia," there are abnormalities of the complement defense system. Together, these deficits predispose patients, especially children, to blood-borne infections with encapsulated organisms. Antimicrobial prophylaxis with penicillin and immunization against these organisms (*S. pneumoniae* and *H. influenzae*) are important strategies to reduce episodes of bacterial sepsis and recurrences of ACS. After age 6 months, annual immunizations against influenza are recommended.

Clinical Presentation. Nearly half of patients with SCD are usually admitted with a diagnosis other than ACS, usually a vaso-occlusive crisis; pain is a prodrome of ACS. The clinical presentation of ACS is similar to that of pneumonia. Cardinal features comprise fever; a new infiltrate on radiograph; symptoms including cough, shortness of breath, and chest pain; signs including tachypnea, crackles, and hypoxia; and pain, including a greater frequency of chest, rib, and abdominal pain in children, and a greater frequency of extremity pain in adolescents and adults. The presenting chest radiograph may be normal, as it may be with clinical pneumonia, so a second radiograph should be obtained as indicated by clinical suspicion. Multilobar involvement, especially of the lower lobes, and effusion are present in two thirds of patients. Upper and middle lobe involvement is more common in children, and isolated lower lobe involvement is more common in adults.[177,178]

Abnormalities seen on radiographs tend to progress. Oxygenation and hemoglobin decrease after diagnosis, despite aggressive intervention. Hypoxia is common, but younger patients are less likely to require oxygen.[174,177]

Bronchoscopy and BAL provide adequate material, and the diagnostic yield is high, but it is associated with risk of complications. The mean hospital stay is 10 days. Adults are more likely to have complications during hospitalization; neurologic events occur in 10% of patients. The most common is altered mental status, although cerebrovascular accidents also are common.[177]

Pathogenesis. The pathogenesis of ACS is the result of a complex series of reactions involving activation of the endothelium, often caused by an infection, and subsequent adherence of sickle erythrocytes. This sequence of events leads to a partial obstruction of microcirculatory flow; prolonged transit allows extensive polymerization of Hb S with its resultant erythrocyte rigidity. Trapping of poorly deformable sickle erythrocytes results in transient or prolonged obstruction, ischemia, and further endothelial activation.[174] Various adhesive proteins expressed on the sickle erythrocyte membrane interact with the corresponding molecules on the endothelial cell and are mediated by plasma ligands, such as thrombospondin and von Willebrand factor.[174] Hb S polymerization generates reactive oxygen species, which activates the transcription factor nuclear factor-κB, which upregulates expression of the adhesion molecule VCAM-1 on the endothelium, facilitating erythrocyte adhesion.

Granulocytes and monocytes also play an important role in microvascular occlusion. Additional vasoactive components also may play a role in the ACS process. Endothelin is a potent vasoconstrictor of the pulmonary vascular bed, and its levels are increased with hypoxemia. In patients with SCD, endothelin-1 levels are increased during the steady state, and increase sharply during the ACS. Nitric oxide, in addition to providing vasodilation of the pulmonary vasculature, downregulates VCAM-1 and inhibits the adherence of normal sickle erythrocytes to vascular endothelium.[174]

Treatment. In the management of ACS, clinicians need to consider the evolving nature of the ACS. Most patients present with pain or develop pain during admission, and in many instances, chest pain may result in hypoventilation, atelectasis, or pneumonia. Incentive spirometry must be started early and be aggressively implemented. A judicious use of opioid analgesics must be implemented early in management.

Dehydration predisposes to vaso-occlusive painful crisis and ACS, and commonly follows episodes of fever, tachypnea, or anorexia. Aggressive rehydration is always indicated in the management of vaso-occlusive crises. Rehydration is often accomplished by the administration of fluids at a rate of 1.5 times maintenance, which is reduced to maintenance when the patient is normovolemic. Overhydration should be avoided because pulmonary edema and worsening of the disease process might ensue. Empiric antibiotic therapy always must include a combination of a macrolide and a second-generation cephalosporin. Vancomycin also is recommended if fever persists, and there is history of infection with penicillin-resistant *S. pneumoniae*, or if the patient resides in an area with a high prevalence of resistance of this organism. Oxygen supplementation also is indicated for decreases in pulse oximetry greater than 4% over baseline, or for values less than 92%.

Oxygenation significantly improves with simple blood transfusion and exchange transfusion. Early transfusions are indicated for patients at high risk of complications; patients presenting with severe anemia, thrombocytopenia, and multilobar pneumonia should receive a transfusion even before respiratory distress develops. A post-transfusion increase in hemoglobin levels greater than 11 g/dL must be avoided, however, because of the risk of sudden increase in blood viscosity that could lead to thrombosis and ischemic episodes. Exchange transfusion is indicated if the patient's baseline hemoglobin is elevated, or the patient has more severe disease, worsening hypoxemia, neurologic abnormalities, or multiorgan failure.

Evidence is mounting that reactive airway disease may play a role as a cause and as a consequence of ACS.[174] Reactive airway disease may occur in almost half of SCD patients, and seems to be a risk factor for the development of ACS and pulmonary hypertension.[181] The concurrent association of reactive airway disease and ACS is associated with more severe exacerbation and prolonged hospitalization. Reactive airway disease is associated with the release of a wider variety of inflammatory mediators and cytokines than with ACS alone, and is associated with airway edema and mucus hypersecretion, factors known to worsen the course of ACS.

Treatment of reactive airway disease exacerbations in the context of ACS is similar to standard acute asthma care. There is a theoretical basis for steroid use because activation of the inflammatory cascade plays a central role in ACS; however, its role is still unclear. A short course of steroids may reduce the length of hospitalization in children and the need for analgesics and oxygen supplementation, but a rebound effect may occur.[179] Bronchoscopy is recommended when patients do not respond to initial therapy. Aggressive mechanical ventilatory support, including extracorporeal membrane oxygenation, may be necessary; nitric oxide also may be used.[174,176,180]

Secondary Complications. As with community-acquired pneumonias, ACS is frequently associated with atelectasis or pleural effusions or both. The pleural fluid is usually sterile and exudative, but may develop empyema. The atelectasis may or may not be associated with retained airway mucus secretions. In some cases, the mucus strings are extensive and dehydrated and may form bronchial casts. Because of their firmness, the syndrome has been referred to as plastic bronchitis. In these cases, fiberoptic bronchoscopy with washes of saline, DNase, or *N*-acetyl cysteine may be useful in clearing the airway obstruction and expediting the resolution of the atelectasis.

Chronic Sickle Cell Lung Disease

Chronic sickle lung disease is a progressive disorder that is insidious in onset during childhood and may be asymptomatic in the absence of frequent exacerbations of ACS. The end stage of progression is characterized by persistent hypoxemia, radiographic evidence of interstitial fibrosis, restrictive lung disease on pulmonary function testing, pulmonary hypertension, and cor pulmonale.

Pulmonary hypertension in patients with SCD has been associated with worsened survival. Close pulmonary and cardiac follow-up are essential to monitor the progression of chronic sickle lung disease.

Pulmonary Hypertension

The obliterative vasculopathy of pulmonary hypertension is evident in one third of post-mortem studies of patients with SCD, but the true prevalence is unknown. This disorder is most frequently recognized in adults, but almost certainly originates earlier in childhood. Although a worsened prognosis for chronic sickle lung disease and pulmonary hypertension is associated with recurrent episodes of ACS, the prevalence of pulmonary hypertension also is high in patients without a history of ACS.

This pathophysiologic predisposition is related to the combination of hemolytic anemia and "functional asplenia."[181] Hemolysis in combination with inadequate splenic clearance results in the accumulation of iron-rich hemoglobin, which functions as a scavenger of nitric oxide and catalyzes the formation of oxygen radical species. Arginase is simultaneously released from erythrocytes and serves to limit the supply of arginine to nitric oxide synthase, limiting the synthesis of nitric oxide. The nitric oxide serves a crucial function in promoting pulmonary vasodilation and limiting the impact of many factors contributing to the vascular remodeling of pulmonary hypertension. The functional asplenia contributes to the remodeling by the failure to clear platelet-derived mediators and cytokines that promote adherence of erythrocytes to the endothelium and cause microthrombosis.

The diagnosis of pulmonary hypertension in SCD is ominous, with a 10-fold increase in the risk for death and survival less than 50% within 4 years. The more recent validation of echocardiography as a diagnostic tool for pulmonary hypertension in SCD should promote earlier detection. Several studies have suggested the potential role for oxygen therapy, red blood cell transfusions, inhaled nitric oxide, intravenous arginine, prostacyclin, and the newer vasodilators. Controlled long-term studies are needed to determine the effectiveness of these and other therapies.[183]

Much of the improved quality of life and survival of patients with SCD is attributed to the details of preventive health care. Because the spleen is a victim of sickle cell vasculopathy in the first few years of life (functional asplenia), functional immunity to encapsulated organisms is impaired, and the risk for sepsis from these organisms is increased. Protective strategies include penicillin prophylaxis and immunizations to *S. pneumoniae* and *H. influenzae*. Penicillin (or erythromycin) is administered twice daily from early infancy to age 5 years in children with the more severe hemoglobinopathies (Hb SS and Hb S/β[0] thalassemia) and through age 3 years in children with less severe variants of SCD, such as Hb SC. Prophylactic antibiotics are given permanently to patients who have undergone splenectomy or have experienced pneumococcal sepsis. The 7-valent pneumococcal vaccine is administered to infants beginning at 2 months of age with four doses administered by the age of 15 months, and the 23-valent vaccine is administered at ages 2 and 5 years and then every 5 to 7 years thereafter. The usual childhood schedule is followed for *H. influenzae* type B immunizations. Immunizations to influenza virus are administered annually after age 6 months. The usual childhood immunization schedule for hepatitis B is emphasized to prevent this potential complication of recurrent red blood cell transfusions.

Therapies to correct the basic genetic or β globin protein defect of SCD and therapies to prevent the progression of SCD do not yet exist. The major current therapeutic strategies are designed to reduce the proportion of erythrocytes carrying predominantly sickle hemoglobin (Hb S) and to delay the progression of pulmonary hypertension.

Of all the new therapies for treating SCD, hydroxyurea is the most promising. Several pediatric and adult trials have reported decreases in pain, the incidence of ACS, and overall mortality.[181] Hydroxyurea therapy was initiated because of the drug's ability to increase Hb F production. This increase in Hb F and a concomitant increase in red blood cell volume effectively reduce the intracellular concentration of Hb S and result in decreased sickling. Hydroxyurea has other beneficial effects, including a decrease in neutrophils and monocytes (intervening in the inflammatory cascade), an increase in red blood cell deformability, and a decrease in the adhesive receptors in the erythrocyte membrane.[181] Trials of increasing length of hydroxyurea therapy in adults and children have shown safety and clinical efficacy, including a reduction in the incidence of ACS.[181]

Other options include therapy with erythropoietin to increase Hb F, but its effectiveness has been suboptimal. Because of this and its substantial expense, use of erythropoietin has been limited. Its primary use is as adjunctive therapy for patients whose response to hydroxyurea is suboptimal or for patients with religious objections to blood transfusions.

Transfusion therapy of normal erythrocytes serves to depress the bone marrow production of erythrocytes expressing sickle hemoglobin.[182] The timing of transfusion may be acute, intermittent, or chronic. Adverse effects of recurrent transfusions include iron overload, blood-borne infections, and alloimmunization, complications that can be reduced by erythrocytopheresis, highly specific crossmatching, and the newer iron-chelating agents. Current indications for red blood cell transfusion therapy in SCD include severe cases of vaso-occlusive painful crisis, recurrent or severe ACS, severe or worsening anemia, and primary and secondary stroke prevention in patients at increased risk.

Because of the potentially serious complications of bone marrow transplantation, in the United States it is offered primarily to patients who have had serious complications, such as stroke or recurrent ACS, and to patients with HLA-matched sibling donors. Its greatest benefit is, however, to patients who have neither experienced significant complications nor developed significant chronic sickle lung disease.

Efforts to develop effective gene therapy or β globin substitution have failed so far. The primary impediment has been the development of a vector suitable for the delivery of the replacement of β globin DNA to bone marrow precursors.

Histiocytic Disorders of the Lung

The histiocytoses are a group of rare hematopoietic disorders characterized by the clonal proliferation and pathologic accumulation of cells of the mononuclear-phagocyte system in tissues. The mononuclear-phagocyte system is a system of cells whose primary functions consist of phagocytosis of foreign material, antigen processing, and antigen presentation to lymphocytes. Mononuclear phagocytes are subclassified into two major classes, macrophages and dendritic cells, based on morphologic and functional characteristics. The most common pulmonary phagocytes are the alveolar and the airway macrophages. They are indistinguishable except for their location within the respiratory tract. These cells are primarily responsible for the sequestering and disposal of inhaled particles and pulmonary surfactant. They play an active role in the maintenance and remodeling of the extracellular connective tissue matrix through the secretion of cytokines that regulate matrix production and degradation. Interstitial macrophages are the second group of pulmonary macrophages with an improved antigen-presenting capability. The second class of mononuclear phagocytes, the dendritic cells, consist of dendritic cells of the lymphoid follicle and Langerhans cells of the skin and other organs.

The histiocytic disorders can be classified into three classes based on the pathologic cells present within the lesions: class I, dendritic cell histiocytosis; class II, non-dendritic cell histiocytosis, and class III, malignant histiocytosis. The rest of this discussion is dedicated to the pathophysiology, clinical presentation, diagnosis, and treatment of Langerhans cell histiocytosis (LCH) and histiocytic disorders involving the lung.

LCH is the most common of the dendritic cell histiocytoses. It is a proliferative disorder of activated Langerhans cells and is characterized by variable biologic behavior and a spectrum of distinct clinical presentations.[184] The pathogenesis of LCH is poorly understood. Because LCH has been shown to be a monoclonal condition, it has been considered a neoplastic disorder.[185,186] Different patterns of clinical involvement indicate other pathogenetic mechanisms, however. The benign histopathologic appearance of the lesions, the occurrence of spontaneous remissions,[187] and the ability to respond to immunomodulation[188] suggest a reactive clonal disorder, rather than a malignant process, at least in some cases. Langerhans cells, similar to other dendritic cells, have a crucial role in the immune system, and it has been suggested that LCH could be the result of immune dysregulation. Although no consistent immunologic abnormalities have been described, there is increasing evidence that LCH may be the result of an uncontrolled and abnormal proliferation of Langerhans cells secondary to immune dysregulation or after exposure to an as-yet-undetermined stimulus.[189,190]

The diagnosis of LCH requires a biopsy with the specimen showing typical pathologic features of Langerhans cell infiltrates and confirmatory positive staining for CD1a and S-100. Alternatively, the demonstration of Birbeck granules by electron microscopy has been used for confirmation of this diagnosis. The diagnosis of pulmonary LCH in children with multisystem disease is usually clinical because the histologic diagnosis is usually made from extrapulmonary lesions. In the rare cases of isolated lung disease, a morphologic confirmation is required, and it can be obtained by lung biopsy or by BAL. In the latter case, the presence of greater than 5% of CD1a-positive cells in the BAL fluid is very suggestive of LCH. BAL also is a good tool for monitoring response and follow-up.[191]

The histopathology of the lesion is uniform, regardless of the clinical severity of the disease. It consists of collections of Langerhans cells, interdigitating cells, and macrophages, accompanied by T lymphocytes with variable numbers of multinucleated giant histiocytes and eosinophils.[192]

In light of the pathologic basis of the diagnosis of LCH and the variable nature of clinical presentations, LCH is now subclassified by the degree of organ involvement: localized single-system disease, multifocal single-system disease, and multisystem disease. Localized LCH, involving skin, lymph node, or bones, usually has a good prognosis. The most common presentation of multifocal

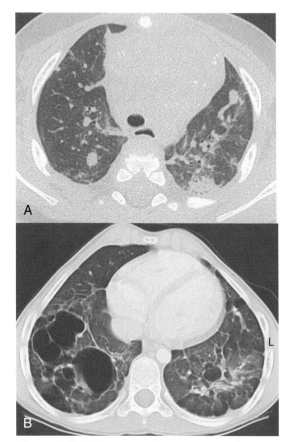

Figure 7-8. Pulmonary involvement in Langerhans cell histiocytosis (LCH). **A,** CT scan shows acute changes in an infant with newly diagnosed LCH and multisystem involvement. Multiple small nodular opacities and cystic changes are seen. Also note enlarged thymus with calcifications. **B,** CT scan of a 6-year-old boy shows chronic fibrosis, air trapping, and bullous disease. This child received treatment for LCH and had lung involvement during infancy.

LCH includes diffuse skin involvement and involvement of multiple bones. The oral cavity; lymph nodes; and, to a lesser extent, lungs, liver, and brain are common sites of involvement in this disease. Lung involvement has been reported to occur in 20% to 50% of patients with multisystem disease. Radiographic changes consistent with past lung involvement are present in 15% to 20% of long-term survivors (Fig. 7-8A).[193,194]

Primary Pulmonary Langerhans Cell Histiocytosis
Primary pulmonary LCH is a disorder that most frequently affects young white adults with an equal sex distribution. LCH in this age group is epidemiologically associated with cigarette smoking; greater than 90% of patients

have a history of smoking, and the disease usually responds to smoking cessation, although systemic chemotherapy also may be needed. An important defining factor is that, in adult cases, Langerhans cell proliferation in primary pulmonary LCH is usually not clonal; this finding is in contrast to that associated with childhood LCH.[195] Although primary pulmonary LCH can occur at any age, it is rarely seen in patients younger than 15 years. Pulmonary involvement as part of systemic LCH is a common feature of multisystem LCH, however, seen in one third of patients.

The pathogenesis underlying primary pulmonary LCH, similar to systemic LCH, is not well defined, but thought to be the result of an abnormal immune reaction to an irritant (i.e., smoke). Primary pulmonary LCH is mostly seen in the third or fourth decade of life. Twenty percent to 25% of patients are asymptomatic at the time of diagnosis, with the disease being detected on a screening chest radiograph. Respiratory symptoms may include chronic cough and dyspnea and, more rarely, hemoptysis or chest pain. Chest pain may be due to pneumothoraces or rib lesions.

Histopathologically, primary pulmonary LCH begins as a proliferation of Langerhans cells along the small airways. These cellular lesions expand to form nodules that can measure 1.5 cm. These nodules include a mixed population of cells with variable numbers of CD1a-positive Langerhans cells, eosinophils, lymphocytes, plasma cells, and fibroblasts. There is progression from cellular nodules to fibrosis, leading to a distinctive honeycomb-like pattern and hyperinflation (Fig. 7-8B). In later stages, fibrosis is the predominant feature, and Langerhans cells are absent from the lesions.[195]

Clinically, acute lung involvement occurs in the context of multisystem disease. Patients usually present during the first 2 years of life, with involvement of multiple systems, such as the bones, skin, lymph nodes, liver, spleen, and hematopoietic system.[193] Children most commonly develop nonproductive cough and dyspnea. Early in the disease, the chest radiograph shows micronodular or reticulonodular and interstitial infiltrates, with superimposed cystic changes predominantly involving the middle and upper lobes, symmetrically. As the disease progresses, nodular lesions are less frequent, and cystic changes are much more prominent, progressing to the appearance of honeycombing and advanced emphysema. Early changes are best seen in high-resolution CT scans. The combination of diffuse cystic changes with small peribronchial nodular opacities on CT is highly suggestive of LCH.[193-195]

Treatment of pulmonary LCH in children needs to be discussed in the context of the degree of involvement of other organs. Lung involvement is considered a poor prognostic feature, however, so these patients need to be treated aggressively, usually with combination chemotherapy, for approximately 12 months. Different regimens have proven to be effective, and different combinations of prednisone, vinblastine, etoposide, mercaptopurine, and methotrexate have been used.[193,194] The optimal therapy for primary pulmonary LCH remains undefined. Smoking cessation is the most important component of therapy. Successful smoking cessation, combined with use of oral corticosteroids, usually results in remission. In cases refractory to corticosteroids, systemic chemotherapy may be required.[195]

Complications of Treatment of Hematologic and Oncologic Disorders

Hematopoietic Stem Cell Transplantation

Hematopoietic stem cell transplantation (HSCT) has been used as a lifesaving procedure in children who have many malignant hematologic, immunologic, and inherited metabolic diseases. Allogeneic and autologous HSCTs are increasingly used. Pulmonary complications depend on various factors, including pretransplant intensive chemotherapy combined with radiation therapy, and post-transplant infectious and noninfectious complications. These complications have been well studied in adults. The pediatric experience is limited, but includes the same respiratory complications.

In one retrospective analysis, severe pulmonary complications occurred in 17 of 138 patients, leading to death in 8 (7%) patients.[196] Three important post-HSCT periods can be identified for lung complications: the first month post-transplant, which is characterized by neutropenia; the second month, in which idiopathic pneumonia syndrome can develop; and the late phase, after the third month, which is characterized by late-onset noninfectious pulmonary complications.

First Phase

The phase that precedes engraftment is typically characterized by prolonged neutropenia and disruption of the mucosal barrier. The combination of neutropenia and mucositis predisposes patients to infectious pulmonary complications. Noninfectious complications (pulmonary edema, diffuse alveolar hemorrhage) also may occur.

Pulmonary edema usually occurs in the second or third week after HSCT.[197] The exact incidence is unknown, but it is a common problem. Patients present with acute onset of dyspnea and clinical findings that include weight gain of rapid onset, bilateral pulmonary crackles, and hypoxemia. The chest radiograph shows mild to severe vascular redistribution and bilateral interstitial infiltrates, with or without pleural effusion. These findings are indistinguishable from other causes of cardiogenic and noncardiogenic pulmonary edema. Overzealous hydration, blood transfusion, and renal and cardiac insufficiency from chemotherapy can contribute to the development of pulmonary edema.[198] The management of post-HSCT pulmonary edema is similar to the management of pulmonary edema resulting from other causes.

Diffuse alveolar hemorrhage (DAH), a serious post-HSCT complication, usually occurs in the second and third week after transplantation.[199] DAH has been reported in 5% of all patients who have undergone HSCT, and is more frequent in autologous HSCT recipients.[200] DAH is characterized by dyspnea of sudden onset, nonproductive cough, fever, and hypoxemia; hemoptysis is rare. Chest radiograph abnormalities include bilateral interstitial infiltrates. The diagnosis is made by BAL that shows a hemorrhagic fluid and

microbiologic results that exclude pulmonary infection. Risk factors for the development of DAH include intensive conditioning chemotherapy, radiation toxicity, solid malignancy, and age older than 40 years. Early diagnosis of DAH and prompt intervention are crucial. High doses of corticosteroids may improve survival and reduce the development of subsequent respiratory failure[201]; however, the prognosis for DAH is very poor.

Second Phase

Between the first and third months post-transplant, as the neutropenia resolves, idiopathic pneumonitis syndrome (IPS) may develop. The diagnosis of IPS is made by exclusion of other causes, including infectious.[202] The incidence of IPS after allogeneic HSCT in adult patients is approximately 10% to 15%, and the median time from transplantation is approximately 45 days.[203] The histologic patterns of IPS are interstitial pneumonitis and diffuse alveolar damage.[203] The usual presenting symptoms include dyspnea, nonproductive cough, fever, hypoxemia, and diffuse pulmonary infiltrates. The risk factor for the development of IPS includes allogeneic HSCT, high-dose radiation, increasing age, chronic myelogenous leukemia, previous splenectomy, and graft-versus-host disease (GVHD). There is no proven effective treatment for IPS after HSCT, although corticosteroids may be helpful in some patients. The prognosis is poor.

Pulmonary complications occurring after the third month post-transplant are usually due to chronic GVHD.[205] The incidence of late-onset noninfectious pulmonary complications after HSCT has been reported to be 10% to 23%.[206,207] The only significant variables associated with such complications were chronic GVHD and complications of GVHD therapy. These obstructive or restrictive pulmonary complications include bronchiolitis obliterans, cryptogenic organizing pneumonia (COP), and toxicity syndrome.

Bronchiolitis obliterans, an obstructive pulmonary disease, affects the small airways and was first described as a late complication of allogeneic HSCT, mostly in long-term survivors who have chronic GVHD, although it can occur at any time. The incidence of bronchiolitis obliterans has been reported to be 2% to 14% in allogeneic HSCT recipients who survive longer than 3 months post-transplant.[208] The cause is unknown. An immunologic mechanism that includes injury of the bronchial epithelia has been suggested, but other causes, such as viral infections, also have been postulated. The pathogenesis is likely to be multifactorial.[209] Patients generally present with dyspnea, wheezing, and nonproductive cough. Chest radiograph findings may be minimal with occasional evidence of hyperinflation. High-resolution CT scan of the chest shows bronchial wall thickening, peripheral vascular pruning, and mosaic lung attenuation with air trapping on expiratory scan.[210]

Airflow obstruction is the hallmark of bronchiolitis obliterans. A reduction in the ratio of forced expiratory volume in 1 second to forced vital capacity is commonly present in patients with GVHD. An obstructive lung disease pattern and the lack of response to bronchodilators form a sufficient basis for making a diagnosis of bronchiolitis obliterans. Although open lung biopsy is required to confirm the diagnosis of bronchiolitis obliterans, it is seldom needed in practice. The diagnosis of bronchiolitis obliterans can be made based on clinical criteria, pulmonary function test abnormalities, and high-resolution CT scan without open lung biopsy. The treatment consists of increasing immunosuppression, usually with prednisone and other agents such as cyclosporine or azathioprine. Bronchiolitis obliterans is often progressive and unresponsive to therapy. A rapid deterioration, as shown on pulmonary function test, and severe obstruction (forced expiratory volume in 1 second <45%) are associated with poor prognosis.

COP is a common late complication; in most cases, the exact etiology is unknown. COP was formerly known as "bronchiolitis obliterans with organizing pneumonia." This condition differs from that of bronchiolitis obliterans. The histologic changes associated with COP are proliferative bronchiolitis and alveolitis, which affect the distal airways. Patients with COP have a characteristically restrictive pattern on pulmonary function tests. Patients with COP have nonproductive cough, low-grade fever, and dyspnea. Chest radiographs are characterized by the presence of patchy pulmonary infiltrates in multiple lobes. Bronchiolitis obliterans manifests with hyperlucency. High-resolution CT shows patchy consolidation, particularly with peribronchovascular or peripheral distribution in immunocompetent patients, in whom ground-glass attenuation and nodules are more frequent.[211] Risk factors for COP include being the recipient of an allogeneic HSCT and the development of GVHD. Corticosteroids are effective in 60% of patients with COP, but infections should be carefully ruled out before initiating treatment with corticosteroids.[206]

Recipients of autologous transplants who receive high-dose chemotherapy or radiotherapy as conditioning for HSCT may experience pulmonary toxicity months to years after the transplantation procedure.[212] Drug-induced and radiation-induced lung toxicity is described in greater detail subsequently. Pulmonary complications are important causes of morbidity and mortality. Chest radiographic changes are nonspecific. High-resolution CT of the chest increases the detection of pulmonary abnormalities, even when results of chest radiographs are normal, and it can help in establishing the diagnosis. It also is helpful in guiding lung biopsy.

Transfusion-Related Acute Lung Injury

Although uncommon, transfusion-related acute lung injury (TRALI) has been increasingly recognized as the leading cause of transfusion-related death in the United States; its development is associated with 1 in 5000 U of transfused blood products.[213] Patients in whom acute onset of bilateral chest infiltrates develops during or within 6 hours of the completion of transfusion of plasma-containing blood products should be evaluated for this condition. In most cases, signs of respiratory distress develop within the first 1 to 2 hours after the transfusion is started. Affected patients usually have hypoxemia (PaO_2/FiO_2 <300 mm Hg) and diffuse lung infiltrates on the chest x-ray suggestive of noncardiogenic pulmonary edema.[214,215]

Blood products implicated in TRALI include whole blood, red blood cells, platelet transfusions (including platelet concentrates and plateletpheresis), fresh frozen plasma, and cryoprecipitate.[216] Although less common, intravenous immunoglobulin preparations also have been implicated in TRALI.[216] The condition has been reported predominantly in patients with cancer or other hematologic diseases such as SCD and in patients undergoing solid organ or stem cell transplantation.[214] Other, less common settings where this adverse transfusion reaction may occur are complement-mediated hemolysis in paroxysmal nocturnal hemoglobinuria and lung damage associated with granulocyte transfusions.[214] Because pulmonary infiltrates may result from various causes, establishing the diagnosis of TRALI may be difficult. The differential diagnosis includes ACS in sickle cell anemia, infections, diffuse alveolar damage after bone marrow recovery, and lung hemorrhage. Patients with TRALI often improve within 48 to 72 hours of onset, but occasional patients die of acute respiratory failure.

TRALI is more common in adults; however, several well-documented pediatric cases have been reported. Neonates, who seem to be protected from TRALI, may develop leukopenia as a complication of transfusion, but not pulmonary problems.[214,217,218] Pediatric oncology patients require frequent and repeated transfusions, so it is not surprising that TRALI has been more frequently reported in this population.[217]

No single test can reliably help make the diagnosis of TRALI, but some clinical clues may be helpful. Patients with TRALI often present with fever, chills, and hypotension. Such patients often have transient leukopenia that resolves within a few hours; this condition may be helpful in making a diagnosis.[219] A complete blood cell count should be obtained in every case in which TRALI is suspected. In patients requiring ventilatory support, a bronchial sample to measure the protein level should be obtained within 15 minutes of intubation to be reliable.[220] An edema fluid protein-to-plasma protein ratio greater than 0.6 is highly suggestive of TRALI. Ratios less than 0.6 may indicate a cardiac source of pulmonary edema.[220] Patients with TRALI also have normal or decreased pulmonary artery wedge pressure and left atrial pressure, although these are rarely measured in children.

The pathophysiology of TRALI is not well understood. Two hypotheses have been postulated. The first one tries to explain TRALI as an antibody-mediated event.[221] These antibodies may bind to the corresponding HLA epitopes on the lung endothelium, resulting in capillary leak and cell damage.[222] Alternatively, some authors hypothesize that a two-event model may explain the occurrence of TRALI. The first event would be host-related predisposing factors, such as the ones described previously, leading to lung sequestration of polymorphonuclear neutrophils.[222] The second event includes the infusion of chemical mediators, including antibodies against polymorphonuclear neutrophils, HLA, or cytokines.[222] Soluble CD40 (a member of the tumor necrosis factor family of receptors) ligands have been reported to accumulate in stored blood components, leading to priming of CD40-dependent granulocyte activation, which ultimately may cause lung injury.[223]

The management of TRALI is largely supportive.[214] Oxygen supplementation and occasional mechanical ventilation should be provided. It is important that clinicians be aware of this potential complication because patients usually do well without long-term sequelae, if they survive the initial insult. The blood bank also should be informed of this complication to avoid repeated exposure of the recipient to the same donor-derived blood products, and if possible, the blood bank can perform anti-HLA antibody detection. These tests are expensive, however, and are not available in many blood banks. If respiratory distress occurs during transfusion, the transfusion should be stopped immediately. Preventing TRALI is a challenge because no test is reliable enough to predict this potential complication.

An increased awareness of this complication may improve the knowledge of its clinical and pathophysiologic features. At present, TRALI can be diagnosed only by excluding other causes, however. TRALI should be included in the differential diagnosis of acute pulmonary problems in pediatric oncology patients.

Chemotherapy-Induced Lung Toxicity

Numerous drugs can cause pulmonary or pleural reactions in children. The most common offenders are certain chemotherapeutic agents used in pediatric oncology (Table 7-1). Other agents with lung toxicity are increasingly reported (Table 7-2). Diffuse interstitial pneumonitis and fibrosis constitute the most frequent clinical presentation. Hypersensitivity lung disease, noncardiogenic pulmonary edema, pleural effusion, bronchiolitis obliterans, and alveolar hemorrhage also are encountered.

Although some drug-induced pulmonary damage is reversible, persistent and even fatal dysfunction may occur. Lung reactions occasionally are temporarily remote from exposure to chemotherapeutic agents. Depending on the agent involved, the reaction may or not be dose-related. The mechanism of toxicity is thought to be direct injury to lung cells in most cases, but immunologic and central nervous system-mediated mechanisms seem to play a role in the toxicity of certain agents. Identified risk factors include patient age, cumulative dose, prior or concurrent radiation, oxygen therapy, and use of other toxic drugs. Most reactions to noncytotoxic drugs seem to develop idiosyncratically. When patients are treated with several potentially toxic drugs or with a toxic drug plus irradiation to the chest or high oxygen concentration, specific offenders cannot be identified. There is little, if any, evidence that children are more susceptible to drug-related lung injury, and they may be less susceptible to some agents, such as bleomycin.

Although better identification of chemotherapy-induced lung toxicity has led to a more judicious use of agents that might cause lung toxicity, the widespread use of higher dose chemotherapy regimens preceding stem cell rescue has improved the chances of survival of high-risk patients who receive a high cumulative dose of chemotherapy and radiotherapy, and who have

Table 7-1	Lung Toxicity Associated with Chemotherapeutic Agents Used in Pediatric Oncology		
DRUG	**PEDIATRIC DISEASES**	**PROPOSED MECHANISM**	**TYPICAL FEATURES**
Bleomycin	Hodgkin disease	Oxidative effect	Most common cause of pulmonary toxicity
	Germ cell tumors	Release of proteases	Dose-related acute and chronic lung toxicity
Busulfan	Bone marrow transplantation	Direct toxicity	Late-onset pulmonary fibrosis
			Radiation may increase toxicity
Carmustine	Bone marrow transplantation	Oxidative damage	Same as bleomycin
Cyclophosphamide	Widely used in several malignancies	Oxidative damage	Lung toxicity is uncommon
			Usually subacute
Methotrexate	Hematologic malignancies	Hypersensitivity or direct effect	Mild and reversible hypersensitivity lung toxicity
	Osteogenic sarcoma		Not related to cumulative dose
Cytarabine	Hematologic malignancies	Not well studied	Capillary leak syndrome
			BO associated with higher doses
Melphalan	Bone marrow transplantation	Similar to busulfan	Similar to busulfan
Fludarabine	Acute myelogenous leukemia	Not well studied	Interstitial pneumonia reported in adults
	Bone marrow transplantation		

BO, bronchiolitis obliterans.
Data from references 224-229, 237, 238, 242.

Table 7-2	Newer Agents Used in Pediatric Cancer Treatment Associated with Lung Toxicity	
DRUG	**PEDIATRIC DISEASE**	**REPORTED LUNG TOXICITY**
Rituximab	Lymphoma, post-transplant lymphoproliferative disease	Acute-onset interstitial pneumonia, lung fibrosis
Imatinib	Chronic myelogenous leukemia	Rare cases of interstitial pneumonia
Filgrastim (G-CSF)	Various diseases, bone marrow transplantation	Pleural effusion and noncardiogenic pulmonary edema and ARDS
Trans-retinoic acid	Acute promyelocytic leukemia	Diffuse pulmonary infiltrates in the setting of retinoic acid syndrome

ARDS, acute respiratory distress syndrome; G-CSF, granulocyte colony-stimulating factor.
Data from references 224, 226, 242-245.

a history of opportunistic infection. This new generation of heavily pretreated survivors constitutes a high-risk population for long-term toxicity, including lung toxicity.

The clinical manifestations of drug-induced lung disease include fever, malaise, dyspnea, and a nonproductive cough. Radiologic studies almost always show diffuse alveolar or interstitial infiltrates, or both. Segmental or lobar disease, particularly if unilateral, should suggest another diagnosis. A restrictive lung pattern in pulmonary function testing may be found before the appearance of radiographic lesions. CT of the chest also may reveal early evidence of parenchymal abnormalities. Hypoxemia is an early and clinically important functional manifestation. Pathologic changes do not distinguish among most drugs and most often consist of interstitial thickening with chronic inflammatory cell infiltrate in the interstitial or alveolar compartment, fibroblast proliferation, fibrosis, and hyperplasia of type II pneumocytes. With hypersensitivity reactions, the interstitial infiltrate includes numerous eosinophils.

The manifestations of drug-induced lung toxicity are usually nonspecific, and so establishing a definitive diagnosis may be difficult. Other diagnoses, such as infection, pulmonary hemorrhage, lung disease related to an underlying disorder, and radiation damage, must be considered in the differential diagnosis. BAL is being increasingly done to provide microbiologic and cytologic information essential to differential diagnosis and as a research tool to identify disease markers and potential pathogenetic mechanisms.

Practical criteria for diagnosing drug-induced lung disease have been suggested.

These include (1) no other likely cause of lung disease, (2) symptoms consistent with the suspected drug, (3) time course compatible with drug-induced lung disease, (4) compatible tissue or BAL findings, and (5) improvement after the drug is discontinued.

Cytotoxic Drugs

Antibiotics—Bleomycin. Bleomycin has been consistently associated with lung toxicity, especially lung fibrosis, in children and adults.[227] Although the drug is active against squamous cell carcinoma and germ cell tumors, its major use in children is in the treatment of HD and other lymphomas.[231,232] Because of the high frequency of lung reactions and the utility of bleomycin for generating animal models of lung fibrosis,[230] this drug has been studied more thoroughly than others. Bleomycin can cause early-onset and late-onset lung injury.[227] Late-onset lung injury, which is initially characterized by interstitial pneumonitis potentially leading to pulmonary fibrosis, is the most common effect and may occur several months or years after exposure to the drug. Early bleomycin toxicity usually manifests as an acute hypersensitivity reaction.[227]

Lung injury secondary to bleomycin occurs in approximately 4% to 7% of all patients receiving the drug,[227] although the reported incidence is 40%. The frequency of reactions in children is not well documented because few children receive this agent. Follow-up data analyses from the Childhood Cancer Survivor Study indicated, however, that the use of bleomycin is significantly associated with pulmonary fibrosis (relative risk 1.7), bronchitis (relative risk 1.4), and chronic cough (relative risk 1.9) at 5 years postdiagnosis.

Bleomycin is metabolized by bleomycin hydrolase, which is lacking in the lungs and skin; the active drug accumulates, giving rise to increased exposure in these tissues.[233] Bleomycin lung toxicity occurs mainly as a result of direct injury to cells and by secondary immunologic reactions.[227,233] Direct toxicity may be mediated by oxidant injury, either through the production of reactive oxygen metabolites or through inactivation of antioxidants.

Bleomycin-induced lung disease can begin insidiously. Asymptomatic patients may have decreases in arterial oxygen saturation and diffusing capacity for carbon monoxide (DLCO). As the illness progresses, there is a decline in vital capacity and total lung capacity, characteristic of restrictive lung disease.[227,234] In interstitial pneumonitis and hypersensitivity lung reactions, patients often present with a dry, hacking cough and dyspnea; these manifestations occur only on exertion in mild cases, but significant respiratory distress accompanies advanced illness. Fever suggests a hypersensitivity reaction. Physical examination reveals tachypnea and crackles. Chest radiographs in symptomatic patients most commonly show diffuse linear densities. CT of the chest is more sensitive for detection of early interstitial disease.

Histopathologic features are nonspecific and similar to the features seen in other cases of diffuse alveolar damage owing to other causes. The diagnosis is established by exclusion. Early features include acute inflammation such as edema, intra-alveolar hemorrhage, desquamation of alveolar cells, and hyaline membrane formation (Fig. 7-9). At a later stage, features of interstitial pneumonitis can be seen, including angiitis and inflammatory infiltrates. Interstitial fibrosis occurs as a final event (Fig. 7-10). The alveolar epithelium discloses morphologic changes including hyperplasia of type II pneumocytes, often with bizarre features. Insult from chemotherapy also may affect the bronchial wall, leading to peribronchial fibrosis. Eosinophil infiltration and granulomatous inflammation have been associated with the use of bleomycin. Features of bronchiolitis obliterans also may occur secondary to bleomycin toxicity. Lung biopsy is sometimes unavoidable in cases of lung fibrosis of unexplained etiology. Some patients also may show pleural thickening leading to fibrosis as a late event.

Risk factors for bleomycin toxicity include age, cumulative dose, and concomitant therapies.[234] Children seem to be less prone to development of bleomycin lung toxicity than older patients.[227,234] There is evidence in animal models and humans that the risk

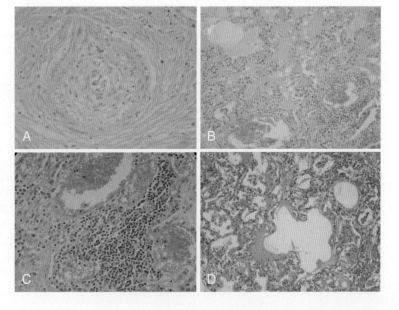

Figure 7-9. Early-onset pathologic pulmonary changes associated with treatment-induced toxicity (hematoxylin-eosin stains). **A**, Vascular changes consisting of thickening of the media and narrowing of the vascular lumen. **B**, Intra-alveolar edema and perivascular mononuclear infiltrates. **C**, Hemorrhage and interstitial mononuclear infiltrate. **D**, Hyaline membrane formation. (See Color Plate)

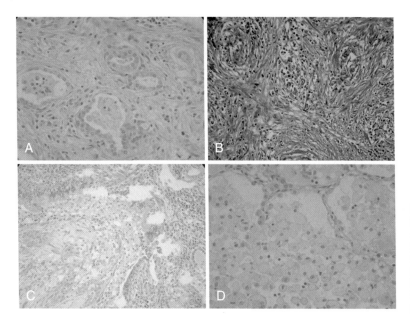

Figure 7-10. Late-onset pathologic pulmonary changes associated with treatment-induced toxicity (hematoxylin-eosin stains). **A,** Increased collagen content in the alveolar septum and epithelial hyperplasia. **B,** Interstitial fibrosis. **C,** Bronchiolitis obliterans. **D,** Organizing pneumonia. (See Color Plate)

of bleomycin lung toxicity increases with dose intensity.[227] Cumulative doses greater than 500 U have been associated with a 20% incidence of interstitial lung toxicity in adults.[227] Lung toxicity, including death resulting from toxicity, may occur with lower doses, however. Patients receiving bleomycin should be monitored by serial determinations of DLCO.[227,235] Bleomycin-induced lung toxicity may occur 6 months after discontinuation of the drug in patients with normal DLCO test results during bleomycin therapy. Although the results of this test can be affected by numerous factors, it is recommended that bleomycin therapy be stopped when the DLCO decreases by greater than 40% to 60% of baseline values.[227] CT of the chest may be useful for monitoring progression of disease. In addition, administration of cumulative doses greater than 400 U should be avoided.

Radiotherapy also can cause lung toxicity by oxidative injury. It may potentiate the risk of lung toxicity by bleomycin. It is currently unknown, however, how much toxicity radiotherapy adds to chemotherapy in these cases. This is an important issue because pediatric patients with HD usually receive both treatment modalities at the same time. Bleomycin toxicity also is more common when bleomycin is combined with another drug than when it is used alone. Bleomycin is not

used in any pediatric therapy as a single agent, however. Other risk factors include a history of oxygen administration and impaired renal function because bleomycin is mainly excreted by the kidneys.[234] There is no method to predict accurately which patients will develop lung toxicity. The most important actions for decreasing the risk of bleomycin lung toxicity are to reduce the total cumulative dose and to encourage patients to avoid exposure to smoking. Current protocols for HD attempt to reduce the total cumulative dose of chemotherapeutic drugs by giving alternating or hybrid regimens, limiting the use of radiotherapy, and reducing the doses.

No established therapy is available for bleomycin lung toxicity. Therapy of bleomycin-induced pneumonitis consists largely of supportive measures. Withdrawal of the drug at the onset of toxicity must be considered. Careful monitoring of oxygen therapy is imperative. The use of steroids is controversial, but reversal of severe toxicity has been documented in some patients after the use of high-dose steroids.[227,236] It has been suggested that responding patients may have hypersensitivity reactions, and that patients with established lung fibrosis may respond less favorably. Patients who experience acute pulmonary symptoms, and who probably have hypersensitivity reactions, should be considered for steroid therapy after infections or other causes of lung disease have been ruled out.[236] Conversely, steroids are of unproven value in patients with a more chronic clinical picture suggesting pulmonary fibrosis.

Other chemotherapeutic agents that have been associated with lung toxicity, but which are seldom used in pediatric oncology, include mitomycin, gemcitabine, paclitaxel, docetaxel, cetuximab, bevacizumab, and chlorambucil. Gemcitabine may be used occasionally for pediatric patients with relapsed or resistant HD.[237] Pulmonary function should be evaluated carefully before gemcitabine is administered to these patients. Drugs often used in pediatric oncology, but which are seldom associated with lung toxicity, include anthracyclines, dactinomycin, vinca alkaloids, and irinotecan.

Antimetabolites—Methotrexate. Methotrexate is a folic acid antagonist used in the treatment of several childhood malignancies, notably leukemias and osteogenic sarcoma, and nonmalignant conditions, such as juvenile rheumatoid arthritis and psoriasis.[238] The clinical features of methotrexate are consistent with a hypersensitivity pneumonitis. Common symptoms include dyspnea and dry cough. Physical examination reveals tachypnea, diffuse crackles, cyanosis, and occasionally skin eruptions. Hypoxemia is observed in 90% to 95% of patients, and mild eosinophilia has been reported in almost half of the patients. Pulmonary function testing may show decreased DLCO. The most common chest radiographic abnormalities are bilateral interstitial infiltrates. Lung biopsy in adults reveals interstitial pneumonitis with lymphocytic and sometimes eosinophilic infiltrates, bronchiolitis, and granuloma formation consistent with a hypersensitivity reaction. Diagnosis of methotrexate-induced pneumonitis is difficult because this condition may mimic other conditions. Therapy consists of withdrawal of the drug and administration of corticosteroids. Clinical improvement precedes radiographic and pulmonary function improvement.

Alkylating Agents—Cyclophosphamide. Cyclophosphamide is widely used in the treatment of leukemias, lymphomas, and nonmalignant illnesses. It frequently produces severe alopecia and hemorrhagic cystitis.

Although pulmonary toxicity is uncommon, it does produce severe and even fatal lung damage. One documented mechanism of lung injury is a cytotoxicity-mediated oxidative process. In experimental animals, cyclophosphamide exposure results in leak of proteins across damaged endothelium and a reduction in lung antioxidant levels. Onset of pulmonary toxicity is usually subacute rather than insidious as with other alkylating agents. Dry cough and dyspnea herald the onset; malaise, anorexia, and weight loss follow. Physical examination reveals tachypnea and diffusely decreased breath sounds. Chest radiographs may show diffuse bilateral infiltrates, sometimes with pleural thickening. Pulmonary function testing reveals hypoxemia and restrictive lung disease. Withdrawal of the drug, supportive therapy, and corticosteroids are the recommended treatment.

Radiation Therapy

The lung is a crucial organ for radiation injury.[239] Clinically, interstitial pneumonitis can occur, and occasionally lung fibrosis. Most radiation lung damage data come from adults with lung and breast cancer; experience in children is more limited. Common malignancies that may include treatment with pulmonary radiotherapy include metastatic Wilms tumor, HD with bulky mediastinal involvement, or, less frequently, Ewing sarcoma-peripheral neuroectodermic tumors of the chest wall and primary lung neoplasms. Children with these types of malignancy often receive a limited dose of lung radiotherapy. Children receiving total body irradiation before HSCT also are at risk of lung toxicity, despite shielding techniques usually undertaken.[240] Severe toxicity may be less frequent in children than in adults.

Risk factors for radiation pneumonitis include dose, lung volume irradiated, fractionation, and radiation planning techniques.[239] Radiation pneumonitis seldom occurs when less than 10% of the lung is irradiated. When doses greater than 20 Gy are used, the risk of radiation pneumonitis increases proportionally, becoming highly likely when doses greater than 60 Gy are used.[241] In contrast to conventional radiotherapy planning, three-dimensional radiotherapy planning effectively allows radiologists to avoid irradiation of surrounding tissues. Fractionation of radiation also may influence the occurrence of pneumonitis; the greater the number of fractions, the lower the likelihood for lung injury.[241]

Radiation can damage the lung through various mechanisms. Although radiation can be toxic to all pulmonary cells, capillary endothelial and type I cells are the most susceptible. Patients with radiation pneumonitis usually present with nonspecific clinical findings 1 to 6 months after the completion of radiotherapy, usually 2 to 3 months later. Patients almost universally present with dyspnea, less frequently with dry cough, and very occasionally with hemoptysis. Radiation lung toxicity is usually self-limited, but severe lung fibrosis may develop occasionally. The diagnosis of radiation pneumonitis is usually made on clinical grounds, based on the clinical findings, the history of radiation to the lungs, and the exclusion of other causes. Lung biopsy is seldom needed, and histopathology is nonspecific, but helps in ruling out other causes of lung injury. Chest x-ray findings also are nonspecific, but they may show focal features within the irradiated field. Early radiographic changes include ground-glass opacification over the irradiated area.[239] Chest x-rays may show alveolar infiltrates at a later stage. As pneumonitis progresses to fibrosis, the radiographic appearance changes accordingly. Pleural effusions are usually absent or small. Asymptomatic patients also present with radiographic changes indistinguishable from those of symptomatic patients. In addition to pneumonitis and lung fibrosis, radiation may cause bronchiolitis obliterans with organizing pneumonia.[239]

Patients with symptomatic radiation pneumonitis benefit from early steroid treatment.[239] Data are based on animal studies, but no reports of controlled clinical trials involving children have been published. There also is clinical evidence that prophylactic use of steroids may be useful in adults. As in chemotherapy-induced damage, steroids have no role in treatment of established lung fibrosis.

Acknowledgments

The authors thank Margaret Carbaugh, for her expert editorial review, and Monica Siminovich, for providing the pathology illustrations and comments on the manuscript.

References

1. Harris NL, et al: Acute myeloid leukemia. In Jaffe ES, et al, eds: World Health Organization Classification of Tumors: Pathology and Genetics of Tumors of Hematopoietic and Lymphoid Tissues. Lyon, France, IARC Press, 2001, p 75.
2. Smith MA, et al: Leukemia. In Ries LAG, et al, eds: Cancer Incidence and Survival among Children and Adolescents: United States SEER Program 1975-1995. Bethesda, MD, National Cancer Institute, 1999, p 17.
3. Percy CL, et al: Lymphomas and reticuloendothelial neoplasms. In Ries LAG, et al, eds: Cancer Incidence and Survival among Children and Adolescents: United States SEER Program 1975-1995. Bethesda, MD, National Cancer Institute, 1999, p 35.
4. Greaves M: Infection, immune responses and the aetiology of childhood leukaemia. Nat Rev Cancer 6:193-203, 2006.
5. Cairo MS, et al: Childhood and adolescent non-Hodgkin lymphoma: New insights in biology and critical challenges for the future. Pediatr Blood Cancer 45:753-769, 2005.
6. Sinfield RL, et al: Spectrum and presentation of pediatric malignancies in the HIV era: Experience from Blantyre, Malawi, 1998-2003. Pediatr Blood Cancer 48(5):515-520, 2006.
7. Uckun FM, et al: Biology and treatment of childhood T-lineage acute lymphoblastic leukemia. Blood 91:735-746, 1998.
8. Mora J, et al: Lymphoblastic lymphoma of childhood and the LSA2-L2 protocol: The 30-year experience at Memorial-Sloan-Kettering Cancer Center. Cancer 98:1283-1291, 2003.
9. White KS: Thoracic imaging of pediatric lymphomas. J Thorac Imaging 16:224-237, 2001.
10. Yellin A, et al: Superior vena cava syndrome associated with lymphoma. Am J Dis Child 146:1060-1063, 1992.
11. McMahon CC, et al: Central airway compression: Anaesthetic and intensive care consequences. Anaesthesia 52:158-162, 1997.
12. Chang SC, et al: Effect of body position on gas exchange in patients with unilateral central airway lesions: Down with the good lung? Chest 103:787-791, 1993.
13. Mathew PM, et al: Clinical, haematological, and radiological features of children presenting with lymphoblastic mediastinal masses. Med Pediatr Oncol 8:193-204, 1980.
14. Cone AM, Stott S: Intermittent airway obstruction during anaesthesia in a patient with an undiagnosed anterior mediastinal mass. Anaesth Intensive Care 22:204-206, 1994.
15. King DR, et al: Pulmonary function is compromised in children with mediastinal lymphoma. J Pediatr Surg 32:294-299, 1997.

16. Rhodes MM, et al: Utility of FDG-PET/CT in follow-up of children treated for Hodgkin and non-Hodgkin lymphoma. J Pediatr Hematol Oncol 28:300-306, 2006.

17. Ribeiro RC, Pui CH: Recombinant urate oxidase for prevention of hyperuricemia and tumor lysis syndrome in lymphoid malignancies. Clin Lymphoma 3:225-232, 2003.

18. Pui CH, et al: Recombinant urate oxidase (rasburicase) in the prevention and treatment of malignancy-associated hyperuricemia in pediatric and adult patients: Results of a compassionate-use trial. Leukemia 15:1505-1509, 2001.

19. Goldman SC, et al: A randomized comparison between rasburicase and allopurinol in children with lymphoma or leukemia at high risk for tumor lysis. Blood 97:2998-3003, 2001.

20. Savage SA, Young G, Reaman GH: Catheter-directed thrombolysis in a child with acute lymphoblastic leukemia and extensive deep vein thrombosis. Med Pediatr Oncol 34:215-217, 2000.

21. Pui CH: Acute lymphoblastic leukemia. In Pui CH, ed: Childhood Leukemias. New York, Cambridge University Press, 2006, p 439.

22. Hann IM, et al: Randomized comparison of DAT versus ADE as induction chemotherapy in children and younger adults with acute myeloid leukemia. Results of the Medical Research Council's 10th AML trial (MRC AML10). Adult and Childhood Leukaemia Working Parties of the Medical Research Council. Blood 89:2311-2318, 1997.

23. Vernant JP, et al: Respiratory distress of hyperleukocytic granulocytic leukemias. Cancer 44:264-268, 1979.

24. Lester TJ, Johnson JW, Cuttner J: Pulmonary leukostasis as the single worst prognostic factor in patients with acute myelocytic leukemia and hyperleukocytosis. Am J Med 79:43-48, 1985.

25. Porcu P, et al: Hyperleukocytic leukemias and leukostasis: A review of pathophysiology, clinical presentation and management. Leuk Lymphoma 39 (1-2):1-18, 2000.

26. Soares FA, Landell GA, Cardoso MC: Pulmonary leukostasis without hyperleukocytosis: A clinico-pathologic study of 16 cases. Am J Hematol 40:28-32, 1992.

27. McKee LC Jr, Collins RD: Intravascular leukocyte thrombi and aggregates as a cause of morbidity and mortality in leukemia. Medicine (Baltimore) 53:463-478, 1974.

28. Bunin NJ, Pui CH: Differing complications of hyperleukocytosis in children with acute lymphoblastic or acute nonlymphoblastic leukemia. J Clin Oncol 3:1590-1595, 1985.

29. Lowe EJ, et al: Early complications in children with acute lymphoblastic leukemia presenting with hyperleukocytosis. Pediatr Blood Cancer 45:10-15, 2005.

30. Roath S, Davenport P: Leucocyte numbers and quality: Their effect on viscosity. Clin Lab Haematol 13:255-262, 1991.

31. Stucki A, et al: Endothelial cell activation by myeloblasts: Molecular mechanisms of leukostasis and leukemic cell dissemination. Blood 97:2121-2129, 2001.

32. Perez-Zincer F, et al: A pulmonary syndrome in patients with acute myelomonocytic leukemia and inversion of chromosome 16. Leuk Lymphoma 44:103-109, 2003.

33. Creutzig U, et al: Early deaths due to hemorrhage and leukostasis in childhood acute myelogenous leukemia: Associations with hyperleukocytosis and acute monocytic leukemia. Cancer 60:3071-3079, 1987.

34. Ventura GJ, et al: Acute myeloblastic leukemia with hyperleukocytosis: Risk factors for early mortality in induction. Am J Hematol 27:34-37, 1988.

35. Resnitzky P, Shaft D: Distinct lysozyme content in different subtypes of acute myeloid leukaemic cells: An ultrastructural immunogold study. Br J Haematol 88:357-363, 1994.

36. Szyper-Kravitz M, et al: Pulmonary leukostasis: Role of perfusion lung scan in diagnosis and follow up. Am J Hematol 67:136-138, 2001.

37. Kaminsky DA, Hurwitz CG, Olmstead JI: Pulmonary leukostasis mimicking pulmonary embolism. Leuk Res 24:175-178, 2000.

38. Cline MJ: Metabolism of the circulating leukocyte. Physiol Rev 45:674-720, 1965.

39. Hess CE, et al: Pseudohypoxemia secondary to leukemia and thrombocytosis. N Engl J Med 301:361-363, 1979.

40. Chillar RK, Belman MJ, Farbstein M: Explanation for apparent hypoxemia associated with extreme leukocytosis: Leukocytic oxygen consumption. Blood 55:922-924, 1980.

41. Lele AV, Mirski MA, Stevens RD: Spurious hypoxemia. Crit Care Med 33:1854-1856, 2005.

42. Fox MJ, Brody JS, Weintraub LR: Leukocyte larceny: A cause of spurious hypoxemia. Am J Med 67:742-746, 1979.

43. Weingarten AE, et al: Pulse oximetry to determine oxygenation in a patient with pseudohypoxemia. Anesth Analg 67:711-712, 1988.

44. Harris AL: Leukostasis associated with blood transfusion in acute myeloid leukaemia. BMJ 1:1169-1171, 1978.

45. Schmidt JE, et al: Pathophysiology-directed therapy for acute hypoxemic respiratory failure in acute myeloid leukemia with hyperleukocytosis. J Pediatr Hematol Oncol 25:569-571, 2003.

46. Hijiya N, et al: Severe cardiopulmonary complications consistent with systemic inflammatory response syndrome caused by leukemia cell lysis in childhood acute myelomonocytic or monocytic leukemia. Pediatr Blood Cancer 44:63-69, 2005.

47. Kang JL, et al: Inhaled nitric oxide attenuates acute lung injury via inhibition of nuclear factor-kappa B and inflammation. J Appl Physiol 92:795-801, 2002.

48. Cuttner J, et al: Therapeutic leukapheresis for hyperleukocytosis in acute myelocytic leukemia. Med Pediatr Oncol 11:76-78, 1983.

49. Zarkovic M, Kwaan HC: Correction of hyperviscosity by apheresis. Semin Thromb Hemost 29:535-542, 2003.

50. Porcu P, et al: Leukocytoreduction for acute leukemia. Ther Apher 6:15-23, 2002.

51. Porcu P, et al: Therapeutic leukapheresis in hyperleucocytic leukaemias: Lack of correlation between degree of cytoreduction and early mortality rate. Br J Haematol 98:433-436, 1997.

52. Giles FJ, et al: Leukapheresis reduces early mortality in patients with acute myeloid leukemia with high white cell counts but does not improve long-term survival. Leuk Lymphoma 42(1-2):67-73, 2001.

53. Bunin NJ, Kunkel K, Callihan TR: Cytoreductive procedures in the early management in cases of leukemia and hyperleukocytosis in children. Med Pediatr Oncol 15:232-235, 1987.

54. Rosen SG, Castleman B, Liebow AA: Pulmonary alveolar proteinosis. N Engl J Med 258:1123-1142, 1958.
55. Trapnell BC, Whitsett JA, Nakata K: Pulmonary alveolar proteinosis. N Engl J Med 349:2527-2539, 2003.
56. Seymour JF, Presneill JJ: Pulmonary alveolar proteinosis: Progress in the first 44 years. Am J Respir Crit Care Med 166:215-235, 2002.
57. deMello DE, Lin Z: Pulmonary alveolar proteinosis: A review. Pediatr Pathol Mol Med 20:413-432, 2001.
58. Teja K, et al: Pulmonary alveolar proteinosis in four siblings. N Engl J Med 305:1390-1392, 1981.
59. Nogee LM, et al: Brief report: Deficiency of pulmonary surfactant protein B in congenital alveolar proteinosis. N Engl J Med 328:406-410, 1993.
60. Dirksen U, et al: Human pulmonary alveolar proteinosis associated with a defect in GM-CSF/IL-3/IL-5 receptor common beta chain expression. J Clin Invest 100:2211-2217, 1997.
61. Nogee LM, et al: A mutation in the surfactant protein C gene associated with familial interstitial lung disease. N Engl J Med 344:573-579, 2001.
62. Shulenin S, et al: *ABCA3* gene mutations in newborns with fatal surfactant deficiency. N Engl J Med 350:1296-1303, 2004.
63. Cordonnier C, et al: Secondary alveolar proteinosis is a reversible cause of respiratory failure in leukemic patients. Am J Respir Crit Care Med 149(3 Pt 1):788-794, 1994.
64. Ruben FL, Talamo TS: Secondary pulmonary alveolar proteinosis occurring in two patients with acquired immune deficiency syndrome. Am J Med 80:1187-1190, 1986.
65. Goldstein LS, et al: Pulmonary alveolar proteinosis: Clinical features and outcomes. Chest 114:1357-1362, 1998.
66. Uchida K, et al: High-affinity autoantibodies specifically eliminate granulocyte-macrophage colony-stimulating factor activity in the lungs of patients with idiopathic pulmonary alveolar proteinosis. Blood 103:1089-1098, 2004.
67. Latzin P, et al: Anti-GM-CSF antibodies in paediatric pulmonary alveolar proteinosis. Thorax 60:39-44, 2005.
68. Price A, et al: Pulmonary alveolar proteinosis associated with anti-GM-CSF antibodies in a child: Successful treatment with inhaled GM-CSF. Pediatr Pulmonol 41:367-370, 2006.
69. Whitsett JA, Weaver TE: Hydrophobic surfactant proteins in lung function and disease. N Engl J Med 347:2141-2148, 2002.
70. Davies J, Turner J, Klein N: The role of the collectin system in pulmonary defence. Paediatr Respir Rev 2:70-75, 2001.
71. Weaver TE, Conkright JJ: Function of surfactant proteins B and C. Annu Rev Physiol 63:555-578, 2001.
72. Hamvas A, et al: Progressive lung disease and surfactant dysfunction with a deletion in surfactant protein C gene. Am J Respir Cell Mol Biol 30:771-776, 2004.
73. Trapnell BC, Whitsett JA: GM-CSF regulates pulmonary surfactant homeostasis and alveolar macrophage-mediated innate host defense. Annu Rev Physiol 64:775-802, 2002.
74. Yoshida M, et al: GM-CSF regulates protein and lipid catabolism by alveolar macrophages. Am J Physiol Lung Cell Mol Physiol 280:L379-L386, 2001.
75. Shibata Y, et al: GM-CSF regulates alveolar macrophage differentiation and innate immunity in the lung through PU.1. Immunity 15:557-567, 2001.
76. Robb L, et al: Hematopoietic and lung abnormalities in mice with a null mutation of the common beta subunit of the receptors for granulocyte-macrophage colony-stimulating factor and interleukins 3 and 5. Proc Natl Acad Sci USA 92:9565-9569, 1995.
77. Nishinakamura R, et al: Mice deficient for the IL-3/GM-CSF/IL-5 beta c receptor exhibit lung pathology and impaired immune response, while beta IL3 receptor-deficient mice are normal. Immunity 2:211-222, 1995.
78. Huffman JA, et al: Pulmonary epithelial cell expression of GM-CSF corrects the alveolar proteinosis in GM-CSF-deficient mice. J Clin Invest 97:649-655, 1996.
79. Reed JA, et al: Aerosolized GM-CSF ameliorates pulmonary alveolar proteinosis in GM-CSF-deficient mice. Am J Physiol 276(4 Pt 1):L556-L563, 1999.
80. Zsengeller ZK, et al: Adenovirus-mediated granulocyte-macrophage colony-stimulating factor improves lung pathology of pulmonary alveolar proteinosis in granulocyte-macrophage colony-stimulating factor-deficient mice. Hum Gene Ther 9:2101-2109, 1998.
81. Lee KN, et al: Pulmonary alveolar proteinosis: High-resolution CT, chest radiographic, and functional correlations. Chest 111:989-995, 1997.
82. Johkoh T, et al: Crazy-paving appearance at thin-section CT: Spectrum of disease and pathologic findings. Radiology 211:155-160, 1999.
83. Wang BM, et al: Diagnosing pulmonary alveolar proteinosis: A review and an update. Chest 111:460-466, 1997.
84. Kajiume T, et al: A case of myelodysplastic syndrome complicated by pulmonary alveolar proteinosis with a high serum KL-6 level. Pediatr Hematol Oncol 16:367-371, 1999.
85. de Blic J: Pulmonary alveolar proteinosis in children. Paediatr Respir Rev 5:316-322, 2004.
86. Mahut B, et al: Pulmonary alveolar proteinosis: Experience with eight pediatric cases and a review. Pediatrics 97:117-122, 1996.
87. Morgan C: The benefits of whole lung lavage in pulmonary alveolar proteinosis. Eur Respir J 23:503-505, 2004.
88. Centella T, et al: The use of a membrane oxygenator with extracorporeal circulation in bronchoalveolar lavage for alveolar proteinosis. Int Cardiovasc Thorac Surg 4:447-449, 2005.
89. Selecky PA, et al: The clinical and physiological effect of whole-lung lavage in pulmonary alveolar proteinosis: A ten-year experience. Ann Thorac Surg 24:451-461, 1977.
90. Venkateshiah SB, et al: An open-label trial of granulocyte macrophage colony stimulating factor therapy for moderate symptomatic pulmonary alveolar proteinosis. Chest 130:227-237, 2006.
91. Dirksen U, et al: Defective expression of granulocyte-macrophage colony-stimulating factor/interleukin-3/interleukin-5 receptor common beta chain in children with acute myeloid leukemia associated with respiratory failure. Blood 92:1097-1103, 1998.
92. Dorfman HD, Czerniak B: Osteosarcoma. In Dorfman HD, Czerniak B, eds: Bone Tumors. St. Louis, Mosby, 1998, p 128.

93. Gurney JG, et al: Incidence of cancer in children in the United States: Sex-, race-, and 1-year age-specific rates by histologic type. Cancer 75: 2186-2195, 1995.

94. Marina NM, et al: Improved prognosis of children with osteosarcoma metastatic to the lung(s) at the time of diagnosis. Cancer 70:2722-2727, 1992.

95. Bacci G, et al: Neoadjuvant chemotherapy for high-grade central osteosarcoma of the extremity: Histologic response to preoperative chemotherapy correlates with histologic subtype of the tumor. Cancer 97:3068-3075, 2003.

96. Meyers PA, et al: Intensification of preoperative chemotherapy for osteogenic sarcoma: Results of the Memorial Sloan-Kettering (T12) protocol. J Clin Oncol 16:2452-2458, 1998.

97. Meyer WH, et al: Carboplatin/ifosfamide window therapy for osteosarcoma: Results of the St Jude Children's Research Hospital OS-91 trial. J Clin Oncol 19:171-182, 2001.

98. Bielack SS, et al: Prognostic factors in high-grade osteosarcoma of the extremities or trunk: An analysis of 1,702 patients treated on neoadjuvant Cooperative Osteosarcoma Study Group protocols. J Clin Oncol 20:776-790, 2002.

99. Parham DM, et al: Childhood multifocal osteosarcoma: Clinicopathologic and radiologic correlates. Cancer 55:2653-2658, 1985.

100. Jaffe N, et al: Adjuvant methotrexate and citrovorum-factor treatment of osteogenic sarcoma. N Engl J Med 291:994-997, 1974.

101. Meyers PA, et al: Osteogenic sarcoma with clinically detectable metastasis at initial presentation. J Clin Oncol 11:449-453, 1993.

102. Kager L, et al: Primary metastatic osteosarcoma: Presentation and outcome of patients treated on neoadjuvant Cooperative Osteosarcoma Study Group protocols. J Clin Oncol 21:2011-2018, 2003.

103. Bacci G, et al: Neoadjuvant chemotherapy for osteosarcoma of the extremities with metastases at presentation: Recent experience at the Rizzoli Institute in 57 patients treated with cisplatin, doxorubicin, and a high dose of methotrexate and ifosfamide. Ann Oncol 14:1126-1134, 2003.

104. Briccoli A, et al: Resection of recurrent pulmonary metastases in patients with osteosarcoma. Cancer 104:1721-1725, 2005.

105. Daw NC, et al: Metastatic osteosarcoma. Cancer 106:403-412, 2006.

106. Goorin AM, et al: Phase II/III trial of etoposide and high-dose ifosfamide in newly diagnosed metastatic osteosarcoma: A Pediatric Oncology Group trial. J Clin Oncol 20:426-433, 2002.

107. Harris MB, et al: Treatment of metastatic osteosarcoma at diagnosis: A Pediatric Oncology Group Study. J Clin Oncol 16:3641-3648, 1998.

108. Bacci G, et al: Neoadjuvant chemotherapy for osteosarcoma of the extremity: Long-term results of the Rizzoli's 4th protocol. Eur J Cancer 37:2030-2039, 2001.

109. Ferrari S, et al: Postrelapse survival in osteosarcoma of the extremities: Prognostic factors for long-term survival. J Clin Oncol 21:710-715, 2003.

110. Su WT, et al: Surgical management and outcome of osteosarcoma patients with unilateral pulmonary metastases. J Pediatr Surg 39:418-423, 2004.

111. McCarville MB, et al: Prognostic factors and imaging patterns of recurrent pulmonary nodules after thoracotomy in children with osteosarcoma. Cancer 91:1170-1176, 2001.

112. Kayton ML, et al: Computed tomographic scan of the chest underestimates the number of metastatic lesions in osteosarcoma. J Pediatr Surg 41:200-206, 2006.

113. Kleinerman ES: Biologic therapy for osteosarcoma using liposome-encapsulated muramyl tripeptide. Hematol Oncol Clin North Am 9:927-938, 1995.

114. Meyers PA, et al: Osteosarcoma: A randomized, prospective trial of the addition of ifosfamide and/or muramyl tripeptide to cisplatin, doxorubicin, and high-dose methotrexate. J Clin Oncol 23:2004-2011, 2005.

115. Duan X, et al: Interleukin-12 enhances the sensitivity of human osteosarcoma cells to 4-hydroperoxycyclophosphamide by a mechanism involving the Fas/Fas-ligand pathway. Clin Cancer Res 10:777-783, 2004.

116. Jia SF, et al: Aerosol gene therapy with PEI: IL-12 eradicates osteosarcoma lung metastases. Clin Cancer Res 9:3462-3468, 2003.

117. Densmore CL, et al: Growth suppression of established human osteosarcoma lung metastases in mice by aerosol gene therapy with PEI-p53 complexes. Cancer Gene Ther 8:619-627, 2001.

118. Knight V, et al: 9-Nitrocamptothecin liposome aerosol treatment of human cancer subcutaneous xenografts and pulmonary cancer metastases in mice. Ann N Y Acad Sci 922:151-163, 2000.

119. Verschraegen CF, et al: Clinical evaluation of the delivery and safety of aerosolized liposomal 9-nitro-20(s)-camptothecin in patients with advanced pulmonary malignancies. Clin Cancer Res 10:2319-2326, 2004.

120. Gurney JG, Swensen AR, Bulterys M: Malignant bone tumors. In: SEER Pediatric Monograph. National Cancer Institute, Bethesda, MD, 1999, p 99.

121. Grier HE, et al: Addition of ifosfamide and etoposide to standard chemotherapy for Ewing's sarcoma and primitive neuroectodermal tumor of bone. N Engl J Med 348:694-701, 2003.

122. Cotterill SJ, et al: Prognostic factors in Ewing's tumor of bone: Analysis of 975 patients from the European Intergroup Cooperative Ewing's Sarcoma Study Group. J Clin Oncol 18:3108-3114, 2000.

123. Paulussen M, et al: Localized Ewing tumor of bone: Final results of the Cooperative Ewing's Sarcoma Study CESS 86. J Clin Oncol 19:1818-1829, 2001.

124. Bacci G, et al: Prognostic factors in nonmetastatic Ewing's sarcoma of bone treated with adjuvant chemotherapy: Analysis of 359 patients at the Istituto Ortopedico Rizzoli. J Clin Oncol 18:4-11, 2000.

125. Miser JS, et al: Treatment of metastatic Ewing's sarcoma or primitive neuroectodermal tumor of bone: Evaluation of combination ifosfamide and etoposide—a Children's Cancer Group and Pediatric Oncology Group study. J Clin Oncol 22: 2873-2876, 2004.

126. Sandoval C, et al: Outcome in 43 children presenting with metastatic Ewing sarcoma: The St. Jude Children's Research Hospital experience, 1962 to 1992. Med Pediatr Oncol 26:180-185, 1996.

127. Craft A, et al: Ifosfamide-containing chemotherapy in Ewing's sarcoma: The Second United Kingdom Children's Cancer Study Group and the Medical Research Council Ewing's Tumor Study. J Clin Oncol 16:3628-3633, 1998.

128. Kolb EA, et al: Long-term event-free survival after intensive chemotherapy for Ewing's family of tumors in children and young adults. J Clin Oncol 21:3423-3430, 2003.

129. Paulussen M, et al: Ewing's tumors with primary lung metastases: Survival analysis of 114 (European Intergroup) Cooperative Ewing's Sarcoma Studies patients. J Clin Oncol 16:3044-3052, 1998.

130. Spunt SL, et al: Selective use of whole-lung irradiation for patients with Ewing sarcoma family tumors and pulmonary metastases at the time of diagnosis. J Pediatr Hematol Oncol 23:93-98, 2001.

131. Paulussen M, et al: Primary metastatic (stage IV) Ewing tumor: Survival analysis of 171 patients from the EICESS studies. European Intergroup Cooperative Ewing Sarcoma Studies. Ann Oncol 9:275-281, 1998.

132. Marina NM, et al: Chemotherapy dose-intensification for pediatric patients with Ewing's family of tumors and desmoplastic small round-cell tumors: A feasibility study at St. Jude Children's Research Hospital. J Clin Oncol 17:180-190, 1999.

133. Nesbit ME Jr, et al: Multimodal therapy for the management of primary, nonmetastatic Ewing's sarcoma of bone: A long-term follow-up of the First Intergroup study. J Clin Oncol 8:1664-1674, 1990.

134. Ladenstein R, et al: A multivariate and matched pair analysis on high-risk Ewing tumor (ET) patients treated by megatherapy (MGT) and stem cell reinfusion (SCR) in Europe. Proc Annu Meet Am Soc Clin Oncol 18:555a, 1999.

135. Schuck A, et al: Hemithorax irradiation for Ewing tumors of the chest wall. Int J Radiat Oncol Biol Phys 54:830-838, 2002.

136. Meyer WH, Spunt SL: Soft tissue sarcomas of childhood. Cancer Treat Rev 30:269-280, 2004.

137. Crist W, et al: The Third Intergroup Rhabdomyosarcoma Study. J Clin Oncol 13:610-630, 1995.

138. Breneman JC, et al: Prognostic factors and clinical outcomes in children and adolescents with metastatic rhabdomyosarcoma—a report from the Intergroup Rhabdomyosarcoma Study IV. J Clin Oncol 21:78-84, 2003.

139. Koscielniak E, et al: Results of treatment for soft tissue sarcoma in childhood and adolescence: A final report of the German Cooperative Soft Tissue Sarcoma Study CWS-86. J Clin Oncol 17:3706-3719, 1999.

140. Sorensen PH, et al: PAX3-FKHR and PAX7-FKHR gene fusions are prognostic indicators in alveolar rhabdomyosarcoma: A report from the Children's Oncology Group. J Clin Oncol 20:2672-2679, 2002.

141. Carli M, et al: European intergroup studies (MMT4-89 and MMT4-91) on childhood metastatic rhabdomyosarcoma: Final results and analysis of prognostic factors. J Clin Oncol 22:4787-4794, 2004.

142. Rodeberg D, et al: Characteristics and outcomes of rhabdomyosarcoma patients with isolated lung metastases from IRS-IV. J Pediatr Surg 40:256-262, 2005.

143. Pappo AS, et al: Metastatic nonrhabdomyosarcomatous soft-tissue sarcomas in children and adolescents: The St. Jude Children's Research Hospital experience. Med Pediatr Oncol 33:76-82, 1999.

144. Ferrari A, et al: Synovial sarcoma: A retrospective analysis of 271 patients of all ages treated at a single institution. Cancer 101:627-634, 2004.

145. Spunt SL, et al: Prognostic factors for children and adolescents with surgically resected nonrhabdomyosarcoma soft tissue sarcoma: An analysis of 121 patients treated at St. Jude Children's Research Hospital. J Clin Oncol 17:3697-3705, 1999.

146. Spunt SL, et al: Clinical features and outcome of initially unresected nonmetastatic pediatric nonrhabdomyosarcoma soft tissue sarcoma. J Clin Oncol 20:3225-3235, 2002.

147. Brecht IB, et al: Grossly-resected synovial sarcoma treated by the German and Italian Pediatric Soft Tissue Sarcoma Cooperative Groups: Discussion on the role of adjuvant therapies. Pediatr Blood Cancer 46:11-17, 2006.

148. Portera CA Jr, et al: Alveolar soft part sarcoma: Clinical course and patterns of metastasis in 70 patients treated at a single institution. Cancer 91:585-591, 2001.

149. Kalapurakal JA, et al: Management of Wilms' tumour: Current practice and future goals. Lancet Oncol 5:37-46, 2004.

150. Dome JS, et al: Treatment of anaplastic histology Wilms' tumor: Results from the fifth National Wilms' Tumor Study. J Clin Oncol 24:2352-2358, 2006.

151. Green DM: The treatment of stages I-IV favorable histology Wilms' tumor. J Clin Oncol 22:1366-1372, 2004.

152. Metzger ML, Dome JS: Current therapy for Wilms' tumor. Oncologist 10:815-826, 2005.

153. Green DM, et al: The treatment of Wilms' tumor patients with pulmonary metastases detected only with computed tomography: A report from the National Wilms' Tumor Study. J Clin Oncol 9:1776-1781, 1991.

154. Cohen M, et al: Lung CT for detection of metastases: Solid tissue neoplasms in children. AJR Am J Roentgenol 139:895-898, 1982.

155. Hidalgo H, et al: The problem of benign pulmonary nodules in children receiving cytotoxic chemotherapy. AJR Am J Roentgenol 140:21-24, 1983.

156. Chang AE, et al: Evaluation of computed tomography in the detection of pulmonary metastases: A prospective study. Cancer 43:913-916, 1979.

157. Green DM, et al: Effect of duration of treatment on treatment outcome and cost of treatment for Wilms' tumor: A report from the National Wilms' Tumor Study Group. J Clin Oncol 16:3744-3751, 1998.

158. de Kraker J, et al: Wilms's tumor with pulmonary metastases at diagnosis: The significance of primary chemotherapy. International Society of Pediatric Oncology Nephroblastoma Trial and Study Committee. J Clin Oncol 8:1187-1190, 1990.

159. Pritchard J, et al: Results of the United Kingdom Children's Cancer Study Group first Wilms' Tumor Study. J Clin Oncol 13:124-133, 1995.

160. Ritchey ML, et al: Preoperative therapy for intracaval and atrial extension of Wilms tumor. Cancer 71:4104-4110, 1993.

161. Riley RD, et al: A systematic review of molecular and biological tumor markers in neuroblastoma. Clin Cancer Res 10(1 Pt 1):4-12, 2004.

162. Cowie F, Corbett R, Pinkerton CR: Lung involvement in neuroblastoma: Incidence and characteristics. Med Pediatr Oncol 28:429-432, 1997.

163. Kammen BF, et al: Pulmonary metastases at diagnosis of neuroblastoma in pediatric patients: CT findings and prognosis. AJR Am J Roentgenol 176:755-759, 2001.
164. Perilongo G, et al: Risk-adapted treatment for childhood hepatoblastoma: Final report of the second study of the International Society of Paediatric Oncology—SIOPEL 2. Eur J Cancer 40:411-421, 2004.
165. Feusner JH, et al: Treatment of pulmonary metastases of initial stage I hepatoblastoma in childhood. Report from the Childrens Cancer Group. Cancer 71:859-864, 1993.
166. Perilongo G, et al: Hepatoblastoma presenting with lung metastases: Treatment results of the first cooperative, prospective study of the International Society of Paediatric Oncology on childhood liver tumors. Cancer 89:1845-1853, 2000.
167. Cohen M, et al: Pulmonary pseudometastases in children with malignant tumors. Radiology 141:371-374, 1981.
168. Robertson PL, Boldt DW, De Campo JF: Paediatric pulmonary nodules: A comparison of computed tomography, thoracotomy findings and histology. Clin Radiol 39:607-610, 1988.
169. McCarville MB, et al: Distinguishing benign from malignant pulmonary nodules with helical chest CT in children with malignant solid tumors. Radiology 239:514-520, 2006.
170. Grampp S, et al: Spiral CT of the lung in children with malignant extra-thoracic tumors: Distribution of benign vs malignant pulmonary nodules. Eur Radiol 10:1318-1322, 2000.
171. Priest JR, et al: Pleuropulmonary blastoma: A clinicopathologic study of 50 cases. Cancer 80:147-161, 1997.
172. Janik JS, et al: Recurrent inflammatory pseudotumors in children. J Pediatr Surg 38:1491-1495, 2003.
173. Karnak I, et al: Inflammatory myofibroblastic tumor in children: Diagnosis and treatment. J Pediatr Surg 36:908-912, 2001.
174. Johnson CS: The acute chest syndrome. Hematol Oncol Clin N Am 19:857, 2005.
175. Koumbourlis AC, et al: Prevalence and reversibility of lower airway obstruction in children with sickle cell disease. J Pediatr 138:188-192, 2001.
176. Minter KR, Gladwin MT: Pulmonary complications of sickle cell anemia: A need for increased recognition, treatment, and research. Am J Respir Crit Care Med 164:2016-2019, 2001.
177. Vichinsky EP, et al: Causes and outcomes of the acute chest syndrome in sickle cell disease. National Acute Chest Syndrome Study Group. N Engl J Med 342:1855-1865, 2000.
178. Gill FM, et al: Clinical events in the first decade in a cohort of infants with sickle cell disease. Cooperative Study of Sickle Cell Disease. Blood 86:776-783, 1995.
179. Bernini JC, et al: Beneficial effect of intravenous dexamethasone in children with mild to moderately severe acute chest syndrome complicating sickle cell disease. Blood 92:3082-3089, 1998.
180. Stuart MJ, Setty BN: Acute chest syndrome of sickle cell disease: New light on an old problem. Curr Opin Hematol 8:111-122, 2001.
181. Vichinsky EP: Perspective: Pulmonary hypertension in sickle cell disease. N Engl J Med 350:857, 2004.
182. Hankins J, et al: Chronic transfusion therapy for children with sickle cell disease and recurrent acute chest syndrome. J Pediatr Hematol Oncol 27:158-161, 2005.
183. Morris CR, et al: Arginine therapy: A novel strategy to induce nitric oxide production in sickle cell disease. Br J Haematol 111:498-500, 2000.
184. Arico M, Egeler RM: Clinical aspects of Langerhans cell histiocytosis. Hematol Oncol Clin North Am 12:247-258, 1998.
185. Yu RC, et al: Clonal proliferation of Langerhans cells in Langerhans cell histiocytosis. Lancet 343:767-768, 1994.
186. Willman CL, et al: Langerhans'-cell histiocytosis (histiocytosis X)—a clonal proliferative disease. N Engl J Med 331:154-160, 1994.
187. Broadbent V, et al: Spontaneous remission of multi-system histiocytosis X. Lancet 1:253-254, 1984.
188. Mahmoud HH, Wang WC, Murphy SB: Cyclosporine therapy for advanced Langerhans cell histiocytosis. Blood 77:721-725, 1991.
189. Kannourakis G, Abbas A: The role of cytokines in the pathogenesis of Langerhans cell histiocytosis. Br J Cancer Suppl 23:S37-S40, 1994.
190. Schultz C, et al: Langerhans cell histiocytosis in children: Does soluble interleukin-2-receptor correlate with both disease extent and activity? Med Pediatr Oncol 31:61-65, 1998.
191. Refabert L, et al: Cd1a-positive cells in bronchoalveolar lavage samples from children with Langerhans cell histiocytosis. J Pediatr 129:913-915, 1996.
192. Schmitz L, Favara BE: Nosology and pathology of Langerhans cell histiocytosis. Hematol Oncol Clin N Am 12:221-246, 1998.
193. Braier J, et al: Outcome in children with pulmonary Langerhans cell histiocytosis. Pediatr Blood Cancer 43:765-769, 2004.
194. Bernstrand C, et al: Pulmonary abnormalities at long-term follow-up of patients with Langerhans cell histiocytosis. Med Pediatr Oncol 36:459-468, 2001.
195. Vassallo R, et al: Pulmonary Langerhans'-cell histiocytosis. N Engl J Med 342:1969-1978, 2000.
196. Griese M, et al: Pulmonary complications after bone marrow transplantation in children: Twenty-four years of experience in a single pediatric center. Pediatr Pulmonol 30:393-401, 2000.
197. Soubani AO, Miller KB, Hassoun PM: Pulmonary complications of bone marrow transplantation. Chest 109:1066-1077, 1996.
198. Dickout WJ, et al: Prevention of acute pulmonary edema after bone marrow transplantation. Chest 92:303-309, 1987.
199. Raptis A, et al: High-dose corticosteroid therapy for diffuse alveolar hemorrhage in allogeneic bone marrow stem cell transplant recipients. Bone Marrow Transplant 24:879-883, 1999.
200. Afessa B, et al: Diffuse alveolar hemorrhage in hematopoietic stem cell transplant recipients. Am J Respir Crit Care Med 166:641-645, 2002.
201. Metcalf JP, et al: Corticosteroids as adjunctive therapy for diffuse alveolar hemorrhage associated with bone marrow transplantation. University of Nebraska Medical Center Bone Marrow Transplant Group. Am J Med 96:327-334, 1994.
202. Kantrow SP, et al: Idiopathic pneumonia syndrome: Changing spectrum of lung injury after marrow transplantation. Transplantation 63:1079-1086, 1997.
203. Clark JG, et al: NHLBI workshop summary: Idiopathic pneumonia syndrome after bone marrow

transplantation. Am Rev Respir Dis 147(6 Pt 1):1601-1606, 1993.

204. Crawford SW, Hackman RC: Clinical course of idiopathic pneumonia after bone marrow transplantation. Am Rev Respir Dis 147(6 Pt 1):1393-1400, 1993.

205. Yen KT, et al: Pulmonary complications in bone marrow transplantation: A practical approach to diagnosis and treatment. Clin Chest Med 25:189-201, 2004.

206. Palmas A, et al: Late-onset noninfectious pulmonary complications after allogeneic bone marrow transplantation. Br J Haematol 100:680-687, 1998.

207. Sakaida E, et al: Late-onset noninfectious pulmonary complications after allogeneic stem cell transplantation are significantly associated with chronic graft-versus-host disease and with the graft-versus-leukemia effect. Blood 102:4236-4242, 2003.

208. Khurshid I, Anderson LC: Non-infectious pulmonary complications after bone marrow transplantation. Postgrad Med J 78:257-262, 2002.

209. Holland HK, et al: Bronchiolitis obliterans in bone marrow transplantation and its relationship to chronic graft-v-host disease and low serum IgG. Blood 72:621-627, 1988.

210. Worthy SA, Flint JD, Muller NL: Pulmonary complications after bone marrow transplantation: High-resolution CT and pathologic findings. Radiographics 17:1359-1371, 1997.

211. Lee KS, et al: Cryptogenic organizing pneumonia: CT findings in 43 patients. AJR Am J Roentgenol 162:543-546, 1994.

212. Wilczynski SW, et al: Delayed pulmonary toxicity syndrome following high-dose chemotherapy and bone marrow transplantation for breast cancer. Am J Respir Crit Care Med 157:565-573, 1998.

213. Kleinman S, et al: Toward an understanding of transfusion-related acute lung injury: Statement of a consensus panel. Transfusion 44:1774-1789, 2004.

214. Sanchez R, Toy P: Transfusion related acute lung injury: A pediatric perspective. Pediatr Blood Cancer 45:248-255, 2005.

215. Fontaine MJ, et al: Diagnosis of transfusion-related acute lung injury: TRALI or not TRALI? Ann Clin Lab Sci 36:53-58, 2006.

216. MacLennan S, Williamson LM: Risks of fresh frozen plasma and platelets. J Trauma 60(6 Suppl):S46-S50, 2006.

217. Fung YL, Williams BA: TRALI in 2 cases of leukemia. J Pediatr Hematol Oncol 28:391-394, 2006.

218. Wallis JP, et al: Transfusion-related alloimmune neutropenia: An undescribed complication of blood transfusion. Lancet 360:1073-1074, 2002.

219. Marques MB, et al: Acute transient leukopenia as a sign of TRALI. Am J Hematol 80:90-91, 2005.

220. Fein A, et al: The value of edema fluid protein measurement in patients with pulmonary edema. Am J Med 67:32-38, 1979.

221. Curtis BR, McFarland JG: Mechanisms of transfusion-related acute lung injury (TRALI): Anti-leukocyte antibodies. Crit Care Med 34(5 Suppl):S118-S123, 2006.

222. Silliman CC: The two-event model of transfusion-related acute lung injury. Crit Care Med 34(5 Suppl):S124-S131, 2006.

223. Khan SY, et al: Soluble CD40 ligand accumulates in stored blood components, primes neutrophils through CD40, and is a potential cofactor in the development of transfusion-related acute lung injury. Blood 108:2455-2462, 2006.

224. Meadors M, Floyd J, Perry MC: Pulmonary toxicity of chemotherapy. Semin Oncol 33:98-105, 2006.

225. Huggins JT, Sahn SA: Drug-induced pleural disease. Clin Chest Med 25:141-153, 2004.

226. Nicolls MR, et al: Diffuse alveolar hemorrhage with underlying pulmonary capillaritis in the retinoic acid syndrome. Am J Respir Crit Care Med 158:1302-1305, 1998.

227. Sleijfer S: Bleomycin-induced pneumonitis. Chest 120:617-624, 2001.

228. Hankins DG, et al: Pulmonary toxicity recurring after a six week course of busulfan therapy and after subsequent therapy with uracil mustard. Chest 73:415-416, 1978.

229. Alessandrino EP, et al: Pulmonary toxicity following carmustine-based preparative regimens and autologous peripheral blood progenitor cell transplantation in hematological malignancies. Bone Marrow Transplant 25:309-313, 2000.

230. Gharaee-Kermani M, Ullenbruch M, Phan SH: Animal models of pulmonary fibrosis. Methods Mol Med 117:251-259, 2005.

231. Martin WG, et al: Bleomycin pulmonary toxicity has a negative impact on the outcome of patients with Hodgkin's lymphoma. J Clin Oncol 23:7614-7620, 2005.

232. Chaudhary UB, Haldas JR: Long-term complications of chemotherapy for germ cell tumours. Drugs 63:1565-1577, 2003.

233. Chen J, Stubbe J: Bleomycins: Towards better therapeutics. Nat Rev Cancer 5:102-112, 2005.

234. Azambuja E, et al: Bleomycin lung toxicity: Who are the patients with increased risk? Pulm Pharmacol Ther 18:363-366, 2005.

235. Wolkowicz J, et al: Bleomycin-induced pulmonary function abnormalities. Chest 101:97-101, 1992.

236. Jensen JL, Goel R, Venner PM: The effect of corticosteroid administration on bleomycin lung toxicity. Cancer 65:1291-1297, 1990.

237. Belknap SM, et al: Clinical features and correlates of gemcitabine-associated lung injury: Findings from the RADAR project. Cancer 106:2051-2057, 2006.

238. Cottin V, et al: Pulmonary function in patients receiving long-term low-dose methotrexate. Chest 109:933-938, 1996.

239. Morgan GW, Breit SN: Radiation and the lung: A reevaluation of the mechanisms mediating pulmonary injury. Int J Radiat Oncol Biol Phys 31:361-369, 1995.

240. Bruno B, et al: Effects of allogeneic bone marrow transplantation on pulmonary function in 80 children in a single paediatric centre. Bone Marrow Transplant 34:143-147, 2004.

241. Tada T, et al: Radiation pneumonitis following multi-field radiation therapy. Radiat Med 18:59-61, 2000.

242. Battistini E, et al: Bronchiolitis obliterans organizing pneumonia in three children with acute leukaemias treated with cytosine arabinoside and anthracyclines. Eur Respir J 10:1187-1190, 1997.

243. Leon RJ, et al: Rituximab-induced acute pulmonary fibrosis. Mayo Clin Proc 79:949, 2004.

244. Bergeron A, et al: Hypersensitivity pneumonitis related to imatinib mesylate. J Clin Oncol 20:4271-4272, 2002.

245. Karlin L, et al: Respiratory status deterioration during G-CSF-induced neutropenia recovery. Bone Marrow Transplant 36:245-250, 2005.

CHAPTER 8

Pulmonary Manifestations of Endocrine and Metabolic Diseases

Carlos Milla

Specific Disorders 170
  Diabetes 170
  Growth Hormone Disorders 172
  Adrenal Disorders 172
  Pseudohypoaldosteronism 172
  Hypothyroidism 174
  Hyperthyroidism 175

Hypoparathyroidism 177
Disorders of the Reproductive System 177
Obesity-Hypoventilation Syndrome and
  Respiratory Complications of Obesity 177
Summary 181
  References 181

Although hormones and growth factors have an influence on the proliferation of lung tissue, especially during early development, there are no significant alterations in lung function or respiratory morbidity associated with the most prevalent endocrine conditions in pediatric patients. Numerous hormones, including corticosteroids and the thyroid hormone, have been shown during the later stages of lung development to stimulate differentiation of type II alveolar epithelial cells and to produce architectural rearrangements of lung connective tissue elements that facilitate gas exchange. Glucocorticoids in the perinatal period delay Clara cell differentiation,[1] elevate surfactant protein mRNA, and have a stimulatory effect on pulmonary cytochrome P-450. These effects translate into the known maturational changes induced by corticosteroids, and consequently they are used antenatally to prevent premature births.

This chapter reviews how endocrine disorders affect the respiratory system. Emphasis is placed on the pulmonary manifestations of diabetes, pseudohypoaldosteronism (PHA), hypothyroidism, hyperthyroidism, and obesity-hypoventilation syndrome. Clinicians should be aware of the potential relationships between endocrine disorders and pulmonary dysfunction.

Specific Disorders

Diabetes

Lung disease is not a major complication for children with diabetes. Barring an infection, it is not a likely threat even when the diabetes has reached a point where other complications are present.[2] Nonetheless, several cross-sectional studies in patients with diabetes have found mild abnormalities in different lung function parameters. In one population cross-sectional study, Lange and colleagues[3] found that forced vital capacity and forced expiratory volume in 1 second were significantly lower in individuals with diabetes than in nondiabetic controls. This finding was especially prominent among patients with insulin-dependent diabetes. Sandler and coworkers[4,5] found mild but significant decreases in lung elastic recoil, diffusing lung capacity, and capillary blood volume in a group of patients with type 1 diabetes compared with healthy controls. The degree of pulmonary dysfunction correlated with the duration of the disease. Other investigators also have reported mild decreases in measures of lung function in patients with diabetes,[6-9] but these results are hardly unanimous.[10]

Experimental data from animal models of diabetes suggest that there are abnormalities in the lung connective tissue synthesis and turnover that are especially prominent in the absence of insulin replacement. Thickening of the alveolar wall from increased deposition of collagen fibers and a reduced degradation of connective tissue have been observed in rats made diabetic by treatment with streptozocin.[11,12] This thickening also has often been noted in the alveolar and endothelial epithelial basement membranes of humans.[13] Such abnormalities in the molecular composition of epithelial basement membranes are well-known complications of diabetes, and they have been extensively studied in the renal glomeruli, with excessive glycosylation of the collagen-like material that confirms the theory being proposed as the underlying pathophysiologic mechanism.[14] As it pertains to the lung, it is possible that hyperglycemia leads to excessive nonenzymatic glycosylation of lung connective tissue, but the consequences of this remain unclear. Animal studies have reported discordant results. Some studies have described irreversible cross-linking of collagen[15] (a form of the protein that is resistant to proteolysis), and a decreased activity of the enzyme calmodulin[16] (which is involved in the regulation of connective tissue remodeling), whereas others have shown interference with the molecular cross-linking of elastin and collagen fibers.[15,17] Regardless, this abnormal accumulation of collagen and elastin fibers alters the lungs' mechanical properties, possibly explaining the decrease in lung tissue elasticity reported in clinical studies.

Notwithstanding the potential effects of diabetes on the lung, children with diabetic ketoacidosis who present with altered consciousness and vomiting are at an increased risk for aspiration. Because aspiration can lead to greater morbidity, the placement of a nasogastric tube and intubation in the presence of altered mental status should be approached with extra caution.

Diabetes is a common complication for patients with cystic fibrosis (CF), typically manifesting in the adolescent and adult years, although its occurrence has been reported in infancy. Because this particular diabetic condition has features of type 1 and type 2 diabetes, it has been named CF-related diabetes to distinguish it as a separate entity. Multiple studies have shown a clear correlation between the presence of CF-related diabetes and shortened survival and increased pulmonary morbidity. Finkelstein and associates[18] reported a significantly shortened survival in CF patients with diabetes,[18] with less than 25% surviving to age 30 years. In addition, clinical deterioration, as assessed by National Institutes of Health score, was apparent 2 years before the diagnosis of diabetes was made. Epidemiologic and registry studies concur in observing greater mortality and pulmonary morbidity among patients with CF-related diabetes. These patients are more likely to be malnourished and to have significant pulmonary dysfunction than CF patients without diabetes.[19-21]

The underlying causes are still not well understood, but these studies raise the question whether it is more likely that a prediabetic state develops insidiously and then contributes to clinical decline, or, alternatively, that sicker patients are simply more susceptible to diabetes. Further longitudinal studies have shown a direct relationship between abnormal glucose tolerance and deteriorating pulmonary function. The annual rate of decline in pulmonary function over a 4-year observation period was found to have a direct correlation with the degree of glucose intolerance at baseline.[22] Notably, the rate of pulmonary decline was inversely related to the magnitude of insulin secretion at baseline; this suggests a relationship between insulin deficiency and clinical deterioration.[22] Because subjects at baseline were no different in terms of pulmonary function and nutritional status, these data strongly support the concept that the insulin-deficient state leads to progressively declining pulmonary function. In addition, female patients with CF-related diabetes have been reported to have worse pulmonary outcomes and an overall disadvantage in survival. The current recommendation is that CF patients older than age 13 should have annual screening for CF-related diabetes through oral glucose tolerance testing.[25]

Infants born to mothers with diabetes are at increased risk for intrauterine or perinatal asphyxia.[26] Maternal vascular disease, manifested primarily by nephropathy, may contribute to the development of fetal hypoxia and subsequent perinatal asphyxia. In addition, respiratory distress syndrome occurs more frequently in infants born to mothers with diabetes than in normal infants at each gestational stage, especially before 38.5 weeks.[27] Hyperinsulinemia causes the delayed maturation of surfactant synthesis; a possible mechanism for this is by interfering with the induction of lung maturation by glucocorticoids.[28,29] Infants born to mothers with diabetes also are at risk for respiratory morbidity from pneumonia, hypertrophic cardiomyopathy, and transient tachypnea of the newborn, which occurs two to three times more commonly in this group than in normal infants.[30]

Growth Hormone Disorders

An increase in lung size has been reported in patients with acromegaly;[31] however, this is not associated with any significant respiratory dysfunction. Obstructive sleep apnea (OSA) is most common in adult patients with either active or treated acromegaly. This condition is believed to be primarily a consequence of upper airway obstruction owing to hypertrophy of the tongue and pharyngeal tissues. In addition, growth hormone-induced changes in central respiratory control have been proposed as a possible mechanism for the disordered sleep pattern found in these patients.[32]

Adrenal Disorders

Only one case has been reported of Cushing syndrome in an infant secondary to a pituitary adenoma who also presented with multicystic lesions in the lungs and kidneys.[33] This infant had elevated serum cortisol levels and nonsuppressed adrenocorticotropic hormone levels and increased urinary steroids. The lung cysts were surgically removed and diagnosed as congenital benign lung cysts.[34] This multicystic lung disease could simply be a coincidental finding because no other similar presentations have been described.

Pseudohypoaldosteronism

The content of body fluid Na^+ is tightly regulated by the epithelial Na^+ channel (ENaC), which is present in apical membranes of many Na^+-absorptive epithelia, such as the renal tubules, distal colon, and lungs (Fig. 8-1). ENaC is specifically inhibited by the diuretic amiloride, and it also is called the amiloride-sensitive Na^+ channel. The major physiologic role of ENaC is to maintain Na^+ homeostasis, blood volume, and blood pressure by providing an apical entry pathway for Na^+ ions to permit rapid transport of Na^+ from the luminal to the interstitial compartment. ENaC consists of three homologous subunits, α, β, and γ. The α subunit is essential for the formation of a functional ion channel, whereas the β and γ subunits can greatly potentiate the level of expressed Na^+ currents.

ENaCs belong to the Degenerin/ENaC superfamily of ion channels. The human ENaC genes have been cloned, and using genetic linkage analysis, it was found that the involvement of ENaC gene mutations results in two distinct human diseases. The autosomal dominant form affects the kidneys only (Liddle syndrome). It is characteristically free from any significant pulmonary involvement and is due to a defect in the function of the aldosterone receptor.[35] The autosomal recessive form is a systemic syndrome that affects the kidneys, colon, sweat and salivary glands, and lungs. As mentioned before, this

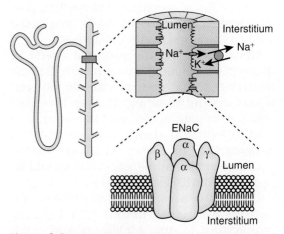

Figure 8-1. Schematic illustration showing the localization of epithelial Na^+ channels (ENaCs) in the collecting duct of the kidney.

syndrome arises from abnormalities in the activity of ENaC. This channel is involved in the apical exchange of Na^+ and movement of water across mucosal surfaces, such as the airway surface.[36] The state of hyperreninism and hyperaldosteronism in patients with systemic PHA type 1 is the result of sustained extracellular fluid volume depletion and is not due to peripheral resistance to mineralocorticoids.

Epithelial Na^+ Channel Mutations

Schaedel and associates[37] looked for ENaC mutations in four patients with PHA type 1 and negative cystic fibrosis transmembrane regulator (*CFTR*) gene analyses: a 2-year-old girl with recurrent bronchopneumonia; an 8-year-old boy with frequent pneumonia colonized with *Pseudomonas aeruginosa*, normal pulmonary function tests, and a normal resting nasal potential difference; his deceased 7-week-old brother; and a 9-year-old boy with recurrent bronchopneumonia. All four patients had mutations of the ENaC α subunit (1449delC, 729delA, C1685→T). The authors suggested that an increase in the Na^+ concentration in the airway surface liquid probably promotes the growth of *P. aeruginosa* and reduces its killing, leading to *P. aeruginosa* lung disease. Lung involvement in patients with PHA type 1 seems to be related to mutations in the α subunit of ENaC, at least based on current evidence. Lung disease seems milder than in CF, however, with no reports of bronchiectasis in patients to date.

The clinical syndrome consists of urinary salt wasting, hyperkalemia, and metabolic acidosis associated with elevated plasma renin activity and aldosterone levels. These manifestations can be present in the neonatal period and lead to death from severe dehydration and electrolyte imbalance. Failure of lung fluid reabsorption at birth has been associated with neonatal respiratory distress syndrome in patients with PHA type 1 and related to ENaC, which is involved in this process.[38] Additional clinical characteristics beyond the neonatal period include persistent clear nasal discharge, frequent lower respiratory infections associated with wheezing and crackles, and failure to thrive.

Hanukoglu and colleagues[39] reported four patients with PHA type 1: an 8-year-old girl

with frequent episodes of cough and lung crackles, who had a forced expiratory volume in 1 second of 91% predicted; an 8-year-old girl with recurrent lower respiratory tract infections and left lower lobe pneumonia, but normal pulmonary function; and twin 4-month-old boys with recurrent episodes of lower respiratory tract infection and wheezing. These patients had sweat chloride values ranging from 70 to 132. The authors noted that up to 4 years of age, respiratory infections usually occurred at times of dehydration. Later in life, the patients' main symptoms were moderately severe cough, wheezing, and crackles.

Marthinsen and coworkers[40] described a 6-year-old boy with PHA type 1. He had a sweat chloride value of 110, and a history of recurrent bronchopneumonia associated with dehydration. Since 18 months of age, sputum cultures were positive for *P. aeruginosa*. A computed tomography scan of his chest showed no evidence of bronchiectasis, and his pulmonary function tests were normal. He was treated with chest physiotherapy and inhaled antibiotics. MacLaughlin[41] noted the similarities between CF and PHA type 1, in terms of pulmonary bacterial infection and sweat chloride concentration. Clinically, PHA type 1 can be indistinguishable from CF, unless serum aldosterone, plasma renin activity, and urinary electrolytes are measured, and genetic studies are performed to rule out the presence of *CFTR* mutations.[36] These similarities are highlighted by the interaction of *CFTR* and ENaC. One of the physiologic functions of *CFTR* is to inhibit the ENaC.[101] If *CFTR* is absent or expressed in reduced quantity, luminal Na^+ absorption through ENaC is enhanced (Fig. 8-2). Na^+ absorption is osmotically drawing water from the airway surface liquid, contributing to depletion of airway surface liquid. Na^+ hyperabsorption could be an important factor in CF pathophysiology because mice overexpressing the β subunit of ENaC do exhibit signs of CF lung disease, such as mucous plugging and neutrophilic inflammation.[102]

An alternative approach to *CFTR* pharmacotherapy would be to inhibit the enhanced Na^+ absorption through ENaC. In the nasal mucosa, the defect in Na^+ reabsorption can be shown by the absence

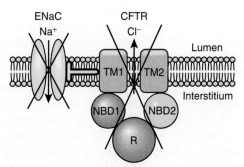

CYSTIC FIBROSIS
SYSTEMIC PSEUDOHYPOALDOSTERONISM TYPE I

Figure 8-2. Cystic fibrosis and systemic pseudohypoaldosteronism type 1. Interaction of *CFTR* and epithelial Na$^+$ channel (ENaC).

of amiloride-sensitive Na$^+$ transport during nasal transepithelial potential difference measurements (Fig. 8-3).

The pulmonary phenotype seems to be related to the absent or severely reduced Na$^+$ transport in airway epithelia, with failure to reabsorb fluid from the airway surface and presence of watery secretions.[42] Despite frequent respiratory manifestations with respiratory exacerbations, patients with PHA type 1 do not experience the destructive process that patients with CF manifest as they age. In addition, airway colonization with pathogens is not as problematic as in patients with CF, which may explain the more benign course of their pulmonary disease.

At present, treatment of these patients is quite similar to the treatment of CF patients. Further research, looking particularly into the electrolyte composition of the airway surface liquid in CF patients, is needed to determine whether airway colonization with *P. aeruginosa* in these two conditions is related to common abnormalities in the electrolyte composition of the airway surface liquid or other host-related abnormalities in these two conditions. Whether patients with PHA type 1 and *P. aeruginosa* lung disease have mucoid *Pseudomonas*, and whether conversion to mucoid also is related to host and environmental factors is unknown.

Hypothyroidism

Many of the manifestations of hypothyroidism are a consequence of the hypometabolic state and accumulation of matrix glycosaminoglycans (myxedema) that are induced by the lack of thyroid hormone.

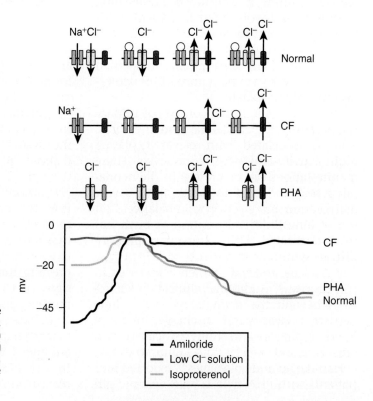

Figure 8-3. Nasal potential difference (PD) in a patient with cystic fibrosis (CF), a patient with pseudohypoaldosteronism (PHA), and a normal subject, illustrating the response to perfusion with amiloride, followed by the addition of chloride-free solution and then isoproterenol.

The hypometabolic state is primarily manifested by weakness, fatigue, cold intolerance, constipation, weight gain, abnormalities in muscle tone, and bradycardia. Myxedema leads to coarseness and induration of the skin, puffy facies, enlargement of the tongue, and hoarseness. Specifically, from a respiratory perspective, respiratory muscle weakness manifests as hypoventilation with shortness of breath and decreased exercise capacity,[43-45] although the presence of cardiovascular disease also could play a role. Abnormal ventilatory responses to hypoxia and hypercapnia can be shown in these patients as well, with the reduction in the ventilatory response to hypoxia being more pronounced.[46,47] Thyroid hormone replacement therapy restores the normal response to hypoxia promptly, whereas the hypercapnic drive is slower to return to normal.[44,47] The reason for the impairment of ventilatory responses in some hypothyroid patients is unknown, but may be related to the decrease in oxygen consumption associated with hypothyroidism.

Muscle weakness, impaired ventilatory responses, and potential upper airway obstruction determine the conditions for the development of significant sleep-disordered breathing. Multiple studies have shown the presence of sleep apnea with central or obstructive components. The obstructive form seems to be more common in these patients. OSA may be caused by an enlarged tongue or reduced oropharynx owing to mucopolysaccharide and protein deposition or by a myopathy involving the muscles of the upper airway. Overweight seems to compound this problem.[48] Based on these findings, it has been proposed that screening for hypothyroidism should be considered during the evaluation of patients with sleep-disordered breathing.[49] In the absence of clinical manifestations of hypothyroidism (i.e., subclinical hypothyroidism), the prevalence of sleep disorders is no different from euthyroid patients, and this needs to be taken into consideration to avoid unnecessary testing. The sleep-disordered breathing is reversible with the institution of appropriate therapy,[50] although the obstructive component may take some time to revert completely.[48]

Bilateral and unilateral pleural effusions have been reported in association with hypothyroidism. The nature of these effusions (transudate or exudate) and their causes is controversial. Changes in capillary permeability in the hypothyroid patient may be related to the development of pleural effusions, however.

The prevalence of hypothyroidism is high among patients with idiopathic pulmonary arterial hypertension, although hypothyroidism is not currently believed to be a risk factor for the condition.[51] The basis of the observed association of the two disorders is unclear.

Hypothyroidism can cause abnormally high sweat electrolyte levels.[52] The presence of elevated sweat electrolyte levels may lead to the misdiagnosis of CF during the evaluation of children with chronic illness.[53-55] The elevated chloride concentrations return to normal with the start of replacement therapy.[55] The abnormality in the ability of the sweat gland to secrete normal sweat is believed to be due to infiltration of the secretory coil with granular material.[56,57]

Hyperthyroidism

The hyperthyroid state does not affect the lung directly, but the increase in metabolism and the development of a hyperthyroid myopathy can affect lung function and cardiopulmonary performance. The hypermetabolic state induced by hyperthyroidism increases the basal metabolic rate and has an associated increase in oxygen consumption and carbon dioxide production.[58] Hyperthyroid patients are typically dyspneic, and show significantly lower resting arterial P_{CO_2} and tidal volume with increased ventilatory responses to carbon dioxide and hypoxia.[59] With exercise, even correcting for carbon dioxide consumption, further increases in ventilatory responses are noted, which are believed to be secondary to an increased central drive and can be blocked by β-blockers.[60] A smaller increment in heart rate between rest and anaerobic threshold, a reduced oxygen consumption at anaerobic threshold, and a reduced oxygen pulse at anaerobic threshold also have been reported.[61,62]

A small study in children with untreated hyperthyroidism found no significant differences at rest compared with a control group in oxygen uptake, minute ventilation, or respiratory rate. During exercise, there were significant differences, however, in oxygen uptake, heart rate, minute ventilation, and respiratory rate.[63] Patients with thyrotoxicosis also have an increased resting reflex hypoxic drive to respiration.[64] These findings suggest an inappropriate increase in respiratory drive, possibly secondary to increased adrenergic stimulation.[60]

Abnormalities in lung function also have been reported in hyperthyroid patients, but a lack of correlation between the severity of dyspnea and abnormalities in lung function suggests that the dyspnea is probably due to extrapulmonary causes.[65,66] The development of myopathy in the hyperthyroid state is known also to affect the respiratory muscles. This muscle weakness, in addition to the above-noted abnormalities, leads to an impaired exercise capacity and increases in breathing effort.[67] In patients with thyrotoxicosis, a linear relationship has been shown between respiratory forces (maximum inspiratory pressure, maximum expiratory pressure) and levels of thyroid hormones (triiodothyronine, thyroxine). In thyrotoxicosis, respiratory muscle weakness affects inspiratory and expiratory muscles and contributes to the dyspnea and exercise abnormalities noted in these patients.[65,68-70] Most of these abnormalities are reversible with therapy, although the pattern of breathing may not return to normal immediately.[71]

Although animal studies suggested an effect of thyroid hormone on bronchial smooth muscle tone and contractility,[72] hyperthyroidism might protect against carbachol-induced bronchospasm.[73] In a study with normal volunteers with induced hyperthyroidism by administration of exogenous triiodothyronine for 3 weeks, no effect on airway reactivity or lung function was noted.[74]

Neonatal Graves disease must be considered in any infant born to a woman with a history of Graves disease. Affected infants are often preterm or low birth weight, appear anxious, and are restless and irritable (Fig. 8-4). They may be febrile, and often the skin is flushed and warm. Tachycardia is a consistent finding and may be accompanied by cardiomegaly and heart failure, with

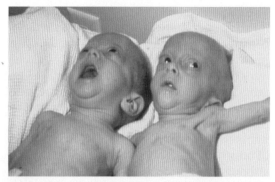

Figure 8-4. Twin boys with neonatal hyperthyroidism confirmed by abnormal thyroid function tests. Clinical features include lack of subcutaneous tissue owing to a hypermetabolic state and a wide-eyed, anxious stare. They were given the diagnosis of neonatal Graves disease, but their mother did not have Graves disease; they had persistent, not transient, hyperthyroidism. At age 8 years, they were treated with radioiodine. They are now believed to have had some other form of neonatal hyperthyroidism, such as a constitutive activation of the thyroid-stimulating hormone receptor. (*From Kliegman RM, et al: Nelson Textbook of Pediatrics, 18th ed. Philadelphia, Saunders, 2007.*)

consequent respiratory distress.[75] Thyromegaly is almost always present and sometimes may cause tracheal compression and added respiratory distress.[76] Persistent pulmonary hypertension of the newborn with the characteristic severe respiratory failure also has been reported in these infants.[77-79] It has been postulated that thyrotoxicosis has effects on pulmonary vascular maturation and the metabolism of endogenous pulmonary vasodilators, contributing to the development of persistent pulmonary hypertension of the newborn.[80]

It also is recognized that some patients with hyperthyroidism may present with variable degrees of pulmonary hypertension and isolated right heart failure.[80] This is reversible when the appropriate therapy for the hyperthyroid state is established.[81,82] The presence of elevated pulmonary pressures in otherwise asymptomatic hyperthyroid patients also has been reported and is reversible after restoration to a euthyroid state.[83] Proposed mechanisms include high cardiac output–induced endothelial injury, increased metabolism of intrinsic pulmonary vasodilating substances resulting in elevated pulmonary vascular resistance, and autoimmune phenomenon.[84]

Hypoparathyroidism

Hypoparathyroidism is an inherited or acquired deficiency of the parathyroid hormone or its action. Parathyroid hormone secretion by the parathyroid glands (prime regulators of serum calcium concentration) maintains serum calcium within a strict range. Biochemical hallmarks of parathyroid hormone insufficiency are hypocalcemia and hyperphosphatemia. Complications of hypoparathyroidism are largely due to hypocalcemia. Laryngospasm, a form of tetany, can lead to stridor and significant airway obstruction and prolongation of the Q-Tc interval. Hypocalcemia also leads to neuromuscular irritability. Affected patients may experience paresthesias, muscle cramping, tetany, or seizures.[85]

Newborns may present with hypoparathyroidism, but it can manifest in individuals of almost any age. Typically, patients with DiGeorge syndrome present during the first few weeks of life. DiGeorge syndrome, which is one manifestation of the 22q11 deletion syndrome, is associated with recurrent infections related to T cell abnormalities and conotruncal defects, such as tetralogy of Fallot and truncus arteriosus. Affected individuals also may have a history of speech delay from velopharyngeal insufficiency. Patients with autoimmune and parathyroid hormone resistance syndromes tend to present in adolescence. Transient hypoparathyroidism is common during the first few days of life in preterm infants, infants of mothers with diabetes mellitus, infants of mothers with hypercalcemia, and infants with prolonged delay in parathyroid gland responsiveness.

Hypocalcemia that produces symptoms, such as seizure, tetany, and laryngospasm, requires intravenous calcium and continuous monitoring for cardiac arrhythmias. Oral calcium and vitamin D are initiated as soon as possible (e.g., when the patient is tolerating oral feeds).

Disorders of the Reproductive System

Disorders of the reproductive system rarely manifest with respiratory abnormalities. Pulmonary metastases are known to occur with granulosa cell tumors, Sertoli-Leydig cell tumors, and choriocarcinoma. Ovarian carcinoma may manifest with pleural effusions. In addition, patients with benign ovarian tumors may present with unilateral pleural effusion (more often right-sided), although bilateral pleural effusions also may occur as part of the Meigs syndrome. Rarely, endometriosis tissue can deposit in the pleural space. During menstruation, this problem may lead to recurrent pneumothorax (catamenial pneumothorax) usually on the right side.

Obesity-Hypoventilation Syndrome and Respiratory Complications of Obesity

Obesity in children is a complex disorder. Its prevalence has increased so significantly in recent years that many consider it a major health concern of the developed world. In the United States, 20% to 27% of all children and adolescents have obesity. Many factors, including genetics, environment, metabolism, lifestyle, and eating habits, are believed to play a role in the development of obesity.[86] Obesity-hypoventilation syndrome is an uncommon finding in children with obesity, with an estimated frequency of 1% to 3%. Stated from a different point of view, 10% of patients with OSA are obese.

No firm diagnostic criteria to define obesity-hypoventilation syndrome exist; this fact, limited pediatric studies, and discrepant definitions of obesity and abnormal pediatric polysomnographic findings make the literature difficult. Obesity, sleep-disordered breathing, and hypercarbia during wakefulness are features generally described with obesity-hypoventilation syndrome. Other features include excessive daytime sleepiness, hyperactivity, poor school performance with difficulty attending to tasks and impaired memory, hypoxia, and signs of cor pulmonale.

In adults, male sex and obesity are common risk factors for OSA. Witnessed apnea, loud disruptive snoring, and daytime sleepiness are frequent presenting complaints. In children, neither these risk factors nor the symptom profile is as predictive for OSA except in children with obesity. Twenty-seven percent of children with OSA have failure to thrive.

In one study, daytime sleepiness occurred with the same overall frequency as in control subjects; in another study, daytime sleepiness was found to be more frequent in obese children with OSA. Mental retardation also has been associated with obesity-hypoventilation syndrome.

The exact mechanism for development of obesity-hypoventilation syndrome is unknown; however, it is believed to be related primarily to abnormalities in ventilatory drive and response to hypoxia and hypercarbia, rather than the mechanical factors related to excessive body weight.[87] Other authors believe that body weight and, more importantly, the distribution of body fat, hormones, and upper airway size and dynamics play important roles.

Associated upper airway obstruction is important in the occurrence of OSA/hypoventilation or hypopnea because OSA/hypoventilation or hypopnea is observed more frequently when the two conditions occur together compared with the simultaneous presentation of OSA/hypoventilation or hypopnea and simple obesity.[88] Other factors that may play a role in the development of airway obstruction during sleep include rapid eye movement (REM) atonia, increased soft tissue and fatty infiltration around the neck, decreased chest wall compliance, and decreased lung volumes (especially in the supine position) secondary to the upward displacement of the diaphragm caused by increased abdominal fat.[88] In children, tonsillar hypertrophy added to obesity seems to be more predictive of abnormal polysomnographic findings.

Higher rates of morbidity and mortality are associated with childhood obesity. Pulmonary consequences observed in children and adolescents include an increased frequency of reactive airway disease, poor exercise tolerance, increased work of breathing, and increased oxygen consumption. The few individuals who develop obesity-hypoventilation syndrome experience right-sided heart failure with right ventricular hypertrophy.

Although pediatricians have long valued a good history and physical examination, studies have indicated that the predictive value of the recorded history and physical examination is only 30% to 50% compared with the overnight polysomnogram. Symptoms during sleep[89] include enuresis (this symptom alone has a predictive value for OSA of 46%) and snoring intensity greater than 30 dB (this symptom has a predictive value for OSA of 60%). Characteristically, snoring tends to worsen during flare-ups of nasal allergies and during upper respiratory infections. Approximately 10% of children who snore have significant sleeping and breathing problems. Other significant symptoms include restless sleep; parasomnias, especially nightmares and sleep walking; witnessed apneas; irregular breathing patterns in sleep; sweating at night; and sleeping with head extended.

During wakefulness, symptoms may include chronic mouth breathing and daytime sleepiness (this symptom occurs much less frequently in children with OSA than in their adult counterparts except in the case of children with obesity). Other important manifestations[89] include hyperactivity (younger children are more likely to show symptoms of sleep deprivation than excessive daytime sleepiness), morning headaches, cardiac rhythm disturbances, systemic or pulmonary hypertension (or both), poor school performance, poor memory, and poor concentration.

Sleep apnea and daytime sleepiness can be aggravated by the use of alcohol, sedating antihistamines, central nervous system depressants, and some over-the-counter cold preparations. Increased incidence of hyperreactive airways (i.e., asthma) is observed in children with obesity (30%). Decreased exercise tolerance also is observed in children with obesity.

Pulmonary function studies may reveal a flow-volume loop with a saw-tooth pattern associated with upper airway obstruction. Most children (58%) in the study by Mallory and colleagues[90] had abnormal pulmonary function studies, primarily obstructive in nature. The data by Fung and associates[91] showed significant changes in forced vital capacity of overweight boys but not girls. These data are consistent with the finding that fat distribution in overweight and obese adolescents differs from that of adults and is gender-specific. Boys tend to accumulate fat in the abdominal area, whereas girls tend to accumulate fat in the subscapular area.

Maximum voluntary ventilation may be decreased. As mentioned, patterns of fat distribution differ in overweight and obese adolescent boys and girls. Because of the impact of the abdominal fat on the diaphragm, the expiratory reserve volume is decreased, and consequently the forced vital capacity is decreased. Adult studies show the expiratory reserve volume to be decreased severely with extreme and morbid obesity. Biring and coworkers[92] found expiratory reserve volume to be the most sensitive indicator of obesity. Many reasons have been offered in addition to the mass effect on the position of the diaphragm. These include decreased diaphragmatic mobility, decreased respiratory compliance, decreased respiratory muscle strength, and fatty infiltration of the respiratory muscles.

Inselman and colleagues[93] reported children with decreased diffusing capacity for carbon monoxide and normal inspiratory and expiratory pressures. By contrast, Biring's group,[92] in subjects 13 to 78 years old, showed the diffusing capacity for carbon monoxide and diffusing capacity for carbon monoxide/alveolar volume ratio to be normal except in subjects with extreme obesity. Airway resistance may be increased.

In the case of children and adolescents, overnight polysomnogram shows morbid obesity can be associated with hypoventilation, hypoxia, and hypercarbia during sleep. Others may present with evidence of OSA.

The multiple sleep latency test can be useful in the evaluation of patients complaining of excessive daytime sleepiness. The multiple sleep latency test is performed on the day after the overnight polysomnogram. Its findings can be used to assess pathologic sleepiness and contribute to a diagnosis of narcolepsy. Cardiac dysrhythmias and right bundle branch block have been reported.

Weight loss is recommended, but often is difficult to achieve and sustain. In addition, although weight loss remains a cornerstone to the treatment of obesity, it may not always improve the symptoms of OSA/hypoventilation or hypopnea. Progesterone, theophylline, protriptyline, and buspirone have been used in limited studies. In some

children, nasal continuous positive airway pressure ventilation has been performed.

Surgical treatment includes tonsillectomy, adenoidectomy, or adenotonsillectomy (may be successful even when weight loss alone does not produce satisfactory resolution of symptoms). Other considerations include tracheostomy, uvulopalatopharyngoplasty, and mandibular advancement surgery. In children with apnea, there is an increased risk of postoperative complications after relief of upper airway obstruction when the patient history includes young age (<2 to 3 years old), morbid obesity, hypotonia, cor pulmonale, or severe OSA. In such patients, one should strongly consider cardiorespiratory monitoring in a pediatric recovery or special care unit. Postoperative pulmonary edema may be observed.

Prader-Willi syndrome is a specific condition resulting from either paternal deletion of 15q11-13 or maternal disomy for chromosome 15. It is characterized by neonatal hypotonia, early childhood obesity, characteristic facial appearance, mental deficiency, hypogonadism, short stature, and behavioral disorders with increased appetite. Restrictive ventilatory impairment resulting primarily from respiratory muscle weakness has been reported. REM sleep-related oxygen desaturations with or without apneas are common sometimes with hypercapnia. Typical obesity-hypoventilation syndrome also has been reported. Hypothalamic dysfunction is probably partly responsible for the sleep abnormalities observed in this syndrome.

Obesity and Asthma Interactions

The relationships, interactions, and association between obesity and asthma are complex, and active sources of hypotheses and research. An association between obesity and asthma incidence or asthma severity or both has been reported in many studies, although there is still considerable discussion about the existence of the association and its meaning.[94] Being overweight has been associated with an increased risk of new-onset asthma in boys and nonallergic children.[95] Asthma is a risk for obesity in urban minority children and adolescents.[96]

In an extensive review of the association between asthma and obesity, Tantisra and Weiss[97] described potential and causal relationships that rely on genetics, immune system modulation, and mechanical mechanisms. Based on current evidence, they reported the following:

1. Obesity has been associated with increases in the incidence and prevalence of asthma in several epidemiologic studies in children.
2. Weight loss in obese subjects results in improvement in the overall pulmonary function and asthma symptoms and decreases in asthma medication usage.
3. Obesity may directly affect the asthma phenotype by mechanical effects, including airway reactivity; cytokine modulation via adipose tissue; common genes or genetic regions; or sex-specific effects, including the hormone estrogen.
4. Obesity also may be related to asthma by genetic interactions with environmental exposures, including physical activity and diet.

In a review of obesity, smooth muscle, and airway hyperreactivity, Shore and Fredberg[98] suggested three possibilities that relate obesity to airway hyperreactivity. The first possibility consists of simple mechanical static and dynamic factors. Static factors include increased abdominal and chest wall mass in an obese individual, which produces lower than normal functional residual capacity. Dynamic factors include the tidal action of spontaneous breathing imposing tidal strains on airway smooth muscle. An obese individual breathes at higher frequencies but smaller tidal volumes compared with a lean individual, resulting in a compromise in the bronchodilating mechanism and predisposing to increased airway reactivity compared with a lean subject (Fig. 8-5).

The second possibility is related to differences in anatomy of the lungs and airways. In children, the mechanical load of obesity might affect lung growth. Obesity also might lead to more accelerated airway remodeling with each asthma exacerbation.

The third possibility for the relationship of obesity to airway hyperreactivity is the inflammatory microenvironment.[99] White adipose tissue, which represents most adipose tissue in humans, is no longer considered an inert tissue devoted to energy storage, but is emerging as an active participant in regulating physiologic and pathologic processes, including immunity and inflammation. Adipose tissue is now considered the largest endocrine organ in the human body.

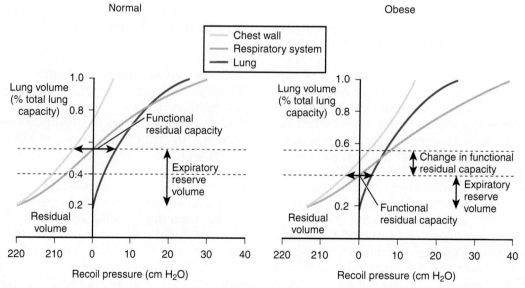

Figure 8-5. Lung, chest wall, and respiratory system pressure-volume curves in normal and obese subjects. Note the effect of the rightward shift in the chest wall curve on the respiratory system pressure-volume curve and on the functional residual capacity and the expiratory reserve volume (as the residual volume is unchanged). (*From Albert RK, Spiro SG, Jett JR: Clinical Respiratory Medicine, 2nd ed. Philadelphia, Mosby, 2004.*)

Exercise Fitness in Overweight Children and Adolescents

A more recent study[100] reported that overweight and nonoverweight adolescents had similar absolute oxygen consumption at the lactate threshold and at maximal exertion, suggesting that overweight adolescents are more limited by the increased cardiorespiratory effort required to move their larger body mass through space than by cardiorespiratory deconditioning. The higher percentage of oxygen consumed during submaximal exercise indicates that overweight adolescents are burdened by the metabolic cost of their excess mass. Their greater oxygen demand during an unloaded task predicted poorer performance during sustained exercise.

A large part of the exercise intolerance observed in overweight adolescents seems to be related to the increased metabolic demands of moving excess mass. Cardiac constraints also may play a role and warrant closer, more detailed evaluation. The clinical implication of understanding how increased load from excess body mass affects exercise tolerance is important for exercise prescriptions for overweight adolescents. Exercise prescriptions may require careful planning to decrease overall body mass in addition to targeting cardiorespiratory conditioning. Although weight-bearing exercise should be used when possible, some severely overweight adolescents require prescriptions for non-weight-bearing exercise to provide a sustainable exercise work intensity that is below the lactate threshold.

Summary

There are many important respiratory manifestations of endocrine diseases in children. Patients with diabetes mellitus are at risk of developing various pulmonary complications. Acute and chronic pulmonary infections are the most common respiratory abnormalities in patients with diabetes mellitus, although cardiogenic and noncardiogenic pulmonary edema can be a complication of their disease.

Hypothyroidism may be associated with respiratory failure that can be caused by a reduction in the central respiratory drive, upper airway obstruction, or associated restrictive pulmonary function from pleural effusions or intrinsic decrease in lung volumes.

Hyperthyroidism can have dyspnea as a major clinical manifestation because of the increase in central respiratory drive associated with the hypermetabolic state. High-output cardiac failure associated with hyperthyroidism can lead to pulmonary edema in some patients.

Hypoparathyroidism may occur associated with hypocalcemia, acute tetany, laryngeal stridor, and muscle weakness.

Benign and malignant ovarian tumors may manifest with unilateral or bilateral pleural effusions.

The interplay between asthma and obesity is clear, but the association between asthma and obesity is less clear regarding cause and effect. The increasing prevalence of both conditions and the significant morbidity and mortality from both make it imperative that practitioners stress the importance of weight management in children and adolescents with and without asthma. Sustained weight loss is difficult. In children with obesity, exercise tolerance also may be limited.

References

1. Sepulveda J and Velasquez BJ, et al: Study of the influence of NA-872 and dexamethasone on the differentiation of Clara cells in albino mice. Respiration 43:363-368, 1982.
2. Hansen LA, et al: Pulmonary complications in diabetes mellitus. Mayo Clin Proc 64:9, 1989.
3. Lange P, et al: Diabetes mellitus, plasma glucose and lung function in a cross-sectional population study. Eur Res J 2:14-19, 1989.
4. Sandler M, et al: Cross-section study of pulmonary function in patients with insulin-dependent diabetes mellitus [erratum in Am Rev Resp Dis 135 (5):1223, 1987]. Am Rev Resp Dis 135:223-229, 1987.
5. Sandler M, et al: Pulmonary function in young insulin-dependent diabetic subjects [erratum in Chest 91:797, 1987]. Chest 90:670-675, 1986.
6. Schuyler MR, et al: Abnormal lung elasticity in juvenile diabetes mellitus. Am Rev Resp Dis 113:37-41, 1976.
7. Schnapf BM, et al: Pulmonary function in insulin-dependent diabetes mellitus with limited joint mobility. Am Rev Resp Dis 130:930-932, 1984.
8. Primhak RA, et al: Reduced vital capacity in insulin-dependent diabetes. Diabetes 36:324-326, 1987.
9. Weir DC, et al: Transfer factor for carbon monoxide in patients with diabetes with and without microangiopathy. Thorax 43:725-726, 1988.

10. Schernthaner G, et al: Lung elasticity in juvenile-onset diabetes mellitus. Am Rev Resp Dis 116:544-546, 1977.
11. Ofulue F, et al: Experimental diabetes and the lung, I: Changes in growth, morphometry, and biochemistry. Am Rev Resp Dis 137:162-166, 1988.
12. Ofulue F, et al: Experimental diabetes and the lung, II: In vivo connective tissue metabolism. Am Rev Resp Dis 138:284-289, 1988.
13. Vracko R, et al: Basal lamina of alveolar epithelium and capillaries: Quantitative changes with aging and in diabetes mellitus. Am Rev Resp Dis 120:973-983, 1979.
14. Brownlee M: Microvascular disease and related abnormalities: Their relation to control of diabetes in Joslin's diabetes mellitus 12th Ed. Marble A, et al, eds: Philadelphia, Lea & Febiger, 1985.
15. Kohn RR, et al: Glycosylation of human collagen. Diabetes 31:5, 1982.
16. Ofulue F, et al: Effects of streptozotocin-induced diabetes on calmodulin and cyclic AMP phosphodiesterase activity in rat lungs. Lung 160:303-310, 1982.
17. Hamlin CR, et al: Apparent accelerated aging of human collagen in diabetes mellitus. Diabetes 24:902-904, 1975.
18. Finkelstein SM, et al: Diabetes mellitus associated with cystic fibrosis. J Pediatr 112:373-377, 1988.
19. Marshall B, et al: Epidemiology of cystic fibrosis-related diabetes. J Pediatr 146:681-687, 2005.
20. Koch C, et al: Presence of cystic fibrosis-related diabetes mellitus is tightly linked to poor lung function in patients with cystic fibrosis: Data from the European Epidemiologic Registry of Cystic Fibrosis. Pediatr Pulmonol 32:343-350, 2001.
21. Liou TG, et al: Predictive 5-year survivorship model of cystic fibrosis. Am J Epidemiol 153:345-352, 2001.
22. Milla C, et al: Trends in pulmonary function in patients with cystic fibrosis correlate with the degree of glucose intolerance at baseline. Am J Resp Crit Care Med 162(3 Pt 1):891-895, 2000.
23. Milla C, et al: Diabetes is associated with dramatically decreased survival in female but not male subjects with cystic fibrosis. Diabetes Care 28:2141-2144, 2005.
24. Sims EJ, et al: Decreased lung function in female but not male subjects with established cystic fibrosis-related diabetes. Diabetes Care 28:1581-1587, 2005.
25. Moran A, et al: Diagnosis, screening and management of cystic fibrosis related diabetes mellitus: A consensus conference report. Diabetes Res Clin Pract 45:61-73, 1999.
26. Miodovnik M, et al: Perinatal asphyxia in infants of insulin-dependent diabetic mothers. J Pediatr 113:9, 1988.
27. Robert MF, et al: Association between maternal diabetes and the respiratory-distress syndrome in the newborn. N Engl J Med 294:4, 1976.
28. Bourbon JR, et al: Fetal lung development in the diabetic pregnancy. Pediatr Res 19:15, 1985.
29. Smith BT, et al: Insulin antagonism of cortisol action on lecithin synthesis by cultured fetal lung cells. J Pediatr 87(6 Pt 1):3, 1975.
30. Persson B, et al: Neonatal morbidities in gestational diabetes mellitus. Diabetes Care 21(Suppl 2):5, 1998.
31. Donelly PM, et al: Large lungs and growth hormone: An increased alveolar number? Eur Respir J 8:10, 1995.
32. Rosenow F, et al: Sleep apnoea in endocrine diseases. J Sleep Res 7:3-11, 1998.
33. Levy SR, et al: Cushing's syndrome in infancy secondary to pituitary adenoma. Am J Dis Child 136:605-607, 1982.
34. Sumner TE, et al: Cushing's syndrome in infancy due to pituitary adenoma. Pediatr Radiol 12:81-83, 1982.
35. Geller DS, et al: Mutations in the mineralocorticoid receptor gene cause autosomal dominant pseudohypoaldosteronism type I. Nat Genet 19:3:279-281, 1998.
36. Edelheit O, et al: Novel mutations in epithelial sodium channel (ENaC) subunit genes and phenotypic expression of multisystem pseudohypoaldosteronism. Clin Endocrinol 62:547-553, 2005.
37. Schaedel C, et al: Lung symptoms in pseudohypoaldosteronism type 1 are associated with deficiency of the alpha-subunit of the epithelial sodium channel. J Pediatr 135:739-745, 1999.
38. Akcay A, et al: Pseudohypoaldosteronism type I and respiratory distress syndrome. J Pediatr Endocrinol 15:1557-1561, 2002.
39. Hanukoglu A, et al: Pseudohypoaldosteronism with increased sweat and saliva electrolyte values and frequent lower respiratory tract infections mimicking cystic fibrosis. J Pediatr 125(5 Pt 1):752-755, 1994.
40. Marthinsen L, et al: Recurrent *Pseudomonas* bronchopneumonia and other symptoms as in cystic fibrosis in a child with type I pseudohypoaldosteronism. Acta Paediatr 87:472-474, 1998.
41. MacLaughlin EF: Pseudohypoaldosteronism and sodium transport. Pediatr Pulmonol Suppl 13:181, 1996.
42. Kerem E, et al: Pulmonary epithelial sodium-channel dysfunction and excess airway liquid in pseudohypoaldosteronism. N Engl J Med 341:156-162, 1999.
43. Laroche CM, et al: Hypothyroidism presenting with respiratory muscle weakness. Am Rev Resp Dis 138:472-474, 1988.
44. Martinez FJ, et al: Hypothyroidism: A reversible cause of diaphragmatic dysfunction. Chest 96:1059-1063, 1989.
45. Siafakas NM, et al: Respiratory muscle strength in hypothyroidism. Chest 102:5, 1992.
46. Zwillich CW, et al: Ventilatory control in myxedema and hypothyroidism. N Engl J Med 292:662-665, 1975.
47. Ladenson PW, et al: Prediction and reversal of blunted ventilatory responsiveness in patients with hypothyroidism. Am J Med 84:5, 1988.
48. Lin CC, et al: The relationship between sleep apnea syndrome and hypothyroidism. Chest 102:1663-1667, 1992.
49. Skjodt NM, et al: Screening for hypothyroidism in sleep apnea. Isr J Resp Crit Care Med 160:732-735, 1999.
50. Jha A, et al: Thyroxine replacement therapy reverses sleep-disordered breathing in patients with primary hypothyroidism. Sleep Med 7:55-61, 2006.
51. Curnock AL, et al: High prevalence of hypothyroidism in patients with primary pulmonary hypertension. Am J Med Sci 318:4, 1999.
52. Hughes DJ: Am J Med 9, 259-260, 1950.
53. Madoff, L: Elevated sweat chlorides and hypothyroidism. J Pediatr 73:244-246, 1968.
54. Strickland AL: Sweat electrolytes in thyroid disorders. J of Pediatr. 1973. 82(2):284-6.
55. Squires L: Abnormal sweat chloride in auto-immune hypothyroidism. Clin Pediatr 28:535-536, 1989.

56. Means MA, Dobson RL, et al: Cytological changes in the sweat gland in hypothyroidism. JAMA 186:113-115, 1963.
57. Dobson RL, et al: Cytologic changes in the eccrine sweat gland in hypothyroidism: A preliminary report. J Invest Dermatol 37:457-458, 1961.
58. Zwillich CW, et al: Thyrotoxicosis: Comparison of effects of thyroid ablation and beta-adrenergic blockade on metabolic rate and ventilatory control. J Clin Endocrinol Metab 46:491-500, 1978.
59. Pino-Garcia JM, et al: Regulation of breathing in hyperthyroidism: Relationship to hormonal and metabolic changes. Eur Resp J 12:400-407, 1998.
60. Small D, et al: Exertional dyspnea and ventilation in hyperthyroidism. Chest 101:1268-1273, 1992.
61. Irace L, et al: Work capacity and oxygen uptake abnormalities in hyperthyroidism. Min Cardioangiol 54:355-362, 2006.
62. Kahaly G, et al: Impaired cardiopulmonary exercise capacity in patients with hyperthyroidism. Chest 109:57-61, 1996.
63. Otsuka H, et al: Exercise performance in children with hyperthyroidism. Acta Paediatr Jap 36:678-682, 1994.
64. Stockley RA, et al: Effect of thyrotoxicosis on the reflex hypoxic respiratory drive. Clin Sci Mol Med 53:93-100, 1977.
65. Mahajan KK, et al: Lung transfer components in hyperthyroidism. J Assoc Physicians India 39:618-620, 1991.
66. Guleria R, et al: Dyspnoea, lung function and respiratory muscle pressures in patients with Graves' disease. Ind J Med Res 104:299-303, 1996.
67. Kahaly G, et al: Cardiovascular hemodynamics and exercise tolerance in thyroid disease. Thyroid 12:473-481, 2002.
68. Ayres J, et al: Thyrotoxicosis and dyspnoea. Clin Endocrinol 16:65-71, 1982.
69. Siafakas NM, et al: Respiratory muscle strength in hyperthyroidism before and after treatment. Am Rev Resp Dis 146:1025-1029, 1992.
70. Mier A, et al: Reversible respiratory muscle weakness in hyperthyroidism. Am Rev Resp Dis 139:529-533, 1989.
71. Kendrick AH, et al: Lung function and exercise performance in hyperthyroidism before and after treatment. QJM 68:615-627, 1988.
72. Nabishah BM, et al: Cyclic adenosine 3′,5′-monophosphate content and bronchial smooth muscle contractility of hyper- and hypothyroid lungs. Clin Exp Pharmacol Physiol 19:839-842, 1992.
73. Israel RH, et al: Hyperthyroidism protects against carbachol-induced bronchospasm. Chest 91:242-245, 1987.
74. Irwin RS, et al: Airway reactivity and lung function in triiodothyronine-induced thyrotoxicosis. J Appl Physiol 58:1485-1488, 1985.
75. Zimmerman, D: Fetal and neonatal hyperthyroidism. Thyroid 9:727-733, 1999.
76. Singer J: Neonatal thyrotoxicosis. J Pediatr 91:5, 1977.
77. Oden J, et al: Neonatal thyrotoxicosis and persistent pulmonary hypertension necessitating extracorporeal life support. Pediatrics 115:e105-e108, 2005.
78. Markham LA, et al: A case report of neonatal thyrotoxicosis due to maternal autoimmune hyperthyroidism [erratum in Adv Neonatal Care 4 (1):41, 2004]. Adv Neonatal Care 3:272-282, 2003.
79. O'Donovan D, et al: Reversible pulmonary hypertension in neonatal Graves's disease. Irish Med J 90:147-148, 1997.
80. Ismail HM: Reversible pulmonary hypertension and isolated right-sided heart failure associated with hyperthyroidism. J Gen Intern Med 22:148-150, 2007.
81. Soroush-Yari A, et al: Pulmonary hypertension in men with thyrotoxicosis. Respiration 72:90-94, 2005.
82. Nakchbandi IA, et al: Pulmonary hypertension caused by Graves' thyrotoxicosis: Normal pulmonary hemodynamics restored by treatment. Chest 116:1483-1485, 1999.
83. Siu CW, et al: Hemodynamic changes in hyperthyroidism-related pulmonary hypertension: A prospective echocardiographic study. J Clin Endocrinol Metab 92:1736-1742, 2007.
84. Marvisi M, et al: Hyperthyroidism and pulmonary hypertension. Resp Med 96:215-220, 2002.
85. Umpaichitra V, et al: Hypocalcemia in children. Clin Pediatr 2001(40):305-312.
86. Strauss R: Childhood obesity. Curr Probl Pediatr 29:1-29, 1999.
87. Zwillich CW, et al: Decreased hypoxic ventilatory drive in the obesity-hypoventilation syndrome. Am J Med 59:343-348, 1975.
88. Rosen CL: Clinical features of obstructive sleep apnea hypoventilation syndrome in otherwise healthy children. Pediatr Pulmonol 27:403-409, 1999.
89. Marcus CL, et al: Evaluation of pulmonary function and polysomnography in obese children and adolescents. Pediatr Pulmonol 21:176-183, 1996.
90. Mallory GB Jr, Fiser DH, Jackson R: Sleep-associated breathing disorders in morbidly obese children and adolescents. J Pediatr 115:892-897, 1989.
91. Fung KP, Harf A, Perlemuter L: Effects of weight on lung function. Arch Dis Child 65:512-515, 1990.
92. Biring MS, et al: Pulmonary physiologic changes of morbid obesity. Am J Med Sci 318:293-297, 1999.
93. Inselman LS, Milanese A, Deurloo A: Effect of obesity on pulmonary function in children. Pediatr Pulmonol 16:130-137, 1993.
94. Ford ES: The epidemiology of obesity and asthma. J Allergy Clin Immunol 115:897-909, 2005.
95. Gilliand FD, et al: Obesity and the risk of newly diagnosed asthma in school age children. Am J Epidemiol 158:406-415, 2003.
96. Gennuso J, et al: The relationship between asthma and obesity in urban minority children and adolescents Arch Pediatr Adolesc Med 152:1197-1200, 1998.
97. Tantisra KG, Weiss ST: Complex interactions in complex traits: Asthma and obesity. Thorax 56 (Suppl 2):64-74, 2001.
98. Shore SA, Fredberg JJ: Obesity, smooth muscle, and hyperresponsiveness. J Allergy Clin Immunol 115:925-927, 2005.
99. Fantuzzi G: Adipose tissue, adipokines, and inflammation. J Allergy Clin Immunol 115:911-919, 2005.
100. Norman A-C, et al: Influence of excess adiposity on exercise fitness and performance in overweight children and adolescents. Pediatrics 115:e690-e696, 2005.
101. Reddy M, Light MJ, Quinton P: Activation of the epithelial Na⁺ channel (ENaC) requires CFTR Cl⁻ channel function. Nature 402:301-304, 1999.
102. Mall M, et al: Increased airway epithelial Na absorption produces cystic fibrosis-like lung disease in mice. Nat Med 10:487-493, 2004.

CHAPTER 9

Pulmonary Manifestations of Neuromuscular Diseases

John R. Bach

Physiology   184
**Assessment of Respiratory Muscle
  Function**   185
  Clinical Evaluation   185
  Laboratory Evaluation   186
**Clinical Manifestations of Respiratory
  Muscle Fatigue**   187
  Neurologic versus Muscular Disease   188
  Clinical Entities   188
  Sleep Evaluation in Neuromuscular
    Diseases   193
  Cardiac Involvement   194
Management   194

Physical Medicine Respiratory Muscle
  Aids   194
Goal One—Maintenance of Lung and Chest
  Wall Mobility   194
Goal Two—Maintain Normal Alveolar
  Ventilation   195
Goal Three—Facilitate Airway Clearance   196
Mechanical Insufflation-Exsufflation   197
Extubation and Decannulation   197
Glossopharyngeal Breathing   198
Perioperative Management   198
Outcomes   198
End-of-Life Care   199
  References   199

Children with neuromuscular disorders have primarily ventilation rather than oxygenation impairment as a result of inspiratory muscle insufficiency. When the respiratory muscles are not assisted, this leads to hypercapnic ventilatory failure or acute respiratory failure mostly owing to ineffective cough during otherwise benign upper respiratory tract infections. Most patients with Duchenne muscular dystrophy (DMD), infantile spinal muscular atrophy (SMA), and other pediatric neuromuscular diseases die prematurely because of failure to use respiratory muscle aids. In large part for this reason, respiratory failure continues to be the most common cause of death for children with severe myopathies, anterior horn cell disorders, and high-level spinal cord injury. The use of inspiratory and expiratory muscle aids can prevent or reverse ventilatory failure, preserve quality of life, and prolong survival for most of these patients. This chapter briefly reviews clinical physiology, presents a diagnostic approach to these diseases, describes some common clinical entities, and concludes with a discussion of the prevention of respiratory failure caused by neuromuscular disease.

Physiology

The three basic components of the respiratory control system are as follows: (1) *sensors*, which gather afferent information and feed it to (2) a central *controller* in the brain, which processes afferent information and sends efferent impulses to the (3) *effectors* (respiratory muscles), which cause ventilation or cough.[1]

The afferent information for ventilation comes from central chemoreceptors located in the medulla, carotid and aortic bodies, and stretch receptors in the lungs. The brainstem is the primary center for the central control of respiratory muscle activity. This control occurs at a subconscious level. The cortex can temporarily override the automatic nature of this mechanism if voluntary control is desired.

For the central commands controlling respiration to operate the ventilatory mechanism, the motor units of the respiratory muscles also must be functioning properly. A motor unit consists of an anterior horn cell, its peripheral nerve axon, the neuromuscular junction, and the muscle fibers it innervates. Normally, when an anterior horn cell fires, the peripheral nerve causes the release of acetylcholine at the terminal axon. Acetylcholine diffuses across the neuromuscular junction, where it binds to receptors on the postjunctional membrane and opens channels for the passage of calcium and sodium ions. The ion influx depolarizes the muscle membrane, which triggers contraction of the myofibrils. Neuromuscular diseases are caused by disorders of the anterior horn cells, peripheral motor nerves, myoneural junction, and muscle fibers.

The muscles of respiration include four groups: the diaphragm, the chest wall muscles, the abdominal muscles, and the muscles of the upper airway (bulbar-innervated). The diaphragm is the principal muscle of inspiration. The phrenic nerves from cervical segments 3, 4, and 5 supply it. The chest wall muscles consist of the internal and external intercostals (T1-T12); the parasternal intercostals (T1-T12); the scalenes (C4-C8); and the accessory inspiratory muscles, including the sternocleidomastoids (cranial nerve XI, C1-C2), trapezoids (cranial nerve XI, C2-C3), and pectoralis major (C5-C7). The abdominal respiratory muscles include the rectus and transverse abdominis and the external and internal obliques (T7-L1). They are the most important muscles of expiration.

The muscles of the upper airway include the muscles of the mouth (cranial nerves IX and X), uvula and palate (XI), tongue (IX and XII), and larynx (C1). Although these muscles do not have a direct action on the chest, they are essential for keeping the upper airway patent, and they affect airway resistance and airflow.

During normal respiration, the most important muscles for breathing in addition to the diaphragm are the parasternal intercostals. Postural muscles such as the external and internal intercostals and the accessory muscles such as scalenes and sternocleidomastoids affect breathing significantly only at high rates of ventilation. Expiration is passive during quiet breathing. The lungs and chest wall are elastic and tend to return to their equilibrium positions after being actively expanded during inspiration. The abdominal muscles are not used during quiet expiration to functional residual capacity. These muscles are contracted during forceful exhalation that deflates lungs to residual volume.

Assessment of Respiratory Muscle Function

Clinical Evaluation

Clinical and laboratory evaluation of the chest wall can provide essential information with regard to chest wall function in a particular patient (Table 9-1). The chest wall configuration and pattern of spontaneous breathing,

Table 9-1	Guidelines for Assessment of Respiratory Muscle Function

Clinical Evaluation
- Chest wall configuration (e.g., scoliosis, overdistention)
- Pattern of spontaneous breathing:
  - Rate and amplitude of breathing
  - Thoracic and/or abdominal breathing
  - Coordination or paradoxic thoracic and abdominal expansion
- Specific maneuvers:
  - Maximal variation in thoracic circumference
  - Maximal excursion of diaphragm (inspection and percussion)
  - Cough maneuver–feeble or strong then objective assessment?

Laboratory Evaluation
- Electromyographic studies of various respiratory muscles
- Roentgenograms (in supine position):
  - Cinefluoroscopic studies of diaphragmatic and rib cage movements
  - Plain roentgenograms in full expiration and inspiration
- Real-time ultrasonography
- Pulmonary function tests:
  - Flows: assisted and unassisted peak cough flows (PCF)
  - Lung volumes
  - Coordination of breathing (respiratory inductance plethysmography)

including rate and amplitude of breathing, thoracic or abdominal breathing, coordinated or paradoxical thoracic and abdominal expansion, maximal variation in chest circumference, maximal diaphragmatic excursion during inspiration, and cough effectiveness, are evaluated.

Careful bedside observation of an at-risk patient usually allows the recognition of clinical signs and symptoms indicating progressive respiratory muscle fatigue. These signs and symptoms include loss of nonbreathing functions of the respiratory system, increased respiratory rate, and pattern of breathing, and other warning signs (Table 9-2).

For an infant and small child, inspection is the most important, and usually the only, evaluation tool that is necessary. The normal movement of chest and abdominal wall is directed outward during inspiration. Inward motion of the chest wall during inspiration is called "paradoxical breathing." This motion is seen when the thoracic cage loses its stability and becomes distorted by the action of the diaphragm. Most infants who present with

Table 9-2	Clinical Manifestations of Respiratory Muscle Failure

Inability to Perform Nonventilatory Functions
  Inability to eat/drink/cry
  Reluctance to pause breathing voluntarily
Major Use of Accessory Muscles
  Sternocleidomastoids and pectoral muscles
Increase in Respiratory Rate to Critical Level
  Adolescents   55 breaths/min
  Children, 4-10 years   70-75 breaths/min
  Infants, 1-3 years   90 breaths/min
  Neonates   120 breaths/min
Signs Reflecting Options Taken to Relieve Fatigue
  Reduced inspiratory time (TI) and decreased Pdi: very shallow breathing
  Deep breaths with a brief pause to rest the muscles
  Respiratory alternans
Signs Indicating Impending Respiratory Arrest
  Cyanotic spell
  Cyanosis with brief cough or brief pause
  Inappropriate pause
  Sustained paradoxic thoracic/abdominal movement
  Drooling in absence of airway obstruction (cannot pause to swallow)
  Central nervous system signs (confusion)

neuromuscular conditions have paradoxical breathing with a seesaw type of thoracoabdominal motion owing to severe intercostal muscle weakness. This is true for all children with SMA type 1 and about 40% with SMA type 2 and for many with severe congenital myopathies and muscular dystrophy.

Respiratory rate is important to monitor. As the work of breathing increases, the patient may opt to use less force per breath, reducing tidal volume with shallow breaths and compensating by taking more breaths per minute to avoid fatigue. A very rapid breathing rate cannot be sustained indefinitely, however, and can lead to respiratory muscle exhaustion. The pattern and regularity of breathing also are helpful to observe for risk of fatigue. Breathing that becomes increasingly more rapid and shallow and is interrupted by a deep breath with a brief pause to rest the muscles can be a sign of fatigue for certain patients with central nervous system disorders. Although pauses are normal in healthy children, they can signal respiratory distress, as does nasal flaring, nocturnal flushing, and perspiration. Cyanotic spells or cyanosis with brief cough or brief pause, sustained paradoxical thoracic/abdominal movement, drooling in the absence of airway obstruction (cannot pause to swallow), and confusion also can be signs of impending respiratory arrest.

Laboratory Evaluation

Longitudinal evaluation of lung function should be obtained in patients older than 6 years of age. Measurements of lung function include forced spirometry, static lung volumes, end-tidal carbon dioxide (CO_2), and oximetry. Measuring maximal inspiratory and expiratory pressures at the mouth also can assess respiratory muscle strength, whereas cough efficacy can be evaluated by measuring peak cough flows (PCFs) using a simple peak flowmeter.

The forced vital capacity (FVC) should be measured in the sitting position. If FVC is less than 80%, it should be measured again in the supine position to investigate for diaphragm weakness.[2] A greater than 20% decrease in FVC when going from sitting to supine indicates diaphragm weakness out of proportion to chest wall muscle weakness. Although

FVC less than 60% indicates a low risk for nocturnal hypoventilation, FVC less than 40% or diaphragm weakness indicates a significant risk for nocturnal hypoventilation. Continuous overnight pulse oximetry and end-tidal or transcutaneous CO_2 should be obtained annually in children too young to perform the FVC maneuver or when FVC is less than 60%, or more often when FVC is less than 40%.

Full overnight polysomnography should be obtained when overnight pulse oximetry is not diagnostic in the presence of symptoms suggestive of hypoventilation or sleep-disordered breathing, and a trial of nocturnal noninvasive ventilation (NIV) is clearly warranted. Polysomnograms are programmed to interpret all abnormalities as being due to central/obstructive apneas and not due to respiratory muscle weakness. For these patients, this is similar to "blaming the brain and throat for what the diaphragm cannot do." It too often results in patients being prescribed continuous positive airway pressure or bilevel positive airway pressure (BiPAP) at inappropriately low spans, rather than sufficient pressure or volume support to correct hypoventilation and rest inspiratory muscles more fully. A nocturnal desaturation pattern, often a smooth one, may indicate alveolar hypoventilation. When the patient has a respiratory tract infection, a sudden nocturnal or diurnal severe desaturation usually indicates mucous plugging.

Arterial blood gases are not routinely needed because of the adequacy of end-tidal CO_2/transcutaneous CO_2 measurement. Pulse oximetry should be reserved for intensive care management only.

PCF also should be measured annually during a steady state and at any episode of respiratory infection; values less than 160 to 200 L/min may indicate that cough is ineffective and may place patients at risk for recurrent respiratory infections and respiratory failure. The assisted PCF–unassisted PCF difference also is an excellent measure of glottic integrity.[3]

Spirometry is equally important for the measurement of maximum insufflation capacity (MIC). The MIC is the measure of the maximum volume of air that the glottis can hold in the lungs by "air stacking"

volumes of air consecutively delivered from a volume-cycled ventilator or manual resuscitator. The MIC–vital capacity difference is a direct function of glottic integrity and an objective measure of bulbar-innervated muscle function. Unassisted PCFs are measured. Then the patient air stacks as deeply as possible, and an abdominal thrust is applied, timed to the glottic opening of a cough effort.

Other qualitative and quantitative measures of respiratory muscle function can be obtained, although they are rarely needed (see Table 9-1). These include electromyographic studies of various respiratory muscles, chest radiographs in supine position, and real-time ultrasonography.[4] Chest radiographs are useful for diagnosing pneumonia and gross atelectasis, but they lag behind oximetry as an indication of these problems (see later). Diaphragmatic strength also can be invasively assessed by measuring transdiaphragmatic pressure[5] and by using a manometer for measuring maximum inspiratory and expiratory pressures at the mouth. The measurement of maximum voluntary ventilation, when possible, can be helpful in determining respiratory muscle endurance.[6] The most important and practical measures continue to be spirometry for FVC and MIC, peak flowmeter for unassisted and assisted PCFs, end-tidal CO_2, and pulse oximetry. The last two also are useful for nocturnal monitoring because they relate to inspiratory muscle dysfunction.

Clinical Manifestations of Respiratory Muscle Fatigue

Acute respiratory muscle fatigue is characterized by exhaustion leading within minutes or hours to respiratory failure. Chronic fatigue is not as easily identified. Symptoms of chronic fatigue are often subtle, and the diagnosis is frequently missed unless specifically considered. Infants with severe neuromuscular disorders often present with tachypnea, nocturnal flushing, profuse perspiration, and frequent arousals. After 6 months of age, these infants develop otherwise benign respiratory tract infections that result in airway mucous plugging because of their ineffective cough. This mucous plugging causes decreases in oxyhemoglobin saturation (Sa_{O_2}) to less than

95%, which, if not quickly reversed by effective assisted coughing, results in pneumonia and respiratory failure with persistent hypoxemia.

In older children, symptoms and signs of chronic respiratory insufficiency include general fatigue and dyspnea on exertion. The first manifestations of chronic respiratory muscle impairment often are symptoms of sleep hypoventilation, however, either nocturnal (frequent nightmares, enuresis, perspiration, frequent awakenings) or daytime symptoms (morning headaches, hypersomnolence, chronic fatigue, impaired concentration, dyspnea, tachycardia, difficulty awakening in the morning, right ventricular failure, peripheral edema, irritability, polycythemia, impaired cognition, anxiety, depression, weight changes, muscle aches, memory impairment), and poor control of upper airway secretions and exacerbation of swallowing difficulties.[7] Often, because many of these patients are wheelchair-bound and inactive, only fatigue, anxiety, and sleeplessness are noted. Small children exhibit increased paradoxical breathing and tachypnea and nasal flaring, and appear distressed.

Neurologic versus Muscular Disease

Some neuromuscular diseases include upper motor neuron involvement. Upper motor neuron lesions result from pathology in the cerebral cortex, brainstem, or spinal cord and are signaled by an increase in muscle tone (spasticity), hyperreflexia, and the persistence or reappearance of primitive reflexes, such as the extensor plantar response (Babinski sign). These patients also may have reflex deep breaths ("sighs") and coughs despite having very low vital capacity and PCFs. Lesions above the foramen magnum also may produce contralateral hemiplegia. Lesions in the cortex or subcortical areas often are associated with disorders of speech or other cortical functions. Lesions in the brainstem usually affect cranial nerve function ipsilateral to the lesion and contralateral hemiplegia. Abnormalities in the spinal cord typically cause bilateral weakness because of the close proximity of the descending tracts. Upper motor neuron disorders can be identified and differentiated further by imaging studies such as computed

tomography, magnetic resonance imaging, and myelography.

The lower motor neuron system includes the anterior horn cell, the peripheral nerve, the neuromuscular junction, and muscle. Manifestations of lower motor neuron involvement include flaccidity, depressed reflexes, fasciculations, and muscle atrophy. Anterior horn cell diseases cause distal weakness without sensory symptoms, whereas disorders of peripheral nerves are almost always accompanied by sensory loss secondary to the involvement of sensory nerves, hyporeflexia, and usually distal weakness. Peripheral nerve weakness can result from damage to either the core axon (axon neuropathies) or the myelin sheath that coats the nerve (demyelinating neuropathies). Disorders of the neuromuscular junction are characterized by fluctuating weakness and frequently involve the extraocular and bulbar-innervated muscles. Sensory symptoms are lacking.

Muscle disorders usually manifest with proximal weakness manifested by inability to rise from a chair or to comb the hair. Sensory symptoms are absent, and reflexes are usually decreased. Serum levels of creatine kinase are frequently elevated. Electrodiagnostic testing may be used to differentiate between anterior horn cell disorders, peripheral neuropathies, neuromuscular junction disorders, and muscle diseases.

Clinical Entities

Table 9-3 lists causes of respiratory muscle dysfunction.

Upper Motor Neuron
Quadriplegia and respiratory compromise can result from acute cervical spinal cord trauma, spinal artery infarction, or compression by tumor. Injuries at or above C3 to C5 involve the phrenic nerves and can cause partial to complete bilateral hemidiaphragmatic paralysis. Intercostal muscle paralysis below the level of the lesion limits the normal outward expansion of the middle and upper rib cage, compromising inspiration further. Expiration also can be reduced because of paralysis of the abdominal and other expiratory muscles. High-level quadriplegics may be unable to generate adequate tidal volumes, and the

Table 9-3	Causes of Respiratory Muscle Dysfunction

SITE OF DEFECT	CAUSES
Central Drive of Breathing	Congenital or acquired
Upper Motor Neuron	Hemiplegia
	Cerebral palsy
	Quadriplegia
Lower Motor Neuron	Poliomyelitis
	Spinal muscular atrophies
	Guillain-Barré syndrome
	Tetanus
	Friedreich's ataxia
	Traumatic nerve lesions
	Phrenic nerve paralysis
Neuromuscular Junction	Myasthenia gravis
	Congenital myasthenic syndromes
	Botulism
	Drugs
Respiratory Muscles	Muscular dystrophies
	Congenital myopathies
	Metabolic myopathies
	Steroid myopathy
	Connective tissue disease
	Diaphragmatic malformation
Nonmuscular, Chest Wall Structures	Scoliosis
	Congenital rib cage abnormality
	Overinflated rib cage
	Connective tissue disease
	Thoracic burns
	Obesity
	Giant exomphalos

accompanying hypoventilation and atelectasis can result in hypoxemia. Low-level cervical quadriplegics with intact phrenic nerves are able to contract their diaphragms. They, too, lack the intercostal muscle activity necessary to stabilize the rib cage for optimal inspiratory function, however. These patients also may lose the use of the abdominal and other expiratory muscles. Combined inspiratory and expiratory weakness can prevent them from effectively coughing and clearing secretions and place them at high risk for pneumonia. Initially, with spinal cord injury, the vital

capacity, maximum inspiratory pressure, and maximum expiratory pressure are reduced. As the initial phase of spinal injury passes, chest wall flaccidity is replaced with spasticity, and there is an improvement in the vital capacity as the more rigid chest wall resists collapse.

Anterior Horn Cell Disorders
SMAs comprise a group of autosomal-recessive degenerative disorders of lower motor neurons classified as type I (Werdnig-Hoffman disease), type II, and type III (Kugelberg-Welander disease), based on the age of onset of muscle weakness and clinical severity. These disorders often manifest in infancy and childhood with an estimated incidence of 1:5000. SMAs are due to a mutation of the survival motor neuron gene located on chromosome 5q13. This mutation is responsible for primary degeneration of the anterior horn cells of the spinal cord and often of the bulbar motor nuclei, which leads to skeletal muscle paralysis and atrophy.

Werdnig-Hoffman disease manifests in the first 6 months of life. Infants with this disease lack head control and are nearly always unable to sit and walk. There is severe hypotonia, generalized weakness, and thin muscle mass. All of these patients have paradoxical inward rib cage movement with each inspiration, the diaphragm being relatively spared. Unless provided with nocturnal high-span BiPAP, they develop pectus excavatum and severe undergrowth of the lungs and chest wall, showing on chest radiography reduced lung volume and a bell-shaped thorax. Unless supported by respiratory muscle aids (described later), more than 90% of patients die by 2 years of age.

In SMA type 2, affected patients are usually able to suck and swallow, and respiration is adequate in early infancy. Swallowing difficulties or choking with feeds becomes apparent in the preschool years, predisposing these patients to recurrent pneumonia and chronic suppurative lung disease. These patients can sit but not walk. About 40% of these patients have paradoxical breathing and require nocturnal high-span BiPAP.

Kugelberg-Welander disease is the mildest SMA (type 3), and patients may appear normal in infancy. The progressive weakness is proximal in distribution, particularly involving shoulder girdle muscles. In the adult-onset form, SMA type 4, patients can walk for some period of time. An X-linked adult-onset type 5 SMA (which affects only men), otherwise known as Kennedy disease, is associated with gynecomastia, temporal atrophy, and endocrine disturbances and hypospermia.

Preliminary data obtained from phase 1 human studies have suggested that sodium valproate may improve anterior horn cell function in SMA. Pharmacologic therapy or gene therapy is unlikely to have a major effect on the course of the disease in older patients with advanced disease, but NIV is effective in many of these patients and may buy time for medical therapies to take effect or even undergo development.

Poliomyelitis is a poliovirus infection of young children that begins with fever and upper respiratory symptoms that are followed by signs of meningeal irritation and asymmetric, flaccid paralysis that can involve the skeletal, respiratory, and bulbar-innervated musculature. The respiratory motor nuclei can be directly involved, resulting in diaphragmatic and accessory respiratory muscle dysfunction. Involvement of lower cranial nerve nuclei can result in upper airway obstruction, pooling of secretions, and aspiration. The medullary respiratory center also can be affected, resulting in irregular respirations and apnea. Many of these patients require ventilatory and hemodynamic support during the acute phase of the illness. Although most patients show substantial muscle recovery over time, they gradually relapse to require ventilatory assistance again later in life with the senescent aging and dropping out of overworked anterior motor neurons with aging.[8]

Disorders of Peripheral Nerves
Hereditary motor and sensorimotor neuropathies are common. The former is often confused with and can be as severe as SMA. The most common is Charcot-Marie-Tooth disease, a demyelinating neuropathy. Almost 15% of patients are left with residual weakness, and an additional 5% experience chronic relapsing (dysimmune) polyneuropathy. Some patients are never weaned from ventilatory support.[8]

Acute idiopathic polyradiculitis, also known as Guillain-Barré syndrome, is the most common peripheral neuropathy causing respiratory failure. It is considered to be an autoimmune disease precipitated by a preceding viral or bacterial infection, such as cytomegalovirus, Epstein-Barr virus, *Mycoplasma pneumoniae*, and *Campylobacter jejuni*. In 80% of these patients, there is a history of a nonspecific viral illness preceding weakness by 2 to 3 weeks. Diagnosis is mainly based on clinical grounds. It usually begins with fine paresthesias in the toes or fingertips followed by progressive muscle weakness in the lower extremities, trunk, upper limbs, and, finally, bulbar-innervated and respiratory muscles. Muscle involvement is relatively symmetric. Facial and oropharyngeal weakness are often impending signs of respiratory failure. Muscle pain is common in the initial stages. Daily bedside evaluation of vital capacity and arterial blood gases is essential for appropriate decisions regarding the need of mechanical ventilatory support, which is required in 20% of affected children. Acute respiratory failure can be avoided with the use of noninvasive aids when bulbar-innervated muscle function is adequate to prevent continuous aspiration of saliva or oxyhemoglobin desaturation. Otherwise, patients need to be intubated for ventilator use and airway secretion management. Early use of high-dose intravenous immunoglobulins or plasma exchange induces a more rapid resolution of the disease. Corticosteroids are now used sparingly because they seem to predispose to the chronic relapsing form of the disease.

Among other peripheral neuropathies leading to respiratory failure, Lyme disease can manifest with a syndrome identical to Guillain-Barré syndrome. In endemic areas, serologic testing for Lyme disease is indicated. Acute intermittent porphyria can cause a neuropathy severe enough to result in respiratory failure. Postdiphtheritic neuropathy, toxic neuropathies (thallium, phosphate, and lead) avitaminosis, paralytic shellfish (saxitoxin) poisoning, and the polyneuropathies associated with systemic lupus erythematosus and polyarteritis nodosa also can cause ventilatory failure.

Disorders of the Neuromuscular Junction

Myasthenia gravis is the most common disorder of the neuromuscular junction. It affects any age group, although clusters of cases are found in adolescent girls. Myasthenia gravis is characterized by fluctuating weakness with a predilection for the ocular muscles (ptosis, diplopia, blurred vision) and bulbar-innervated muscles (dysphagia, dysphasia, and aspiration). The pupillary response to light is preserved. Similar to the adult form, juvenile myasthenia gravis is an acquired immunologic disorder of neuromuscular transmission associated with circulating antibodies against postsynaptic acetylcholine receptors. These antibodies can be detected in the serum of 90% of patients with generalized myasthenia gravis.

Diagnosis of juvenile myasthenia gravis is based on clinical symptoms, electrophysiologic studies, a positive finding of circulating acetylcholine receptor autoantibodies, and transient improvement with anticholinesterase medication. Most patients in whom this disease is suspected but undiagnosed show a dramatic response to intravenous edrophonium chloride, a short-acting acetylcholinesterase inhibitor. Benign thymic hyperplasia or thymoma occurs in 90% of these patients. Management is primarily based on anticholinesterase medication (pyridostigmine bromide). Improvement with anticholinesterase medication is often incomplete, however, and most patients require further therapeutic measures, including thymectomy, which results in improvement or remission in 80% of patients without thymomas. Immunosuppressive drugs (prednisone, azathioprine, or cyclosporine) are frequently recommended. Other autoimmune diseases, such as rheumatoid arthritis, systemic lupus erythematosus, and thyrotoxicosis, commonly complicate the clinical picture.

Transient neonatal myasthenia gravis is a syndrome that affects 30% of infants born to mothers with autoimmune myasthenia gravis. Clinical features are usually noted within hours of birth and include feeding and respiratory difficulties, hypotonia, weak cry, facial weakness, and palpebral ptosis. Respiratory difficulties are related to feeding problems causing aspiration pneumonia, upper airway obstruction owing to inability to handle oropharyngeal secretions, or respiratory muscle weakness. Some patients may require ventilatory support during this period. After the abnormal antibodies disappear, the infants have normal strength and are not at increased risk for developing myasthenia gravis in later childhood. The syndrome of transient neonatal myasthenia gravis is to be distinguished from a rare, often hereditary, and often permanent, congenital myasthenia gravis not related to maternal myasthenia gravis. This disorder is characterized by an abnormality of the acetylcholine receptor, manifested as high conductance and excessively fast closure, and is probably due to a mutation affecting a single amino acid residue. Therapy for acute attacks (myasthenia crisis) includes mechanical ventilation in combination with plasma exchange, acetylcholinesterase inhibitors (pyridostigmine), and corticosteroids or other immunosuppressants.

Botulism is a rare disorder of the neuromuscular transmission blockade caused by the binding of one of the neurotoxins (A, B, E, and F) produced by *Clostridium botulinum*. The toxin that is carried in the bloodstream prevents the release of acetylcholine from the presynaptic terminal and affects nicotinic and muscarinic synapses. Botulism occurs in three forms: infantile botulism, the most common, in which the organism and its spores are ingested in honey or other foods, or from the environment; food-borne (classic) botulism, in which preformed toxin is ingested in nonacidic home-canned or factory-canned vegetables or meat; and wound botulism (very rare), in which *C. botulinum* and its spores contaminate traumatic or surgical wounds.[9]

Infant botulism is most commonly seen in the first 4 months of life. Constipation is usually the first symptom; thereafter, neuromuscular dysfunction results in progressive descending muscle weakness, with early bulbar involvement and hypotonia. Acute respiratory failure develops in 90% of affected infants. Respiratory failure results from respiratory muscle weakness and paralysis, causing hypoventilation; bulbar palsy and upper airway muscle weakness, leading to aspiration pneumonia or upper airway obstruction; and inability to clear secretions, resulting in pneumonia and atelectasis. Endotracheal intubation is performed as soon as depression of the gag reflex is noted.

In older children with food-borne or wound botulism, the onset of neurologic symptoms follows a characteristic pattern of diplopia, blurred vision, ptosis, dry mouth, dysphagia, dysarthria, decreased gag reflex, and decreased corneal reflex followed by flaccid descending paralysis that often progresses to affect the respiratory muscles. The diagnosis should be considered if a previously healthy infant, usually younger than 6 months, has a history of constipation and then acutely develops weakness with difficulty in sucking, swallowing, crying, or breathing. It is suggested by electromyographic changes of brief, small, abundant motor unit potentials in response to high rates of stimulation similar to that seen in aminoglycoside toxicity. The diagnosis is confirmed by showing neurotoxin in the serum, stool, or contaminated food. Treatment includes positioning the head backward to open the airway and improve respiratory mechanics. Respiratory muscle aids are often required, and pneumonia is a common complication and a major cause of death. Antibiotic therapy is not part of the treatment of uncomplicated infantile or food-borne botulism because the toxin is primarily an intracellular molecule. Antibiotics are reserved for the treatment of complications. Wound botulism requires aggressive use of antibiotics and antitoxin.

The neuromuscular junction is perhaps the most common site adversely affected in drug-induced neuropathies. Several drugs have been reported to produce or potentiate unwanted neuromuscular blockade, including aminoglycosides, clindamycin, polymyxin, colistin, propranolol, calcium channel blockers, quinidine, lidocaine, corticosteroids, chlorpromazine, and lithium.

Disorders of Muscles

DMD is the most common and severe of the muscular dystrophies that affect humans. Inherited as an X-linked recessive trait, it has an estimated incidence of 1:3000 male births. The gene responsible for DMD and Becker muscular dystrophy has been localized on the short arm of the X chromosome (Xp21). The dystrophin gene regulates the expression of dystrophin, a protein that links the normal contractile apparatus to the sarcolemma in skeletal muscle. DMD usually manifests in boys with proximal muscle weakness at 2 to 4 years of age. Poor head control in infancy may be an early sign of weakness. Clinical diagnosis is made after consideration of history, physical findings, and elevated serum creatine kinase level. Diagnosis is confirmed by finding an abnormality in the dystrophin gene by mutation analysis of blood leukocyte DNA. By inducing specific exon skipping during messenger RNA splicing, antisense compounds were shown to correct the open reading frame of the *DMD* gene and to restore dystrophin expression *in vitro* and in animal models *in vivo*.[32]

Respiratory disease in DMD is the major cause of morbidity and mortality. Loss of lung function progresses linearly after the initiation of wheelchair use; increasing hypoxemic dips are seen during sleep in subsequent teenage years, and respiratory failure occurs between 18 and 20 years of age. Unless properly managed with respiratory muscle aids, these patients invariably die before age 30. The deterioration in pulmonary function in DMD parallels the progression of the disease. A FVC of less than 1 L is a predictor of poor outcome, with a 5-year survival rate of only 8% if assisted ventilation is not provided. Death is due to respiratory failure in 80% of cases or to cardiac failure in 10% to 20% of cases.[10]

A restrictive syndrome secondary to muscle weakness characterizes the pulmonary compromise in patients with DMD. When daytime hypercapnia develops in DMD patients, life expectancy without noninvasive ventilatory assistance is approximately 9 to 10 months. Chest wall muscle weakness and contractures, spinal deformity, and vertebrocostal ankylosis also occur. When assisted PCF decreases to less than 300 L/min, a pulse oximeter and Cough-Assist™ (JH Emerson Company, Cambridge, MA) are prescribed for the oximetry protocol as described subsequently. Patients with DMD eventually require 24-hour use of noninvasive inspiratory muscle aids, but can live well into their 40s using them.[21]

Congenital myotonic dystrophy is the second most common muscular dystrophy. Myotonic dystrophy is an autosomal dominant inherited disease that occurs with an estimated frequency of 1:7500 to 1:18,500. The mutation responsible is an expansion of trinucleotide (CTG) repeats in the region of the myotonic dystrophy protein kinase (*DMPK*) gene, on the long arm of chromosome 19. Myotonia, a very slow relaxation of muscle after contraction, and muscle weakness are the prominent clinical features, but many organ systems can be affected, including the cardiac, endocrine, and ophthalmologic systems. Involvement of the respiratory system is the major contributor to morbidity and mortality.

Neonatal myotonic dystrophy is a severe form of myotonic dystrophy that develops in a few infants born to mothers, and rarely to fathers, with myotonic dystrophy. Prominent manifestations include hypotonia without myotonia, feeding difficulties, and respiratory distress. Respiratory failure is common and may result in death in the neonatal period. Examining the parents and finding the repeat segment of DNA on the myotonic dystrophy gene can confirm the diagnosis.[11] Polyhydramnios and decreased fetal movements are common. Prematurity, hydrops fetalis with pleural effusions, and pulmonary hypoplasia can increase respiratory difficulties owing to diaphragmatic weakness at birth. Fifty percent of neonates with congenital myotonic dystrophy need respiratory support at birth.

The diagnosis of this disease is suspected when the newborn is recognized to be difficult to wean from the ventilator for unknown reasons. Thin ribs and an elevated right diaphragm on the chest radiograph may hint at the diagnosis. The breathing pattern of these patients is similar to that of any patient with a restrictive syndrome secondary to respiratory muscle weakness—increased rate with small tidal volumes at rest. Myotonia and weakness of the respiratory muscles and the muscles of deglutition, decreased ventilatory drive, and failure of myotonic muscles to benefit from inspiratory muscle support (ventilatory assistance) make these patients very prone to chronic hypoventilation and cor pulmonale.

Sleep Evaluation in Neuromuscular Diseases

Neuromuscular diseases are frequently associated with sleep-disordered breathing and alveolar hypoventilation. Onset of respiratory insufficiency can be subtle. Symptoms of sleep hypoventilation include gradually increasing headache, somnolence, and, rarely, vomiting. Patients with some neuromuscular disorders also are at risk for upper airway obstruction.

Children with DMD may go through an early phase of latent or occult nocturnal hypoxemia before there is evidence of daytime respiratory impairment. Such episodes of hypoxemia can result in a disrupted sleep pattern and impair daytime cognitive performance. The sleep laboratory is an ideal site to diagnose occult episodes of nocturnal hypoxemia in patients with most types of significant restrictive lung disease.

The timing and necessity of polysomnography to detect sleep hypoventilation have not been determined in patients with neuromuscular disorders. Sleep hypoventilation correlates with an awake $PaCO_2$ of 45 mm Hg or greater and a base excess 4 mmol/L or greater. Ambulatory monitoring at home with recording of cardiac and respiratory variables has been suggested as the first diagnostic step in testing for sleep-disordered breathing in patients with DMD. These devices can detect the presence of decreases in sleep-related oxyhemoglobin saturation. A negative test result does not rule out the diagnosis of sleep-disordered breathing and must be followed by polysomnography.

It is recommended to review sleep quality and symptoms of sleep-disordered breathing at every patient encounter, and an annual evaluation for sleep-disordered breathing should be obtained in patients with DMD starting from the time they are wheelchair users or when clinically indicated. Overnight pulse oximetry with continuous CO_2 monitoring provides useful information about nighttime gas exchange, although central or obstructive events not associated with desaturation or

CO_2 retention would not be detected. A simple capillary blood gas measurement on arousal in the morning can show CO_2 retention, although not as sensitively as continuous capnography.

Cardiac Involvement

Cardiac involvement is universal in individuals with DMD. Cardiac disease is the second most common cause of death in individuals with DMD.[16] Dilated cardiomyopathy primarily involves the left ventricle, and can lead to dyspnea and other symptoms of congestive heart failure. Conversely, right ventricular failure can result from respiratory failure and pulmonary hypertension. Individuals with DMD also are at risk for ventricular arrhythmias. Although some studies have suggested that the respiratory and peripheral muscle weakness tend to be inversely related to the risk of cardiac failure, other studies suggest that left heart and respiratory failure tend to occur in parallel. It is recommended that all individuals with DMD obtain regular cardiac evaluation with annual electrocardiograms and echocardiograms, starting at least by school age.

Management

The three goals of management are to (1) provide insufflations to expand the lungs and chest walls optimally to maintain compliance and promote lung growth in children, (2) maintain normal alveolar ventilation around-the-clock, and (3) maximize PCF. The use of inspiratory and expiratory muscle aids attains these goals. Many patients become continuous ventilator users for years without ever being hospitalized.[12-14]

It is surprising that a treatment applied at night can have the sustained effect of correcting arterial blood gas tensions during the day. Over the years, it has been hypothesized that this improvement is mediated by many possible mechanisms. It has been suggested[30] that NIV may work by (1) improving ventilatory mechanics; (2) resting fatigued respiratory muscles, improving strength and endurance; or (3) enhancing ventilatory sensitivity to CO_2.

As mentioned earlier, numerous neuromuscular disorders are associated with cardiomyopathy or conduction defects or both. The consequences of cardiac disease are worsened by hypoxemia and hypercapnia. NIV therapy may have direct cardioprotective effects.

Physical Medicine Respiratory Muscle Aids

Inspiratory and expiratory muscle aids are devices and techniques that involve the application of forces to the body or pressure changes to the airway to assist inspiratory or expiratory muscle function. Body ventilators act on the body to assist inspiration just as an abdominal thrust can assist coughing. Negative pressure applied to the airway during expiration also assists the expiratory muscles for coughing, just as positive pressure applied to the airway during inhalation, or noninvasive intermittent positive-pressure ventilation (NPPV), assists the inspiratory muscles. Continuous positive airway pressure assists neither inspiratory nor expiratory muscles and should rarely, if ever, be used for these patients.

Goal One—Maintenance of Lung and Chest Wall Mobility

As the vital capacity decreases, the largest breath can expand only a small fraction of the lungs. Similar to limb articulations, the lungs and chest wall require regular mobilization. Use of incentive spirometry or deep breathing can expand the lungs no greater than the vital capacity and is useless. Lung mobilization can be achieved by air stacking, by providing deep insufflations, or by nocturnal high-span (inspiratory–expiratory positive airway pressure >10) BiPAP for infants (Fig. 9-1).[13]

The patient uses a mouthpiece to "air stack" consecutively delivered volumes from a volume-cycled ventilator or a manual resuscitator multiple times, three times daily. If the lips or cheeks are too weak to permit air stacking via a mouthpiece, it is done via a nasal interface or Bennett Lipseal (Puritan-Bennett Inc. Boulder, CO) (Fig. 9-2). Most patients can learn to use glossopharyngeal breathing (GPB) for lung expansion to or

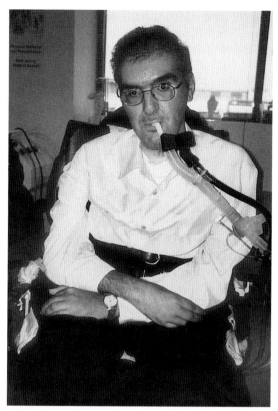

Figure 9-1. This 25-year-old man with Duchenne muscular dystrophy and severe scoliosis required 24-hour noninvasive intermittent positive-pressure ventilation (NIPPV) for more than 5 years. Here he is seen using mouthpiece NIPPV for daytime ventilatory support.

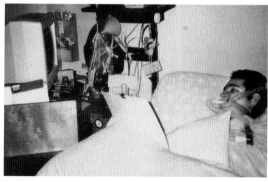

Figure 9-2. This 30-year-old Duchenne muscular dystrophy patient has required 24-hour ventilatory support since he was 14 years old. He uses simple mouthpiece intermittent positive-pressure ventilation during daytime hours and mouthpiece with lip seal retention (seen here) for nocturnal ventilatory support.

beyond the MIC.[15,16] If the bulbar-innervated muscles are too weak for deep air stacking, single deep insufflations are provided via a Cough-Assist™ (Philips Respironics) at 40 to 70 cm H_2O three times daily.

Lung expansion can increase MIC, maximize PCF, improve pulmonary compliance, prevent atelectasis, and provide mastery of NIV. Anyone who can air stack can use NIV as opposed to requiring tracheotomy.

The chest wall develops abnormally in patients with some congenital neuromuscular diseases, such as type 1 SMA and some inherited myopathies. In patients with type 1 SMA, the relative preservation of diaphragm strength in the face of marked weakness of the intercostal muscles commonly leads to a characteristic sternal recession and a small chest. These chest wall deformities restrict pulmonary development. Over and above this effect on thoracic configuration, lung growth is heavily influenced by chest wall respiratory motion. Although infants cannot air stack, nocturnal use of high-span BiPAP has been shown to prevent pectus excavatum and promote lung and chest wall growth for infants with SMA.[17]

Some experts have advocated for many years the use of NIV therapy to hyperinflate the chest wall to preserve mechanical function. This stretching action of NIV may have an additional effect on chest wall expansion and compliance and on underlying pulmonary expansion and growth.

Any patient capable of air stacking who loses breathing tolerance during chest colds can use NIV continuously or be extubated directly to it. This is extremely important for avoiding a tracheotomy because such patients are extubated without being ventilator weaned.

Goal Two—Maintain Normal Alveolar Ventilation

Inspiratory Muscle Aids
NPPV, delivered via volume-cycled machines, can be noninvasively delivered via Lipseals, Oracles, and nasal and oronasal interfaces for ventilatory support during sleep, with the patients trained and equipped in the outpatient setting. Lipseals and Oracles (Fisher-Paykell, Laguna Hills, CA) can provide essentially closed systems of ventilatory support.[17]

Patients requiring around-the-clock support use simple 15- or 22-mm angled mouthpieces (4-730-00, Puritan-Bennett Inc, Boulder, CO) held between the teeth for NPPV

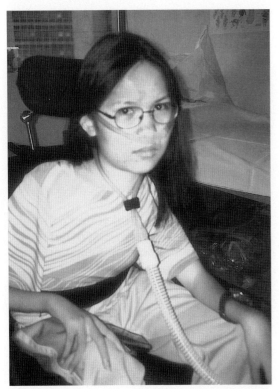

Figure 9-3. This patient with spinal muscular atrophy required nocturnal noninvasive intermittent positive-pressure ventilation (NIPPV) for 18 years. She switched from lip seal to nasal NIPPV in 1984.

drive is not depressed, even patients with little or no measurable vital capacity can be safely ventilated day and night by nasal or oral ventilation.

Besides continuous dependence on NIV, benefits from part-time use include respiratory muscle rest, increased tidal volumes, improved alveolar ventilation and blood gases, improved lung compliance and chemotactic sensitivity, and possibly improved ventilation/perfusion matching by reducing atelectasis and small airway closure. A reasonable peak inspiratory pressure to start with is 8 cm H_2O, with the expectation to increase this in increments as necessary to reduce the work of breathing. Peak inspiratory pressure levels of 10 to 16 cm H_2O suffice for most children. Positive end-expiratory pressure should be set at a level to accomplish two goals: increase functional residual capacity and maintain the patency of the upper airway at end expiration. The positive end-expiratory pressure setting is generally adjusted in the range of 4 to 10 cm H_2O. To accomplish optimal rest, high volumes or pressure spans should be used—inspiratory to expiratory positive airway pressure spans of 10 to 12 for BiPAP users. Patients vary the volume of air taken to adjust tidal volume, speech volume, and cough flows, and to air stack.

Respiratory impairment initially manifests as sleep hypoventilation. When symptomatic and treated, pulmonary hypertension and right ventricular failure can be prevented. There are no significant complications of NPPV and continuous users who learn GPB need not worry about accidental disconnection or ventilator failure.

(Fig. 9-3) during the day. To use mouthpiece NPPV effectively and conveniently, adequate neck rotation and oral motor function are necessary to grab the mouthpiece and receive NPPV without air leakage.

When the lips are too weak to grab a mouthpiece, the patient can use an intermittent abdominal pressure ventilator[18] or continue nocturnal nasal NPPV through daytime hours, alternating nasal interfaces to vary skin pressure. A popular interface for daytime use is the Nasal-Aire (InnoMed Technologies, Boca Raton, FL) because this interface permits the use of glasses and does not obstruct vision.

The use of oronasal interfaces seems to be unnecessary. Using a Lipseal and placing cotton pledgets in the nostrils, and then sealing the nostrils with a Band-Aid can provide a closed system of ventilatory support. It is crucial to avoid the depression of ventilatory drive by the use of sedative medications or oxygen, or daytime hypercapnia that results in oxyhemoglobin desaturation to less than 95%. As long as ventilatory

Goal Three—Facilitate Airway Clearance

Chest percussion and vibration are not substitutes for coughing. Bulbar-innervated inspiratory and expiratory muscles and respiratory aids are needed for coughing. The oximetry feedback respiratory aid protocol consists of using a pulse oximeter for feedback to maintain Sao_2 greater than 94% by maintaining effective alveolar ventilation and airway secretion elimination by using inspiratory or expiratory aids, or both—up to continuous NPPV and assisted coughing. This is most important during respiratory tract infections and when extubating patients with little or no breathing tolerance.

Normal Cough

Adequate expiratory muscle function is crucial for creating the PCF necessary to clear airway secretions and bronchial mucous plugs. A normal cough requires a precough inspiration or insufflation to about 85% of total lung capacity.[22] This is followed by the development of thoracoabdominal pressures sufficient to generate an explosive decompression of the chest at glottic opening and PCF exceeding 5 L/sec.[23] Total expiratory volume during normal coughing is about 2.3 ± 0.5 L.[24] Normal values are unavailable for small children.

Assisted Coughing

Patients with less than 5 L/sec of unassisted PCF benefit from assisted coughing. Techniques of manually assisted coughing involve the use of a manually applied abdominal thrust, which may be combined with an anterior chest wall compression timed to glottic opening.[22] For small children, one hand or only a few fingers can be used. For adolescents or adults with less than 1.5 L of vital capacity, a maximal insufflation or air stacking precedes the manual assist. Manually assisted coughing is less effective in the presence of scoliosis, marked obesity, or abdominal distention, and should not be used for 1 hour after meals. Abdominal thrusts are not used for patients after abdominal trauma or surgery, and anterior chest compression is avoided in elderly patients.

Mechanical Insufflation-Exsufflation

Currently available mechanical insufflator-exsufflators can cycle automatically between positive and negative pressure, or the cycling can be done manually. The insufflation and exsufflation pressures are usually set at $+40$ cm H_2O to -40 cm H_2O. Similar pressures have been used without untoward effects on children 4 months old, although children are often not optimally cooperative with it until age $2\frac{1}{2}$ years. An abdominal thrust applied during exsufflation increases PCF.[3]

One treatment consists of about five cycles of mechanical insufflation-exsufflation followed by a period of normal breathing or ventilator use for 20 to 30 seconds to avoid hyperventilation. Five or more treatments are given in one sitting, and the treatments are repeated until no further secretions are expelled, and mucous plug-triggered hemoglobin desaturations are reversed. Mechanical insufflation-exsufflation sessions can be repeated every 5 to 10 minutes as needed. Although usually applied via oronasal interface, mechanical insufflation-exsufflation also can be applied via endotracheal or tracheostomy tubes to clear secretions without the airway irritation and discomfort caused by tracheal suctioning. Also, in contrast to most attempts at bronchial suctioning,[25] mechanical insufflation-exsufflation eliminates airway secretions from the bronchial tree. Transtracheal use of mechanical insufflation-exsufflation rather than suctioning seems to be associated with a decrease in the production of airway secretions caused by the irritative effects of invasive airway suctioning.

The use of mechanical insufflation-exsufflation permits clinicians to extubate consistently patients with little ventilator-free breathing ability, and convert them to the use of NPPV. It also permits clinicians to avoid intubation, or to extubate quickly patients with neuromuscular diseases with profuse airway secretions in acute respiratory failure during intercurrent respiratory tract infections. No significant pulmonary complications have been reported with the use of mechanical insufflation-exsufflation.[26]

Extubation and Decannulation

Patients who are intubated and who then undergo tracheotomy during an acute hospitalization can be evaluated for possible transition to NPPV.[27] Although 94% of conventionally managed children with SMA type 1 fail extubation, the success rate using a noninvasive extubation protocol is about 90%.[13] In this protocol, children are extubated only when Sao_2 remains greater than 94% in ambient air, and they are extubated directly to high-span BiPAP. Manually and mechanically (Cough-Assist) assisted coughing is used

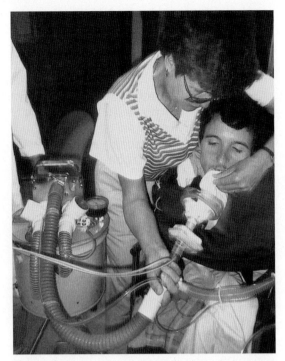

Figure 9-4. This 11-year-old boy with Duchenne muscular dystrophy was extubated after spinal instrumentation for scoliosis reduction despite requiring continuous ventilatory support. He was switched to 24-hour noninvasive intermittent positive-pressure ventilation and required aggressive mechanical insufflation-exsufflation (seen here) to clear his airway secretions.

aggressively after extubation.[13] Although children can be decannulated and switched to using NIV 24 hr/day, because of anxiety and inability to cooperate, we have not done this for any continuously ventilator-dependent patients younger than age 12 (Fig. 9-4).

Glossopharyngeal Breathing

Inspiratory and, indirectly, expiratory muscle activity can be assisted by GPB.[15] This technique involves the glottis projecting air into the lungs. One breath usually consists of six to nine gulps of 60 to 100 mL each. GPB can provide an individual who has little or no measurable vital capacity with normal lung ventilation throughout daytime hours and perfect safety in the event of ventilator failure day or night. The safety and versatility afforded by GPB are key reasons to eliminate tracheotomy in favor of noninvasive aids.

Perioperative Management

Patients with vital capacity less than 40% to 60% of normal or hypercapnia have a risk of failing ventilator weaning in the postoperative period. These patients should be trained in NPPV via simple 15-mm angled mouthpieces and nasal interfaces preoperatively. Patients with assisted PCF less than 300 L/m have a high risk of developing pneumonia and other complications because of difficulties in postoperative airway secretion expulsion. They should be trained in manually and mechanically assisted coughing. These patients can be routinely extubated and decannulated with no autonomous ability to breathe whether in the postoperative period or otherwise. Extubation of untrained patients to NIV who are unable to sustain their breathing autonomously often results in panic and extubation failure.

Outcomes

NPPV is overwhelmingly preferred over tracheotomy for speech, sleep, swallowing, comfort, appearance, security, and use of GPB.[19] NIV also has favorable impact on respiratory infectious complications in children with neuromuscular disorders.[33] Another study showed 200% cost savings by using NIV support methods for patients with no ventilator-free breathing by facilitating community living.[12] Infants with SMA type 1 who undergo tracheotomy lose all ability to breathe unaided and do not develop the ability to speak, whereas infants with the same disease severity who are maintained by noninvasive methods usually require only nocturnal high-span BiPAP and develop the ability to speak.[20]

Many patients have become continuous ventilator users for years without ever being hospitalized.[21] Hundreds of hospitalizations have been avoided by using continuous ventilatory support along with mechanical insufflation-exsufflation and assisted coughing at home.[12,13,17,18,21]

Virtually all patients with neuromuscular disease can be managed without resorting to tracheotomy. The exceptions are patients who are unable to cooperate because of coma or mental retardation and patients whose bulbar-innervated musculature is so severely impaired that speech and swallowing have become impossible, and saliva is continuously aspirated. The latter situation is rare in pediatric neuromuscular disease. Even patients with severe SMA type 1 (who can never breathe autonomously or swallow) can be managed safely without resorting to tracheotomy.[13] Patients can become continuously dependent on NPPV without ever being hospitalized, intubated, tracheotomized, or bronchoscoped.[21] These methods enhance quality of life; permit the use of GPB for security in the event of ventilator failure; and can drastically decrease morbidity, mortality, and cost.[12,28,29]

End-of-Life Care

Care for someone in the late stages of a progressive chronic illness focuses on enhancement of quality of life for the patient and their family. A multidisciplinary approach is required, including primary and specialist physicians, hospice/palliative care specialists, and social services, and spiritual care, family members, and others appropriate to the patient's cultural or religious background.[31]

The goals of end-of-life care for patients with neuromuscular disorders include the following:
1. Treating conditions (pain, dyspnea) that cause distress (palliative care)
2. Attending to the psychosocial and spiritual needs of the patient and family
3. Respecting the patient and family's choice concerning testing and treatment

References

1. West JB: Respiratory Physiology—The Essentials. Baltimore, Williams & Wilkins, 2005.
2. Kang SW, Bach JR: Maximum insufflation capacity: The relationships with vital capacity and cough flows for patients with neuromuscular disease. Am J Phys Med Rehabil 79:222-227, 2000.
3. Praud J-P, Canet E: Chest wall function and dysfunction in children. In Chernick V, et al, eds: Kendig's Disorders of the Respiratory Tract in Children, 7th ed. Philadelphia, WB Saunders, 2006.
4. Bach JR: Mechanical insufflation-exsufflation: Comparison of peak expiratory flows with manually assisted and unassisted coughing techniques. Chest 104:1553-1562, 1993.
5. Kelly BJ, Luce JM: The diagnosis and management of neuromuscular diseases causing respiratory failure. Chest 99:1485-1494, 1991.
6. Bennett DA, Black TP: Recognizing impending respiratory failure from neuromuscular causes. J Crit Illness 3:46-60, 1988.
7. Bach JR, Alba AS: Management of chronic alveolar hypoventilation by nasal ventilation. Chest 97:52-57, 1990.
8. Bach JR, et al: Mouth intermittent positive pressure ventilation in the management of post-polio respiratory insufficiency. Chest 91:859-864, 1987.
9. Thilo EH, Townsend SF, Deacon J: Infant botulism at 1 week of age: Report of two cases. Pediatr 92:151, 1993.
10. Smith DE, et al: Practical problems in the respiratory care of patients with muscular dystrophy. N Engl J Med 316:1197-1204, 1987.
11. Bergoffen JA, et al: Paternal transmission of congenital myotonic dystrophy. J Med Genet 31:518-520, 1994.
12. Bach JR, et al: The ventilator individual: Cost analysis of institutionalization versus rehabilitation and in-home management. Chest 101:26-30, 1992.
13. Bach JR, et al: Spinal muscular atrophy type 1: Management and outcomes. Pediatr Pulmonol 34:16-22, 2002.
14. Bach JR, et al: Neuromuscular ventilatory insufficiency: The effect of home mechanical ventilator use vs. oxygen therapy on pneumonia and hospitalization rates. Am J Phys Med Rehab 77:8-19, 1998.
15. Bach JR, et al: Glossopharyngeal breathing and non-invasive aids in the management of post-polio respiratory insufficiency. Birth Defects 23:99-113, 1987.
16. Kang SW, Bach JR: Maximum insufflation capacity. Chest 118:61-65, 2000.
17. Bach JR: Prevention of pectus excavatum for children with spinal muscular atrophy type 1. Am J Phys Med Rehab 82:815-819, 2003.
18. Bach JR, Alba AS: Intermittent abdominal pressure ventilator in a regimen of noninvasive ventilatory support. Chest 99:630-636, 1991.
19. Bach JR: A comparison of long-term ventilatory support alternatives from the perspective of the patient and care giver. Chest 104:1702-1706, 1993.
20. Bach JR, Chaudhry SS: Management approaches in muscular dystrophy association clinics. Am J Phys Med Rehab 79:193-196, 2000.
21. Gomez-Merino E, Bach JR: Duchenne muscular dystrophy: Prolongation of life by noninvasive respiratory muscle aids. Am J Phys Med Rehab 81:411-415, 2002.
22. Leith DE: Cough. In Brain JD, Proctor D, Reid L, eds: Lung Biology in Health and Disease: Respiratory Defense Mechanisms, Part 2. New York, Marcel Dekker, 1977, pp 545-592.
23. Bach JR, et al: Airway secretion clearance by mechanical exsufflation for post-poliomyelitis ventilator assisted individuals. Arch Phys Med Rehab 74:170-177, 1993.
24. Aldrich JK, et al: Weaning from mechanical ventilation: Adjunctive use of inspiratory muscle resistive training. Crit Care Med 17:143-147, 1989.
25. Fishburn MJ, Marino RJ, Ditunno JF: Atelectasis and pneumonia in acute spinal cord injury. Arch Phys Med Rehab 71:197-200, 1990.
26. Bach JR: Update and perspectives on noninvasive respiratory muscle aids, part 2: The expiratory muscle aids. Chest 14:158-174, 1991.

27. Bach JR: Alternative methods of ventilatory support for the patient with ventilatory failure due to spinal cord injury. J Am Paraplegia Soc 105:1538-1544, 1994.

28. Tzeng AC, Bach JR: Prevention of pulmonary morbidity for patients with neuromuscular disease. Chest 118:1390-1396, 2000.

29. Bach JR: The Management of Patients with Neuromuscular Disease. Philadelphia, Elsevier, 2003.

30. Simonds AK: Recent advances in respiratory care for neuromuscular disease. Chest 130:1879-1886, 2006.

31. Wolfe L: Should parents speak with a dying child about impending death. N Engl J Med 351:1251-1253, 2004.

32. Van Deutekom JC, et al: Local dystrophin restoration with antisense oligonucleotide PRO051. N Engl J Med 357:2677-2686, 2007.

33. Dohna-Schwake C, et al: Non-invasive ventilation reduces respiratory tract infections in children with neuromuscular disorders. Pediatr Pulmonol 43: 67-71, 2008.

CHAPTER 10

Pulmonary Manifestations of Rheumatoid Diseases*

C. Egla Rabinovich, Edward Fels, Joseph Shanahan, J. Marc Majure, and Thomas M. Murphy

Systemic Lupus Erythematosus 202
Drug-Induced Lupus 211
Mixed Connective Tissue Disease 212
Sjögren Syndrome 215
Juvenile Rheumatoid Arthritis 217
Scleroderma 220
Juvenile Dermatomyositis 225
Ankylosing Spondylitis 226
Sarcoidosis 228

**Pneumonitis Resulting from
  Antirheumatic Therapy** 232
  Methotrexate Pneumonitis 232
  Tumor Necrosis Factor-α Blockade and
    Tuberculosis 233
  Other Rheumatology Medications Associated
    with Pulmonary Disease 233
Summary 233
Acknowledgments 234
    References 234

Arthritis is the most commonly recognized manifestation of rheumatic disease, but pulmonary manifestations can occur in nearly all disorders and are found in various age groups in children. Symptoms of pulmonary disease in children may be subtle or absent, and children at elevated risk should be screened for pulmonary involvement.

The combination of well-developed vascularity, exposure to external stimuli and toxins in ambient air, and a covering (the pleura) that shares structures and functions analogous to joint synovia contributes to the susceptibility of the lungs to rheumatic and vasculitic inflammatory expression. Although the mechanisms of the pulmonary inflammation of rheumatologic disorders differ by etiology, common patterns of sequence and expression are seen. The initial inflammatory lesions usually lack an identifiable etiology and behave as though the child's pulmonary tissue is foreign (hence the term "autoimmunity"). Genetic susceptibility or genetic modifiers are now well established for many disorders. Although acute expression with resolution sometimes occurs, chronic and relapsing scenarios are more common. The general sequence is as follows:

Acute inflammation $\Rightarrow$ Amplification $\Rightarrow$ Failure of repair, resolution $\Rightarrow$ Relapse

Genetic predisposition	Cellular	Chronic vasculitis
	Humoral	Remodeling
	Lytic enzymes	Chronic interstitial pneumonitis
	Oxidant stress	Fibrosis
	Immune complexes	

In some disorders, such as systemic lupus erythematosus (SLE), bleeding and infection are integral participants in the expression of the chronic inflammation. The cycle of immune-mediated inflammation, vascular leakage, and attempts at repair recurs with progressive organ damage, leading to loss of organ function. Available pharmacologic therapies directed at alleviating the inflammation in

---

*This chapter is dedicated to the life and contributions of Deborah Kredich, MD, a founder and developer of the field of pediatric rheumatology and holder of certificate number one from the American Sub-Board of Rheumatology of the American Board of Pediatrics.

these disorders inhibit, but do not yet arrest the inflammatory process enough to prevent further organ damage.

The list of childhood rheumatologic disorders is long. This chapter reviews the most common conditions and their associated pulmonary manifestations.

Systemic Lupus Erythematosus

SLE is an autoimmune disease characterized by multisystem inflammation and tissue damage. It commonly develops in young women, but patients of either gender or any age may be affected. In pediatric populations, SLE prevalence is similar in prepubescent boys and girls, but female predominance increases steadily after puberty.[1] The prevalence of SLE increases with age, and SLE can develop in individuals of any race or ethnicity. Neonatal lupus occurs rarely and is caused by the passage of autoantibodies (anti-Ro, SSA and anti-La, SSB) across the placenta that cause congenital heart block or a self-limited lupus rash that manifests shortly after delivery and persists until maternal antibodies disappear, usually in the first year of life.

Pulmonary manifestations are common. Excluding common pulmonary infections, the pleura is the most frequently involved tissue of the pulmonary system.[2-4] Other parenchymal complications—acute lupus pneumonitis (ALP), alveolar hemorrhage (AH), pulmonary embolism, and pulmonary arterial hypertension (PAH)—occur less frequently, but are potentially lethal. Although the clinical literature of SLE is focused on adult studies, the reported pediatric literature suggests similar arrays of pulmonary manifestations and clinical syndrome courses.[1,5,6] The prevalence of pulmonary involvement is difficult to estimate because of selection bias related to methodologies that are retrospective or case-series in nature.[5-8] Pediatric data are insufficient to draw inferences regarding the variation in disease expression based on age or physical development. A large histopathologic study of lung involvement with SLE in children suggests that these lesions do not differ from the lesions in

adults.[9] These and other studies confirm that the more uncommon cases of chronic lung disease develop in children as well, including symptomatic chronic interstitial lung disease (ILD) and shrinking lung syndrome. Drug-induced lupus (DIL) is often characterized by lung involvement. Infection remains a leading cause of death in patients with SLE, however. In view of the risk of pulmonary infection associated with immunosuppressive treatments for SLE, the clinical approach to patients with pulmonary complaints should always include a thorough search for infection. Initial treatment regimens for acutely ill patients should incorporate empiric antibiotic therapy until the precise cause of the pulmonary disease is ascertained.

Noninfectious pulmonary complications of SLE are summarized in Table 10-1. Pleuritis is the most common pulmonary manifestation of SLE. Symptoms include pleuritic chest pain and dyspnea in association with other features of lupus disease activity, such as fever, fatigue, rash, and arthritis. Chest radiographs may show small to moderate pleural effusions. Large effusions are unusual (Figs. 10-1 and 10-2). When pleural effusion is noted in SLE, diagnostic thoracentesis for pleural fluid aspiration and analysis is indicated. These effusions are typically serous or serosanguineous exudates. Hemorrhagic effusions associated with hypoxemia can occur with pulmonary infarcts and infection. These entities should always be considered in the differential diagnosis of pleuritis, particularly in the absence of coexisting features of systemic lupus activity. Pleural pathology in SLE consists of local inflammation with immunoglobulin and complement deposition.[10] In some cases, pleural fibrosis is observed, although the fibrosis is infrequently considered clinically important.

Mild pleuritis is usually treated effectively with nonsteroidal anti-inflammatory drugs (NSAIDs). In more severe cases, such as large symptomatic effusions, corticosteroids are indicated. If the pleural effusions are not associated with significant multisystem activity, efforts should be made to limit corticosteroid exposure, especially in children, by using short pulses of therapy instead of prolonged tapers. Recurrent episodes of pleurisy may respond to treatment with

Table 10-1	Noninfectious Pulmonary Complications of Systemic Lupus Erythematosus						
PULMONARY MANIFESTATION	**ESTIMATED PREVALENCE**	**ONSET**	**PRESENTING SIGNS AND SYMPTOMS**	**RADIOGRAPHIC CHANGES**	**PROGNOSIS**	**TREATMENT**	**DIFFERENTIAL DIAGNOSIS**
Pleuritis	50-80%	Acute	Pleurisy, dyspnea, orthopnea, pleural rub	Pleural effusion	Good	NSAIDs, corticosteroids	Infection, PE, ALP, AH, PTX, drug toxicity
ALP	≤10%	Acute	Dyspnea, cough, fever, chest pain, pleurisy, hemoptysis; often preceded by or associated with infection, hypoxemia	Patchy acinar infiltrates with bibasilar predominance	Poor; mortality 50%	Corticosteroids, plasmapheresis, CYC, AZA	Infection, PE, AH, pleuritis
AH	≤2%	Acute	Dyspnea, cough, chest pain, decrease in hemoglobin, pleurisy, hypoxemia	Patchy acinar infiltrates with bibasilar predominance	Mortality 50%	Corticosteroids, plasmapheresis, CYC, AZA	Infection, ALP, PE, vasculitis, Goodpasture syndrome, IPH
Acute reversible hypoxemia	<1%	Acute/chronic	Dyspnea, low FVC, low DLCO	Normal	Good	Corticosteroids	Infection, PE, early ALP or AH, shrinking lung syndrome
Chronic interstitial pneumonitis	3%	Chronic, may be long-term complication of ALP	Dyspnea, cough, low FVC, low DLCO, fibrosis	CXR—reticular interstitial infiltrates: ground glass, honeycombing	Poor to good	Corticosteroids, CYC, AZA	Infection, LIP, drug toxicity, chronic aspiration

(Continued)

Table 10-1	Noninfectious Pulmonary Complications of Systemic Lupus Erythematosus—Cont'd						
PULMONARY MANIFESTATION	ESTIMATED PREVALENCE	ONSET	PRESENTING SIGNS AND SYMPTOMS	RADIOGRAPHIC CHANGES	PROGNOSIS	TREATMENT	DIFFERENTIAL DIAGNOSIS
Shrinking lung disease	<1%	Chronic	Dyspnea, orthopnea, low FVC, low DLCO	Normal or basilar atelectasis, elevated diaphragm	Good	Corticosteroids	Respiratory muscle weakness from myopathies
Thromboembolic disease	—	Acute	Dyspnea, pleurisy, hemoptysis, fever, pleural rub	CXR—normal or effusion	Variable	Anticoagulation	Infection, pleurisy, PTX, AH or ALP
Pulmonary hypertension	5-14%	Chronic	Dyspnea, chest discomfort, right heart failure, pericardial effusion, elevated BNP, low DLCO with stable FVC	CXR—normal or perfusion	Variable	Pulmonary vasodilators (ETRA, prostanoids, phosphodiesterase type 5 inhibitors, anticoagulants; CYC and corticosteroids in select cases	Infection, interstitial lung disease

AH, alveolar hemorrhage; ALP, acute lupus pneumonitis; AZA, azathioprine; BNP, brain natriuretic peptide; CXR, chest radiograph; CYC, cyclophosphamide; DLCO, diffusing capacity for carbon monoxide; ETRA, endothelin receptor antagonist; FVC, forced vital capacity; IPH, idiopathic pulmonary hemosiderosis; LIP, lymphocytic interstitial pneumonia; NSAIDs, nonsteroidal anti-inflammatory drugs; PE, pulmonary embolus; PTX, pneumothorax.

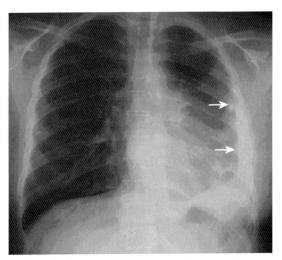

Figure 10-1. A 15-year-old girl with systemic lupus erythematosus. Posteroanterior chest radiograph shows left-sided pleural effusion (*arrows*). The remainder of the examination was normal.

hydroxychloroquine or methotrexate. More aggressive immunosuppressants are needed infrequently.

ALP is a rare complication of SLE, commonly manifesting with an acute, profound loss of respiratory function. ALP occurs in 1% to 4% of patients and accounts for nearly 4% of SLE hospital admissions.[2-3] Although ALP may be a forme fruste of SLE, it most frequently occurs in patients with established disease.[11] The clinical presentation includes acute onset of dyspnea, cough, fever, and hypoxemia. Coexisting infection is a common observation, suggesting that bacterial or viral infections may trigger ALP. Many patients report pleuritic chest pain. Hemoptysis occurs occasionally, but less frequently than the AH syndrome of pulmonary lupus. Chest radiographs show a diffuse or patchy acinar infiltrate with lower lobe predominance. With a rapidly progressive respiratory

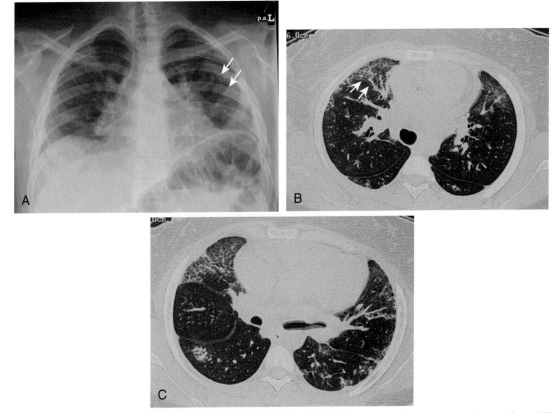

Figure 10-2. A 17-year-old girl with systemic lupus erythematosus. **A,** Posteroanterior chest x-ray shows bilateral ill-defined nodular opacities, two of which (*arrows*) are evident in the left lung. **B** and **C,** Axial high-resolution chest CT scans at the level of the carina (**B**) and slightly more inferiorly (**C**) show peripheral patchy fibrotic changes with scattered nodular opacities; note subtle bronchiectasis (*arrows* in **B**).

decline, many patients require mechanical ventilation. Bronchoscopy is suggested to exclude underlying infection, but because of the frequent coexistence of pulmonary infection with ALP, the discovery of a pathogen does not obviate the need for aggressive immunosuppressive therapy. Culture and antimicrobial sensitivity testing of bronchoscopic or open lung biopsy specimens is helpful in directing antibiotic therapy.

The histopathologic features of ALP appear similar to diffuse alveolar damage. Inflammatory cellular infiltrates involve the interstitium and alveolar wall.[11-13] Nonspecific features, including edema, hemorrhage, and hyaline membranes, are commonly observed. Complement and immunoglobulin deposition may be shown by direct immunofluorescent staining, but vasculitic lesions are uncommon.

Treatment of ALP is based primarily on retrospective analyses of clinical cohorts, case series, and anecdotal reports.[2,13,14] Typical treatment incorporates high dose, intravenous corticosteroids (1 to 2 mg/kg/day of prednisone or equivalent, usually to a maximum of 60 mg/day) and supportive respiratory care. Because mortality rates approach 50%,[11] rapidly progressive respiratory decline indicates a need for more aggressive interventions, such as pulse intravenous methylprednisolone (30 mg/kg/day up to 1000 mg/day for 3 days) and plasmapheresis. Additional immunosuppressive agents, including azathioprine and cyclophosphamide, should be considered in patients who have persistent or recurrent disease. Some centers advocate early initiation of azathioprine or cyclophosphamide in patients who are seriously ill.

ALP is usually expressed as a severe, but self-limited, monophasic inflammation. Chronic interstitial disease[11] may rarely develop in survivors of the acute illness, however. The incidence of chronic progression of ALP seems to be low enough that prolonged corticosteroid or immunosuppressive use is not usually necessary in patients who recover quickly from the initial onset of ALP. These patients should be monitored closely for pulmonary decline by determining serial pulmonary function every 3 to 6 months.

AH in SLE occurs rarely,[6] but it may account for 3.7% of all SLE-related hospitalizations.[15] Although AH can be the initial manifestation of SLE, most patients have an established diagnosis. AH most often occurs in patients who have high anti-dsDNA titers. Coexisting renal disease is seen in 60% to 90% of patients with AH. Most patients are young women who present with dyspnea, sometimes fever and pleurisy, and acute hypoxemia. Frank hemoptysis occurs in more than 50% of patients. Most patients with AH exhibit hemoptysis at some point during their illness, helping to differentiate AH from ALP. Pulmonary bleeding is usually substantial with an average hemoglobin decrease of approximately 7%.[15] Chest radiographs show diffuse, bilateral acinar infiltrates that may progress rapidly over hours and in some cases just as rapidly resolve. The respiratory compromise in more than half of patients is rapid and profound, resulting in a need for supplemental oxygen and assisted ventilation. With assisted ventilation, the addition of positive end-expiratory pressure should theoretically be beneficial, impeding alveolar bleeding and maintaining alveolar expansion. Occasional cases of mild AH may be managed more conservatively. Because of the propensity for acute decompensation, all suspected cases of AH should be managed with caution, preferably with hospitalization. Mortality rates with AH are 40% to 90% in published series, with many fatalities occurring early.[2,3,15,16]

Pulmonary infection may coexist in some cases.[15] The relevance of infection as a causal agent is uncertain. The frequency of coexisting infection makes bronchoscopy a useful approach to the evaluation of these patients, however. As in ALP, the presence of a pulmonary pathogen in bronchoalveolar lavage (BAL) or biopsy specimens does not obviate the need for immunosuppression, but it helps guide the choice of antibiotics. Most patients have evidence of frank hemorrhage on BAL. In patients without bloody lavage fluid, the presence of hemosiderin-laden macrophages is evidence of recent hemorrhage.[16,17] Bronchoscopic and open lung biopsy specimens show nonspecific interstitial and alveolar wall infiltrates of lymphocytes and neutrophils, edema, and hyaline membranes.[15] Hemosiderin-laden macrophages or inflammation of small pulmonary arterioles or capillaries (known as capillaritis) helps distinguish AH from ALP. Direct immunofluorescent staining may show granular interstitial or endothelial staining for complement and immunoglobulins.[18] This differentiates AH from Goodpasture syndrome, in which the histopathology is characterized by a pattern of linear immunofluorescence.

The prognosis of AH is similar to ALP and relates proportionately to the severity at presentation.[2,3,15-17,19] Treatment recommendations are based on case series and anecdotal reports, although the early use of plasmapheresis in severe cases is based on the success of this therapy in Goodpasture syndrome, which is similarly characterized by recurrent AH. The core initial therapy is aggressive intravenous corticosteroid dosing (1 to 2 mg/kg/day of prednisone or equivalent) or may begin with intravenous pulse methylprednisolone (1000 mg/day × 3 days). Early initiation of cyclophosphamide is advocated by some centers. Even the addition of this potent immunosuppressant is not uniformly effective at reversing respiratory failure, however. Some patients hemorrhage recurrently at variable intervals. Plasmapheresis may be indicated in patients who have recurrent hemorrhages even after starting corticosteroids because this may provide a more rapid onset of immunosuppression than cyclophosphamide. Nonetheless, efficacy data for plasmapheresis therapy are lacking. Even the published data for cyclophosphamide are conflicting. Some analyses have suggested that cyclophosphamide use is a risk factor for AH-associated mortality; however, these results probably reflect referral bias because cyclophosphamide is more likely to be used in patients who are more seriously ill.

The frequency and range of expression of chronic ILD in patients with SLE is not well documented. Chronic ILD probably affects less than 2% of lupus patients, and many of these patients probably have clinically mild illness.[20-22] Some authors have reported chronic ILD developing as a consequence of ALP.[11,14] In some cases, interstitial scarring and restrictive changes on pulmonary function tests (PFTs) probably reflect injury from the acute pulmonary inflammation. Progressive dyspnea and pulmonary function decline in a subset of patients, however, probably reflecting more classically chronic progressive ILD. Reports from other authors have described a few

patients with chronic ILD presenting typically with cough, dyspnea, radiographic interstitial infiltrates or honeycomb changes, and restrictive lung disease pattern on PFTs. Histologic data are sparse, but include nonspecific interstitial inflammation with changes of fibrosis.[10-12,21] Some patients with chronic ILD apparently respond to corticosteroids, rarely with marked improvement.

In our center, we have observed patients with two different histologic patterns of ILD. A young African-American woman with a history of antiphospholipid antibody syndrome presented with persistent dyspnea and cough over 12 months. Repeated high-resolution computed tomography (CT) scans performed during this period showed transient patchy interstitial infiltrates. Initially, the concern was for recurrent pulmonary emboli, even though she was being aggressively anticoagulated. Lung tissue obtained by video-assisted thoracoscopy open lung biopsy showed changes consistent with nonspecific interstitial pneumonitis, however, without any evidence of thrombosis or of fibroblastic foci or honeycomb changes. This patient was treated with oral corticosteroids for several months. Her respiratory symptoms and scan findings completely resolved.

In a second case, an older white woman with inflammatory arthritis and subacute cutaneous lupus presented with progressive dyspnea, chronic cough, and restrictive lung disease pattern on PFTs. High-resolution CT scan revealed patchy ground-glass findings and honeycomb changes with a peripheral and basilar predominance. A lung biopsy performed by video-assisted thoracoscopy revealed changes consistent with nonspecific interstitial pneumonia with fibroblastic foci. In addition, areas of heterogeneous honeycomb scar were noted on lower lobe specimens. The patient was treated with corticosteroids and 12 months of intravenous pulse cyclophosphamide because the lung pathology was most characteristic of ILD seen in scleroderma (systemic sclerosis). Substantial improvements in respiratory function (including elimination of her initial dependence on supplemental oxygen) in addition to reductions in ground-glass opacities on scanning were observed. After a course of cyclophosphamide, the patient was transitioned to oral azathioprine for maintenance therapy and has not experienced relapse of ILD after 1 year.

Although chronic forms of ILD are rare in SLE, they occur occasionally and may be misdiagnosed as manifestations of SLE. Careful evaluation, including serial PFTs and using prone imaging, can increase diagnostic sensitivity. Most patients should undergo open lung biopsy to confirm the diagnosis; determine the degree of fibrosing interstitial disease; and exclude other pathology, such as thrombosis, malignancy, and chronic infection. Treatment may be limited to a course of corticosteroids in patients with pathology limited to nonspecific interstitial pneumonitis,[22] but prolonged courses of cyclophosphamide,[23] methotrexate,[24] or azathioprine should be considered in patients with changes of fibrosis on biopsy.

Patients with SLE are at risk for the development of venous thrombosis and thromboembolism. Approximately 30% to 40% of patients with SLE have circulating antiphospholipid antibodies. These antibodies are associated with an increased risk for venous and arterial thrombosis and pregnancy wastage, particularly late first-trimester and second-trimester pregnancy loss.[25] In patients with antiphospholipid syndrome (defined as the presence of anticardiolipin antibodies or lupus anticoagulant and thrombosis or defined pregnancy loss), recurrent thrombosis is common.[26,27] Treatment following a thrombosis requires lifelong anticoagulation, and subsequent pregnancies after a loss should be managed with heparin through 3 to 6 months postpartum.

Venous thrombosis and thromboembolism are the most common thrombotic complications of antiphospholipid antibody syndrome. Lupus patients presenting with acute dyspnea, with or without pleurisy or hemoptysis, should undergo immediate evaluation for pulmonary embolus, including ventilation/perfusion or spiral CT and lower extremity Doppler ultrasound to detect deep vein thrombosis. The absolute risk for clot in patients with antiphospholipid antibodies and no prior history of thrombosis is unknown. Procoagulant risk factors, including cigarette smoking, estrogen-based contraceptive use, and nephrotic-range proteinuria from renal disease, likely increase the risk.[28] In rare cases, chronic thromboembolism can lead to the development of PAH. In patients presenting with PAH complicating SLE, careful ventilation/perfusion scanning is necessary to exclude chronic pulmonary thromboembolic disease.

PAH is not as rare in SLE as previously thought, and is characterized by progressive dyspnea and hypoxemia that progresses rapidly to right heart failure. PAH may be an idiopathic condition typically occurring in healthy young women or may develop secondary to other conditions, including autoimmune disease (most commonly seen in scleroderma), chronic venous thromboembolism, congenital heart defect resulting in arterial-to-venous shunts, human immunodeficiency virus (HIV), sickle cell disease, prior history of anorexigenic weight loss drugs, and portopulmonary disease of liver failure. Originally considered a rare SLE complication, PAH is now recognized to develop in 1% to 14% of patients.[3,29,30] As with scleroderma patients, lupus-associated PAH has a poor prognosis, with mortality rates of 50% within 2 years of diagnosis.[2]

PAH often is unrecognized in early stages. Patients typically present with dyspnea on exertion. By the time more alarming signs and symptoms develop, most patients have progressed to substantial, and in some cases irreversible, right heart failure. Risk factors for the development of PAH in SLE patients are not well defined, although a greater percentage of these patients with PAH report Raynaud phenomenon and have measurable antiphospholipid antibodies. Significant right heart failure is suggested by a constellation of any of the following signs: syncope, ascites, lower extremity edema, right ventricular heave, or a right-sided S_3 auscultatory sound. Careful evaluation of diagnostic testing increases the sensitivity for detecting early PAH. Echocardiogram is the primary screening tool and should be performed in all SLE patients presenting with dyspnea. Estimated peak right ventricular pressures are often elevated. Signs of right heart strain, such as right atrial or ventricular enlargement and dyskinetic septal motion, strongly suggest PAH, but are more common in advanced disease. PFTs may show a disproportionate decrease in diffusing capacity for carbon monoxide (DLCO) compared with decreases in lung volumes.[31] In scleroderma patients, serum brain natriuretic peptide seems to be a sensitive and specific marker of PAH in patients with normal left ventricular function.[32] Histopathologic remodeling in PAH in SLE patients is nonspecific. Vascular lesions include intimal thickening, medial smooth muscle hypertrophy, and plexiform pathology, lesions also seen in scleroderma and idiopathic PAH.[3]

The diagnosis of PAH is suggested by dyspnea (in the absence of an alternative cardiopulmonary explanation) in conjunction with an elevated peak right ventricular systolic pressure on echocardiogram, accompanied by possible elevations of the forced vital capacity (FVC)-DLCO ratio and serum brain natriuretic peptide levels. The confirmatory diagnostic test that is considered a gold standard is a right heart catheterization. The catheterization findings outlined in Table 10-2 confirm the diagnosis of PAH. Because of the co-occurrence of shunts resulting from congenital heart disease in children, an experienced pediatric cardiologist or critical care specialist should perform the right heart catheterization. Echocardiograms are insensitive instruments to detect shunts; a careful right heart catheterization is crucial in all patients with suspected PAH.

When SLE patients are diagnosed with PAH, chronic venous thromboembolic disease should be carefully considered. Standard treatment of all SLE patients with PAH includes anticoagulation, but the level of anticoagulation may need to be increased for patients with antiphospholipid antibodies who have developed clots. Treatment for SLE-associated PAH differs from treatment of PAH in patients with scleroderma. In the scleroderma group, no benefit has been observed from the use of immunosuppressive therapy.[33] Evidence from case reports and retrospective studies in SLE suggest, however, that a subset of patients improve or experience reversal of PAH with aggressive immunosuppressive therapy incorporating corticosteroids and cyclophosphamide.[33,34]

In our adult rheumatology clinic, all patients with SLE who develop PAH, excluding PAH resulting from congenital heart disease or chronic venous thromboembolic disease, are treated with six monthly doses of intravenous pulse cyclophosphamide (1 g/m^2/dose) and tapering doses of corticosteroids. Concomitant treatment with standard PAH drugs is initiated in all patients with significant clinical symptoms (World Health Organization class III and IV) or with 6-minute walk distance test less than 320 meters. In patients with mild disease (World Health Organization class I and II) who have good 6-minute walk distance test, PAH drugs may be held while the patient is treated with immunosuppression, provided that the patient is followed carefully with monthly visit, quarterly echocardiograms, and 6-minute walk tests.

Shrinking lung syndrome is a rare complication of SLE, although it is possible that mild cases may go undiagnosed.[35,36] Patients characteristically present with progressive dyspnea and a restrictive lung pattern on PFTs.[36] Orthopnea is a unique clinical feature of shrinking lung syndrome. DLCO may or may not be decreased. Chest radiographs reveal elevated diaphragms and bibasilar atelectasis. This finding may be present, however, even when there is no evidence of parenchymal or pleural disease. The differential diagnosis includes

Table 10-2 Diagnostic Features of Pulmonary Artery Hypertension on Right Heart Catheterization

RIGHT HEART CATHETERIZATION MEASUREMENT	RESULT CONFIRMING PULMONARY ARTERY HYPERTENSION*
Elevated mean pulmonary arterial pressure	>25 mm Hg at rest (>30 mm Hg with exercise)
Normal pulmonary capillary wedge pressure	<15 mm Hg
Elevated pulmonary vascular resistance	>3 Wood units

*All features are necessary to confirm diagnosis of pulmonary artery hypertension.

ILD; this does not show inflammatory or fibrotic changes, however. ILD is not a feature of shrinking lung syndrome. The cause of shrinking lung syndrome is likely to be multifactorial. In a few cases, progressive pleural fibrosis results in restrictive lung disease. More recent studies suggest that at least some patients have reduced lung volumes secondary to diaphragmatic and intercostal muscle weakness.[37,38]

Although this condition was previously considered relentlessly progressive, most cases of shrinking lung syndrome seem to have a good prognosis, stabilizing or sometimes spontaneously improving over time. For symptomatic patients, a trial of corticosteroids is indicated, although the response rates from limited published data are uncertain.[36,39] Occasionally, progressive dyspnea and loss of lung volumes requires cytotoxic treatments, such as azathioprine or cyclophosphamide.[40] Little is known about shrinking lung syndrome in pediatric SLE, with only a few cases reported.[40] In our clinic, we care for a boy with shrinking lung syndrome and concomitant valvulitis requiring a valvular replacement.

The airways are infrequently affected in SLE (Table 10-3). Rare cases of bronchiolitis obliterans with organizing pneumonia (BOOP) have been reported.[2,3,41,42] BOOP lesions are characterized histologically by inflammatory changes within the distal airways and alveoli associated with nonspecific bronchiolar inflammation. Patients present with dyspnea caused by a restrictive ventilatory deficit. Fever, interstitial infiltrates, and cough may be part of the initial presentation. In most cases, open lung biopsy is needed to confirm the diagnosis. Treatment typically is initiated with corticosteroids, which are usually effective.[2,41] The etiology of BOOP in SLE is uncertain, but may be induced by infection.

Primary upper airway disease in SLE is extremely rare. A few authors have suggested an increased risk for postintubation subglottic stenosis. Extra care may be required for SLE patients after extubation. Obstructive lung disease is uncommon in SLE. Some patients develop esophageal dysmotility, however, similar to that seen in scleroderma. As a result, the lower esophagus can become patulous, resulting in an increased risk for aspiration, particularly at night when the patient sleeps prone. Common symptoms of aspiration include nocturnal cough and wheezing. PFTs may show a decreased forced expiratory volume in 1 second (FEV_1)/FVC ratio. A decreased DLCO in the setting of preserved lung volumes also may suggest chronic aspiration. Esophageal dysmotility is often evident on barium swallow, although incidental detection of a patulous esophagus may occur with chest CT scans ordered to exclude ILD. High-resolution CT may show patchy ground-glass opacities in the right lower lobe. Treatment includes aggressive acid-reducing therapy, preferably with proton-pump inhibitors. In addition, antiaspiration interventions (Table 10-4) and prebedtime doses of metoclopramide to enhance lower esophageal and gastric emptying may benefit some patients.

Patients with SLE have immunocompromise, placing them at risk for respiratory tract infection, often with opportunistic organisms. Compromised immune responsiveness in

Table 10-3	Rare Airway Diseases in Systemic Lupus Erythematosus	
	PATHOLOGY	ESTIMATED PREVALENCE
Upper airway	Laryngeal inflammation	Rare
	Epiglottitis	Rare
	Subglottic stenosis	Rare, may be risk in postextubation period
Lower airway	Reactive airway disease	Rare, may be associated with reflux and aspiration in patients with esophageal dysmotility
	Bronchiolits obliterans with organizing pneumonia	Probably rare

Table 10-4	Managing Aspiration Associated with Esophageal Dysmotility

PATHOLOGY	INTERVENTION
Acid reflux and aspiration	Proton-pump inhibitor; may require dose titration to eradicate symptoms of heartburn
Aspiration	Raise the head of the bed 2-4 inches
	Avoid bed wedges, multiple pillows
	Nothing to eat or drink within 3-4 hr of going to bed
	Avoid caffeinated beverages after dinner
Esophageal dysmotility	Prokinetic therapy, preferably metoclopramide, taken before bedtime; additional dose of metoclopramide before dinner may be necessary

SLE is a result of abnormalities of complement or cell-mediated immunity, reduced pulmonary macrophage and phagocytic function, treatment with medications (corticosteroids and immunosuppressive agents), and compromised airway clearance resulting from airway inflammation and weak cough (respiratory muscle weakness). The most common organisms responsible for respiratory tract infection in SLE patients include *Klebsiella aerobacter*, *Escherichia coli*, and β-hemolytic streptococcus. *Candida albicans*, *Aspergillus* species, and *Pneumocystis jiroveci* (formerly *Pneumocystis*

carinii) also have been cultured from the lungs of these patients. Patients with immune dysfunction and patients receiving immunosuppressive therapy should receive routine trimethoprim-sulfamethoxazole prophylaxis.

Drug-Induced Lupus

The development of DIL syndromes has been most strongly associated with procainamide, hydralazine, and phenytoin. Through various mechanisms, these agents induce autoreactive immune responses in some patients, resulting in clinical lupus-like disease. Other agents have been associated with lupus-like conditions (Table 10-5) that are more heterogeneous than classic DIL. Pleuropulmonary manifestations, particularly pleurisy and pleural effusions, are the most common clinical features of DIL; other features include arthralgia, fever, and, less commonly, rash.[43] Most affected patients also develop autoantibodies, including antinuclear antibodies (ANAs) and antihistone antibodies. After discontinuation of the offending drug, the clinical manifestations are self-limited in most cases. Treatment is typically conservative, using NSAIDs and occasionally corticosteroids to manage symptoms.

Chronic SLE and internal organ involvement, particularly central nervous system

Table 10-5	Agents Associated with Drug-Induced Lupus Syndromes	
STRENGTH OF ASSOCIATION WITH DRUG-INDUCED LUPUS	AGENT	PLEUROPULMONARY MANIFESTATIONS (%)
Strong	Procainamide	75
	Hydralazine	25
	Phenytoin	Probably uncommon
Moderate	Isoniazid	Uncommon
	Methyldopa	Uncommon
	Penicillamine	Uncommon
	Quinidine	Uncommon
	Minocycline	Uncommon
	Tumor necrosis factor-α inhibitors	Uncommon
Weak	Statins	Uncommon
	Interferons	Uncommon
	Terbinafine	Uncommon
	Zafirlukast	Uncommon

or renal disease, are very unusual complications of DIL. Antihistone antibody titers often decrease as DIL wanes, but ANA titers may remain elevated indefinitely and are not worthy of serial assessment. In rare cases, usually with procainamide, pulmonary parenchymal disease may develop and even be associated with pulmonary fibrosis. Aggressive immunomodulatory therapy is not typically indicated, however, even in these settings. Because DIL may take weeks to months (rarely up to a year) to resolve, patients with pulmonary manifestations, particularly dyspnea or abnormal PFTs, should be monitored on a regular basis. Pulmonary manifestations with drugs less traditionally associated with DIL, such as minocycline, are less common and should be viewed as potential manifestations of another pulmonary process or evidence of chronic SLE that has been unmasked by the drug.

Mixed Connective Tissue Disease

Mixed connective tissue disease (MCTD) is categorized as an overlap syndrome because patients manifest features that are characteristic of multiple defined autoimmune disorders (Table 10-6). They often develop a mixture of features of SLE, rheumatoid arthritis, and dermatomyositis. The defining serologic feature of MCTD is the presence of antiribonucleoprotein autoantibodies. Table 10-7 lists the most common clinical findings.[44-50] In MCTD, serious complications of lupus, such as nephritis or central nervous system pathology, are unusual. Consequently, MCTD is generally regarded as having a better prognosis, provided that inflammatory muscle disease and deforming synovitis can be controlled with immunomodulatory therapy.[13] Prospective cohort studies now suggest, however, that the insidious development of ILD or PAH results in a substantial increase in morbidity and mortality for a subset (approximately 20% to 30%) of patients with MCTD.[51]

There are many reported pleuropulmonary manifestations of MCTD. ILD, pleuritis,

Table 10-6	Kasukawa Criteria for Diagnosis of Mixed Connective Tissue Disease*

1. Raynaud phenomenon or swollen fingers or hands, or both
2. Antiribonucleoprotein antibody positive
3. At least one feature from two of the following three categories
    SLE features
        Polyarthritis
        Facial rash
        Serositis
        Lymphadenopathy
        Leukopenia
        Thrombocytopenia
    Scleroderma features
        Sclerodactyly
        Esophageal dysmotility
        Pulmonary fibrosis
        Vital capacity <80% of normal
        Diffusing capacity <70% of normal
    Dermatomyositis features
        Muscle weakness
        Elevated serum muscle enzymes
        EMG abnormalities of myositis

*Must meet all three criteria to be diagnosed with mixed connective tissue disease.
EMG, electromyogram; SLE, systemic lupus erythematosus.
From Kasukawa R, Tojo T, Miyawaki S: Preliminary diagnostic criteria for classification of mixed connective tissue disease. In Kasukawa R, Sharpe G, eds: Mixed Connective Tissue Disease and Antinuclear Antibodies. Amsterdam, Elsevier, 1987, pp 41-47.

and PAH are the most common and clinically important forms (Table 10-8).[51,53-59] Pleuritis occurs occasionally, a distinct difference from SLE, but rarely MCTD can be associated with large, symptomatic pleural effusions.[60] Patients typically are managed with NSAIDs for mild to moderate pleuritis or corticosteroids for large symptomatic effusions. Rarely, venous thromboembolic disease associated with antiphospholipid antibodies may occur. Progressive esophageal dysmotility is far more common in MCTD than in SLE, and increases the risk for aspiration pneumonia or chronic aspiration–associated bronchoconstriction or mild pulmonary fibrosis. The management of antiphospholipid antibody syndrome and esophageal dysmotility in MCTD is identical to that in SLE patients.

Table 10-7	Clinical Manifestations of Mixed Connective Tissue Disease	
CLINICAL FEATURE	**FREQUENCY IN ADULTS (%)**	**FREQUENCY IN CHILDREN (%)**
Inflammatory arthritis	95	82-93
Myositis	63	47-61
Pulmonary disease	20-80	35-60
Raynaud phenomenon	85	85-94
Skin rash	38	33-38
Esophageal dysmotility	67	21-41
Hepatosplenomegaly	15-19	29
Serositis	43	23-28
Antiribonucleoprotein antibody	100	100
Rheumatoid factor	70	57-68

Inflammatory and fibrosing ILD affects 66% of patients with MCTD.[61] Most patients with abnormally low lung volume or DLCO on PFTs are asymptomatic, although an unknown subset of these patients develop progressive interstitial inflammation and pulmonary fibrosis. The lower rate of progressive pulmonary fibrosis differentiates lung disease in MCTD from ILD in scleroderma, which progresses to marked fibrosis and severe pulmonary functional decline in a greater portion of patients.[62] Patients with MCTD who develop ILD typically present with progressive dyspnea on exertion. Dry cough also is reported. PFTs most commonly show a restrictive pattern with reduced lung volumes and decreases in DLCO. PFTs are considered to be more sensitive technology for detecting ILD. Characteristic high-resolution CT scan findings include septal thickening and ground-glass opacities with peripheral and basilar lung zone predominance. Traction bronchiectasis and honeycomb changes form later in the disease process, typically with a basilar, subpleural distribution. As in scleroderma-associated ILD, rare cases of ILD associated with MCTD may manifest with dyspnea and abnormal PFTs, but normal-appearing chest x-ray. BAL may be a useful diagnostic tool in this setting. Most patients with ILD show a neutrophilic or eosinophilic predominance in the cell count differential.

Treatment of ILD in patients with MCTD depends on the severity of the process at the time of diagnosis. Most cases seem to be mild, so corticosteroids are the initial immunosuppressant of choice. In patients without symptomatic improvement and decreased lung volumes and DLCO on follow-up PFTs (within 3 months), the addition of cyclophosphamide should be considered. Mostly small, retrospective reports and case studies seem to support the efficacy of cyclophosphamide.[57,61,63] In patients presenting with significant pulmonary functional loss, substantial fibrosis, and intensely inflammatory BAL fluid, or a rapidly progressing course, the clinician should consider combination therapy with corticosteroids and cyclophosphamide at the outset of treatment.

Our center uses the same treatment regimen in scleroderma-associated ILD and moderate to severe ILD associated with MCTD, which incorporates intravenous pulses of cyclophosphamide (0.5 to 1 mg/kg/mo) with tapering doses of corticosteroids. The most appropriate duration of cyclophosphamide therapy is unknown at this time for ILD associated with MCTD. Our center administers 6 to 12 monthly doses depending on the severity of the lung disease and the quality of the initial clinical response. Corticosteroids may induce scleroderma-renal crisis; their use in scleroderma lung disease should be minimized or used cautiously. Because of the low risk of scleroderma renal crisis in MCTD, initial corticosteroid doses are more aggressive, beginning at 1 mg/kg/day and tapering over 3 to 6 months. Patients should be monitored closely with at least quarterly PFTs and scans at least every 6 months. Serial 6-minute walk tests provide a useful measure of changes in functional capacity. In addition, measuring pulse oximetry during the test can assess the need for supplemental oxygen.

Table 10-8   Pulmonary Manifestations of Mixed Connective Tissue Disease

PLEUROPULMONARY DISEASE	FREQUENCY (%)	CLINICAL FEATURES	DIAGNOSTIC TESTING	DIFFERENTIAL DIAGNOSIS	TREATMENT
Pleuritis and pleural effusion	≤20	Pleurisy, dyspnea	CXR	PE, angina, chest wall disease, infection	NSAIDs, corticosteroids
ILD	20-50	Often asymptomatic; cough, dyspnea	PFTs, BAL, open-lung biopsy	PAH, aspiration, infection	Corticosteroids with or without CYC
PAH	20-30	Dyspnea, right heart failure	Echocardiogram, PFTs, BNP	ILD, pulmonary venous hypertension (left heart disease, pulmonary fibrosis), CVTED	Vasodilators and antiproliferative agents (ETRAs, prostanoids, phosphodiesterase type 5 inhibitors)
Venous thromboembolic disease	Rare	Acute dyspnea, pleurisy, cough, hemoptysis	Spiral CT, ventilation/perfusion scan, D-dimer, antiphospholipid antibody testing	Infection, vasculitis, pleuritis	Immunosuppression—corticosteroids with or without CYC Anticoagulation
Aspiration pneumonitis	Rare	Acute dyspnea with cough, classically right lower lobe infiltrate, fever; can progress to ARDS	CXR, PFTs, BAL, barium swallow	Infection, ILD	Aspiration/reflux therapy, antibiotics
Alveolar hemorrhage	Rare	Acute dyspnea, patchy acinar infiltrates with bibasilar predominance, fever, hemoptysis, rapid decline in hemoglobin	CXR, BAL, serial hemoglobin	Infection, PE, Goodpasture syndrome, SNV	Corticosteroids, CYC
Pulmonary vasculitis	Rare	Dyspnea, hemoptysis, patchy interstitial or alveolar infiltrates	PFTs, open-lung biopsy	Alveolar hemorrhage, PE, infection, SNV; may be cause of PAH	Corticosteroids, CYC
Obstructive airways disease	Rare	Wheezing, cough; nocturnal symptoms may predominate if aspiration is the cause	PFTs, barium swallow	Likely associated with reflux/aspiration from esophageal dysmotility	Aspiration/reflux therapy, bronchodilators, consider corticosteroids

BAL, bronchoalveolar lavage; BNP, brain natriuretic peptide; CVTED, chronic venous thromboembolic disease; CXR, chest radiograph; CYC, cyclophosphamide; ETRAs, endothelin receptor antagonists; ILD, interstitial lung disease; NSAIDs, nonsteroidal anti-inflammatory drugs; PAH, pulmonary arterial hypertension; PE, pulmonary embolism; PFTs, pulmonary function tests; SNV, systemic necrotizing vasculitis.

In children, ILD has been reported in mild and severe forms. There is no evidence for a difference in the prevalence or clinical characteristics of ILD in children compared with adults with ILD. Because ILD in this disease tends toward pulmonary fibrosis, it is important to monitor all patients for ILD with frequent PFTs, preferably every 3 to 6 months in the first few years after diagnosis, and then annually. Patients who develop dyspnea and restrictive pattern on PFTs should undergo or experience a decrease in DLCO. If the result is unremarkable, and no other explanation is available for the pulmonary decline, BAL is indicated to confirm the presence of interstitial inflammation. In these cases, BAL also may be a useful outcome measure, especially if the scan fails to show changes.

The leading cause of death in MCTD is PAH.[51] PAH is now recognized to develop in nearly one third of MCTD patients and has been reported in children and adults.[47,51,64-69] Postmortem studies have shown intimal proliferation and medial smooth muscle hypertrophy in the small vessels of the lungs, occasionally associated with superimposed thrombosis and plexiform lesions.[70] The histologic features in MCTD are identical to the features observed in PAH patients with scleroderma. Because antiphospholipid antibody syndrome is far less common in patients with MCTD, PAH developing as a consequence of chronic venous thromboembolic disease is unlikely. In all patients who develop PAH, routine screening for underlying causes of secondary PAH should be done, including screening for chronic venous thromboembolic disease, HIV, sickle cell disease, and congenital heart disease. The natural history of PAH in MCTD is unclear. Although there are rare reports of remission in patients treated with immunosuppressive and other drugs, progressive PAH followed by right heart failure is the leading cause of death in MCTD. PAH progresses more rapidly in patients with underlying connective tissue disorders than in patients with idiopathic PAH. Annual screening with echocardiogram, PFTs, serum brain natriuretic peptide, and 6-minute walk test is a key component

in MCTD management. PAH may develop 20 years after diagnosis.[71]

PAH in patients with MCTD has rarely been reported to improve with immunomodulatory therapy.[33,34,67,69] Because responsiveness to immunosuppression is not characteristic of PAH in scleroderma, it is possible that some patients with MCTD may develop PAH as a consequence of an immune-mediated inflammatory process, such as a vasculitis. To date, there are no substantiating pathologic data to support this hypothesis. The rate of response to immunosuppressive therapy suggests, however, that treatment of PAH in patients with MCTD should incorporate a course of corticosteroids and intravenous pulse cyclophosphamide for 3 to 6 months.[34] In our center, all patients with MCTD are concomitantly treated with standard vasoactive medications, such as endothelin receptor antagonists or phosphodiesterase type 5 inhibitors. We may initiate parenteral prostanoid therapy (continuous subcutaneous treprostinil or continuous intravenous epoprostenol) in patients with rapidly progressing PAH, fulminant or severe right heart failure, or extremely poor functional status. At present, there is no clear evidence of efficacy or safety favoring any single PAH treatment in MCTD.

Sjögren Syndrome

Sjögren syndrome is a chronic autoimmune disease that primarily affects the lacrimal and salivary glands. The cardinal clinical features are parotitis, keratoconjunctivitis sicca, and xerostomia; there is variable systemic involvement. Clinical manifestations include dry eyes, dry mouth with oral ulcerations, dental caries, salivary gland swelling, difficulty swallowing, vulvovaginitis, and gastrointestinal problems. The hallmark autoantibody findings include a positive ANA, Ro (SS-A), La (SS-B), and rheumatoid factor (RF). Additionally, patients with Sjögren syndrome often have an elevated erythrocyte sedimentation rate and hypergammaglobulinemia. Similar to other autoimmune diseases, it affects females significantly more often than males, with a ratio of approximately 9:1. Sjögren syndrome may occur alone (primary) or in association with other connective tissue diseases, such as rheumatoid arthritis, SLE, and systemic sclerosis (secondary).

In the pediatric population, Sjögren syndrome is extraordinarily rare with a mean age of onset of 10 years.[72] A review of 145 pediatric cases revealed parotid enlargement in 70%, eye involvement in 66%, and xerostomia in 43%. A positive ANA was detected in 78%. Antibodies to Ro, La, and RF were positive in 74%, 65%, and 66% of patients. Depending on which modality is used, pulmonary involvement in adult Sjögren syndrome has been estimated at 9% to 75%. In contrast to adults, pulmonary involvement is rare in children.

Pulmonary involvement can manifest clinically with progressive dyspnea and dry cough. Physical examination may reveal bibasilar crackles; digital clubbing is usually absent. PFTs typically reveal a restrictive pattern with diminished DLCO. Chest radiographs are less sensitive than high-resolution CT, but may show reticular or nodular opacities. Findings include ground-glass opacities, honeycombing, lung cysts, consolidation, and bronchiectasis. A CT scan from a patient with Sjögren syndrome is shown in Figure 10-3. Although BAL is not routinely warranted, it may assist in excluding an infectious etiology. BAL can show evidence of lymphocytic or neutrophilic alveolitis, the latter associated with more progressive disease. Various histopathologic patterns are seen, including lymphocytic interstitial pneumonia, nonspecific interstitial pneumonia, usual interstitial pneumonia, cryptogenic organizing pneumonia, primary pulmonary lymphoma, and fibrosis. The hallmark finding on lung histopathology is a CD4[+] polyclonal lymphocytic and plasma cell infiltrate. Figure 10-4 shows pulmonary histopathology from a patient with Sjögren syndrome who shows a lymphocytic interstitial pneumonia pattern.

Treatment of ILD in Sjögren syndrome centers on immunosuppression, usually with systemic corticosteroids. No controlled trials have examined the efficacy of alternative immunosuppressive agents, such as azathioprine, cyclosporine, and cyclophosphamide. Treatment needs to be adjusted depending on the severity of disease and the presence or absence of other systemic features.

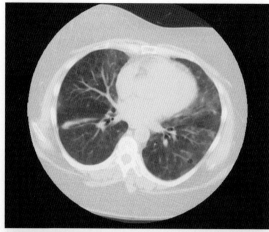
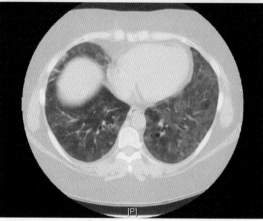

Figure 10-3. CT scan of the chest shows diffuse ground-glass opacities with parenchymal cysts in a patient with Sjögren syndrome and interstitial lung disease.

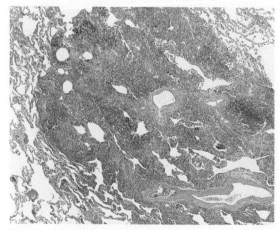

Figure 10-4. Lung biopsy histopathology specimen from a patient with Sjögren syndrome. The pattern is that of a patchy and nodular diffuse lymphoid interstitial pneumonitis. (See Color Plate)

Juvenile Rheumatoid Arthritis

Juvenile rheumatoid arthritis (JRA) is a chronic inflammatory disease of unclear etiology, which can manifest with articular and extra-articular involvement. The American College of Rheumatology (ACR) has classified JRA into three subtypes[73]: (1) polyarthritis characterized by involvement of five or more inflamed joints, (2) oligoarthritis with involvement of fewer than five inflamed joints, and (3) systemic onset with features of arthritis and characteristic fever.[73] Systemic-onset JRA is most commonly associated with extra-articular manifestations, but the other subtypes may be complicated by nonarticular organ involvement. Lung involvement, although uncommon, can have deleterious consequences when not recognized and treated.

The pleuropulmonary manifestations of JRA can be classified as involvement of the parenchyma, airways, pleura, and pulmonary vasculature.[74,75] These manifestations include parenchymal or pleural infection, interstitial pneumonia/pneumonitis (IP), interstitial fibrosis, BOOP, rheumatoid nodules, bronchiectasis, chronic obstruction, obstructive bronchiolitis, pleuritis, pleurisy, pulmonary vasculitis, and PAH.[74,75] When referring to the involvement of lung parenchyma, the term "interstitial lung disease" has been applied. The pulmonary toxicities of medications used to treat JRA (discussed subsequently) can add a level of complexity when assessing the impact of the disease.

In contrast to adults with rheumatoid arthritis, lung involvement in JRA historically has been seen with much less frequency.[76-78] Pleuropulmonary involvement has been reported in 1% to 40% of adults with rheumatoid arthritis.[79] This range is influenced by the method used to detect evidence of lung disease. Earlier studies relied on data obtained from chest x-rays and PFTs.[79] The use of high-resolution CT of the chest has improved our ability to identify lung disease.[80-82] In a prospective assessment of 150 rheumatoid arthritis patients, 20% had findings on CT consistent with ILD.[81] Data on the prevalence of pleuropulmonary involvement in children with JRA are sparse. A study of 191 patients with JRA at a single academic center identified evidence of lung or pleural involvement in 4% of children.[4] Most of the children (75%) had systemic-onset JRA.[76] A smaller study examined the prevalence of PFT abnormalities in patients with JRA and found asymptomatic abnormal PFTs in 60%, half of whom had subnormal DLCO.[77] Only one patient had an abnormal chest radiograph. In contrast, PFT measurements in a separate population of JRA patients did not identify any differences between DLCO, total lung capacity (TLC), or FEV_1 compared with controls.[83] Children with JRA had lower FVC and peak expiratory flow rates, which were attributed to respiratory muscle weakness rather than intrinsic lung disease.

Pleuropulmonary manifestations of JRA can manifest indolently and can precede the onset of arthritis.[78,84-90] Data, particularly those obtained from PFTs, suggest that there may be a prodromal period of asymptomatic disease.[77,83] No longitudinal studies have assessed the significance of abnormal PFT measurements in children with JRA. The available data suggest that the prevalence of lung disease remains low in these patients.[76]

In circumstances where pleuropulmonary involvement precedes onset of arthritis, patients can present with cough, dyspnea, and tachypnea.[84,85,87,90] A prior history of recurrent pulmonary infiltrates, often treated as infections, has been reported.[85,90] Patients with a known diagnosis of JRA can present with similar subjective symptoms of cough, dyspnea, and tachypnea in addition to chest pain.[76,78,86,88,91,92] Physical examination findings may reveal digital clubbing, cyanosis, bibasilar crackles on chest auscultation, nasal flaring, tachycardia, tachypnea, and hypoxia.[76,78,84-88,90-92] The presence of clubbing is often an indicator of prolonged disease.

Occasionally, the objective physical examination findings can be difficult to interpret in the setting of active arthritis, especially in patients with systemic-onset JRA. These patients can have a febrile illness associated with arthritis, rash, lymphadenopathy, hepatosplenomegaly, elevated inflammatory markers erythrocyte sedimentation rate, and C-reactive protein, leukocytosis, and serositis.[73] Under these circumstances, it is important to be vigilant for other mimics of chronic inflammatory arthritis, such as infection and malignancy. If the physical examination suggests a pleuropulmonary process, it is advisable to assess the problem thoroughly.

The use of PFTs for diagnosing and screening for pleuropulmonary disease in JRA is of paramount importance. A diminished DLCO has been observed in 0% to 30% of children with JRA.[77,83] In controlled studies, significant decreases of FVC and peak expiratory flow have been observed, but were attributed to respiratory muscle weakness.[83] Most PFT abnormalities can be described as restrictive lung defects with impaired DLCO.[78,84,85,87-90] An isolated depression of DLCO can be seen independently of restrictive or obstructive lung physiology.[86] The lack of longitudinal PFT assessment studies in JRA has limited the ability to interpret these findings. Several case reports have documented improvement or stabilization of PFTs in children with JRA over time, many of whom were treated with immunosuppressive therapy.[76,86,87,90,92] Progressively worsening PFTs portend greater morbidity and mortality.[85,87]

An additional use of PFTs is to focus on the assessment of PAH. Although uncommon in patients with JRA, primary PAH has been seen in a child with systemic-onset JRA.[86] In this patient, all parameters of pulmonary function were normal except for DLCO, which was 35% of normal. The authors have seen two patients whose course of systemic-onset JRA was complicated by PAH. Both patients died as a result of their disease. Although PFTs may suggest PAH, the diagnosis is confirmed by direct measurement of pulmonary arterial pressure by a right heart catheterization.

Chest radiographs have frequently failed to provide important qualitative descriptions or indications of disease severity in rheumatoid arthritis.[74,81] Of 28 adults with rheumatoid arthritis with evidence of ILD, only 36% had abnormal chest radiographs. Multiple case reports of children with active pleuropulmonary manifestations of JRA showed objective abnormal findings on chest radiographs, however.[76,78,84,87,88,90-92] Using a chest radiograph to screen for JRA in an asymptomatic child may be of limited clinical utility.

Findings include pleural effusions, patchy pulmonary infiltrates, reticulonodular infiltrates, and alveolar infiltrates with air bronchograms.[76,78,84,85,87,88,90,91,93] One patient presented with a pneumomediastinum in the setting of organizing bronchiolitis.[93] Other findings include ground-glass opacities, reticular lesions, honeycombing, intralobular septal thickening, bronchiectasis, consolidations, pleural effusions, pleural irregularities, and mediastinal lymphadenopathy.[80,91,93]

Studies using high-resolution CT scan of the chest have shown the greater sensitivity of this diagnostic study compared with conventional chest radiographs in detecting ILD.[80,81] High-resolution CT provides the opportunity to detect ILD at an earlier stage and potentially to improve long-term prognosis.

The pleuropulmonary manifestations of JRA can be categorized as manifestations involving the pleura, parenchyma, airways, or vasculature. In contrast to adults with rheumatoid arthritis–related ILD, pulmonary rheumatoid nodules are rare in children with JRA.[73,78,94] Rheumatoid nodules, which are usually present at the elbows and distally, are classically seen in patients who are RF-positive. Histologic examination of a rheumatoid nodule is characterized by a central area of fibrinoid necrosis surrounded by palisading epithelioid histiocytes, which is surrounded further by a matrix of lymphocytes, plasma cells, and fibroblasts.[75,95] Most children with JRA are RF-negative.[73] Population-based estimates have documented positive RF in 3% to 42% of children with JRA.[96,97] The greater presence of positive RF was seen in an aboriginal Canadian population with a known HLA association with rheumatoid arthritis.[97] Of children who have a positive RF, most are adolescents and have a polyarticular course that mimics adult rheumatoid arthritis.[73]

When feasible, pleural fluid assessment can help identify the underlying cause of pleuritis. Pleural fluid suggestive of an exudative rheumatoid effusion is often characterized as follows: lymphocyte-predominant leukocytosis (100 to 7000 cells/L), low glucose (<50 mg/dL), elevated lactate dehydrogenase (>1000 IU/L), elevated protein (>4 g/dL), and depressed complements.[75,95] It is necessary to exclude infection because this is also one of the few conditions associated with low pleural fluid glucose levels. In patients with systemic-onset JRA, pleuritis is the most common pleuropulmonary complication.[73,76]

BAL offers potential advantages in assessing ILD in JRA. It allows for analysis of inflammatory cells, and can aid in excluding infectious etiologies in acute and chronic processes. Compared with open lung biopsy, it is less invasive. Studies in adults with rheumatoid arthritis–related ILD have shown poor correlation between BAL findings and PFTs.[80,82] There was a trend toward increased numbers of neutrophils in patients with usual interstitial pneumonia compared with nonspecific interstitial pneumonia. Overlap was noted on BAL findings, however, in patients with usual interstitial pneumonia and patients with inflammatory airway disease with organizing pneumonia. These findings highlight the difficulty in interpreting BAL specimens, but do not obviate the utility of BAL to exclude infection.

Lung biopsy remains the gold standard for assessing pleuropulmonary disease in JRA. An appropriate sample can provide information about parenchymal, pleural, airway, and vascular involvement. Although a lung biopsy is not necessary in every JRA patient with an acute pulmonary process, it should be considered in circumstances in which therapy is predicated on discerning between an aseptic inflammatory process, an infectious process, and a vascular process.

Most, but not all, children with JRA with biopsy-proven pleuropulmonary disease are RF-positive.[76,84-88,90,91] Lung biopsy specimens were obtained in patients who had radiographic evidence of parenchymal disease.[76,84,85,87,88,90,91] In one patient who was diagnosed with primary PAH, a lung biopsy specimen was obtained to exclude vasculitis in the setting of normal imaging studies.[86] The predominance of lung biopsy specimens obtained from patients with parenchymal disease adds an element of selection bias, particularly with regard to assessing pleural disease.

Findings on lung biopsy have shown lymphoid interstitial pneumonitis, IP with

lymphoid bronchiolitis, isolated lymphoid bronchiolitis, BOOP, IP with thickened alveolar septa, and septal lymphocytic IP with prominent lymphoid follicles and germinal centers.[76,84,85,88,90,93] An adolescent girl with seropositive JRA complicated by small vessel vasculitis developed ILD with evidence of severe pulmonary fibrosis and arteritis of the pulmonary vessels on lung biopsy specimen.[87] The family history was positive for seropositive JRA with ILD in the patient's mother. One child with systemic-onset JRA who was RF-negative developed pulmonary interstitial and intra-alveolar cholesterol granulomas, also called "lipoid" pneumonia.[91] Whether this pneumonia was related to the underlying disease or therapy was unclear because the patient had been treated with chlorambucil, cyclophosphamide, and methotrexate. A child with sero-negative systemic-onset JRA underwent lung biopsy with objective evidence of PAH.[86] Histology showed pulmonary vascular obstruction with findings of intimal fibrosis of the small and medium-sized pulmonary arteries. Postmortem pleuropulmonary evaluation of 16 patients with a known diagnosis of JRA found radiographically and clinically detectable pulmonary lesions in 70%.[94] Gross assessment showed lung edema in 13 patients, pleural effusions in 3 patients, and pulmonary amyloidosis in 3 patients, and no pulmonary nodules. Most of the patients died of complications of amyloidosis, and many had multiorgan failure that may have contributed to the pulmonary findings at autopsy.

The pathogenesis of pleuropulmonary disease in JRA is incompletely understood. Data collected from adults with rheumatoid arthritis suggest aberrant T cell and B cell activation in patients with extra-articular disease.[98,99] Patients with rheumatoid arthritis with interstitial pneumonitis (usual interstitial pneumonia or nonspecific interstitial pneumonia) have significantly greater levels of CD4+ T cells and, to a lesser extent, CD3+ cells on lung biopsy specimens compared with patients with idiopathic IP, suggesting a possible crucial role of CD4+ T cells in the pathogenesis of rheumatoid arthritis–associated IP.[98] Similarly, patients with rheumatoid arthritis with IP have increased numbers of CD20$^+$ B cells on lung biopsy specimens.[99] Aggregates of CD20$^+$ B cells were found predominantly in a peri-bronchiolar distribution. The central role of B lymphocytes in the pathogenesis of rheumatoid arthritis has been well described and is supported by the effectiveness of targeted B cell therapy in patients with rheumatoid arthritis.[100-103] Whether these findings suggest a direct role of B cells in the pathogenesis of rheumatoid arthritis–related IP remains to be determined. In addition, patients with rheumatoid arthritis with IP have greater numbers of mast cells on lung biopsy specimens.[104] It is unclear whether the increased presence of mast cells is secondary to elevated CD4$^+$ T cells or underlying pulmonary fibrosis. It is possible that mast cells or mast cell mediators induce the release of transforming growth factor-β, which is associated with the development of pulmonary fibrosis. The elucidation of these pathways is key to the identification of novel therapeutic targets.

To date, no randomized trials have shown the efficacy or superiority of immuno-suppressive agents in treating rheumatoid arthritis–associated ILD. Limited experience in treating children with pleuropulmon-ary disease and JRA produced variable results.[76,84,85,87,88,90,91,93] Although some patients had complete resolution of their lung disease, others had chronic or pro-gressive ILD as evidenced objectively and subjectively.

Glucocorticoids have been the mainstay of therapy for pleuropulmonary disease in JRA. Additional immunosuppressive agents that have been used with variable success include cyclophosphamide, cyclosporine, intravenous immunoglobulin, salicylates, parenteral gold, methotrexate, etanercept, penicillamine, and hydroxychloroquine.[76,84,85,87,88,90,91,93] The evidence does not indicate clearly whether prognosis may correlate with initiation of therapy early in the course of lung disease. When monitored serially, patients with baseline evidence of restrictive lung disease often continue to have a component of restrictive lung function.[76,85,90,93] Complete resolution of radiographic abnormalities might be predictive of a good pulmonary prognosis.[76,84,88] When isolated PAH is

found with JRA, it should be treated similarly to PAH associated with scleroderma, with emphasis on the use of pulmonary vaso-dilators used in idiopathic PAH. Even with advances in therapeutics, however, it is important for care providers and families to recognize that the pleuropulmonary mani-festations of JRA can be fatal despite aggres-sive immunosuppressive therapy.[87,91,94]

Scleroderma

The cardinal clinical characteristic of sclero-derma (also known as systemic sclerosis) is fibrous involvement of skin. Scleroderma in children is divided into two distinct clinical categories, juvenile localized sclero-derma (JLS) and juvenile systemic sclerosis (JSSc).[105] Although the more common man-ifestation is JLS,[106,107] it is estimated that 10% of all cases of systemic sclerosis have had onset in the pediatric age group.[108,109] The incidence of JLS has been estimated to be 2.7 per 100,000.[110] The incidence of JSSc has not been reliably reported in the literature, and it is recognized as being rare. It has been estimated that less than 1% of all children followed in pediatric rheumatol-ogy clinics have JSSc.[111] There is not a clear gender or racial predilection for JSSc, in con-trast to adult scleroderma, in which women, African Americans, and Native Americans are more likely to be affected.[112]

Classification of JLS is generally divided into five categories: plaque morphea, generalized morphea, bullous morphea, deep morphea, and linear scleroderma, including scleroderma *en coup de sabre* and Parry-Romberg syndrome (Table 10-9). Pulmonary manifestations usu-ally do not occur in the JLS subtypes, but are common in JSSc. Provisional criteria for the diagnosis of JSSc were determined by an international expert consensus conference comprising the Pediatric Rheumatology Euro-pean Society, the ACR, and the European League Against Rheumatism and have been approved by the ACR (Table 10-10).[113,149]

The presence of proximal skin sclerosis/induration of the skin is the required major criterion needed for diagnosis of JSSc (see Table 10-10). At least 2 of 20 minor cri-teria also need to be present, of which the

Table 10-9	Classification of Juvenile Localized Scleroderma (JLS)	
SUBTYPE	**CLINICAL CHARACTERISTICS**	**% OF JLS**
Plaque morphea	Discrete patch, confined to dermis with occasional involvement of subcutaneous tissue	26
Generalized morphea	Multiple plaque morphea lesions in at least 3 anatomic sites or multiple confluent patches	7
Bullous morphea	Multiple bullae most common in lower extremities associated with lymphatic dilatation	
Linear scleroderma	Involvement of subcutaneous tissue, muscle, bone	65
Limb	Linear plaques that follow dermatome pattern, hyperpigmented, depressed when healed, may involve underlying muscle or bone, causing atrophy of limb, limb-length discrepancy	
Coup de sabre	Linear lesions on face, commonly unilateral, may cause alopecia of scalp or eyebrows with asymmetric facial development	
Parry-Romberg syndrome	Progressive hemifacial atrophy	
Deep morphea	Least common but most disabling, primary site of involvement in panniculus or subcutaneous tissue	2

three possible pulmonary manifestations are evidence of pulmonary fibrosis by chest radiograph or high-resolution CT scan, decreased DLCO, or PAH.[113] Skin involvement is characterized by skin that is initially edematous, followed by thickening and eventual fibrosis and thinning of skin. Defining the extent of skin involvement is important because it has become recognized that patients with diffuse scleroderma have a greater risk of cardiac and renal disease, although a similar risk of pulmonary disease. It also is recognized that patients with sclerodermatous induration of the torso have significantly increased risk of severe organ damage and death.[114] Scleroderma primarily progresses within the first 5 years of disease, at which time it may enter a period of relative quiescence.[115] There are case reports, however, of pulmonary fibrosis occurring more than 10 years after onset of scleroderma.[116] Pulmonary manifestations of systemic sclerosis can be from intrinsic lung pathology, from effects of PAH, or from fibrosis of the skin of the torso resulting in restriction of the chest wall and lungs.

The etiologies and pathogenesis of scleroderma, JSSc, and JLS are unknown. The basic pathology of scleroderma is threefold: There is a widespread vasculopathy, an autoimmune and inflammatory reaction, and progressive fibrosis.[117] The vasculopathy manifests as endothelial cell injury and

activation, and may be the first manifestation of SSc.[118] This vasculopathy is seen clinically as Raynaud phenomenon, periungual telangiectasias with capillary dropout, cutaneous telangiectasias, PAH, gastric antral vascular ectasia, and scleroderma renal crisis with malignant hypertension. Microvascular injury leads to vascular remodeling with eventual progressive narrowing and obliteration of the vascular lumen. The vasculopathy is thought to induce autoimmunity and an inflammatory reaction.[117]

The inflammatory reaction is initially seen as a perivascular monocyte and a macrophage infiltrate that progresses to involve multiple inflammatory cell types. An altered balance between T helper subtype 1 and T helper subtype 2 cytokines may be the basis for the pathogenesis of the inflammatory response.[119] Autoimmunity is evidenced by the findings of scleroderma-specific autoantibodies (see Table 10-10). A role for B cells in the pathogenesis of scleroderma also has been postulated. Depletion of B cells resulted in reduction of skin fibrosis, autoantibody production, and hypergammaglobulinemia when given to newborn mice in a mouse model for scleroderma.[120] Adult mice with established disease undergoing B cell depletion did not have any improvement in these measures, suggesting that when the inflammatory reaction is established, it triggers irreversible fibrosis.

Table 10-10	Classification Criteria for Juvenile Systemic Sclerosis
Major Criterion (required)	Proximal skin sclerosis/ skin induration
Minor Criteria (at least 2 of 20 required)	
Cutaneous	Sclerodactyly
Peripheral vascular	Raynaud phenomenon
	Nail-fold capillary abnormalities
	Digital tip ulcers
Gastrointestinal	Dysphagia
	Gastroesophageal reflux
Cardiac	Arrhythmias
	Heart failure
Renal	Renal crisis
	New-onset arterial hypertension
Respiratory	Pulmonary fibrosis (by BAL or HRCT)
	Decreased DLCO
	Pulmonary arterial hypertension
Neurologic	Neuropathy
	Carpal tunnel syndrome
Musculoskeletal	Tendon friction rubs
	Arthritis
	Myositis
Serologic	Antinuclear antibodies
	SSc-selective autoantibodies
	Anticentromere, anti–topoisomerase I (Scl70)
	Antifibrillarin, anti-PMScl
	Anti–RNA polymerase I or III

DLCO, diffusing capacity for carbon monoxide.
Data from references 1, 52.

The fibrosis in scleroderma accounts for most of the morbidity. The fibrosis tends to increase as the inflammatory cellular infiltrates decrease, and then may ultimately regress.[121] Various cells upregulate profibrotic soluble factors; these include transforming growth factor-β, interleukin-4, platelet-derived growth factor, monocyte chemoattractant protein-1, and CTGF. These soluble factors activate fibroblasts and related mesenchymal cells to increase the production of extracellular matrix (especially collagen) that replaces normal tissue.[117] After fibrosis has progressed, it tends to be irreversible and refractory to treatment.

Pulmonary involvement is currently the leading cause of death in scleroderma, given the progress in managing the previously lethal scleroderma renal crisis with the introduction of angiotensin-converting enzyme inhibitors and reduced reliance on long-term therapy with high-dose corticosteroids. The period of most rapid decline in lung function in adults is in the first 4 years of disease.[122] Clinical manifestations occur late in the progression of lung disease, so it is imperative that children with scleroderma be screened for pulmonary involvement. Given the paucity of data in the pediatric population, current knowledge is derived from available adult studies. In addition to the more common manifestations of scleroderma, such as alveolitis and ILD (discussed subsequently), less common phenotypes include shrinking lung syndrome[123] and pulmonary-renal syndrome with renal failure and diffuse AH.[124]

The lung pathology of scleroderma is that of an initial alveolitis that eventually progresses to fibrosis and is seen clinically as ILD. Early changes include interstitial edema and patchy inflammation of alveolar walls, primarily with lymphocytes and monocytes, leading to a combination of inflammatory reaction and fibroblast proliferation.[125-127] An increase in memory T cells also is seen, likely contributing in the long term to the evolution of pulmonary injury and remodeling.[128] With progressive thinning and rupture of alveolar walls, numerous tiny cysts form in association with interstitial and peribronchial fibrosis.[129] Consequently, lung volumes and DLCO progressively decrease. Lung inflammation has been shown to be associated with the evolution of progressive restrictive lung disease.[130-132]

The diagnosis of the initial lesion, the alveolitis, remains a clinical challenge. In a group of 13 children with scleroderma examined for lung disease, only 2 had dyspnea on exertion, even though 11 had ILD by high resolution CT scan of the chest.[132] The most common clinical manifestation of lung involvement in another study of

13 children was a chronic nonproductive cough.[133] Chest radiographs are often normal until late in the disease, when irreversible fibrosis has already occurred.[132] A combination of PFTs and BAL may be the best way to detect pulmonary involvement and follow treatment response.[134] PFTs show decreased FVC and decreased DLCO. A decreased FVC has been shown to correlate with the presence of honeycombing and ground-glass appearance.[132] A decreased DLCO has been found to reflect best the extent of fibrosing alveolitis, but also can be reflective of pulmonary vascular disease.[135,136] Other findings on examination in children with scleroderma include subpleural micronodules and linear opacities.[137] An autopsy in a child with scleroderma correlated ground-glass attenuation on high resolution CT scan of the chest with extensive interstitial fibrosis.[132]

BAL has been proposed as an approach to tracking and predicting the evolution of pulmonary inflammation in patients with scleroderma. In adults with scleroderma, an increased percentage of polymorphonuclear leukocytes and eosinophils or both on BAL have been correlated with a decline in FVC over time and increased early mortality.[131,138,139] A polymorphonuclear count of 4% or greater and eosinophils 2% or greater of total white blood cells recovered on BAL has been defined as evidence of active alveolitis.[140,141] Thus defined, active alveolitis on BAL has been found to correlate with abnormalities and tracks with a future decrease in FVC.

Controversy persists because BAL abnormalities have been found more recently not to be predictive of long-term disease progression or treatment response, although increased polymorphonuclear leukocytes were linked to early mortality.[142,143] The selection of the site of sampling of BAL fluid (right middle lobe versus site of abnormality on diagnostic imaging) may explain some of the differences in prognostic utility.[144] Technique in BAL fluid acquisition and analysis also has been a potential explanation for the disparity in studies. Despite the lack of consistent prediction of treatment response, alveolitis on BAL does correlate with abnormalities on high-resolution CT scan.[143] Lack of

normalization of BAL abnormalities after cyclophosphamide therapy did not differentiate clinical response in a group of 25 patients who underwent BAL before and after cyclophosphamide therapy.[145]

Although abnormal BAL fluid analysis with increased polymorphonuclear leukocytes and eosinophils suggests alveolitis and predicts changes on high-resolution CT scan, at present there is no good rationale for repeating the BAL after therapy for scleroderma lung disease. The utility of early BAL is for early diagnosis of alveolitis (often before findings emerge on the chest radiograph) and for excluding potential infection.

The development of high-resolution CT as an imaging tool has improved the detection of alveolitis in scleroderma. The prevalence of pulmonary fibrosis in scleroderma, as detected by high-resolution CT, has been described to be present in 90% of adults with scleroderma. Plain chest radiographs are not sensitive for diagnoses of alveolitis or fibrosis. Common findings include ground-glass opacities, reticular linear opacities, honeycombing, nodules, cylindrical bronchiectasis, and parenchymal bands. Ground-glass appearance is more indicative of cellular infiltration, whereas a reticular pattern is correlated with fibrosis.[146] Serial studies in patients with fibrosing alveolitis have shown that ground-glass appearance regresses with treatment when it is the predominant finding. If this appearance is seen in a mixed pattern with reticular opacities, however, treatment is often ineffective.[147] Mediastinal adenopathy is present in more than 50% of patients with scleroderma; a significant relationship has been described between mediastinal adenopathy and the presence of interstitial disease.[148]

The development of PAH in scleroderma remains an ominous sign because PAH is a major cause of morbidity and mortality. PAH is a pathologic state accompanied by a progressive increase in pulmonary vascular resistance leading to right-sided heart failure and premature death. It is characterized by a mean arterial pressure greater than 25 mm Hg at rest or greater than 30 mm Hg during exercise.[149] PAH in patients with scleroderma is encountered most commonly as part of the vasculopathy of the microcirculation.[150,151] Other causes of PAH in scleroderma include thrombotic disease and underlying cardiopulmonary disease. The prevalence of PAH in scleroderma is 50%, whereas its clinical presence is apparent in only 20% to 30%.[152,153]

The frequency of symptoms and signs of PAH have been determined by a national registry. The most common initial symptom was dyspnea (60%) followed by fatigue (19%), syncope or near-syncope (13%), chest pain (7%), palpitations (5%), and edema (3%).[154] Signs of PAH can be subtle and include accentuated second heart sound (S_2) in 93%, right-sided S_4 in 38%, right-sided S_3 in 23%, peripheral edema in 32%, and cyanosis in 20%. Other clinical signs of PAH include a left parasternal right ventricular heave and signs of elevated jugular venous pressure.

Clinical signs of PAH can be subtle, leading to delay in diagnosis and treatment. A right-sided heart catheterization with measurement of pulmonary arterial pressure is the gold standard for determination of PAH and should be done if clinical suspicion arises. A decreased DLCO is associated with PAH, although this also can be a sign of pulmonary alveolitis or fibrosis. A DLCO less than 53% predicted, or a DLCO that declines over time has been shown to be a predictor of subsequent development of PAH.[155] Electrocardiogram may suggest the diagnosis if signs of right ventricular hypertrophy or strain are seen. Generally, the electrocardiogram is too insensitive and nonspecific as a tool to be used for screening for PAH.[156] Findings on chest radiograph that suggest PAH include prominence of the main pulmonary artery, enlarged hilar vessels, and decreased peripheral vessels. Right atrial and ventricular enlargement also may be seen in more advanced cases.[149,157] A normal chest radiograph does not rule out PAH.

The most commonly used screening test for PAH is transthoracic Doppler echocardiography. Although echocardiograms have reasonable sensitivity and specificity for detecting moderate to severe PAH, their role as a screening tool for early or mild disease has not been established.[158] Indirect signs of PAH include right ventricular hypertrophy and enlargement, right atrial enlargement, paradoxical motion of the interventricular septum, and diastolic left ventricular compression. Right ventricular systolic pressure is estimated by the echocardiogram and is used as a surrogate measure of systolic pulmonary arterial pressure. Some authors have advocated for a combination of DLCO measurement with echocardiographic estimate of pulmonary arterial pressure, but these screening methods have been poorly validated.[159,160]

Treatment of scleroderma lung disease should be initiated when an active alveolitis (compared with lung fibrosis) is the dominant histopathology. Cyclophosphamide given daily at a dose up to 2 mg/kg orally has been the only effective agent shown in a prospective multicenter trial to slow the loss of FVC over time, while improving dyspnea, skin scores, and health-related quality of life.[161,162] Whether to add low-dose prednisone to cyclophosphamide is controversial and unproven. Smaller studies and retrospective cohort studies have suggested that mycophenolate mofetil may be effective; however, prospective randomized data are unavailable to date.[163,164] Clinical trials of drug therapy to date have not targeted the pediatric population.

Aggressive and early treatment of PAH has dramatically increased life expectancy in PAH associated with systemic sclerosis. General supportive measures for management of PAH include correction of hypoxia with oxygen therapy, regulation of intravascular volume status with fluid/sodium restriction or diuretics, digitalis (although efficacy is unproven), anticoagulation, and prevention of pulmonary infections with vaccinations for influenza and pneumococcal pneumonia.[165]

Medical treatment of PAH in childhood is more often targeted to children with congenital heart defects; scleroderma-specific treatments are lacking. Medical treatment of PAH includes calcium channel blockers, prostacyclin analogues, endothelin receptor antagonists, phosphodiesterase type 5 inhibitors, and combination therapies (Table 10-11).[157,165] The dual endothelin receptor antagonist bosentan has been reported to be efficacious in treating PAH in children.[166] Combination therapies with bosentan and iloprost or sildenafil and bosentan have been attempted.[157] Lung transplantation is an option for patients in whom medical therapy ceases to be effective.

Table 10-11	Treatment of Pulmonary Arterial Hypertension in Scleroderma			
DRUG CATEGORY	**MECHANISM OF ACTION**	**EXAMPLES**	**ADMINISTRATION**	**SPECIAL NOTES**
Prostacyclins	Pulmonary and systemic vasodilator, platelet aggregation inhibition	Epoprostenol	Continuous intravenous	
		Treprostinil	Continuous subcutaneous	
		Iloprost	Inhaled q3-4h	
Calcium channel blockers	Long-term vasodilator	Nifedipine Diltiazem	Oral	Use only in patients proven to have pulmonary vasodilator response on right heart catheterization
Endothelin receptor antagonists	Block receptors for endothelin, a potent endogenous vasoconstrictor	Bosentan	Oral	Two receptors described, ET_A, ET_B. Bosentan: inhibits both receptors; selective blockers are in development
Phosphodiesterase type 5 inhibitor	Inhibits phosphodiesterase type 5, which inactivates cGMP, which relaxes pulmonary vascular smooth muscle cells. Phosphodiesterase type 5 inhibitors dilate pulmonary arterial beds	Sildenafil	Oral	

cGMP, cyclic guanosine monophosphate.

Juvenile Dermatomyositis

Juvenile dermatomyositis (JDMS) manifests as a chronic autoimmune inflammatory disorder of skin and muscle typically characterized by a rash, proximal muscle weakness, and elevation of muscle enzymes. The clinical hallmarks are listed in Table 10-12. If the rash is absent, the term "polymyositis" is applied. Polymyositis is rare in the pediatric age group, however, and children with a polymyositis syndrome without a rash should be investigated for various metabolic, neurologic, and endocrine disorders, and for potential toxin exposure. Pulmonary involvement with JDMS in children is relatively rare. The characteristic histopathology of the disease is a generalized vasculitis, which produces the characteristic rash and a typical pattern of proximal muscle weakness. When the expression of the proximal weakness is profound, respiratory

failure from thoracic muscle fatigue may result. The onset of respiratory failure is often not heralded by classic signs of respiratory distress, such as retractions or tachypnea. Children with severe weakness should be monitored for respiratory muscle weakness (negative inspiratory force in younger children), breathing capacity (vital capacity in older children), or carbon dioxide retention (end-tidal capnography or blood gas measurements).

Blood markers of JDMS are unhelpful. The presence of ANAs is not required for the diagnosis of JDMS, but they may be present in 50% of pediatric cases.

The pulmonary pathology is largely extrapolated from adults with dermatomyositis because 30% to 50% of adults have ILD, whereas the pulmonary expression of JDMS is rare in children.[167,168] The histopathology is devoid of vasculitic contribution. The characteristic lung fibrosis can manifest either as

Table 10-12 — Characteristics of Juvenile Dermatomyositis

FINDINGS	
Organ Involvement	
Skin	Heliotrope rash
	Purple, swollen eyelids
	Gottron papules (scaly lesions on knuckles)
	Malar rash
	Shawl rash (upper anterior/posterior thorax)
	Calcinosis may affect skin
Muscles	Proximal myopathy
	Lymphocytic inflammation early
	Calcinosis late
	Electromyography has typical changes
	Muscle biopsy
	Perivascular infiltrates
	Small vessel occlusion
	Fibrillar degeneration
	Perifibrillar mononuclear cell cuffing
	Sarcolemma nuclear proliferation
	Elevation of muscle enzymes
Lung Disease*	*Not* a vasculitis
Histopathology	Usual interstitial pneumonitis
	Bronchiolitis obliterans with organizing pneumonia
	Capillary leak syndrome
Lung disease marker	Antibody to Jo-1 associated with pulmonary complications such as fibrosis
Radiographic changes	Pulmonary fibrosis
	Pneumothorax or pneumomediastinum (less common)
	Patchy alveolar infiltrates (less common)
Therapy	Corticosteroids standard (oral or intravenous)
	Hydroxychloroquine for skin disease, may be steroid-sparing
	Methotrexate (some use as standard; some use only for drug-resistant disease)
	Alternative anti-inflammatory agents
	Azathioprine
	Cyclophosphamide
	Cyclosporine
	Rituximab (ongoing trial)

*Rare in childhood; data are from adults.

interstitial/alveolar (usual interstitial pneumonitis) or small airways obstruction (BOOP). An alternative presentation is that of acute respiratory distress syndrome with the pathophysiologic processes associated with vascular leak, such as alveolar edema and the formation of hyaline membranes. Antibodies to the Jo-1 tissue antigen, unusual in childhood, are associated with the evolution of pulmonary complications, such as fibrosis. The histocompatibility antigens HLA-DQA1*0501 and HLA-DQA1*0401 have been reported to have increased expression in white patients. A single case of lipoproteinosis has been reported in a child with dermatomyositis.

Although much progress has been made in the therapy of JDMS, treatment strategies are not grounded in prospective, controlled data from pediatric clinical trials. Before the use of corticosteroids, the mortality from JDMS was 30%, and another 30% had chronic illness. After the implementation of corticosteroid therapy in the 1960s, the mortality has diminished to less than 10%. This therapy remains the mainstay for skin and muscle disease and is administered either orally or intravenously. More severe disease, such as weakness of the thoracic musculature, is often treated with pulse methylprednisolone (30 mg/kg up to 1 g given intravenously over 1 hour). Hydroxychloroquine is used to control skin manifestations and may permit a more rapid taper of therapy with corticosteroids. Methotrexate is increasingly used as a first-line agent; some centers still reserve its use for therapy of resistant disease. Alternative immunomodulatory therapies for JDMS have included azathioprine, cyclophosphamide, and cyclosporine. A National Institutes of Health–sponsored trial of rituximab for the treatment of refractory JDMS is ongoing (http://www.clinicaltrials.gov).

Ankylosing Spondylitis

Juvenile ankylosing spondylitis (JAS) is one of the rarest spondyloarthropathies, a group of disorders that share the following features: inflammation of the axial skeleton (especially sacroiliitis) and inflammation of the entheses (the insertion points on bone of tendons and ligaments), RF-seronegative, absence of rheumatoid nodules, infrequency of other autoantibodies, genetic association with the histocompatibility antigen HLA-B27, and family clustering of the related disorders (inflammatory bowel disease, psoriatic arthritis, and reactive arthritis).[169] Extra-articular manifestations cross these disease lines and include iritis and psoriatic-like rashes.

Although the criteria for the diagnosis of ankylosing spondylitis in adults are well worked out and require a confirmation of sacroiliitis, a major challenge for pediatricians is that the expression of arthritis in the axial skeleton is often not the earliest manifestation, which can evolve slowly over years. Progress in the classification of these disorders was achieved with the recognition of the seronegative enthesitis and arthritis syndrome.[170] The seronegative enthesitis and arthritis syndrome classification system allowed the identification of children with enthesitis or peripheral arthritis or both who lacked the classic finding of arthritis of the axial skeleton. Follow-up studies[171] revealed that many of these children subsequently developed spine or sacroiliac joint involvement that completed the diagnostic criteria of JAS. Because the criteria for adult ankylosing spondyloarthropathy fail to discern children who are developing JAS or are at risk of developing JAS, criteria[172] for the related disorder, enthesitis-related arthritis, have become popular among pediatricians caring for these children (Table 10-13). In this scheme, a diagnosis of enthesitis-related arthritis is confirmed by the presence of arthritis and enthesitis. Alternatively, a diagnosis of enthesitis-related arthritis can be confirmed by the presence or either arthritis or enthesitis, provided that two of the following five criteria are met: (1) sacroiliac joint tenderness or inflammatory spinal pain or both, (2) HLA-B27 seropositive, (3) positivity of HLA-B27-associated disease in a first-degree or second-degree relative, (4) anterior uveitis, or (5) onset of arthritis in a boy older than 8 years. The diagnosis of enthesitis-related arthritis is excluded by the presence of either a dermatologist-confirmed diagnosis of psoriatic

Table 10-13	Enthesitis-Related Arthritis
Required Features	
Arthritis and enthesitis *or*	
Arthritis or enthesitis plus at least two of the following	
Sacroiliac joint tenderness and/or inflammatory spinal pain	
Positive for HLA-B27	
Family history positive for one or more first-degree or second-degree relatives with HLA-B27-confirmed disease	
Anterior uveitis usually associated with erythema, pain, or photophobia	
Onset of arthritis in a boy >8 years old	
Exclusions	
Dermatologist-confirmed psoriasis in a first-degree or second-degree relative	
Presence of systemic arthritis	

From Petty RE, et al: Revision of the proposed classification criteria for juvenile idiopathic arthritis. Durban, 1998. J Rheumatol 25:1991-1994, 1998.

arthritis in a first-degree or second-degree relative or the presence of systemic arthritis.

Because of the tendency of JAS to evolve over time, most patients with this diagnosis are in late childhood or adolescence. Some children with enthesitis-related arthritis are diagnosed with ankylosing spondylitis or related arthropathy in adulthood. The male-to-female ratio is approximately 7:1. The frequency of diagnoses of ankylosing spondylitis is low in African Americans and in native Japanese.

The precise etiology of the disorder is unknown. The association of the disease with the HLA-B27 antigen suggests a molecular genetic pathway. T helper subtype 1 lymphocytes, $CD8^+$ and $CD14^+$ inflammatory cells, and the cytokine tumor necrosis factor (TNF)-α all have been implicated in the etiology.

Respiratory complications of JAS are rare.[173-188] Chest wall restriction results from arthritis or ankylosis of sternocostal or costovertebral joints, and manifests most frequently as a reduced TLC or a reduced FVC. It most often is not associated with dyspnea. In a series of more than 1000 adults with ankylosing spondylitis, approximately 1% were shown to have pleuropulmonary manifestations.[173] Pleural thickening (but not pleural effusion) was relatively common, and fibrous and bullous disease was seen. Pleural thickening, when observed, would usually become bilateral. Symptoms of inflammatory or fibrotic disease were uncommon. High-resolution CT scans show a greater sensitivity in detecting pulmonary parenchymal abnormalities. Infrequent findings in adults include ILD, bronchiectasis, paraseptal emphysema, and apical fibrosis.

The most common pulmonary function changes in a group of asymptomatic adults with a history of normal chest radiographs were a reduced TLC and FVC. Flow rates, DLCO, elastic recoil, and exercise tolerance were normal except in the patients with the most severely restricted lung capacities.[174] Studies of pulmonary function in patients with JAS are few and show slightly different patterns.[175,177] Of 18 older children and adolescents with JAS, none had respiratory symptoms. All had chest radiographs that were initially normal. Six had abnormalities of pulmonary function, of which a reduced vital capacity was most common. A few showed an elevation of the FRC or a reduced DLCO.

Sarcoidosis

Sarcoidosis is a chronic multisystem inflammatory disorder of unknown etiology characterized by the expression in a wide range of tissues of noncaseating granulomas in lesions that lack infections that might ordinarily cause them. Because of the broad range of potential tissue sites, sarcoidosis, similar to tuberculosis, can mimic an expansive array of clinical disorders and can be asymptomatic or organ-threatening or life-threatening. Commonly affected organs include thoracic lymph nodes, lungs, liver, spleen, eyes, bones, joints, salivary and lacrimal glands, central nervous system, and skin. Less commonly affected organs include the heart, blood vessels, other lymph nodes, kidneys, gut, and peripheral nerves.[189-191]

Sarcoidosis may occur in the preschool age group with a triad of a granulomatous skin rash, uveitis, and arthritis,[192,193] originally described as Blau syndrome,[194] a syndrome of early-onset systemic granulomatosis, similar to early-onset sarcoidosis,

accompanied by a strong family history.[195] Fifty percent to 90% of familial and nonfamilial versions[196] of early-onset systemic granulomatous syndromes manifest one of several mutations in the caspase recruitment domain-15 (CARD15)/nucleotide-binding oligomerization domain-2 (NOD2) proteins, members of the NOD family of proteins, located on chromosome 16.[197] These mutations are associated with the activation of nuclear factor κB, a nuclear transcription factor associated with the upregulated expression of numerous inflammatory cytokines. These patients frequently develop hypertension, fever, hepatosplenomegaly, and parotid swelling with a risk of cardiac or cerebral sequelae. Only infrequently do they develop lung disease,[194,198] including when a mutation occurs in the CARD15 gene family.[199] These cases are often refractory to therapy, including the use of systemic corticosteroids.

The more common presentation of sarcoidosis (which is not associated with mutations in the CARD15/NOD2 gene complex[200-202]) occurs most frequently in the third and fourth decades of life, and includes combinations of lung disease, lymphadenopathy, fever, weight loss, and hypercalcemia.[203] Variations of this phenotype occur throughout the school-age years and are more common in adolescents. School-age children are more likely to have pulmonary parenchymal involvement in addition to hilar or paratracheal adenopathy compared with adults with sarcoidosis.[204-219] Although multiorgan disease expression in children is typical (commonly in unexpected combinations), isolated involvement of a wide range of organs is described in numerous case reports that include infants and younger children.

Sarcoidosis apparently affects boys and girls equally.[204] The true incidence of the disease is unknown because of the absence of screening programs and the frequency of asymptomatic disease, but is estimated to be 5 per 100,000 in whites and 40 per 100,000 in African Americans in the United States.[204,232] Most reported U.S. cases are located in the southeastern United States. In Europe, sarcoidosis is more apparent in northern countries, such as Sweden, where autopsy-derived data suggest a prevalence of 641 per 100,000.[220,221] The prevalence also is greater throughout Scandinavia and Great Britain and in ethnic Japanese compared with the United States.[190] Although several HLA associations have been suggested, no definitive genetic etiology has emerged. Several familial clusters nonetheless have been reported.

The classic lesion suggesting a diagnosis of sarcoidosis in a tissue biopsy specimen is a noncaseating granuloma.[191] This lesion is seen in various disorders other than sarcoidosis, such as certain toxic exposures (beryllium) and certain viral and fungal infections, and in lymph node–draining sites of cancer, so a careful analysis of the clinical context and an expert pathologic review of the entire specimen are crucial.[190] Noncaseating granulomas also can be seen in specimens from patients with disorders such as tuberculosis that are characterized by caseating and necrotizing granulomas. A typical lesion consists of an organized ring of epithelioid cells that are compact and radially arranged, are populated with Langerhans-type giant cells (also arranged circularly around a central granular zone), and are surrounded by lymphocytes.[191,205] There is no evidence of caseation in lesions of patients with sarcoidosis, and necrotizing features are unusual.

The immune inflammatory response believed to be responsible for the evolution of the granulomas is thought to originate with the presentation of antigens by a macrophage to T lymphocytes, which then elaborate the activating cytokine interleukin-1.[191,222,223] This serves to recruit CD4+ lymphocytes from peripheral blood to the site of activation (the lung), where they induce the differentiation of B lymphocytes that secrete IgM, IgA, and IgG. Local T cells elaborate interleukin-2, a cytokine important for lymphocyte proliferation. Additional cytokines and chemokines activate macrophages and recruit blood monocytes to the lung, where they differentiate into additional macrophages and amplify the response. Other inflammatory cells are activated, and various humoral factors are produced with a resulting robust and complex inflammatory response that may resolve spontaneously or may persist and intensify. If the granulomatous response persists, its

natural course is hyalinization and generation of collagen and other ground substances to form fibrous and otherwise remodeled tissue.

The exact mechanisms that drive these differential paths of inflammation resolution or progression are unknown. Although this process lacks the full expression of T helper subtype 2 orchestration that characterizes an allergic inflammatory response, the critical participation of CD4+ T lymphocytes in the generation of the granulomas helps explain the usually dependable response of the lesions to treatment with systemic corticosteroids, which is the mainstay of therapy for more severe or risk-loaded cases of sarcoidosis.[222,224] The granulomas are known to be capable of secreting and activating vitamin D,[189,191] which helps to explain the frequently observed complications of hypercalcemia and hypercalciuria and their frequently positive response to treatment with corticosteroid therapy.

The clinical expression of sarcoidosis depends on the intensity of the inflammatory response, its level of generalization, and whether or not the granulomatous process interferes critically with organ function. In most children, multiple organs are involved, regardless of symptoms.[204] Because there is widely disseminated inflammation, many children present with nonspecific complaints, such as malaise, weight loss, lethargy, anorexia, headache, and, less commonly, fever, abdominal pain, or nausea. If the inflammation is focused, there may be organ-localizing symptoms or signs, such as pain or swelling, but it is common for such symptoms to be absent. Even cutaneous lesions may be asymptomatic. Because any organ or multiple organs might be involved, a thorough physical examination directed to uncommon findings is mandated.

Respiratory symptoms, if present, include cough, dyspnea, chest pain, or sputum production.[222] Signs often are absent, but might include unequal, coarse, or muffled breath sounds or wheezing or crackles. In contrast, most chest radiographs of children with sarcoidosis are positive. In a series published from Duke University[225] of 19 children with sarcoidosis, all the radiographs showed abnormalities. Nearly all cases show parabronchial ("hilar") adenopathy, and most show paratracheal adenopathy. Parenchymal involvement is usually present with or without evidence of adenopathy. Typical features include reticulonodular and interstitial patterns. Less typical features include alveolar filling processes; distinct nodules; fibrotic phenotypes; or more dramatic changes, such as pneumothorax, pleural effusion, calcification, pleural thickening, or atelectasis.[225,226]

The adult radiographic staging process has been adopted for use in evaluating children.[190,191,222,227,239] Stage 0 is a normal chest radiograph. Stage 1 indicates the presence of bilateral parabronchial adenopathy. Stage 2 criteria include the presence of parabronchial adenopathy and pulmonary parenchymal infiltrates. A stage 3 radiograph shows parenchymal infiltrates without the perihilar adenopathy. The presence of fibrotic lesions and bullous emphysema is considered to indicate either late stage 3 or stage 4 sarcoidosis. The utility of this staging paradigm has been validated in multiple studies in adults, and the experience with children seems consistent with these results.

Generally, disease progression follows the sequence of the radiographic staging, and the prognosis worsens with the more advanced stages. When the hilar or paratracheal adenopathy is not evident, it does not generally reappear at a later time. Most patients with either stage 1 or stage 2 disease undergo remissions, whereas the rate of remission declines with the progression of the stages. Despite the fact that patients with stage 1 disease may have granulomas on lung biopsy or parenchymal disease on high-resolution CT scans,[226] the better prognosis remains linked to the appearance of the plain radiographic appearance, despite its apparent lack of sensitivity in detecting subtle parenchymal disease.

The most consistently shown abnormality[226,228-230] of pulmonary function (50% of children in one large series) is a restrictive pattern in which the TLC and FRC are reduced. DLCO abnormalities also are seen. Less common are obstructive patterns, in which the FEV_1-to-FVC ratio is reduced; this accounted for 15% of the abnormalities in the same

study. Syndromes of airway hyperresponsiveness[231] and airway obstruction are common in sarcoidosis. It is unknown whether these syndromes result from endobronchial granulomatous lesions,[232] airway compression by enlarged lymph nodes,[189] altered airway growth, inflammation-directed airway hyperresponsiveness, or an overlap syndrome with childhood asthma. For children with these syndromes, a trial of bronchodilators and asthmatic anti-inflammatory therapy may be helpful. For the few children with airway compression from enlarged paratracheal or parabronchial lymph nodes, a trial of systemic corticosteroids to reduce the mass of the nodes may be warranted.

In rare cases, granulomas may involve any of the structures of the larynx and upper airway, producing hoarseness, stridor, dyspnea, obstructive sleep apnea, cough, or dysphagia.[190] If the symptoms are significant, treatment with oral or systemic corticosteroids may bring needed relief.

The diagnosis of sarcoidosis is based on criteria published in a joint consensus statement of the American Thoracic Society and European Respiratory Society in 1999.[227] The diagnostic criteria for children do not differ from those for adults. The diagnosis requires (1) a compatible clinical profile, (2) histologic evidence of noncaseating granulomas without pathologic evidence of another etiologic process, and (3) exclusion of other disease processes that might manifest with a similar clinical profile or histopathology (notably infections and toxins). The crucial parts of the diagnosis are the requirement of tissue confirmation and the elimination by careful history, physical examination, and laboratory evaluation of confounding candidates.

The performance of lung cultures via bronchoscopy is sometimes necessary to complete the analysis. The tissue source can be a suspicious lesion anywhere on the body, such that superficial targets, such as skin or conjunctival lesions, are often preferred to avoid the necessity of general anesthesia.[190] One series from Turkey determined that biopsy of the minor salivary glands yielded a 48% positive yield for noncaseating granulomatous lesions in patients with confirmed sarcoidosis with no positive lesions in children with tuberculosis.[233] The feasibility of fine needle aspiration of lung or mediastinal lymph nodes has been shown in adolescent patients. Other sites of biopsy that frequently yield a diagnosis include peripheral muscles and liver.

Supportive diagnostic studies that are not entirely specific are often useful and necessary because of potentially confounding clinical presentations. The erythrocyte sedimentation rate is usually elevated in active sarcoidosis. Levels of serum angiotensin-converting enzyme are elevated in 80% of children with sarcoidosis; the angiotensin-converting enzyme is synthesized in the epithelioid cells of the granulomas.[191,234] The level of the angiotensin-converting enzyme also can be used as a marker of disease activity in patients who have elevations with disease activity that decline with remission. For many patients, this is a very helpful marker. Many diseases, including diabetes, liver disease, and several neoplasms, also are associated with elevated angiotensin-converting enzyme levels, however.[235] Angiotensin-converting enzyme levels in children younger than 15 years can be 50% greater than their adult counterparts, so pediatric-specific normal values should be applied.

Serum chitotriosidase has been proposed as a disease marker for sarcoidosis activity, but its sensitivity, specificity, and utility have not yet been confirmed.[236] For children whose diagnosis or management includes bronchoscopy, the determination of a BAL fluid ratio of CD4+-to-CD8+ lymphocytes of greater than 3.5, although insensitive (53% detection), has been determined to be highly specific (94%) for the diagnosis of sarcoidosis.[237] In addition, criteria have been determined that are characteristic for pulmonary parenchymal sarcoidosis and help to confirm the diagnosis.

The hallmark of therapy for sarcoidosis is oral or parenteral corticosteroids.[189,222,238] Several trials have shown improvement in clinical symptoms and pulmonary function with the daily administration of oral corticosteroids, but despite more than 50 years of use, data are still lacking for evidence of their impact in modifying the trajectory of the underlying disease or preventing death. Many patients with mild disease

recover without intervention, raising questions about the need for therapy for many patients. Nonetheless, many shorter term studies in adults have shown the effectiveness in improving symptoms, pulmonary function, and radiographic appearance. Typical treatment strategies include an initial oral dose of prednisone or prednisolone of 1 mg/kg/day to a usual maximum of 60 mg/day.[222] When the desired treatment effect is achieved (improvement in symptoms, pulmonary function, or radiograph), usually in several weeks, the daily dose is tapered over several weeks to a few months. Therapy typically lasts approximately 6 months, but longer treatment intervals are sometimes required. As doses decline, alternate-day therapy usually sustains the positive effects until the patient can be weaned off the medication. A less studied but often effective alternative therapy is chloroquine, given as 250 mg by mouth twice daily for 2 weeks and then once daily for long-term suppression of inflammation. To minimize the risk of chloroquine-associated retinopathy, the maximal maintenance dosage should not be greater than 3.5 to 4 mg/kg of ideal body weight each day.[222] Sarcoidosis that is refractory to usual therapy may respond to methotrexate or to pharmacologic blockade of TNF-α, such as etanercept or infliximab. The response to therapy for early-onset sarcoidosis (Blau syndrome) is often disappointing and challenging.

A more recently published approach[238] suggests an alternative treatment decision paradigm designed to limit the use of systemic corticosteroids to those satisfying preset standards in the following categories: (1) severity of disease expression, (2) progression of the disease, (3) risk to vulnerable organs, or (4) unacceptability of the quality of life with untreated disease. The specific criteria for respiratory-related issues are listed in Table 10-14. The paradigm also specifies that corticosteroid therapy should be administered to patients with disease localization to heart or central nervous system; to patients with sight-threatening ocular disease uncontrolled by local measures; to patients with severe hypercalcemia (≥ 3 mM·L^{-1} ionic calcium); to patients

Table 10-14	Criteria for Corticosteroid Therapy of Pulmonary Sarcoidosis

Absolute Criteria

Severe restriction or diffusion impairment on presentation (FVC <50% or DLCO <50% predicted)

Severe airway obstruction on presentation (FEV$_1$ <50% predicted)

Progressive pulmonary disease (decrease of FVC >10% or DLCO >15% from baseline)

Evidence for severe or progressive lung fibrosis with active disease

Relative Criteria

Symptomatic pulmonary disease with mild-to-moderate lung function impairment

Symptoms cause unacceptable quality of life (e.g., dyspnea, fatigue, or weight loss)

DLCO, diffusing capacity for carbon monoxide; FEV$_1$, forced expiratory volume in 1 second; FVC, forced vital capacity. Adapted from Grutters JC, van den Bosch JMM: Corticosteroid treatment in sarcoidosis. Eur Resp J 28:627-636, 2006.

with hypercalciuria with nephrocalcinosis and renal dysfunction; to patients with granulomatous interstitial nephritis; to patients with liver involvement with intrahepatic cholestasis, portal hypertension, or hepatic failure; or to patients with bone marrow involvement with pancytopenia. The relative criteria also would apply to patients with disfiguring skin involvement.

With or without therapy, the outcome for most school-age children seems to be favorable. The prognoses for school-age children with more advanced pulmonary disease and for preschool-age children with the more difficult-to-control triad of skin lesions, ocular disease, and arthropathy are more guarded.[210] Because several features of disease expression in this younger group differ, including the general absence of respiratory system involvement, this seems to be a different disease whose criteria for therapy and follow-up need sharper definition.

For patients with pulmonary disease, there is a need for adequately controlled trials of therapy with corticosteroids,[238] and alternative candidate therapies in children whose disease is well characterized and for whom the treatment protocols allow for stage-specific evaluations of outcomes. There is a special need for better defined therapy for early-onset sarcoidosis. Because of the variability of expression, these multiple phenotypes need characterization by large, multicenter trials. Only with these data can the treatment guidelines be rationalized.

Pneumonitis Resulting from Antirheumatic Therapy

Methotrexate Pneumonitis

Methotrexate has emerged as an important therapy for JRA and other rheumatic diseases.[240,241] At doses commonly used in children and adolescents, 0.5 to 1 mg/kg or 10 to 15 mg/m^2/wk, methotrexate is efficacious and well tolerated. An uncommon but concerning pulmonary complication of methotrexate therapy is hypersensitivity pneumonitis. Methotrexate pneumonitis is more prevalent in adult patients than in children. Estimates of pneumonitis in adults using low doses of methotrexate ($\leq$25 mg/wk) range from 0.5% to 14%.[242-246] Risk factors include older age, preexisting lung disease, previous use of disease-modifying antirheumatic drugs, and hypoalbuminemia.[247]

Symptoms of methotrexate pneumonitis include dyspnea, dry cough, and fever.[244,246,248,249] Peripheral eosinophilia can be found, but is neither sensitive nor specific.[245,246] The physical examination may reveal bibasilar crackles and tachypnea.[246,249] Chest radiographs rarely appear normal, and frequently reveal interstitial or alveolar infiltrates or both.[246,249] High-resolution CT scans of the chest often identify ground-glass opacities, interstitial infiltrates, or alveolar infiltrates.[246] BAL fluid with a predominance of CD4$^+$ lymphocytes supports a diagnosis of methotrexate pneumonitis.[243,246,250,251] Lung pathology is nonspecific, but findings include interstitial infiltrates, fibrosis, granulomas, and diffuse alveolar damage.

Serial PFTs in children with JRA have shown that there is no relationship between the development of pulmonary disease and methotrexate exposure.[252-255] Cron and colleagues[248] reported a girl with polyarticular JRA who presumably developed methotrexate pneumonitis. The patient had a diminished FVC, but DLCO was not assessed, and a chest radiograph was normal. These abnormalities resolved with discontinuation of methotrexate and initiation of systemic corticosteroids.

The signs and symptoms of methotrexate pneumonitis are frequently indistinguishable from an infectious process. Searles and McKendry[256] proposed diagnostic criteria for methotrexate pneumonitis that are based on the absence of an infectious etiology as determined by blood or sputum cultures or histopathologic examination of a lung biopsy specimen. If methotrexate pneumonitis is suspected, methotrexate should be discontinued. Systemic corticosteroids are often required, and can be tapered over weeks to months.[246,248,249] Resumption of methotrexate is generally not recommended.

Tumor Necrosis Factor-α Blockade and Tuberculosis

Therapies aimed at inhibiting the proinflammatory effects of TNF-α have emerged as promising treatment options for children with JRA.[257,258] TNF-α inhibitors, such as etanercept, adalimumab, and infliximab, increase the risk of reactivation of latent tuberculosis.[259-262] This potential complication can be minimized with appropriate screening for tuberculosis. The clinical use of infliximab has been associated with rare reports of interstitial pneumonitis.[263,264]

Other Rheumatology Medications Associated with Pulmonary Disease

Cyclophosphamide, a cytotoxic agent that has been used in the treatment of organ-threatening rheumatic disease, can rarely cause interstitial pneumonitis.[265] Cases of cyclophosphamide-induced pulmonary fibrosis are confounded by the presence of an underlying disease with known pulmonary manifestations independent of medication exposure.[266] Leflunomide and sulfasalazine, drugs historically used in the treatment of inflammatory arthritis, are linked with the development of interstitial pneumonitis.[267-270] Similarly, azathioprine has been associated with interstitial pneumonitis, bronchiolitis, and diffuse alveolar

damage.[271] There have been reports of interstitial pneumonitis in patients with lymphoproliferative disease who were treated with the B cell–depleting agent rituximab.[272] Bronchiolitis has been described in patients exposed to penicillamine, a medication that is less commonly used today because of the availability of safer and more effective medications.[273,274] Gold salts, which are rarely prescribed in today's biologic era, have been associated with a pulmonary hypersensitivity reaction characterized by pulmonary infiltrates and peripheral eosinophilia.[274,275] Such complications are rare, and infectious processes are more frequently implicated as causing acute pulmonary exacerbations with accompanying radiographic changes.

Summary

The array of pediatric pulmonary complications of the various rheumatologic disorders illustrates the complexities and challenges of the underlying disorders and the continuing lack of detailed knowledge of the pathophysiology and optimal treatment paradigms in children. Although the vertical transfer of information of disease pathogenesis and management has made much progress from adult studies, such as with the diagnosis and management of PAH, there also is abundant evidence that in many instances the underlying disorders may differ in important and fundamental respects between children and adults. Recognition of pulmonary complications of rheumatic disorders in children is often more difficult and requires enlightened anticipation and a high index of suspicion. Further progress in understanding and treating the various pediatric disorders is hampered by the lack of pediatric-specific information.

Crucial to further progress are the expansion of orphan childhood disease databases and the expansion of the current pediatric rheumatology research groups to include a national clinical trials and outcomes effort. In this way, a comprehensive approach to determining basic natural history, risks, and outcomes and to defining the next generation of therapies in a disease-specific and age-specific manner can be achieved.

Acknowledgments

The authors gratefully acknowledge the assistance of Donald Frush, MD, in the preparation of the radiograph reproductions, and Alexander Spock, MD, in the preparation of the manuscript.

References

1. Delgado E, et al: The pulmonary manifestations of childhood onset systemic lupus erythematosus. Semin Arthritis Rheum 19:285-293, 1990.
2. Orens JB, Martinez FJ, Lynch JP 3rd: Pleuropulmonary manifestations of systemic lupus erythematosus. Rheum Dis Clin North Am 20:159-193, 1994.
3. Murin S, Wiedemann HP, Matthay RA: Pulmonary manifestations of systemic lupus erythematosus. Clin Chest Med 19:641-665, 1998.
4. Cervera R, et al: Systemic lupus erythematosus: Clinical and immunologic patterns of disease expression in a cohort of 1000 patients. Medicine 72:113-124, 1993.
5. Beresford MW, et al: Cardio-pulmonary involvement in juvenile systemic lupus erythematosus. Lupus 14:152-158, 2005.
6. Ciftci E, et al: Pulmonary involvement in childhood-onset systemic lupus erythematosus: A report of five cases, Rheumatology 43:587-591, 2004.
7. de Jongste JC, et al: Respiratory tract disease in systemic lupus erythematosus. Arch Dis Childhood 61:478-483, 1986.
8. Lilleby V, et al: Pulmonary involvement in patients with childhood-onset systemic lupus erythematosus. Clin Exp Rheumatol 24:203-208, 2006.
9. Nadorra RL, Landing BH: Pulmonary lesions in childhood onset systemic lupus erythematosus: Analysis of 26 cases, and summary of literature. Pediatr Pathol 7:1-18, 1987.
10. Miller LR, Greenberg SD, McLarty JW: Lupus lung. Chest 88:265-269, 1985.
11. Matthay RA, et al: Pulmonary manifestations of systemic lupus erythematosus: Review of twelve cases of acute lupus pneumonitis. Medicine 54:397-409, 1975.
12. Haupt HM, Moore GW, Hutchins GM: The lung in systemic lupus erythematosus: Analysis of the pathologic changes in 120 patients. Am J Med 71:791-798, 1981.
13. Inoue T, et al: Immunopathologic studies of pneumonitis in systemic lupus erythematosus, Ann Intern Med 91:30-34, 1979.
14. Matthay RA, Hudson LD, Petty TL: Acute lupus pneumonitis: Response to azathioprine therapy. Chest 63:117-120, 1973.
15. Zamora MR, et al: Diffuse alveolar hemorrhage and systemic lupus erythematosus: Clinical presentation, histology, survival, and outcome. Medicine 76:192-202, 1997.
16. Lee CK, et al: Pulmonary alveolar hemorrhage in patients with rheumatic diseases in Korea. Scand J Rheumatol 29:288-294, 2000.
17. Santos-Ocampo AS, Mandell BF, Fessler BJ: Alveolar hemorrhage in systemic lupus erythematosus: Presentation and management. Chest 118:1083-1090, 2000.
18. Eagen J, et al: Pulmonary hemorrhage in systemic lupus erythematosus. Medicine 57:545-560, 1978.
19. Boumpas DT, et al: Systemic lupus erythematosus: Emerging concepts, part 1: Renal, neuropsychiatric, cardiovascular, pulmonary, and hematologic disease. Ann Intern Med 122:940-950, 1995.
20. Holden M: Massive pulmonary fibrosis due to systemic lupus erythematosus. N Y State J Med 73:462-465, 1973.
21. Eisenberg H, et al: Diffuse interstitial lung disease in systemic lupus erythematosus. Ann Intern Med 79:37-45, 1973.
22. Weinrib L, Sharma OP, Quismorio FP Jr: A long-term study of interstitial lung disease in systemic lupus erythematosus. Semin Arthritis Rheum 20:48-56, 1990.
23. Eiser AR, Shanies HM: Treatment of lupus interstitial lung disease with intravenous cyclophosphamide. Arthritis Rheum 37:428-431, 1994.
24. Fink SD, Kremer JM: Successful treatment of interstitial lung disease in systemic lupus erythematosus with methotrexate. J Rheumatol 22:967-969, 1995.
25. Harris N: Antiphospholipid syndrome. In Klippel J, Dieppe P, eds: Rheumatology, Vol 2. London, Mosby, 1998, p 7351.
26. Khamashta M, et al: The management of thrombosis in the antiphospholipid-antibody syndrome. N Engl J Med 332:993-998, 1995.
27. Campos LM, et al: Antiphospholipid antibodies and antiphospholipid syndrome in 57 children and adolescents with systemic lupus erythematosus, Lupus 12:820-826, 2003.
28. Myones BL, McCurdy D: The antiphospholipid syndrome: Immunologic and clinical aspects: Clinical spectrum and treatment. J Rheumatol 27:20-28, 2000.
29. Gladman D, Sternberg L: Pulmonary hypertension in systemic lupus erythematosus. J Rheumatol 12:365-367, 1985.
30. Pan TL, Thumboo J, Boey ML: Primary and secondary pulmonary hypertension in systemic lupus erythematosus. Lupus 9:338-342, 2000.
31. Steen V, Medsger TA Jr: Predictors of isolated pulmonary hypertension in patients with systemic sclerosis and limited cutaneous involvement. Arthritis Rheum 48:516-522, 2003.
32. Allanore Y, et al: N-terminal pro-brain natriuretic peptide as a diagnostic marker of early pulmonary artery hypertension in patients with systemic sclerosis and effects of calcium-channel blockers. Arthritis Rheum 48:3503-3508, 2003.
33. Sanchez O, et al: Immunosuppressive therapy in connective tissue diseases-associated pulmonary arterial hypertension. Chest 130:182-189, 2006.
34. Jais X, et al: Immunosuppressive therapy in lupus- and mixed connective tissue disease-associated pulmonary arterial hypertension: A retrospective analysis of twenty-three cases. Arthritis Rheum 58:521-531, 2008.
35. Gibson G, Edmonds J, Hughes G: Diaphragm function and lung involvement in systemic lupus erythematosus. Am J Med 63:926-932, 1977.
36. Karim MY, et al: Presentation and prognosis of the shrinking lung syndrome in systemic lupus erythematosus. Semin Arthritis Rheum 31:289-298, 2002.
37. Hawkins P, et al: Diaphragm strength in acute systemic lupus erythematosus in a patient with

paradoxical abdominal motion and reduced lung volumes. Thorax 56:329-330, 2001.

38. Hardy K, et al: Bilateral phrenic paralysis in a patient with systemic lupus erythematosus. Chest 119:1274-1277, 2001.

39. Oud KT, et al: The shrinking lung syndrome in systemic lupus erythematosus: Improvement with corticosteroid therapy. Lupus 14:959-963, 2005.

40. Ferguson PJ, Weinberger M: Shrinking lung syndrome in a 14-year-old boy with systemic lupus erythematosus. Pediatr Pulmonol 41:194-197, 2006.

41. Min JK, et al: Bronchiolitis obliterans organizing pneumonia as an initial manifestation in patients with systemic lupus erythematosus. J Rheumatol 24:2254-2257, 1997.

42. Gammon RB, et al: Bronchiolitis obliterans organizing pneumonia associated with systemic lupus erythematosus. Chest 102:1171-1174, 1992.

43. Richardson B, Yung R: Drug-induced lupus. Rheum Dis Clin North Am 20:61-86, 1994.

44. Tiddens HA, et al: Juvenile-onset mixed connective tissue disease: Longitudinal follow-up. J Pediatr 122:191-197, 1993.

45. Singsen BH: Mixed connective tissue disease in childhood. Pediatr Rev 7:309-315, 1986.

46. Oetgen WJ, Boice JA, Lawless OJ: Mixed connective tissue disease in children and adolescents. Pediatrics 67:333-337, 1981.

47. Michels H: Course of mixed connective tissue disease in children. Ann Med 29:359-364, 1997.

48. Mier R, et al: Long term follow-up of children with mixed connective tissue disease. Lupus 5:221-226, 1996.

49. Hoffman RW, et al: U1-70-kd autoantibody-positive mixed connective tissue disease in children: A longitudinal clinical and serologic analysis. Arthritis Rheum 36:1599-1602, 1993.

50. Venables PJ: Mixed connective tissue disease. Lupus 15:132-137, 2006.

51. Burdt MA, et al: Long-term outcome in mixed connective tissue disease: Longitudinal clinical and serologic findings. Arthritis Rheum 42:899-909, 1999.

52. Kasukawa R, Tojo T, Miyawaki S: Preliminary diagnostic criteria for classification of mixed connective tissue disease. In Kasukawa R, Sharpe G, eds: Mixed Connective Tissue Disease and Antinuclear Antibodies. Amsterdam, Elsevier, 1987, p 41.

53. Prakash UB, Luthra HS, Divertie MB: Intrathoracic manifestations in mixed connective tissue disease. Mayo Clin Proc 60:813-821, 1985.

54. Prakash UB: Respiratory complications in mixed connective tissue disease. Clin Chest Med 19:733-746, 1998.

55. Prakash UB: Lungs in mixed connective tissue disease. J Thorac Imaging 7:55-61, 1992.

56. Bull TM, Fagan KA, Badesch DB: Pulmonary vascular manifestations of mixed connective tissue disease. Rheum Dis Clin North Am 31:451-464, 2005.

57. Derderian SS, et al: Pulmonary involvement in mixed connective tissue disease. Chest 88:45-48, 1985.

58. Sullivan WD, et al: A prospective evaluation emphasizing pulmonary involvement in patients with mixed connective tissue disease. Medicine 63:92-107, 1984.

59. Girod C: The lung in mixed connective tissue disease. Semin Respir Crit Care Med 20:99-108, 1999.

60. Ilan Y, et al: Mixed connective tissue disease presenting as a left sided pleural effusion. Ann Rheum Dis 51:1157-1158, 1992.

61. Bodolay E, et al: Evaluation of interstitial lung disease in mixed connective tissue disease (MCTD). Rheumatology 44:656-661, 2005.

62. Saito Y, et al: Pulmonary involvement in mixed connective tissue disease: Comparison with other collagen vascular diseases using high resolution CT. J Comput Assist Tomogr 26:349-357, 2002.

63. Wiener-Kronish JP, et al: Severe pulmonary involvement in mixed connective tissue disease. Am Rev Respir Dis 124:499-503, 1981.

64. Wigley FM, et al: The prevalence of undiagnosed pulmonary arterial hypertension in subjects with connective tissue disease at the secondary health care level of community-based rheumatologists (the UNCOVER study). Arthritis Rheum 52:2125-2132, 2005.

65. Kotajima L, et al: Clinical features of patients with juvenile onset mixed connective tissue disease: Analysis of data collected in a nationwide collaborative study in Japan. J Rheum 23:1088-1094, 1996.

66. Guit GL, et al: Mediastinal lymphadenopathy and pulmonary arterial hypertension in mixed connective tissue disease. Radiology 154:305-306, 1985.

67. Friedman DM, Mitnick HJ, Danilowicz D: Recovery from pulmonary hypertension in an adolescent with mixed connective tissue disease. Ann Rheum Dis 51:1001-1004, 1992.

68. Mier RJ, et al: Pediatric-onset mixed connective tissue disease. Rheum Dis Clin North Am 31:483-496, 2005.

69. Rosenberg AM, et al: Pulmonary hypertension in a child with mixed connective tissue disease. J Rheumatol 6:700-704, 1979.

70. Hosada T, et al: Mixed connective tissue disease with pulmonary hypertension: A clinical and pathological study. J Rheumatol 14:826-830, 1987.

71. Vegh J, et al: Clinical and immunoserological characteristics of mixed connective tissue disease associated with pulmonary arterial hypertension. Scand J Immunol 64:69-76, 2006.

72. Talal N: Sjögren's syndrome: Historical overview and clinical spectrum of disease. Rheum Dis Clin North Am 18:507-515, 1992.

73. Cassidy JT, Petty RE: Chronic arthritis in childhood. In Cassidy JT, Petty R, eds: Textbook of Pediatric Rheumatology, 5th ed. Philadelphia, WB Saunders, 2005, pp 206-260.

74. Horton MR: Rheumatoid arthritis associated interstitial lung disease. Crit Rev Comput Tomogr 45(5-6):429-440, 2004.

75. Shiel WC Jr, Prete PE: Pleuropulmonary manifestations of rheumatoid arthritis. Semin Arthritis Rheum 13:235-243, 1984.

76. Athreya BH, et al: Pulmonary manifestations of juvenile rheumatoid arthritis: A report of eight cases and review. Clin Chest Med 1:361-374, 1980.

77. Wagener JS, et al: Pulmonary function in juvenile rheumatoid arthritis. J Pediatr 99:108-110, 1981.

78. Yousefzadeh DK, Fishman PA: The triad of pneumonitis, pleuritis, and pericarditis in juvenile rheumatoid arthritis. Pediatr Radiol 8:147-150, 1979.

79. Tanoue LT: Pulmonary manifestations of rheumatoid arthritis. Clin Chest Med 19:667-685, 1998.

80. Biederer J, et al: Correlation between findings, pulmonary function tests and bronchoalveolar lavage cytology in interstitial lung disease associated with rheumatoid arthritis. Eur Radiol 14:272-280, 2004.

81. Dawson JK, et al: Fibrosing alveolitis in patients with rheumatoid arthritis as assessed by high resolution computed tomography, chest radiography, and pulmonary function tests. Thorax 56:622-627, 2001.

82. Lee HK, et al: Histopathologic pattern and clinical features of rheumatoid arthritis-associated interstitial lung disease. Chest 127:2019-2027, 2005.

83. Knook LM, et al: Lung function abnormalities and respiratory muscle weakness in children with juvenile chronic arthritis. Eur Respir J 14:529-533, 1999.

84. Lovell D, Lindsley C, Langston C: Lymphoid interstitial pneumonia in juvenile rheumatoid arthritis. J Pediatr 105:947-950, 1984.

85. Noyes BE, et al: Early onset of pulmonary parenchymal disease associated with juvenile rheumatoid arthritis. Pediatr Pulmonol 24:444-446, 1997.

86. Padeh S, et al: Primary pulmonary hypertension in a patient with systemic-onset juvenile arthritis. Arthritis Rheum 34:1575-1579, 1991.

87. Rohayem J, et al: Pulmonary fibrosis and other clinical manifestations of small vessel vasculitis in a family with seropositive juvenile rheumatoid arthritis. Pediatr Pulmonol 33:65-70, 2002.

88. Sohn DI, et al: Juvenile rheumatoid arthritis and bronchiolitis obliterans organized pneumonia. Clin Rheumatol 26:247-250, 2007.

89. Thomas E, et al: National study of cause-specific mortality in rheumatoid arthritis, juvenile chronic arthritis, and other rheumatic conditions: A 20 year followup study. J Rheumatol 30:958-965, 2003.

90. Uziel Y, et al: Lymphocytic interstitial pneumonitis preceding polyarticular juvenile rheumatoid arthritis. Clin Exp Rheumatol 16:617-619, 1998.

91. Schultz R, et al: Development of progressive pulmonary interstitial and intra-alveolar cholesterol granulomas (PICG) associated with therapy-resistant chronic systemic juvenile arthritis (CJA). Pediatr Pulmonol 32:397-402, 2001.

92. Zaglul H, Carswell F, Simpson RM: A case of persistent pulmonary functional abnormalities in systemic-onset juvenile chronic polyarthritis. Eur J Pediatr 138:315-316, 1982.

93. Dikensoy O, et al: Bronchiolitis obliterans in a case of juvenile rheumatoid arthritis presented with pneumomediastinum. Respiration 69:100-102, 2002.

94. Romicka A, Maldyk E: Pulmonary lesions in the course of rheumatoid arthritis in children. Pol Med Sci Hist Bull 15:263-268, 1975.

95. Harris ED, Ruddy S, Kelley WN, eds: Kelley's Textbook of Rheumatology. Philadelphia, WB Saunders, 2005.

96. Bowyer S, Roettcher P; for the Pediatric Rheumatology Database Research Group: Pediatric rheumatology clinic populations in the United States: Results of a 3 year survey. J Rheumatol 23:1968-1974, 1996.

97. Oen K, et al: Juvenile rheumatoid arthritis in a Canadian First Nations (aboriginal) population: Onset subtypes and HLA associations. J Rheumatol 25:783-790, 1998.

98. Turesson C, et al: Increased CD4[+] T cell infiltrates in rheumatoid arthritis-associated interstitial pneumonitis compared with idiopathic interstitial pneumonitis. Arthritis Rheum 52:73-79, 2005.

99. Atkins SR, et al: Morphologic and quantitative assessment of CD20[+] B cell infiltrates in rheumatoid arthritis-associated nonspecific interstitial pneumonia and usual interstitial pneumonia. Arthritis Rheum 54:635-641, 2006.

100. Cohen SB, et al: Rituximab for rheumatoid arthritis refractory to anti-tumor necrosis factor therapy: Results of a multicenter, randomized, double-blind, placebo-controlled, phase III trial evaluating primary efficacy and safety at twenty-four weeks. Arthritis Rheum 54:2793-2806, 2006.

101. Edwards JC, et al: Efficacy of B-cell-targeted therapy with rituximab in patients with rheumatoid arthritis. N Engl J Med 350:2572-2581, 2004.

102. Emery P, et al: The efficacy and safety of rituximab in patients with active rheumatoid arthritis despite methotrexate treatment: Results of a phase IIB randomized, double-blind, placebo-controlled, dose-ranging trial. Arthritis Rheum 54:1390-1400, 2006.

103. Lindenau S, et al: Aberrant activation of B cells in patients with rheumatoid arthritis. Ann N Y Acad Sci 987:246-248, 2003.

104. Atkins SR, et al: Morphological and quantitative assessment of mast cells in rheumatoid arthritis associated non-specific interstitial pneumonia and usual interstitial pneumonia. Ann Rheum Dis 65:677-680, 2006.

105. Foeldvari I, Wulffraat N: Recognition and management of scleroderma in children. Paediatr Drugs 3:575-583, 2001.

106. Vancheesware R, et al: Childhood onset scleroderma. Arthritis Rheum 39:1041-1049, 1996.

107. Zulian F, et al: Juvenile localized scleroderma: Clinical and epidemiological features in 750 children. Rheumatology 45:614-620, 2006.

108. Warrick JH, et al: High resolution computed tomography in early scleroderma lung disease. J Rheumatol 18:1520-1528, 1991.

109. Uziel Y, Miller ML, Laxer RM: Scleroderma in children. Pediatr Clin North Am 42:1171-1203, 1995.

110. Peterson LS, et al: The epidemiology of morphea (localized scleroderma) in Olmsted County 1960-1993. J Rheumatol 24:73-80, 1997.

111. Cassidy JT, et al, eds: Textbook of Pediatric Rheumatology. Philadelphia, WB Saunders, 2005.

112. Mayes MD: Scleroderma epidemiology. Rheum Dis Clin North Am 29:239-254, 2003.

113. Zulian F, et al: The Pediatric Rheumatology European Society/American College of Rheumatology/European League Against Rheumatism provisional classification criteria for juvenile systemic sclerosis. Arthritis Rheum 57:203-212, 2007.

114. Clements PJ, Medsger TA: Organ involvement: Skin. In Clements PJ, Furst DE, eds: Systemic Sclerosis. Baltimore, Williams & Wilkins, 1995, p 51.

115. Steen BD, Medsger TA: Severe organ involvement in systemic sclerosis with diffuse scleroderma. Arthritis Rheum 43:2437-2444, 2000.

116. Benan M, Hande I, Gul O: The natural course of progressive systemic sclerosis patients with interstitial lung involvement. Clin Rheumatol 26:349-354, 2007.

117. Varga J, Abraham D: Systemic sclerosis: A prototypic multisystem fibrotic disorder. J Clin Invest 117:557-567, 2007.

118. Kahaleh MC, Sherer GK, LeRoy EC: Endothelial injury in scleroderma. J Exp Med 149:1326-1335, 1979.

119. Wynn TA: Fibrotic disease and the T(H)1/T(H)2 paradigm. Nat Rev Immunol 4:583-594, 2004.

120. Hasegawa M, et al: B-lymphocyte depletion reduces skin fibrosis and autoimmunity in the tight-skin mouse model for systemic sclerosis. Am J Pathol 169:954-966, 2006.

121. Sakkas LI: New developments in the pathogenesis of systemic sclerosis. Autoimmunity 38:113-116, 2005.

122. Clements PJ: Systemic sclerosis (scleroderma) and related disorders: Clinical aspects. Balliere Clin Rheumatol 14:1-16, 2000.

123. Scire CA, et al: Shrinking lung syndrome in systemic sclerosis. Arthritis Rheum 48:2999-3000, 2003.

124. Naniwa R, Banno S, Suguira Y: Pulmonary-renal syndrome in systemic sclerosis: Report of three cases and review of the literature. Mod Rheumatol 17:37-44, 2007.

125. Harrison NK, et al: Pulmonary involvement in systemic sclerosis: The detection of early changes by thin section CT scan, bronchoalveolar lavage and 99mTc-DTPA clearance. Respir Med 83:403-414, 1989.

126. Harrison NK, et al: Evidence for protein oedema, neutrophil influx, and enhanced collagen production in lungs of patients with systemic sclerosis. Thorax 45:606-610, 1990.

127. Harrison NK, et al: Structural features of interstitial lung disease in systemic sclerosis. Am Rev Respir Dis 144:706-713, 1991.

128. Wells AU, et al: Fibrosing alveolitis in systemic sclerosis: Increase in memory T-cells in lung interstitium. Eur Respir J 8:266-271, 1995.

129. Lamblin C, et al: Interstitial lung diseases in collagen vascular diseases. Eur Respir J 18(Suppl 32):69s-80s, 2001.

130. Silver RM, et al: Evaluation and management of scleroderma lung disease using bronchoalveolar lavage. Am J Med 88:470, 1990.

131. White B, et al: Cyclophosphamide is associated with pulmonary function and survival benefit in patients with scleroderma and alveolitis. Ann Intern Med 132:947-954, 2000.

132. Seely JM, et al: Systemic sclerosis: Using high-resolution CT to detect lung disease in children. AJR Am J Roentgenol 170:691-697, 1998.

133. Garty BZ, et al: Pulmonary function in children with progressive systemic sclerosis. Pediatrics 88:1161-1167, 1991.

134. Remy-Jardin M, et al: Pulmonary involvement in progressive systemic sclerosis: Sequential evaluation with CT, pulmonary function tests and bronchoalveolar lavage. Radiology 188:499-506, 1993.

135. Wells AU, et al: Fibrosing alveolitis in systemic sclerosis. Arthritis Rheum 40:1229-1236, 1997.

136. White B: Interstitial lung disease in scleroderma. Rheum Dis Clin North Am 29:371-390, 2003.

137. Koh DM, Hansell DM: Computed tomography of diffuse interstitial lung disease in children. Clin Radiol 55:659-667, 2000.

138. Whitt C, et al: Pulmonary involvement in diffuse cutaneous systemic sclerosis: Bronchoalveolar fluid granulocytosis predicts progression of fibrosing alveolitis. Ann Rheum Dis 58:635-640, 1999.

139. Peterson MW, Monick M, Hunninghake GW: Prognostic role of eosinophils in pulmonary fibrosis. Chest 92:51-56, 1987.

140. BAL Cooperative Group Steering Committee: Bronchoalveolar lavage constituents in healthy individuals, idiopathic pulmonary fibrosis, and selected comparison groups. Am Rev Respir Dis 141:S169-S202, 1990.

141. Tashkin DP, et al: Cyclophosphamide versus placebo in scleroderma lung disease. N Engl J Med 354:2655-2666, 2006.

142. Goh NS, et al: Bronchoalveolar lavage cellular profiles in patients with systemic sclerosis-associated interstitial lung disease are not predictive of disease progression. Arthritis Rheum 56:2005-2012, 2007.

143. Strange C, et al: Bronchoalveolar lavage and response to cyclophosphamide in scleroderma interstitial lung disease. Am J Respir Crit Care Med 177:91-98, 2008.

144. Baughman RP, Raghu G: Bronchoalveolar cellular analysis in scleroderma lung disease: Does Sutton's law hold? Am J Respir Crit Care Med 177:2-3, 2008.

145. Mittoo S, et al: Persistence of abnormal bronchoalveolar lavage findings after cyclophosphamide treatment in scleroderma patients with interstitial lung disease.Arthritis Rheum 56:4195-4202, 2007.

146. Wells AU, et al: High resolution computed tomography as a predictor of lung histology in systemic sclerosis. Thorax 47:738-742, 1992.

147. Wells AU, et al: Serial CT in fibrosing alveolitis: Prognostic significance of the initial pattern. AJR Am J Roentgenol 161:1159-1165, 1993.

148. Wechsler RJ, et al: The relationship of thoracic lymphadenopathy to pulmonary interstitial disease in diffuse and limited systemic sclerosis: CT findings. AJR Am J Roentgenol 167:101-104, 1996.

149. Galie N, et al; for the Task Force on Diagnosis and Treatment of Pulmonary Arterial Hypertension of the European Society of Cardiology: Guidelines on diagnosis and treatment of pulmonary arterial hypertension. Eur Heart J 25:2243-2278, 2004.

150. Launay D, et al: High resolution computed tomography in fibrosing alveolitis associated with systemic sclerosis. J Rheumatol 34:1005-1011, 2007.

151. Silver RM: Scleroderma clinical problems: The lungs. Rheum Dis Clinic North Am 22:825-840, 1996.

152. Fagan KA, Badesch DB: Pulmonary hypertension associated with connective tissue disorders. Prog Cardiovasc Dis 45:225-234, 2002.

153. Mehta S, Little S: Screening for pulmonary hypertension in scleroderma: How and when to look. J Rheumatol 33:204-206, 2006.

154. Rich S, et al: Primary pulmonary hypertension: A national prospective study. Ann Intern Med 107:216-223, 1987.

155. Steen V, Medsger TA: Predictors of isolated pulmonary hypertension in patients with systemic sclerosis and limited cutaneous involvement. Arthritis Rheum 48:516-522, 2000.

156. Ahearn GS, et al: Electrocardiography to define clinical status in primary pulmonary hypertension and pulmonary arterial hypertension secondary to collagen vascular disease. Chest 122:524-527, 2002.

157. Bull TM: Screening and therapy of pulmonary hypertension in systemic sclerosis. Curr Opin Rheumatol 19:598-603, 2007.

158. Mukerjee D, et al: Echocardiography and pulmonary function as screening tests for pulmonary arterial hypertension in systemic sclerosis. Rheumatology 43:461-466, 2004.

159. Zulian F: Systemic sclerosis and localized scleroderma in childhood. Rheum Dis Clin North Am 34:239-255, 2008.

160. Hsaio SH, et al: Right heart function in scleroderma: Insights from myocardial Doppler tissue imaging. J Am Soc Echocardiogr 19:507-514, 2006.

161. Tashkin DP, et al: Cyclophosphamide versus placebo in scleroderma lung disease. N Engl J Med 354:2655-2666, 2006.

162. Khanna D, et al: Impact of oral cyclophosphamide on health-related quality of life in patients with active scleroderma lung disease. Arthritis Rheum 56:1676-1684, 2007.

163. Gerbina AJ, Goss CH, Molitor JA: Effect of mycophenolate mofetil on pulmonary function in scleroderma-associated interstitial lung disease. Chest 133:455-460, 2008.

164. Liossis SNC, Bounas A, Andonopoulos AP: Mycophenolate mofetil as first-line treatment improves clinically evident early scleroderma lung disease. Rheumatology 45:1005-1008, 2006.

165. Galie N, et al: Guidelines on the diagnosis and treatment of pulmonary arterial hypertension. Eur Heart J 25:2243-2278, 2004.

166. Beghetti M: Current treatment options in children with pulmonary arterial hypertension and experiences with oral bosentan. Eur J Clin Invest 36 (Suppl 3):25-31, 2006.

167. Fathi M, et al: Interstitial lung disease, a common manifestation of newly diagnosed polymyositis and dermatomyositis. Ann Rheum Dis 63: 297-301, 2004.

168. Schnabel A, et al: Interstitial lung disease in polymyositis and dermatomyositis: Clinical course and response to treatment. Semin Arthritis Rheum 32:273-284, 2003.

169. Cassidy JT, Petty RE: Juvenile ankylosing spondylitis. In Cassidy JT, Petty R, eds: Textbook of Pediatric Rheumatology, 5th ed. Philadelphia, WB Saunders, 2005, p 304.

170. Rosenberg AM, Petty RE: A syndrome of seronegative enthesopathy and arthropathy in children. Arthritis Rheum 25:1041-1047, 1982.

171. Cabral DA, Oen KG, Petty RE: SEA syndrome revisited: A long term followup of children with a syndrome of seronegative enthesopathy and arthropathy. J Rheumatol 19:1282-1285, 1992.

172. Petty RE, et al: Revision of the proposed classification criteria for juvenile idiopathic arthritis: Durban, 1998. J Rheumatol 25: 1991-1994, 1998.

173. Rosenow EC, et al: Pleuropulmonary manifestations of ankylosing spondylitis. Mayo Clin Proc 52:641-649, 1977.

174. Feltelius N, et al: Pulmonary involvement in ankylosing spondylitis. Ann Rheum Dis 45:736-740, 1986.

175. Camiciottoli G, et al: Pulmonary function in children affected by juvenile spondyloarthropathy. J Rheumatol 26:1382-1386, 1999.

176. Cabral DA, Malleson PN, Petty RE: Spondyloarthropathies of childhood. Pediatr Clin North Am 42:1051-1070, 1995.

177. Camiciottoli G, et al: Pulmonary function in children affected by juvenile spondyloarthropathy. J Rheumatol 26:1382-1386, 1999.

178. Sampaio-Barros PD, et al: Pulmonary involvement in ankylosing spondylitis. Clin Rheumatol 26: 225-230, 2007.

179. Ayhan-Ardic FF, et al: Pulmonary involvement in lifelong non-smoking patients with rheumatoid arthritis and ankylosing spondylitis without respiratory symptoms. Clin Rheumatol 25:213-218, 2006.

180. Kiris A, et al: Lung findings on high resolution CT in early ankylosing spondylitis. Eur J Radiol 47: 71-76, 2003.

181. Baser S, et al: Pulmonary involvement starts in early stage ankylosing spondylitis. Scand J Rheumatol 325-327, 2006.

182. Maghraoui AE, et al: Lung findings on thoracic high-resolution computed tomography in patients with ankylosing spondylitis: Correlations with disease duration, clinical findings and pulmonary function testing. Clin Rheumatol 23: 123-128, 2004.

183. Altin R, et al: Comparison of early and late pleuropulmonary findings of ankylosing spondylitis by high-resolution computed tomography and effects on patients' daily life. Clin Rheumatol 24:22-28, 2005.

184. Feltelius N, et al: Pulmonary involvement in ankylosing spondylitis. Ann Rheum Dis 45:736-740, 1986.

185. Cohen AA, Natelson EA, Fechenr RE: Fibrosing interstitial pneumonitis in ankylosing spondylitis. Chest 59:369-371, 1971.

186. Lee C-C, et al: Spontaneous pneumothorax associated with ankylosing spondylitis. Rheumatology 44:1538-1541, 2005.

187. Quismorio FP: Pulmonary involvement in ankylosing spondylitis. Curr Opin Pulm Med 12:342-345, 2006.

188. Kchir MM, et al: Bronchoalveolar lavage and transbronchial biopsy in spondyloarthropathies. J Rheumatol 913-916, 1992.

189. DeRemee RA: Concise review for primary care physicians: Sarcoidosis. Mayo Clin Proc 70: 177-181, 1995.

190. Henry MM, Noah TL: Sarcoidosis. In Chernick V, et al, eds: Kendig's Disorders of the Respiratory Tract in Children, 7th ed. Philadelphia, WB Saunders, 2006, p 927.

191. Abernathy RS: Sarcoidosis. In Hilman B, ed: Pediatric Respiratory Disease. Philadelphia, WB Saunders, 1993, p 305.

192. Harris C, et al: Rare diagnosis: Sarcoid arthritis in four children. JAMA 197:31, 1966.

193. Hetherington S: Sarcoidosis in young children. Am J Dis Child 136:13-15, 1982.

194. Blau EB: Familial granulomatous arthritis, iritis and rash. J Pediatr 107:689-693, 1985.

195. Becker ML, Rosé CD: Blau syndrome and related genetic disorders causing childhood arthritis. Curr Rheumatol Rep 7:427-433, 2005.

196. Rosé CD, et al: Pediatric granulomatous arthritis: An international registry. Arthritis Rheum 54:3337-3344, 2006.

197. Kanazawa N, et al: Early-onset sarcoidosis and CARD15 mutations with constitutive nuclear factor-κB activation: Common genetic etiology with Blau syndrome. Blood 105:1195-1197, 2004.

198. Tsagris VA, Liapi-Adamidou G: Sarcoidosis in infancy: A case with pulmonary involvement as a cardinal manifestation. Eur J Paediatr 158: 258-260, 1999.

199. Becker ML, et al: Interstitial pneumonitis in Blau syndrome with documented mutation in CARD15. Arthritis Rheum 56:1292-1294, 2007.

200. Milman N, et al: Blau-syndrome associated mutations in exon 4 of the caspase activating recruitment domain (CARD 15) gene are not found in ethnic Danes with sarcoidosis. Clin Respir J 1:74-79, 2007.
201. Schürmann M, et al: CARD15 gene mutations in sarcoidosis. Eur Respir J 22:748-754, 2003.
202. Akahoshi M, et al: Mutation screening of the CARD15 gene in sarcoidosis. Tissue Antig 71:564-567, 2008.
203. Lindsley CB, Laxer RM: Granulomatous vasculitis, giant cell arteritis and sarcoidosis. In Cassidy JT, Petty R, eds: Textbook of Pediatric Rheumatology, 5th ed. Philadelphia, WB Saunders, 2005, p 539.
204. Patishall EN, Kendig EL Jr: Sarcoidosis in children. Pediatr Pulmonol 22:195-203, 1996.
205. James DG, ed: Sarcoidosis and Other Granulomatous Disorders. New York, Marcel Dekker, 1994.
206. McGovern JP, Merritt DH: Sarcoidosis in childhood. Adv Pediatr 8:97-135, 1956.
207. Robinson PJ, Olinsky A: Sarcoidosis in children. Compr Ther 8:63-68, 1982.
208. Abernathy RS: Childhood sarcoidosis in Arkansas. South Med J 78:435-439, 1985.
209. Heatherington SV: Sarcoidosis in children. Compr Ther 8:63-68, 1982.
210. Kendig EL, Brummer DL: The prognosis of sarcoidosis in children. Chest 70:351-353, 1976.
211. Jasper PL, Denny FW: Sarcoidosis in children: With special emphasis on the natural history and treatment. J Pediatr 73:499-512, 1968.
212. Siltzbach LE, Greenberg GM: Childhood sarcoidosis—a study of 18 patients. N Engl J Med 279:1239-1245, 1968.
213. Hoffman AL, Milman N, Byg K-E: Childhood sarcoidosis in Denmark 1979-1994: Incidence, clinical features and laboratory results at presentation in 48 children. Acta Paediatr 93:30-36, 2004.
214. Patishall EN, et al: Childhood sarcoidosis. J Pediatr 108:169-177, 1986.
215. Patishall EN, Kendig EL Jr: Sarcoidosis in children. In James DG, ed: Sarcoidosis and Other Granulomatous Disorders. New York, Marcel Dekker, 1994, p 387.
216. Ibid.
217. Conron M, DuBois RM: Immunological mechanisms in sarcoidosis. Clin Exp Allergy 31:543-554, 2001.
218. Cimaz R, Ansell BM: Sarcoidosis in the pediatric age. Clin Exp Rheumatol 20:231-237, 2002.
219. Baculard A, et al: Pulmonary sarcoidosis in children: A follow-up study. Eur Respir J 17:628-635, 2001.
220. Sharma OP: Sarcoidosis. Dis Monthly 36:471-535, 1990.
221. James DG, et al: A world view of sarcoidosis. Ann N Y Acad Sci 278:321-332, 1976.
222. Kravitz RM: Sarcoidosis. In Burg FB, et al, eds: Gellis and Kagan's Current Pediatric Therapy, 2nd ed. Philadelphia, WB Saunders, 1999, p 547.
223. Conron M, Du Bois RM: Immunologic mechanisms in sarcoidosis. Clin Exp Allergy 31:543-554, 2001.
224. Baughman PR: Therapeutic options for sarcoidosis: New and old. Curr Opin Pulm Med 8:464-469, 2002.
225. Marcille R, et al: Long-term outcome of pediatric sarcoidosis with emphasis on pulmonary status. Chest 102:1444-1449, 1992.
226. Abehsara M, et al: Sarcoidosis with pulmonary fibrosis: CT patterns and correlation with pulmonary function. AJR Am J Roentgenol 174:1751-1757, 2000.
227. Statement on sarcoidosis: Joint Statement of the American Thoracic Society (ATS), the European Respiratory Society (ERS) and the World Association of Sarcoidosis and other Granulomatous Disorders (WASOG) adopted by the ATS Board of Directors and by the ERS Executive Committee, February 1999. Am J Respir Crit Care Med 160:736-755, 1999.
228. Winterbauer RH, Hutchinson JF: Use of pulmonary function tests in the management of sarcoidosis. Chest 78:640-647, 1980.
229. Levinson RS, et al: Airway function in sarcoidosis. Am J Med 62:51-59, 1977.
230. Pattishall EN, Strope GL, Denny FW: Pulmonary function in children with sarcoidosis. Am Rev Respir Dis 133:94-96, 1986.
231. Bechtel JJ, et al: Airway hyperreactivity in patients with sarcoidosis. Am Rev Respir Dis 124:759-761, 1981.
232. Torrington KG, Shorr AF, Parker JW: Endobronchial disease and racial differences in pulmonary sarcoidosis. Chest 111:619-622, 1997.
233. Tabak L, et al: The value of labial biopsy in the differentiation of sarcoidosis from tuberculosis. Sarcoidosis Vasc Diffuse Lung Dis18:191-195, 2001.
234. Lieberman J: Angiotensin-converting enzyme and serum lysozyme. In Lieberman J, ed: Sarcoidosis. Orlando, Grune & Stratton, 1986, p 145.
235. Schorr AF, Torrington KG, Parker JM: Serum angiotensin converting enzyme does not correlate with radiographic stage at initial diagnosis of sarcoidosis. Respir Med 91:399-401, 1997.
236. Brunner J, School-Burgi S, Zimmerhackl L-B: Chitotriosidase as a marker of disease activity in sarcoidosis. Rheumatol Int 27:1171-1172, 2007.
237. Costabel U: Sensitivity and specificity of BAL findings in sarcoidosis. Sarcoidosis 9(Suppl 1):211-214, 1992.
238. Grutters JC, van den Bosch JMM: Corticosteroid treatment in sarcoidosis. Eur Resp J 28:627-636, 2006.
239. Merten DF, Kirks DR, Grossman H: Pulmonary sarcoidosis in childhood. AJR Am J Roentgenol 135:673-679, 1980.
240. Silverman E, et al: Leflunomide or methotrexate for juvenile rheumatoid arthritis. N Engl J Med 352:1655-1666, 2005.
241. Wallace CA: The use of methotrexate in childhood rheumatic diseases. Arthritis Rheum 41:381-391, 1998.
242. Cottin V, et al: Pulmonary function in patients receiving long-term low-dose methotrexate. Chest 109:933-938, 1996.
243. Hilliquin P, et al: Occurrence of pulmonary complications during methotrexate therapy in rheumatoid arthritis. Br J Rheumatol 35:441-445, 1996.
244. Imokawa S, et al: Methotrexate pneumonitis: Review of the literature and histopathological findings in nine patients. Eur Respir J 15:373-381, 2000.
245. Ohosone Y, et al: Clinical characteristics of patients with rheumatoid arthritis and methotrexate induced pneumonitis. J Rheumatol 24:2299-2303, 1997.
246. Zisman DA, et al: Drug-induced pneumonitis: The role of methotrexate. Sarcoidosis Vasc Diffuse Lung Dis 18:243-252, 2001.

247. Alarcon GS, et al: Risk factors for methotrexate-induced lung injury in patients with rheumatoid arthritis: A multicenter, case-control study. Methotrexate-Lung Study Group. Ann Intern Med 127:356-364, 1997.
248. Cron RQ, Sherry DD, Wallace CA: Methotrexate-induced hypersensitivity pneumonitis in a child with juvenile rheumatoid arthritis. J Pediatr 132: 901-902, 1998.
249. Kremer JM, et al: Clinical, laboratory, radiographic, and histopathologic features of methotrexate-associated lung injury in patients with rheumatoid arthritis: A multicenter study with literature review. Arthritis Rheum 40:1829-1837, 1997.
250. Schnabel A, et al: Bronchoalveolar lavage cell profile in methotrexate induced pneumonitis. Thorax 52:377-379, 1997.
251. White DA, et al: Methotrexate pneumonitis: Bronchoalveolar lavage findings suggest an immunologic disorder. Am Rev Respir Dis 139:18-21, 1989.
252. Camiciottoli G, et al: Effect on lung function of methotrexate and non-steroid anti-inflammatory drugs in children with juvenile rheumatoid arthritis. Rheumatol Int 18:11-16, 1998.
253. Graham LD, et al: Morbidity associated with long-term methotrexate therapy in juvenile rheumatoid arthritis. J Pediatr 120:468-473, 1992.
254. Pelucchi A, et al: Lung function and diffusing capacity for carbon monoxide in patients with juvenile chronic arthritis: Effect of disease activity and low dose methotrexate therapy. Clin Exp Rheumatol 12:675-679, 1994.
255. Schmeling H, et al: Pulmonary function in children with juvenile idiopathic arthritis and effects of methotrexate therapy. Z Rheumatol 61:168-172, 2002.
256. Searles G, McKendry RJ: Methotrexate pneumonitis in rheumatoid arthritis: Potential risk factors: Four case reports and a review of the literature. J Rheumatol 14:1164-1171, 1987.
257. Horneff G, et al: The German etanercept registry for treatment of juvenile idiopathic arthritis. Ann Rheum Dis 63:1638-1644, 2004.
258. Lovell DJ, et al; for the Pediatric Rheumatology Collaborative Study Group: Etanercept in children with polyarticular juvenile rheumatoid arthritis. N Engl J Med 342:763-769, 2000.
259. Gomez-Reino JJ, et al: Treatment of rheumatoid arthritis with tumor necrosis factor inhibitors may predispose to significant increase in tuberculosis risk: A multicenter active-surveillance report. Arthritis Rheum 48:2122-2127, 2003.
260. Keane J, et al: Tuberculosis associated with infliximab, a tumor necrosis factor alpha-neutralizing agent. N Engl J Med 345:1098-1104, 2001.
261. Wallis RS, et al: Granulomatous infectious diseases associated with tumor necrosis factor antagonists. Clin Infect Dis 38:1261-1265, 2004.
262. Winthrop KL, et al: Tuberculosis associated with therapy against tumor necrosis factor alpha. Arthritis Rheum 52:2968-2974, 2005.
263. Takeuchi T, et al: Postmarketing surveillance of the safety profile of infliximab in 5000 Japanese patients with rheumatoid arthritis. Ann Rheum Dis 67:189-194, 2008.
264. Villeneuve E, St-Pierre A, Haraoui B: Interstitial pneumonitis associated with infliximab therapy. J Rheumatol 33:1189-1193, 2006.
265. Spector JI, Zimbler H, Ross JS: Early-onset cyclophosphamide-induced interstitial pneumonitis. JAMA 242:2852-2854, 1979.
266. Stentoft J: Progressive pulmonary fibrosis complicating cyclophosphamide therapy. Acta Med Scand 221:403-407, 1987.
267. Hamadeh MA, Atkinson J, Smith LJ: Sulfasalazine-induced pulmonary disease. Chest 101:1033-1037, 1992.
268. McCurry J: Japan deaths spark concerns over arthritis drug. Lancet 363:461, 2004.
269. Suissa S, Hudson M, Ernst P: Leflunomide use and the risk of interstitial lung disease in rheumatoid arthritis. Arthritis Rheum 54:1435-1439, 2006.
270. Wolfe F, Caplan L, Michaud K: Rheumatoid arthritis treatment and the risk of severe interstitial lung disease. Scand J Rheumatol 36:172-178, 2007.
271. Ananthakrishnan AN, et al: Severe pulmonary toxicity after azathioprine/6-mercaptopurine initiation for the treatment of inflammatory bowel disease. J Clin Gastroenterol 41:682-688, 2007.
272. Wagner SA, Mehta AC, Laber DA: Rituximab-induced interstitial lung disease. Am J Hematol 82:916-919, 2007.
273. Murphy KC, et al: Obliterative bronchiolitis in two rheumatoid arthritis patients treated with penicillamine. Arthritis Rheum 24:557-560, 1981.
274. O'Duffy JD, et al: Bronchiolitis in a rheumatoid arthritis patient receiving auranofin. Arthritis Rheum 29:556-559, 1986.
275. Podell TE, et al: Pulmonary toxicity with gold therapy. Arthritis Rheum 23:347-350, 1980.

CHAPTER 11

Pulmonary Manifestations
of Systemic Vasculitis

BRIAN P. O'SULLIVAN AND TED KREMER

Definition of Vasculitis 241
Specific Vasculitis Syndromes 244
  Pulmonary-Renal Syndromes 244
  Henoch-Schönlein Purpura 246
  Wegener Granulomatosis 247
  Microscopic Polyangiitis 249

Churg-Strauss Syndrome 250
Behçet Disease 251
Takayasu Arteritis 252
Idiopathic Pulmonary-Renal Syndrome 253
Summary 254
  References 254

The pulmonary vasculitides are a heterogeneous group of primary or secondary diseases, in which there is inflammation that may lead to progressive destruction of the pulmonary microvasculature. Pulmonary involvement may develop because the lung has an extensive vascular and microvascular network, sensitizing antigens can easily reach the lung, and there are large numbers of vasoactive and activated immune cells in the lung. Primary or isolated pulmonary vasculitis is extremely rare in children. Pulmonary vasculitis is an unusual condition in children and is almost always seen in conjunction with a systemic vasculitis syndrome. This chapter reviews common systemic vasculitides associated with pulmonary disease and discusses presentation, diagnosis, and therapy.

Definition of Vasculitis

Before embarking on a discussion of specific illnesses associated with inflammation of blood vessels and pulmonary involvement, clarifying what is meant by "vasculitis," how vasculitides may manifest systemically, and some of the serologic markers associated with these diseases is in order. Simply defined, vasculitis is inflammation of the walls of blood vessels. Perivascular cuffing is not a vasculitis. The involved vessels may be arteries, veins, or capillaries; large,

medium-sized, or small arteries may be involved; the infiltrate may be neutrophils, lymphocytes, eosinophils, or plasma cells; the inflammation may be necrotizing or granulomatous; there may or may not be immune complex deposition or antineutrophil antibodies. All of these characteristics determine the specific type of vasculitis.

A definite diagnosis cannot be made without tissue biopsy, although several clinical syndromes are fairly typical and should suggest what type of pathology one is likely to see. The clinical and pathologic features vary, and depend on the site and type of blood vessel involved. Although many vasculitides affect adults and children, some, such as Kawasaki disease, occur almost exclusively in children. Other vasculitides, such as temporal arteritis, rarely, if ever, occur in childhood, and others, such as polyarteritis and Wegener granulomatosis, have different etiologic, clinical, and prognostic characteristics in children.[1] It was thought inappropriate to continue applying the adult classification criteria to vasculitis occurring in childhood. The newly adopted classification for childhood vasculitides comes from the consensus criteria endorsed by the European League Against Rheumatism and the Pediatric Rheumatology European Society (Table 11-1).[1]

Despite extensive investigation, the pathogenesis of vascular inflammation is unknown in most cases. Vasculitis probably results from

Table 11-1	New Classification of Childhood Vasculitis

I. Predominantly large vessel vasculitis
   A. Takayasu arteritis
II. Predominantly medium-sized vessel vasculitis
   A. Kawasaki disease
   B. Childhood polyarteritis nodosa
   C. Cutaneous polyarteritis
III. Predominantly small vessel vasculitis
   A. Granulomatous
      1. Wegener granulomatosis
      2. Churg-Strauss syndrome
   B. Nongranulomatous
      1. Henoch-Schönlein purpura
      2. Microscopic polyangiitis
      3. Isolated cutaneous leukocytoclastic vasculitis
      4. Hypocomplementemic urticarial vasculitis
IV. Other vasculitides
   A. Behçet disease
   B. Vasculitis secondary to infection (including hepatitis B–associated polyarteritis nodosa), malignancies, and drugs (including hypersensitivity vasculitis)
   C. Vasculitis associated with connective tissue diseases
   D. Isolated vasculitis of the central nervous system
   E. Cogan syndrome
   F. Unclassified

the combination of multiple risk factors, including genetic predisposition, environmental factors (infection and inhalation of particulate matter), and chance. Figure 11-1 shows the distribution of vasculitis type in vessels of various sizes. There is a great deal of overlap regarding which vessels are involved in some common vasculitides, notably Wegener granulomatosis and microscopic polyangiitis.[2] Large vessel vasculitides, such as giant cell arteritis and Takayasu arteritis, do not cause much pulmonary disease because the intrapulmonary vessels are medium-sized arteries or smaller. Medium-sized vessel arteritides include polyarteritis nodosa. Classic polyarteritis nodosa is uncommon in children and generally not associated with lung disease,[3] although case reports of lung disease in association with polyarteritis

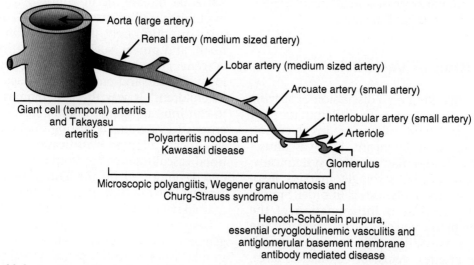

Figure 11-1. Spectrum of systemic vasculitides organized according to predominant size of vessels affected. (*From Savage COS, et al: ABC of arterial and vascular disease: Vasculitis. BMJ 320:1325-1328, 2000.*)

nodosa and Kawasaki disease have been published.[4-6] The small vessel variant of polyarteritis nodosa, microscopic polyangiitis, is associated with lung disease and is discussed in detail subsequently.

Typically, patients with small vessel vasculitides present with pulmonary manifestations. These include Wegener granulomatosis, microscopic polyangiitis, Henoch-Schönlein purpura, Churg-Strauss syndrome, and Goodpasture syndrome.

Systemic manifestations of vasculitides include malaise, fever, weight loss, joint pain, kidney disease, and skin rash.[2] Diagnosis of a specific vasculitis syndrome depends on clinical and serologic characteristics.

Typical vasculitis syndromes are associated with deposition of immune complexes in blood vessel walls.[7] Goodpasture syndrome is the classic example of IgA-related complex deposition. A subset of small vessel vasculitides has minimal immune-complex deposition in vessel walls. These so-called pauci-immune vasculitides include Wegener granulomatosis, microscopic polyangiitis, Churg-Strauss syndrome, and renal-limited vasculitis. Small amounts of immune complexes form on the surfaces of blood vessels in these diseases, but differ from larger vessel vasculitides in that there is not the gross accumulation of immune complexes seen in the large vessel diseases; also, the small vessel vasculitides are associated with a greater degree of necrotizing injury. The precise cause of tissue injury in Wegener granulomatosis and microscopic polyangiitis is uncertain, but there is a strong association between disease activity and the presence of antineutrophil cytoplasmic antibodies (ANCA).

There is mounting evidence that ANCA play a causative role in Wegener granulomatosis and microscopic polyangiitis (Fig. 11-2).[7] A strong case can be made that the presence of ANCA directly leads to disease based on several lines of evidence. First, an infant who was born to a mother with high circulating levels of ANCA developed pulmonary hemorrhage and glomerulonephritis within days of birth.[8] The infant's serum was ANCA-positive. Treatment with corticosteroids and exchange transfusion brought the disease into remission. Second, neutrophils that have been activated by ANCA-IgG kill cultured endothelial cells.[9] Third, monocytes and neutrophils interact with ANCA, and monocyte-derived mediators of inflammation can damage vessel walls further.[10] Finally, glomerulonephritis has been precipitated in several murine models with transfer of ANCA-IgG.[7] Taken together, these findings indicate that the presence of ANCA may be toxic to blood vessels and precipitate disease.

ANCA come in two forms, and the nomenclature has become confused as more has been learned about these antibodies. Initially, the designations used for ANCA-IgG were P-ANCA (for perinuclear staining) and C-ANCA (for cytoplasmic staining) when anti-ANCA antibodies were used to detect the presence and location of intracellular ANCA (Fig. 11-3). These older terms have been replaced by more precise terms based on the specific antigens against which ANCA is directed. The target for P-ANCA is

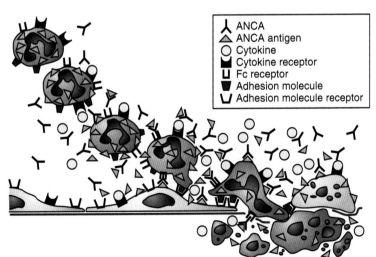

ANCA	ANCA
ANCA antigen	ANCA antigen
Cytokine	Cytokine
Cytokine receptor	Cytokine receptor
Fc receptor	Fc receptor
Adhesion molecule	Adhesion molecule
Adhesion molecule receptor	Adhesion molecule receptor

Figure 11-2. Events in the pathogenesis of antineutrophil cytoplasmic antibody (ANCA) small vessel vasculitis that have been observed in vitro. Beginning in the top left and moving to the right, cytokines or other priming factors induce neutrophils to express more ANCA antigens at the cell surface, where they are available for binding to ANCA, which activates neutrophils. Neutrophils that have been activated by ANCA interact with endothelial cells via adhesion molecules and release toxic factors that cause apoptosis and necrosis. (*From Jennette JC, Xiao H, Falk RJ: Pathogenesis of vascular inflammation by anti-neutrophil cytoplasmic antibodies. J Am Soc Nephrol 17:1235-1242, 2006.*)

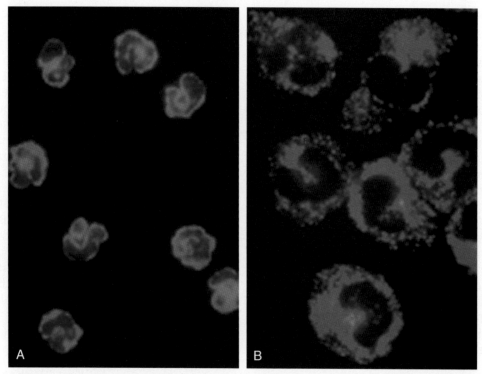

Figure 11-3. A and **B,** Indirect immunofluorescence staining showing perinuclear antineutrophilic cytoplasmic antibody (**A**) and cytoplasmic antineutrophilic cytoplasmic antibody (**B**) distribution. (See Color Plate)

most frequently myeloperoxidase (MPO) (although some other antigens have been reported), and the target for C-ANCA is proteinase-3 (PR3).[7,11] On activation, neutrophil cytoplasmic granules move to the cell surface where expression of MPO and PR3 antigens allows association with circulating ANCA. ANCA activation of neutrophils requires antigen binding and Fc-receptor engagement. Levels of PR3 antigen expression may be genetically determined, making some individuals more prone to ANCA-associated diseases than others.[12]

Consistent with the association of these two ANCA with different disease processes, internalization of MPO-ANCA and PR3-ANCA causes different cellular responses. MPO-ANCA causes generation of intracellular oxidants, whereas PR3-ANCA causes endothelial cell apoptosis.[7] MPO-ANCA and PR3-ANCA activate neutrophils to release mediators of acute inflammation.

Indirect immunofluorescence and enzyme-linked immunosorbent assay tests for ANCA are available. It is recommended that a combination of these tests be used if the diagnosis of an ANCA-associated vasculitis is suspected.

Positive ANCA by indirect immunofluorescence alone is not specific for systemic vasculitis; a positive indirect immunofluorescence test can be seen in patients with systemic lupus erythematosus, rheumatoid arthritis, Felty syndrome, ulcerative colitis, and other multisystem conditions.[13] It is imperative also to employ the enzyme-linked immunosorbent assay test, which differentiates PR3-ANCA from MPO-ANCA. This distinction is important because, as noted before, different ANCA may be associated with various disease processes. ANCA-associated diseases are the same in children as in adults.[14]

Specific Vasculitis Syndromes

Pulmonary-Renal Syndromes

Numerous disorders affect the small vessels of the lungs and the kidneys. These conditions are associated most often with a combination of pulmonary hemorrhage and nephritis. Pulmonary hemorrhage may not be obvious, and can manifest simply as diffuse, patchy pulmonary infiltrates on a chest radiograph in a child who has unexplained anemia. Although easy to diagnose when the lungs and kidneys are affected simultaneously, in all of these syndromes there may be temporal separation of specific organ involvement.

The pulmonary-renal syndromes consist of Henoch-Schönlein purpura, Wegener granulomatosis, microscopic polyangiitis, Churg-Strauss syndrome, Goodpasture syndrome, and systemic lupus erythematosus.[15] All of these entities are associated with an inflammatory component, and children affected by them generally have an elevated erythrocyte sedimentation rate and other serum markers of inflammation. Table 11-2 highlights the clinical and laboratory features of these syndromes. The pulmonary manifestations of systemic lupus erythematosus are discussed in detail in Chapter 10 and are not reiterated here.

All of the pulmonary-renal syndromes occur with a low frequency in childhood. The most common small vessel vasculitis in childhood, Henoch-Schönlein purpura, has the lowest incidence of associated pulmonary disease, and all the other forms of vasculitis in childhood are quite rare in general, so despite the fact that they are commonly associated with lung disease, they are still unusual causes of pulmonary hemorrhage. When a pulmonary-renal syndrome does occur, however, it can be devastating. Pulmonary hemorrhage can be massive and life-threatening, and usually

manifests as anemia in association with pulmonary infiltrates on chest radiographs (Fig. 11-4). Glomerulonephritis can be sudden and severe with little prodrome. Early treatment with anti-inflammatory agents is lifesaving, so a high degree of suspicion for and rapid recognition of this syndrome are key.[16]

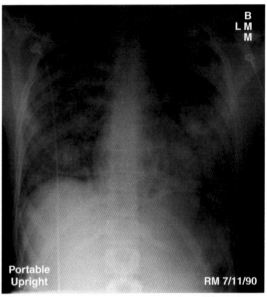

Figure 11-4. Chest x-ray shows patchy infiltrates caused by pulmonary hemorrhage in a 16-year-old boy with perinuclear antineutrophilic cytoplasmic antibody-positive pulmonary-renal syndrome. The patient had a hemoglobin of 4.1 g/dL with a hematocrit of 11.5% at the time of presentation.

Table 11-2	Clinical and Serologic Findings in Patients with Pulmonary-Renal Syndromes*				
	HSP	**GPS**	**WG**	**MPA**	**SLE**
Pulmonary hemorrhage	0 to +	++++	+++	+++	+ to ++
Glomerulonephritis	++++	++++	++++	++++	+++ to ++++
Upper airway involvement	0	0	++++	++	+ to ++
Skin rash	++++	0 to +	+++	+++	++++
Arthralgia	++++	0	+++	+++	++++
Elevated ESR	+	0	++++	++++	++++
Abdominal involvement	++++	0	0	0	0
Serology	IgA positive, IgM positive	Anti-GBM (rarely P-ANCA)	C-ANCA (rarely P-ANCA)	P-ANCA, C-ANCA	ANA, anti–double-stranded DNA (rarely P-ANCA)

*0 = not present; increasing association with increasing number of + signs.
ANA, antinuclear antibody; C-ANCA, cytoplasmic antineutrophilic cytoplasmic antibody; ESR, erythrocyte sedimentation rate; GBM, glomerular basement membrane; GPS, Goodpasture syndrome; HSP, Henoch-Schönlein purpura; MPA, microscopic polyangiitis; P-ANCA, perinuclear antineutrophilic cytoplasmic antibody; SLE, systemic lupus erythematosus; WG, Wegener granulomatosis.

Any child with anemia and pulmonary infiltrates must be suspected of having pulmonary hemorrhage, be it idiopathic, traumatic, or due to small vessel vasculitis.[17] The skin also should be examined for signs of cutaneous vasculitis (palpable purpura, erythema nodosum, ulceration, splinter hemorrhages),[18] and the nose, ears, and nasopharynx and oropharynx should be examined for the presence of bleeding or granuloma. When the diagnosis of small vessel vasculitis is being considered, urine sediment must be evaluated for the presence of cellular casts and protein. Serum creatinine levels can be maintained in the normal range even in the face of glomerular injury, so waiting for an increase in serum urea and creatinine unduly delays the diagnosis.

Henoch-Schönlein Purpura

Henoch-Schönlein purpura is the most common form of small vessel vasculitis in childhood. Its incidence is estimated to be 10 to 14 per 100,000, with boys affected twice as frequently as girls. In the United States, the prevalence peaks in children 5 years old. Approximately 75% of cases occur in children 2 to 11 years old. Henoch-Schönlein purpura is rare in infants and young children.

The etiology of Henoch-Schönlein purpura is largely unknown, although it commonly follows an upper respiratory tract infection. Group A streptococcus has been implicated as a trigger for Henoch-Schönlein purpura because many patients with Henoch-Schönlein purpura have elevated antistreptolysin O antibodies. The pathophysiology of Henoch-Schönlein purpura is not fully understood, but IgA plays a crucial role in the immunopathogenesis, as evidenced by increased serum IgA concentrations, IgA-containing circulating immune complexes, and IgA immune complex deposition in vessel walls and renal mesangium. Henoch-Schönlein purpura is almost exclusively associated with abnormalities involving IgA1, rather than IgA2. IgA-negative biopsies occur in 10% to 25% of cases of Henoch-Schönlein purpura, although it is possible that these IgA-negative cases represent other, unidentified vasculitic syndromes misdiagnosed as Henoch-Schönlein purpura because of overlapping features.

The classic presentation includes erythematous papules followed by nonthrombocytopenic palpable purpura in the lower extremities, trunk, and face; arthralgia or arthritis; abdominal pain; gastrointestinal bleeding; and nephritis. Renal involvement occurs in approximately 60% of cases and leads to a significant degree of morbidity (Table 11-3).

Although renal abnormalities in Henoch-Schönlein purpura are common, the classic pulmonary manifestations, such as diffuse alveolar hemorrhage and interstitial pneumonitis, are thought to be infrequent. Subclinical pulmonary manifestations, including diffusion defects and radiographic anomalies, seem to be quite frequent in patients with Henoch-Schönlein purpura, but are not commonly reported. Other respiratory manifestations include pleural effusion and chylothorax. Diffuse alveolar hemorrhage is the most frequent pulmonary complication associated with Henoch-Schönlein purpura, but, as previously noted, pulmonary hemorrhage is rare in these patients, although it has been reported.[19,20]

Pulmonary hemorrhage is secondary to disruption of the alveolar-capillary membranes by circulating immune complexes. In a series reported from the Mayo Clinic of 28 patients with pulmonary involvement in Henoch-Schönlein purpura, 18 patients were 20 years old or younger. Of these patients, 26 had diffuse alveolar hemorrhage, 5 of whom had associated pleural effusions; 9 patients died (3 children).[21] The youngest reported patient with pulmonary disease associated with Henoch-Schönlein purpura was a 5-month-old infant who died

Table 11-3	Classification Criteria for Henoch-Schönlein Purpura

At least one of the following four conditions should be present
  Diffuse abdominal pain
  Any biopsy specimen showing predominant IgA deposition
  Arthritis or arthralgia
  Renal involvement (any hematuria or proteinuria or both)
In the presence of palpable purpura (*mandatory criterion*)

of complications associated with diffuse alveolar hemorrhage and interstitial fibrosis.[22]

The clinical presentation of patients with Henoch-Schönlein purpura complicated by diffuse alveolar hemorrhage may vary. Typically, these patients are diagnosed with Henoch-Schönlein purpura before the onset of pulmonary symptoms. Some patients may develop milder pulmonary symptoms, such as cough, which may be associated with blood-tinged sputum and crackles on lung auscultation. Other patients progress to dyspnea at rest, hemoptysis, and occasionally respiratory failure requiring intubation and ventilatory support. Blood loss into the lungs may be severe enough to require transfusion therapy. Chest radiographs show diffuse pulmonary infiltrates secondary to alveolar hemorrhage. Bronchoscopy is useful only if uncertainty exists regarding pulmonary hemorrhage versus infection as the cause of the physical examination and radiologic abnormalities. Lung biopsy is rarely needed because affected tissue generally can be obtained from less dangerous biopsy sites (skin or kidney).

Treatment of Henoch-Schönlein purpura almost always includes the use of corticosteroids. Prednisone, 1 to 2 mg/kg/day, is the initial choice. Cyclophosphamide, 2 to 3 mg/kg/day, commonly is added in cases involving severe pulmonary hemorrhage. Length of therapy depends on the time to resolution of symptoms and radiographic clearance of pulmonary infiltrates. Supportive care, including mechanical ventilation, is often necessary in cases with severe alveolar damage.

Although clinically important pulmonary disease is rare in Henoch-Schönlein purpura, even patients without respiratory symptoms have objective signs of mild lung abnormalities. In a cohort of children with Henoch-Schönlein purpura free of clinical pulmonary symptoms, patients were noted to have an impaired diffusing capacity for carbon monoxide. In this study, 70% of the patients had radiographic evidence for mild interstitial lung changes.[23] In another group of children with Henoch-Schönlein purpura who had no evidence for lung disease clinically or radiographically, the finding of an abnormal diffusing capacity for carbon monoxide was again seen.[24]

Wegener Granulomatosis

Wegener granulomatosis is a necrotizing granulomatous vasculitis with a broad spectrum of findings and progression. Wegener granulomatosis and microscopic polyangiitis are extremely similar diseases with great overlap in clinical and pathologic presentations. As such, it has been suggested now to combine these diseases under the rubric, "ANCA-associated small vessel vasculitis." These two entities are discussed separately here partly for historical reasons and partly because there remain many clinical studies that focus on either one or the other of these entities. Practically, it might be impossible to distinguish Wegener granulomatosis from microscopic polyangiitis, however, even with tissue biopsy. What looks to be microscopic polyangiitis initially may prove to be Wegener granulomatosis later, when manifestations in other organs become apparent, and granulomas are present. The overlap in serology between these two entities is highlighted in Table 11-3.

Wegener granulomatosis is uncommon in children; its peak incidence is in adults in their 60s and 70s. The etiology of Wegener granulomatosis is unknown, and it does not have specific genetic markers. In adults, systemic Wegener granulomatosis is noted for its severity and high mortality.[25] Still, Wegener granulomatosis has been reported in children; as in adults, it generally manifests with the triad of upper airway, lower airway, and renal involvement. Children frequently present with cough, sinus pain, fever, arthralgias or arthritis, hemoptysis, and skin rashes or ulceration. Cutaneous manifestations may precede other systemic symptoms by months and occur most commonly on the legs. The predominant skin finding is palpable purpura, but lesions may be vesicular, papular, or nodular, and even urticaria has been reported.[18] Upper airway manifestations of Wegener granulomatosis include rhinorrhea, purulent or bloody discharge, persistent otitis media, sinusitis, saddle-nose deformity, subglottic stenosis, and tracheal stenosis.[26] Renal involvement may occur early or late in the course, and when present, it requires aggressive management to avoid rapid progression to end-stage renal disease.

The American College of Rheumatology criteria require the presence of two of the following four criteria for the diagnosis of Wegener granulomatosis: nasal-oral inflammation, abnormal findings on chest radiograph, abnormal urinalysis, and granulomatous inflammation on biopsy specimen.[1] The presence of subglottic, tracheal, or endobronchial stenosis, and the presence of a high titer of PR3 or positive C-ANCA staining have been included more recently in the diagnostic criteria.[1] The new classification of a child as having Wegener granulomatosis requires the presence of three of the newly established criteria of six (Table 11-4).

Pulmonary disease develops in nearly 75% of children with Wegener granulomatosis.[27] The clinical spectrum of pulmonary involvement in Wegener granulomatosis includes cough, sinusitis, chest pain, pleuritis, or hemoptysis. In children, densities on the chest radiograph of an asymptomatic patient may be the first sign of disease. One third of all abnormal chest radiographs in children with Wegener granulomatosis are not associated with pulmonary symptoms. Radiographic findings frequently include transient or persistent infiltrates and nodules, whereas focal atelectasis, pleural effusion, pulmonary hemorrhage, and mediastinal or hilar lymph node enlargement are less common.[28]

The precise radiographic findings in children are difficult to state because there are no large case series in children younger than 18 years old. Wadsworth and colleagues[29] reported diffuse interstitial and alveolar infiltrates secondary to diffuse alveolar hemorrhage as the most consistent finding in a group of 11 children with Wegener granulomatosis (7 of 11). Of the other four, one child had a thick-walled cavitary lesion, and another child had bilateral nodules. Computed tomography (CT) scans of the sinuses and of the chest are helpful for diagnosis. CT virtual bronchoscopy (high-resolution helical CT with three-dimensional reconstruction) allows visualization of central airway stenosis with high specificity, but low sensitivity; it does not eliminate the need for bronchoscopy.

The diagnosis of Wegener granulomatosis may be made histologically or serologically in the right clinical setting. Histologic changes are patchy, making false-negative biopsy results owing to sampling error possible. The accuracy of the biopsy depends on the site, disease activity, and amount of tissue obtained. Given the presence of skin, kidney, or upper airway lesions in many patients with Wegener granulomatosis, biopsy of these areas, where diagnostic findings may occur and where the risk of the procedure is low, is preferred. In some cases, lung biopsy may be necessary, however. Bronchoscopic transbronchial biopsy is not recommended because the likelihood of obtaining a diagnostic specimen is low. Open lung biopsy always is risky, and this may be especially true in the pulmonary vasculitides. Surgical pathology of the lung in Wegener granulomatosis shows three characteristic changes: (1) parenchymal necrosis, (2) vasculitis, and (3) granulomatous inflammation.[31] Figure 11-5 shows the pathogenesis of the vasculitis and granuloma formation in Wegener granulomatosis.

Serologic diagnosis of Wegener granulomatosis depends on testing for ANCA. ANCA directed at PR3 are found in 70% to 90% of patients with active Wegener granulomatosis.[32] In the appropriate clinical setting, the positive predictive value of positive PR3 ANCA approaches 99%. In the appropriate circumstance, patients can be treated for Wegener granulomatosis on the basis of positive ANCA without obtaining tissue for diagnosis.[33] MPO-ANCA may be positive in Wegener granulomatosis, although this is much less common. The accuracy of any diagnostic test is based on pretest

Table 11-4	Classification Criteria for Wegener Granulomatosis

Three of the following six conditions should be present
  Abnormal urinalysis*
  Granulomatous inflammation on biopsy specimen
  Nasal-sinus inflammation
  Subglottic, tracheal, or endobronchial stenosis
  Abnormal chest x-ray or CT scan of the chest
  High titer of proteinase-3 or positive C-ANCA staining

*If kidney biopsy is performed, it characteristically shows necrotizing pauci-immune glomerulonephritis.
C-ANCA, cytoplasmic antineutrophilic cytoplasmic antibody.

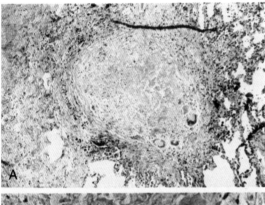

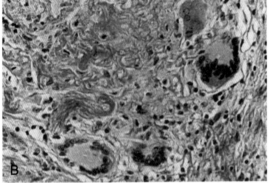

Figure 11-5. Photomicrographs of lung biopsy specimen from a patient with Wegener granulomatosis. **A,** Necrotizing granulomatous vasculitis with destruction of vessel wall and obliteration of lumen. **B,** Granulomatous inflammation with multinucleated giant cells. (*From Curg A, Brallas, Metal. Am Rev Respir Dis 134:149-166, 1986.*)

probability. Positive ANCA in a patient with few or no clinical signs or symptoms of Wegener granulomatosis or microscopic polyangiitis should be interpreted with caution.

Wegener granulomatosis shows significant pulmonary morbidity. Pulmonary function tests may show obstructive defects in 55% of cases; such defects are often caused by endobronchial lesions and scarring, whereas restrictive defects and reduced lung volumes or diffusing capacity for carbon monoxide may be found in 30% to 40% of cases. Sinus or pulmonary infections may mask the diagnosis or be found at the time of the initial evaluation. Similar findings often occur during treatment. Pneumonia accounts for 40% of serious infections and is associated with significant mortality.

The effective management of Wegener granulomatosis requires early diagnosis, close patient follow-up, and careful attention to potential treatment complications. Therapy is usually initiated with high-dose

prednisone (2 mg/kg/day) and oral daily cyclophosphamide (2 mg/kg/day). High-dose prednisone is maintained until active disease manifestations have decreased, and then it is tapered, depending on disease activity. Therapy with cyclophosphamide is continued for at least 1 year after achieving complete remission, and is then tapered. Intravenous gamma globulin has been used successfully in some cases refractory to above-mentioned therapy.[34] If the disease is in remission, further switching of therapy to azathioprine has proved efficacious in adults and is worth trying in children.[34]

Prophylaxis with trimethoprim-sulfamethoxazole is now commonly prescribed for children with Wegener granulomatosis. Use of such an aggressive regimen has improved the prognosis for adults and children with Wegener granulomatosis. It seems that Wegener granulomatosis associated with the presence of PR3-ANCA has an earlier response to therapy than MPO-ANCA-associated disease.[35] A significant portion of pediatric patients are still subject to chronic morbidity and mortality.[27] Persistence of granuloma may be the root of relapses in Wegener granulomatosis, and much work is ongoing to uncover the driving force behind this persistence and means of eradicating the granuloma.[25]

Microscopic Polyangiitis

Microscopic polyangiitis is a necrotizing pauci-immune vasculitis affecting predominantly small vessels and is often associated with a high titer of MPO-ANCA or positive P-ANCA staining.[1] Microscopic polyangiitis, similar to Wegener granulomatosis, can be associated with crescentic glomerulonephritis and hemorrhagic pulmonary capillaritis. Microscopic polyangiitis has an incidence of approximately 1:100,000 in the general population with mean age of onset of about 50 years.[36] Microscopic polyangiitis is more prevalent than Wegener granulomatosis,[37] although both are quite rare in adults and rarer yet in children.

Pulmonary involvement occurs in one quarter to one third of patients with microscopic polyangiitis.[38] There may be a long delay between onset of symptoms and diagnosis because of the nonspecific characteristic of many of the symptoms.[39] In one case series of adults with microscopic polyangiitis selected for the presence of alveolar hemorrhage, renal signs were present in 97% of patients, showing a strong concordance between renal and lung disease when the latter is present.[39]

Microscopic polyangiitis can present very similarly to Wegener granulomatosis, but without granuloma formation or nasopharyngeal/large airway involvement. As with any patient with vasculitis, systemic manifestations, such as fever, weight loss, asthenia, myalgias, and arthralgias, are common. Isolated pulmonary hemorrhage may occur, but most patients with alveolar-capillary hemorrhage have extrathoracic manifestations.[38] Interstitial fibrosis may predate the onset of pulmonary vasculitis by years and can be the initial manifestation of microscopic polyangiitis.[40] In classic microscopic polyangiitis, chest radiographic abnormalities reflect pulmonary hemorrhage with the major finding being patchy, bilateral airspace opacities. The nodules seen in Wegener granulomatosis are not present in microscopic polyangiitis because of the lack of granuloma formation. A study looking at CT findings in 51 patients who had MPO-ANCA-positive microscopic polyangiitis showed ground-glass attenuation in greater than 90% with areas of consolidation and bronchovascular thickening in many of these patients. Pathologic correlation showed that these findings were due to pulmonary hemorrhage, interstitial inflammation, and fibrosis.[41]

Serologic diagnosis is less certain with microscopic polyangiitis than with Wegener granulomatosis. Although most patients with microscopic polyangiitis are MPO-ANCA-positive, PR3-ANCA may be present in 40%, and 10% of patients with microscopic polyangiitis may be ANCA-negative (Table 11-5).[38]

Treatment of microscopic polyangiitis is the same as for Wegener granulomatosis—a combination of corticosteroids, cyclophosphamide, and azathioprine. Disease relapses are common within the first 2 years of diagnosis. The risk of death from microscopic polyangiitis is greater in patients who are PR3-ANCA-positive and is increased if pulmonary hemorrhage is present.[39]

Churg-Strauss Syndrome

Churg-Strauss syndrome is another pauci-immune pulmonary-renal syndrome. Churg-Strauss syndrome is defined as an ANCA-associated, eosinophil-rich granulomatous disease involving the respiratory tract, notably the lungs and sinuses. The hallmark of Churg-Strauss syndrome is its association with peripheral blood eosinophilia and asthma; this is accompanied by extravascular granulomas and a necrotizing vasculitis affecting small to medium-sized vessels.[1,42] The triad of tissue infiltration by eosinophils, necrotizing vasculitis, and extravascular granulomas is rarely seen simultaneously, and the three are found together in only a few patients.[42] Because of its rarity, the prevalence and incidence of Churg-Strauss syndrome in children are unknown.

Diagnosis of Churg-Strauss syndrome is based on criteria developed by the American College of Rheumatology (Table 11-6). For classification purposes, a patient is said to have Churg-Strauss syndrome if at least four of these six criteria are positive. The presence of any four or more of the six criteria yields a diagnostic sensitivity of 85% and a specificity of greater than 99%.[43]

Churg-Strauss syndrome occurs in phases, with the prodromal phase including rhinitis and asthma, the second phase including

Table 11-5	Distribution of ANCA Serology in Wegener Granulomatosis and Microscopic Polyangiitis	
ANCA RESULT	**WEGENER GRANULOMATOSIS**	**MICROSCOPIC POLYANGIITIS**
Positive PR3 ANCA/C-ANCA	65–70%	35–45%
Positive MPO ANCA/P-ANCA	15–25%	45–55%
Negative ANCA	10–20%	10–20 %

ANCA, antineutrophilic cytoplasmic antibody; C-ANCA, cytoplasmic antineutrophilic cytoplasmic antibody; MPO, myeloperoxidase; P-ANCA, perinuclear antineutrophilic cytoplasmic antibody; PR3, proteinase-3.

Table 11-6	Criteria for the Classification of Churg-Strauss Syndrome

Asthma
Eosinophilia >10%
Neuropathy—mononeuropathy or polyneuropathy
Pulmonary infiltrates, nonfixed
Paranasal sinus abnormality
Extravascular eosinophils

peripheral blood and tissue eosinophilia, and the third phase consisting of systemic vasculitis. Asthma and sinusitis may precede the onset of vasculitis by many years. Pericarditis, myocarditis, and tamponade may be seen in the vasculitis phase of the disease, and occur in approximately half of all patients with Churg-Strauss syndrome. In one series, congestive heart failure and myocardial infarction were responsible for nearly half of deaths from Churg-Strauss syndrome.[44]

Boyer and colleagues[45] reported two pediatric patients with Churg-Strauss syndrome presenting with prominent pulmonary involvement. One, a 16-year-old with a previous history of asthma, presented with pleuritic chest pain and a peripheral pulmonary nodule complicated by an eosinophilic pleural effusion. The other patient presented at age 6 with cough, weight loss, and radiographic infiltrates. Lung biopsy specimens revealed elements characteristic of Churg-Strauss syndrome, including eosinophilic microabscesses and vasculitis. There has been an increase in reported cases of pediatric Churg-Strauss syndrome in more recent years, but whether this reflects a true increased incidence or rather heightened diagnostic suspicion is unclear. The youngest children reported to have Churg-Strauss syndrome were 2 years old.[45] In contrast to adult patients with Churg-Strauss syndrome, in whom MPO-ANCA positivity is common, children with Churg-Strauss syndrome are generally ANCA-negative. ANCA testing should be done in any child for whom the diagnosis is considered, but a negative test does not exclude the diagnosis.

Cutaneous findings are common in Churg-Strauss syndrome, occurring in one half to three quarters of patients.[42] These lesions

represent the small vessel involvement, with purpura and subcutaneous nodules being most common. Such lesions are a common early presenting symptom of the vasculitis phase in children.[45] Mononeuritis multiplex is seen in many adults with Churg-Strauss syndrome; optic neuritis also is reported.

Pulmonary findings beyond the presence of asthma include abnormal chest radiographs with patchy infiltrates. During the second phase of the illness, when tissue eosinophilia is present, radiographs may have the appearance of chronic eosinophilic pneumonia. Pleural effusion has been reported in 25% to 50% of adults.[42] Renal involvement in Churg-Strauss syndrome is less severe and prominent than in Wegener granulomatosis. Although pulmonary vasculitis is present, diffuse alveolar hemorrhage is not as prominent in Churg-Strauss syndrome as in the other pulmonary-renal syndromes.[46]

Asthma and eosinophilia are common findings in children. The diagnosis of Churg-Strauss syndrome is considered when more involved pulmonary disease (including pleuritis) occurs, or when other signs of systemic vasculitis, such as cutaneous lesions, cardiomyopathy, nephritis, or neuropathy, become manifest. Laboratory studies suggestive of Churg-Strauss syndrome include eosinophilia, elevated erythrocyte sedimentation rate, and, in some patients, positive MPO-ANCA. Because of the lack of specificity of these findings, tissue diagnosis is often necessary. Biopsy of low-risk, easily accessible lesions such as skin lesions is preferable. If the only organ involved with systemic vasculitis is the lung, a transbronchial biopsy can be performed, but the small sample of tissue obtained from a child should not be considered sufficient to rule out the diagnosis if it is negative for eosinophilic vasculitis or granuloma. In these rare cases, a video-assisted thoracoscopic biopsy may be necessary.

Behçet Disease

Behçet disease is a chronic, multisystem, inflammatory disease that classically manifests with a clinical triad of relapsing ulcers of the mouth, genital ulcers, and uveitis/iritis.[34] It also may manifest with systemic features, including arthritis, thrombophlebitis migrans, erythema nodosum, meningoencephalitis, and arterial aneurysms. The incidence in the United States is estimated at 7.5 per 100,000 with approximately 1% to 2% of patients being children. Behçet disease may be diagnosed at any age, but the peak age of onset is between the second and fourth decades of life. Male-to-female ratio is equal. An important feature for making the diagnosis in children is a positive family history.[34] Multiple organs are usually involved, including the skin, central nervous system, gastrointestinal tract, genitourinary system, joints, heart, and lungs. Histologically, an extensive vasculitis occurs, affecting arteries and veins of all sizes. Immune complex disease in large vessels leads to aneurysm formation or thrombosis. Pulmonary artery involvement is the most severe complication of the disease.

The etiology of Behçet disease is unknown, although a genetic predisposition associated with a trigger such as an infectious agent or environmental exposure likely results in the onset of the disease. The finding of HLA-B51 immunogenetics supports the diagnosis.[47] More severe cases are noted in young men diagnosed before age 25 years. Typically, the course is relapsing and remitting.

Lung disease occurs in 1% to 5% of cases.[48] Pulmonary involvement in Behçet disease varies greatly and includes findings such as pulmonary artery aneurysm, pulmonary artery thrombosis, and pleural and parenchymal abnormalities. Pulmonary artery aneurysm is a rare complication of Behçet disease, but the lung is the second most common site for aneurysms after the aorta. The most common clinical presentation is hemoptysis resulting from rupture of the aneurysm and erosion into a bronchus. Other clinical findings include cough, chest pain, and dyspnea. Hemoptysis can be misdiagnosed as a pulmonary embolism because deep venous thrombosis and abnormal ventilation/perfusion scans are often seen in patients with Behçet disease. Embolism of thrombi to the lung is actually quite rare in Behçet disease because thrombi in inflamed veins are highly adherent to the vessel wall and rarely migrate.

Thrombosis of aneurysms in the pulmonary artery may occur, leading to infarction of downstream pulmonary parenchyma. Thrombus formation may occur in other major vessels, including the superior and inferior vena cavae.

Chest radiographs are abnormal in 90% of cases, with pleural effusion in 70%, diffuse bilateral infiltrates in 37%, right lower lobe infiltrate in 28%, hilar vascular prominence in 14%, and round densities in 10% of cases.[48] Pulmonary artery aneurysms appear as hilar enlargement on radiographic studies. Helical CT of the chest is the preferred method for diagnosis of aneurysms because angiography may cause trauma to arteries and lead to additional aneurysm formation.

Pulmonary parenchyma and pleural involvement in Behçet disease are usually attributed to pulmonary hemorrhage or infarction or both. Findings include focal or diffuse alveolar infiltrates, wedge-shaped or linear shadows, volume loss, and ill-defined reticular or nodular opacities of the parenchyma or pleura. Pleural effusions secondary to pulmonary infarction, pleural vasculitis, or superior vena cava thrombosis may occur. The literature includes one case report of organizing pneumonia associated with pulmonary artery aneurysm.

Treatment for patients with Behçet disease and pulmonary complications often involves a combination of corticosteroids and cyclophosphamide. Anticoagulant and thrombolytic therapy should be used with caution because hemorrhage from an existing pulmonary artery aneurysm is a risk. Autologous stem cell transplantation has been used successfully for therapy of Behçet disease in two patients (32 years old and 49 years old) with pulmonary involvement presenting with hemoptysis and pulmonary artery aneurysms resistant to conventional therapy.[49] The duration of remission at the time of this report was greater than 5 years.

Takayasu Arteritis

Takayasu arteritis is a chronic inflammatory and obliterative disease of large vessels, with preference for the aorta and its major branches. Table 11-7 lists more recently

Table 11-7	Classification Criteria for Takayasu Arteritis

At least one of the following four conditions should be present

   Decreased peripheral artery pulses or claudication of extremities or both

   Blood pressure difference >10 mm Hg

   Bruits over aorta or its major branches or both

   Hypertension (related to childhood normative data)

In the presence of angiographic abnormalities (on radiography, CT, or MRI) of aorta or its main branches (*mandatory criterion*)

published diagnostic criteria.[1] This vasculitis is more commonly found in Asian and Indian populations, with a female-to-male ratio of 2.5:1, and is rarely found in other populations. One third of cases occur before age 20 years, and symptoms usually appear after age 10 years.

Early disease manifestations (pre-pulseless phase) include night sweats, weight loss, myalgias, and arthritis, often followed by unexplained hypertension. During the pulseless phase, systemic symptoms are very common. Skin manifestations include erythema nodosum, malar rash, and erythema induratum. Cardiac involvement includes dilated cardiomyopathy, myocarditis, and pericarditis. Other associated conditions include interstitial lung disease and pneumonic consolidation. Pulmonary artery involvement may occur, but is an infrequent presenting sign.

The presence of intermittent unexplained systemic symptoms of variable duration with a significantly elevated erythrocyte sedimentation rate (≥ 60 mm/hr) and a hypochromic microcytic anemia with leukocytosis should prompt periodic auscultation of large arteries and blood pressure measurements in all four limbs. A polyclonal hypergammaglobulinemia is present in one third of the cases. Complement activation results in elevated levels of C3a and C5a, which may be used to guide therapy.

The diagnosis is confirmed by angiography, which often outlines a massively dilated aortic arch, with aneurysmal dilation and stenosis of various large vessels—carotid, subclavian, or abdominal aorta. Magnetic resonance angiography may be helpful as a noninvasive test for subsequent monitoring of affected vessels.

Early identification and surgical resection of the predominant lesions are essential, in conjunction with appropriate immunosuppressive therapy. Prevention of chronic hypertension and decreased perfusion sometimes can be accomplished by excision of a stenotic area with graft replacement or stent insertion to prevent restenosis.

Idiopathic Pulmonary-Renal Syndrome

The term "idiopathic pulmonary-renal syndrome" has been applied to a group of poorly defined disorders characterized by unexplained pulmonary hemorrhage and rapidly progressive glomerulonephritis without other organ involvement.[52] Pulmonary capillaritis with diffuse alveolar hemorrhage is almost always present in these patients. Many of these cases are associated with P-ANCA and no other identifying markers. Idiopathic pulmonary renal syndrome likely represents many different disease processes not clearly defined. Although an uncommon association, pulmonary fibrosis and hemorrhage can occur with juvenile rheumatoid arthritis and is presumably secondary to rheumatoid-associated small vessel vasculitis.[53,54]

Cases of diffuse alveolar hemorrhage with isolated pulmonary vasculitis *without* evidence of systemic disease and *without* positive ANCA serology have been reported.[55] In this one case series, eight patients had pulmonary capillaritis, but none of the eight had glomerulonephritis or other systemic disease, and none had remarkable serologic studies (i.e., all relevant serologies were negative). We provide care for one child with a similar presentation. She had isolated pulmonary hemorrhage with profound anemia and respiratory failure at age 3. Open lung biopsy showed the presence of small vessel vasculitis. She has had mildly elevated erythrocyte sedimentation rate (26 to 34 mm/hr) and multiple negative ANCA studies without any signs of kidney disease. She has done well on long-term anti-inflammatory therapy, initially consisting of corticosteroids and cyclophosphamide, which has been successfully changed to azathioprine (unpublished report). Not all small vessel vasculitis need be associated with systemic disease or positive ANCA serology.

Summary

Vasculitis is an infrequent but serious cause of lung disease in children. When present, it can have a fulminating, life-threatening course. Diagnosis often can be made on the basis of clinical presentation and serologic studies, but biopsy of skin, nose, kidney, or lung may be necessary to ascertain the precise syndrome. Pulmonary vasculitis is generally seen in association with systemic disease; however, primary pulmonary vasculitis has been reported.

The respiratory system may be involved in all systemic vasculitides, although with a variable frequency. Lung disease is an important feature of the ANCA-associated systemic vasculitides, such as Wegener granulomatosis, Churg-Strauss syndrome, and microscopic polyangiitis. In Wegener granulomatosis, almost all patients have either upper airway or lower respiratory tract disease. Solitary or multiple nodules and masses are the most common findings on chest radiograph. Asthma is a cardinal symptom of Churg-Strauss syndrome, often preceded by allergic rhinitis, frequently complicated by sinusitis. Pulmonary transient and patchy alveolar infiltrates are the most common radiographic findings. In microscopic polyangiitis, diffuse alveolar hemorrhage owing to alveolar capillaritis is the most frequent manifestation of the respiratory involvement, with clinical signs of hemoptysis, respiratory distress, and anemia. Diffuse alveolar hemorrhage may be subclinical, however, and has to be suspected when chest radiograph shows new unexplained bilateral alveolar infiltrates, in the face of declining hemoglobin levels.

References

1. Ozen S, et al: EULAR/PRES endorsed consensus criteria for the classification of childhood vasculitides. Ann Rheum Dis 65:936-941, 2006.
2. Savage COS, et al: ABC of arterial and vascular disease: Vasculitis. BMJ 320:1325-1328, 2000.
3. Ozen S, et al: Juvenile polyarteritis: Results of a multicenter survey of 110 children. J Pediatr 145:517-522, 2004.
4. Nick J, et al: Polyarteritis nodosa with pulmonary vasculitis. Am J Respir Crit Care Med 153:450-453, 1996.
5. Guo X, et al: Hepatitis B-related polyarteritis nodosa complicated by pulmonary hemorrhage. Chest 119:1608-1610, 2001.
6. Uziel Y, et al: "Unresolving pneumonia" as the main manifestation of atypical Kawasaki disease. Arch Dis Child 88:940-942, 2003.
7. Jennette JC, Xiao H, Falk RJ: Pathogenesis of vascular inflammation by anti-neutrophil cytoplasmic antibodies. J Am Soc Nephrol 17:1235-1242, 2006.
8. Bansal PJ, Tobin MC: Neonatal microscopic polyangiitis secondary to transfer of maternal myeloperoxidase-antineutrophil cytoplasmic antibody resulting in neonatal pulmonary hemorrhage and renal involvement. Ann Allergy Asthma Immunol 93:398-401, 2004.
9. Savage CO, et al: Autoantibodies developing to myeloperoxidase and proteinase 3 in systemic vasculitis stimulate neutrophil cytotoxicity toward cultured endothelial cells. Am J Pathol 141:335-342, 1992.
10. Falk R, Jennette J: Anti-neutrophil cytoplasmic autoantibodies with specificity for myeloperoxidase in patients with systemic vasculitis and idiopathic necrotizing and crescentic glomerulonephritis. N Engl J Med 318:1651-1657, 1988.
11. Sullivan EJ, Hoffman GS: Pulmonary vasculitis. Clin Chest Med 19:759-775, 1998.
12. Morgan MD, et al: Anti-neutrophil cytoplasm-associated glomerulonephritis. J Am Soc Nephrol 17:1224-1234, 2006.
13. Merkel PA, et al: Prevalence of antineutrophil cytoplasmic antibodies in a large inception cohort of patients with connective tissue disease. Ann Intern Med 126:866-873, 1997.
14. Ellis EN, Wood EG, Berry P: Spectrum of disease associated with anti-neutrophil cytoplasmic autoantibodies in pediatric patients. J Pediatr 126:40-43, 1995.
15. von Vigier R, et al: Pulmonary renal syndrome in childhood: A report of twenty-one cases and a review of the literature. Pediatr Pulmonol 29:382-388, 2000.
16. Fullmer JJ, et al: Pulmonary capillaritis in children: A review of eight cases with comparison to other alveolar hemorrhage syndromes. J Pediatr 146:376-381, 2005.
17. Godfrey S: Pulmonary hemorrhage/hemoptysis in children. Pediatr Pulmonol 37:476-484, 2004.
18. Stone J, Nousari H: "Essential" cutaneous vasculitis: What every rheumatologist should know about vasculitis of the skin. Curr Opin Rheumatol 13:23-34, 2001.
19. Vats KR, et al: Henoch-Schönlein purpura and pulmonary hemorrhage: A report and literature review. Pediatr Nephrol 13:530-534, 1999.

20. Al-Harbi NN: Henoch-Schönlein nephritis complicated with pulmonary hemorrhage but treated successfully. Pediatr Nephrol 17:762-764, 2002.
21. Nadrous H, Yu A, et al: Involvement in Henoch-Schönlein purpura. Mayo Clin Proc 79:1151-1157, 2004.
22. Paller AS, Kelly K, et al: Pulmonary hemorrhage: An often fatal complication of Henoch-Schönlein purpore. Pediatr Dermatol 14:299-302, 1997.
23. Godfrey S: Pulmonary hemorrhage/hemoptysis in children pediatric. Pulmonology 37:476-484, 2004.
24. Cazzato S, Bernardi F, et al: Pulmonary function abnormalities in children with Henoch-Schönlein purpore. Eur Respir J 13:597-601, 1999.
25. Bacon PA: The spectrum of Wegener's granulomatosis and disease relapse. N Engl J Med 352:330-332, 2005.
26. Dinwiddie R, Snapper S: Systemic diseases and the lung. Pediatr Respir Rev 6:181-189, 2005.
27. Rottem M, et al: Wegener granulomatosis in children and adolescents: Clinical presentation and outcome. J Pediatr 122:26-31, 1993.
28. Hall SL, et al: Wegener's granulomatosis in pediatric patients. J Pediatr 106:739-744, 1985.
29. Wadsworth D, Siegel M, Day D: Wegener's granulomatosis in children: Chest radiographic manifestations. AJR Am J Roentgenol 163:901-904, 1994.
30. Summers RM, Aggarwal NR, Sneller MC: CT virtual bronchoscopy of the central airways in patients with Wegener's granulomatosis. Chest 121:242-250, 2002.
31. Travis WD, et al: Surgical pathology of the lung in Wegener's granulomatosis: Review of 87 open lung biopsies from 67 patients. Am J Surg Pathol 15:315-333, 1991.
32. O'Sullivan BP, Erickson LA, Niles JL: Case 30-2002: An eight-year-old girl with fever, hemoptysis, and pulmonary consolidations. N Engl J Med 347:1009-1017, 2002.
33. Falk R, Jennette J: ANCA small-vessel vasculitis. J Am Soc Nephrol 8:314-322, 1997.
34. Ozen S: The spectrum of vasculitis in children. Best Pract Res Clin Rheumatol 16:411-425, 2002.
35. Stangou M, et al: Factors influencing patient survival and renal function outcome in pulmonary-renal syndrome associated with ANCA (+) vasculitis: A single-center experience. J Nephrol 18:35-44, 2005.
36. Jennette JC, Thomas DB, Falk RJ: Microscopic polyangiitis (microscopic polyarteritis). Semin Diagn Pathol 18:3-13, 2001.
37. Gonzalez-Gay M, et al: The epidemiology of the primary systemic vasculitides in northwest Spain: Implications of the Chapel Hill Consensus Conference definitions. Arthritis Care Res 49:388-393, 2003.
38. Collins CE, Quismorio FP Jr: Pulmonary involvement in microscopic polyangiitis. Curr Opin Pulm Med 11:447-451, 2005.
39. Lauque D, et al: Microscopic polyangiitis with alveolar hemorrhage: A study of 29 cases and review of the literature. Medicine 79:222-233, 2000.
40. Eschun GM, Mink SN, Sharma S: Pulmonary interstitial fibrosis as a presenting manifestation in perinuclear antineutrophilic cytoplasmic antibody microscopic polyangiitis. Chest 123:297-301, 2003.
41. Ando YMD, et al: Thoracic manifestation of myeloperoxidase-antineutrophil cytoplasmic antibody (MPO-ANCA)-related disease: CT findings in 51 patients. J Comput Assist Tomogr 28:710-716, 2004.
42. Lhote F, Cohen P, Guillevin L: Polyarteritis nodosa, microscopic polyangiitis and Churg-Strauss syndrome. Lupus 7:238-258, 1998.
43. Masi AT, et al: The American College of Rheumatology 1990 criteria for the classification of Churg-Strauss syndrome (allergic granulomatosis and angiitis). Arthritis Rheum 33:1094-1100, 1990.
44. Lanham JG, et al: Systemic vasculitis with asthma and eosinophilia: A clinical approach to the Churg-Strauss syndrome. Medicine 63(2):65-81, 1984.
45. Boyer D, et al: Churg-Strauss syndrome in children: A clinical and pathologic review. Pediatrics 118:e914-e920, 2006.
46. Specks UMD: Diffuse alveolar hemorrhage syndromes. Curr Opin Rheum 13:12-17, 2001.
47. Mizuki N, Inoko H, Ohno S: Pathogenic gene responsible for the predisposition of Behçet's disease. Int Rev Immunol 14:33-48, 1997.
48. Erkan F, Kiyan E, Tunaci A: Pulmonary complications of Behçet's disease. Clin Chest Med 23:493-503, 2002.
49. Maurer B, et al: Autologous haematopoietic stem cell transplantation for Behçet's disease with pulmonary involvement: Analysis after 5 years of follow up. Ann Rheum Dis 65:127-129, 2006.
50. Miller ML, Pachman LM: Vasculitis syndromes. In Behrman R, Kliegman R, Jenson HB, eds: Nelson's Textbook of Pediatrics, 17th ed. Philadelphia, WB Saunders.
51. Jain S, et al: Takayasu arteritis in children and young Indians. Int J Cardiol 75(Suppl 1):S153-S157, 2000.
52. Sanchez M, et al: Idiopathic pulmonary-renal syndrome with antiproteinase 3 antibodies. Respiration 61:295-299, 1994.
53. Glass D, Soter NA, Schur PH: Rheumatoid vasculitis. Arthritis Rheum 19:950-951, 1976.
54. Rohayem J, et al: Pulmonary fibrosis and other clinical manifestations of small vessel vasculitis in a family with seropositive juvenile rheumatoid arthritis. Pediatr Pulmonol 33:65-70, 2002.
55. Jennings C, et al: Diffuse alveolar hemorrhage with underlying isolated, pauciimmune pulmonary capillaritis. Am J Respir Crit Care Med 155:1101-1109, 1997.

CHAPTER 12

Pulmonary Manifestations of Dermatologic Diseases

ROBERT SIDBURY AND NELSON L. TURCIOS

Yellow Nail Syndrome   256
Neurofibromatosis Type 1   258
Tuberous Sclerosis Complex   259
Hereditary Hemorrhagic
   Telangiectasia   261
Klippel-Trénaunay-Weber
   Syndrome   263
Cutis Laxa (Generalized
   Elastolysis)   264

Ehlers-Danlos Syndrome   264
Pseudoxanthoma Elasticum   265
Xanthoma Disseminatum and
   Erdheim-Chester Disease   266
Hermansky-Pudlak Syndrome   267
Erythema Multiforme   267
Mastocytosis   269
Dyskeratosis Congenita   271
   References   272

Systemic diseases often manifest with cutaneous findings. Many pediatric conditions with prominent skin findings also have significant pulmonary morbidity. These conditions include inherited multisystem genetic disorders, such as yellow nail syndrome, neurofibromatosis type 1 (NF1), tuberous sclerosis complex (TSC), hereditary hemorrhagic telangiectasia (HHT), Klippel-Trénaunay-Weber syndrome, and Ehlers-Danlos syndrome (EDS), and reactive processes, such as xanthoma disseminatum and mastocytosis. This chapter discusses the common presentations and pulmonary manifestations of these disorders.

Yellow Nail Syndrome

Yellow nail syndrome was described first in 1964 in a group of 13 patients with lymphedema and distinctive nail findings.[1] Yellow nail syndrome is mostly a disease of early middle age, affecting women more commonly than men by 1.6:1[2]; however, neonatal chylothorax has been described in association with yellow nail syndrome.[3] It also has been reported in a male infant born with congenital lymphedema, who developed bilateral pleural effusions and a pericardial effusion at 6 months of age.[4] The classic clinical presentation includes yellowish nail discoloration and dystrophy (89%), lymphedema (80%), and pleuropulmonary disease (63%).[2] Two of the three clinical manifestations are required for the diagnosis of yellow nail syndrome. The cause of this syndrome remains unknown, although a few cases apparently followed episodes of pneumonia. Many cases have been attributed to congenital lymphatic hypoplasia, similar to that occurring in primary lymphedema.[3] Yellow nail syndrome has been associated with numerous malignancies and immunodeficiencies.[5]

Yellow nail syndrome is characterized by thickened, yellowish gray, slow-growing nails that are excessively curved along both axes. Nail changes are insidious in onset, are bilateral, and affect hands and feet (Fig. 12-1). Nail changes may occur before or after other physical findings. Cuticles and lunula may be absent, and fragility and separation from the nail plate (onycholysis) may be seen. These findings may easily be confused with onychomycosis. Nail cultures are negative, and systemic antifungal therapy is unhelpful. Histopathologic changes in the nail matrix and bed show dense fibrous tissue, which replaces subungual stroma with numerous ectatic,

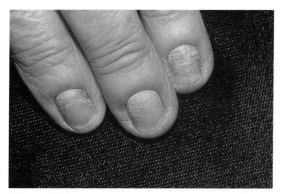

Figure 12-1. Yellowish discoloration and thickening of the nail plate. (See Color Plate)

endothelium-lined vessels that are similar to the pleural abnormalities found in yellow nail syndrome.[6]

Primary lymphedema typically involves the upper and lower extremities. The lymphedema is believed to be secondary to congenital atresia or hypoplasia of the lymphatics.[7] Lymphoscintigraphy is diagnostic.

The pleuropulmonary manifestations include pleural effusions and bronchiectasis. Pleural effusion may precede the onset of nail changes by several years. Pleural effusions range from small, unilateral, and asymptomatic to large, bilateral, and recurrent (Fig. 12-2). The fluid can be an exudate or transudate.[7] Empyema has been reported as a complication of yellow nail syndrome. The pleural effusion may be due to defective lymphatic drainage, rather than excess production of pleural fluid. Electron microscopy has revealed the presence of dilated lymphatic capillaries in the visceral pleura, suggesting an obstruction to the lymph drainage.[8] Yellow nail syndrome associated with bilateral cystic lung disease was reported in a 4-year-old girl, which suggests that normal lymphatic drainage is essential for normal lung development.[9]

There also is an increased incidence of sinusitis, bronchiectasis, and lower respiratory tract infections in patients with yellow nail syndrome, possibly related to an inherent immunodeficiency.[10] Bronchiectasis affects mostly the upper lobes, and the cause is unknown.[11] High-resolution computed tomography (CT) of the chest is diagnostic.

Other features that have been described in yellow nail syndrome include Raynaud phenomenon, keratosis obturans involving the external ear, excess cerumen, nephrotic syndrome, pericardial effusions, chylous ascites, intestinal lymphangiectasia, and selective antibody deficiency. Several cases of yellow nail syndrome in association with cancer of the breast, lung, and larynx have been reported. The nail changes are related to lymphatic obstruction, which is caused by the underlying malignancy.

Large, recurrent pleural effusions may require repeated thoracentesis, pleuroperitoneal shunting, chemical or surgical pleurodesis, or pleurectomy.[12] Chylous effusions are more difficult to treat and may require

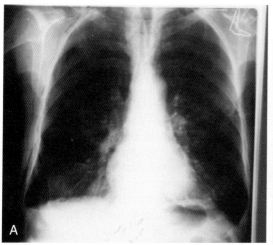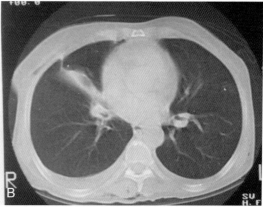

Figure 12-2. A, Chest x-ray of a patient with yellow nail syndrome reveals right-sided pleural effusion. **B,** CT scan reveals bronchiectasis and fibrotic changes in anterior segment of right upper lobe and right-sided pleural effusion in a patient with yellow nail syndrome.

dietary restriction of fat and supplements of medium-chain triglycerides.[13] Treatment of the pulmonary disease or malignancy has resulted in resolution of nail changes.

Neurofibromatosis Type 1

NF1, also called von Recklinghausen disease or peripheral NF, is a common autosomal dominant neurocutaneous disorder. Virtually every organ system may be affected. These protean features may be present at birth or in early childhood, but complications are generally delayed for years.[14]

NF1 occurs in 1 in 3000 individuals; there is no ethnic or gender predilection. NF1 has a high spontaneous mutation rate (50%) and variable expression.[15] The gene responsible for NF1 is located on chromosome 17. The gene product, neurofibromin, subserves a tumor suppressor function, and loss of heterozygosity results in the hamartomatous multiorgan growth that accounts for the clinical heterogeneity seen in NF1.

Café au lait macules are the hallmark cutaneous finding in NF1 and are present in almost 100% of patients (Fig. 12-3). Other cutaneous features may manifest slightly later in infancy or childhood, including axillary (Crowe sign) or inguinal freckling, or both, and neurofibromas. Rubbery discrete neurofibromas do not tend to occur until adolescence or later, although plexiform neurofibromas are generally present at birth (Fig. 12-4). Plexiform neurofibromas grow indolently and have a distinctive "bag of worms" texture, and often have overlying hyperpigmentation and hypertrichosis. Deeper plexiform neurofibromas may cause asymmetry or localized gigantism.

Noncutaneous features include asymptomatic iris hamartomas (Lisch nodules). These nodules are present in 95% of NF1 patients by 10 years of age.[14] Optic gliomas occur in 15%, but most are asymptomatic and nonprogressive. Skeletal features of NF1 include scoliosis, long bone dysplasia, nonossifying cyst formation, and short stature. A distinctive tibial anteromedial bowing manifests often in the first year of life, with medullary sclerosis and cortical thinning seen radiographically.

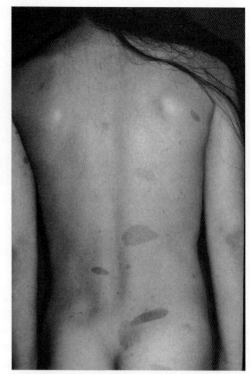

Figure 12-3. Multiple café au lait macules in a child with neurofibromatosis type 1. (See Color Plate)

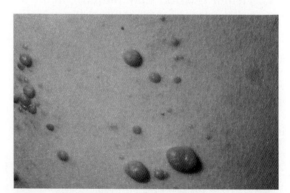

Figure 12-4. Cutaneous neurofibromas. (See Color Plate)

Neuropsychiatric disability is common, with 50% of NF1 patients having attention-deficit/hyperactivity disorder, learning disability, and verbal or nonverbal disability. Other features described in NF1 include hypertension secondary to renal artery stenosis or, less commonly, pheochromocytoma, macrocephaly, and increased malignancy risk for pilocytic astrocytomas, peripheral nerve sheath tumors, and leukemia.[15]

Diagnosis is based on established clinical criteria (Table 12-1). Gene testing also is available, and newer techniques have improved

Table 12-1	Diagnostic Criteria for Neurofibromatosis

Six or more café au lait macules >5 mm in greatest diameter in prepubertal individuals and >15 mm in greatest diameter in postpubertal individuals

Axillary or inguinal freckling

Two or more iris Lisch nodules

Two or more neurofibromas or one plexiform neurofibroma

Distinctive osseous lesion such as sphenoid wing dysplasia or cortical thinning of long bones

Optic pathway gliomas

First-degree relative with neurofibromatosis type 1 whose diagnosis was based on aforementioned criteria

mutation detection rates to around 90%. Brain magnetic resonance imaging (MRI) may reveal unidentified bright objects, but these have unclear diagnostic and prognostic significance, and no established recommendation exists for routine brain imaging. Genetic evaluation of suspected patients and family members, ophthalmologic evaluation annually until 10 years of age for diagnostic screening in suspected patients, and annual dermatologic examinations with a Wood light are helpful.

Pulmonary involvement resulting from NF1 is uncommon and manifests later in childhood or early adulthood. Pulmonary manifestations include diffuse pulmonary fibrosis, bullous lung disease, endobronchial neurofibromas, and mediastinal masses.[16] Pulmonary fibrosis is usually seen in the basal areas of the lungs, whereas bullous lesions occur predominantly in the apical areas.[17] When mediastinal lesions are located in the posterior mediastinum, they may manifest as "dumbbell" tumors with intraspinal extension. MRI of the involved spinal area is helpful in assessing the anatomic relationships of such tumors. Primary pulmonary neurofibromas are rare. Affected patients typically present with dyspnea on exertion.[16]

Chest radiographs and chest CT scans reveal reticulonodular infiltrates in the bases and bullous lesions in the apices.[18] Histologically, alveolar septal fibrosis and alveolitis lead to a mixed obstructive and restrictive lung dysfunction. In 5% of patients with NF, the neurofibromas, regardless of their location, may undergo malignant degeneration and commonly metastasize to the lungs.[17] "Scar" cancer of the lung can complicate long-standing NF1 pulmonary involvement.

Tuberous Sclerosis Complex

TSC is a neurocutaneous disorder characterized by intracranial abnormalities and distinctive skin markings. Historically, this disease was thought to consist of facial angiofibromas and disabling neurologic disorders, including epilepsy, mental retardation, and autism, but it is now acknowledged to affect many organ systems, including the eye, kidneys, heart, and lungs. Its incidence is approximately 1 in 6000.[19]

TSC is a disorder of cellular differentiation and proliferation that is inherited as an autosomal dominant trait with variable expression and a high spontaneous mutation rate.[20] Molecular genetic analysis has implicated two causal mutations in the genesis of TSC: *TSC1*, on chromosome 9q34, encodes hamartin, and *TSC2*, on chromosome 16p13, encodes tuberin.[21]

The diagnostic criteria for TSC consist of major and minor features (Table 12-2).[21] Younger patients generally present with neurologic manifestations, whereas pulmonary manifestations are more common in later life. Cutaneous findings are age-related with 90% of affected patients having hypopigmented macules at birth or very early in infancy and childhood. The signature "ash-leaf macule" is most characteristic, but TSC-related hypopigmentation may be polygonal, confetti-like, or segmental (Fig. 12-5). Three or more hypopigmented macules suggest TSC and should initiate a thorough family history and diagnostic work-up. Connective tissue nevi (Shagreen patch) typically occur on the trunk or face (fibrous forehead plaque) and may be seen at birth or early in life. Ungual fibromas (Koenen tumors) (Fig. 12-6) and facial angiofibromas manifest later in childhood or early adolescence. Other organ systems involved include the eyes ("mulberry tumors" and retinal hamartomas), heart (rhabdomyomas), kidneys (cysts, angiomyolipomas), and lungs (lymphangiomyomas).

Table 12.2	Diagnostic Criteria for Tuberous Sclerosis Complex	
MAJOR FEATURES	**MINOR FEATURES**
• Facial angiofibromas or forehead plaque	• Multiple randomly distributed pits in dental enamel
• Nontraumatic ungual or periungual fibroma	• Hamartomatous rectal polyps
• Hypomelanotic macules—more than three	• Bone cysts
• Shagreen patch (connective tissue nevus)	• Cerebral white-matter "migration tracts"
• Cortical tuber	• Gingival fibromas
• Subependymal nodule	• Nonrenal hamartoma
• Subependymal giant cell astrocytoma	• Retinal achromic patch
• Multiple retinal nodular hamartomas	• "Confetti" skin lesions
• Cardiac rhabdomyoma, single or multiple	• Multiple renal cysts
• Lymphangiomyomatosis	
• Renal angiomyolipoma	

Adapted and reprinted with permission from Roach et al., 1998.
Source: J. Pediatr Health Care © 2007. Mosby, Inc.

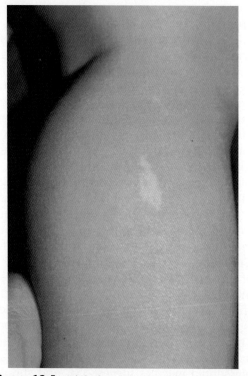

Figure 12-5. Ash-leaf macule in a child with tuberous sclerosis. (See Color Plate)

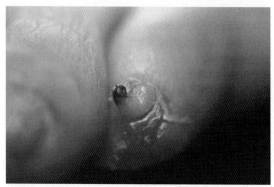

Figure 12-6. Periungual fibromas (Koenen tumors) in tuberous sclerosis. (See Color Plate)

Pulmonary involvement in TSC is uncommon, typically occurring in adolescent girls or women. Respiratory symptoms include chronic cough, progressive dyspnea, hemoptysis, and recurrent pneumothoraces.[21] Pulmonary involvement is extremely rare in men or children. Unilateral lung cysts and a large pneumothorax were described in a 7-year-old boy with TSC.[22] Recurrent acute respiratory distress syndrome secondary to TSC was reported in a 4-year-old boy.[23]

Histopathologically, two patterns of lung involvement have been described: lymphangiomyomatosis, also called lymphangioleiomyomatosis, and micronodular pneumocyte hyperplasia/multifocal alveolar hyperplasia. Lymphangiomyomatosis occurs exclusively in women of childbearing age and is characterized by widespread proliferation of abnormal smooth muscle cells surrounding lymphatic and blood vessels and small airways.[24]

Angiomyolipomas may produce generalized cystic or fibrotic changes in the lung and lead to spontaneous pneumothorax. Lymphatic obstruction may cause chylous effusion, and venous obstruction may lead to alveolar hemorrhage and hemoptysis. Bronchiolar obstruction results in air trapping and later lung cyst formation.

Radiographic evidence indicates that the incidence of lymphangiomyomatosis among women with TSC is 26% to 39%.[25] Chest radiography may be normal or reveal diffuse interstitial lung disease or multifocal cysts. Thoracic CT may show variable thin-walled cysts scattered in all parts of the lungs, with normal-appearing lung tissue between cysts.

A thorough diagnostic evaluation should include a dermatologic examination with Wood light to assess subclinical pigmentary change and renal and cardiac ultrasound. Cardiac rhabdomyomas are congenital and may regress spontaneously by several years of age. Consequently, two-dimensional echocardiography in the newborn period is indicated if TSC is suspected. Renal angiomyolipomas and cysts are present in 15% of patients, and ultrasound or abdominal CT can detect even asymptomatic lesions. Although benign, renal lesions are the second most common cause of morbidity because of growth and parenchymal destruction resulting in hematuria, hypertension, and renal failure. An ophthalmologic examination may detect the pathognomonic retinal hamartomas, which occur in 76% of patients. A dental examination can identify enamel pits and craters in permanent teeth and gingival fibromas. Evaluation of the central nervous system is essential, including a thorough neurologic examination and contrast-enhanced CT or MRI.

Treatment for TSC is symptomatic. Many physical findings are generally stable and nonprogressive, such as the pigmentary and connective tissue changes in the skin. Other findings, such as cardiac rhabdomyomas, recede spontaneously.

Therapy for pulmonary TSC is similar to that for lymphangiomyomatosis, which some consider a forme fruste of TSC.[24] Hormonal factors may play a role in the pathogenesis of lymphangiomyomatosis/TSC, which is consistent with typical presentation in premenopausal women, and are a potential therapeutic target. Medroxyprogesterone has been recommended when the disease becomes symptomatic or shows deterioration on pulmonary function tests. Oophorectomy, radiotherapy, or a combination of these has been beneficial. Other therapies that have shown some benefit include chemotherapeutic agents, such as cyclophosphamide. Tamoxifen has yielded mixed results to date, and corticosteroids are ineffective. Surgery has a role in pulmonary tuberous sclerosis to obtain a lung biopsy specimen for diagnosis, and to treat complications such as pneumothorax, to excise bullae, and to perform pleurodesis.

Because tumor cells from patients with TSC activate mammalian target of rapamycin (mTOR), mTOR inhibitor (sirolimus) has been identified as a potential therapeutic agent. The drug sirolimus suppresses mTOR signaling. The results of a clinical trial of sirolimus in patients with TSC and in patients with lymphangiomyomatosis revealed that lymphangiomyomatosis regressed during sirolimus therapy, but tended to increase in volume after therapy was stopped. Suppression of mTOR signaling might constitute an ameliorative treatment in patients with TSC or sporadic lymphangioleiomyomatosis.[21]

The prognosis for patients with pulmonary TSC is generally one of progressive decline as a result of lymphatic obstruction, alveolar hyperplasia, pleural thickening, and cyst formation. In severe cases, progressive respiratory insufficiency and death may occur. These patients may be considered for lung transplantation, but they are not candidates, given the coexisting conditions from TSC.

Hereditary Hemorrhagic Telangiectasia

HHT, also known as Osler-Weber-Rendu syndrome, is an autosomal dominantly inherited condition characterized by telangiectasias of the skin and mucous membranes, and intermittent bleeding from vascular abnormalities. Angiomas of the skin and oral, nasal, and conjunctival mucosa become evident in the second or third decade of life.[26] They appear bright red, punctate or linear, and blanch on pressure (Fig. 12-7).

HHT occurs in 1 in 10,000 individuals and has wide ethnic and geographic distribution.[26] Phenotypic heterogeneity exists with

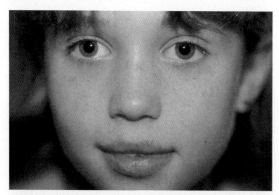

Figure 12-7. Facial angiomas in tuberous sclerosis (i.e., adenoma sebaceum). (See Color Plate)

variable age of onset, organ involvement, and severity even within families. Two separate loci have been identified—endoglin (*HHT-1*), on chromosome 9, and *ALK-1* (*HHT-2*), on chromosome 12—and this correlates with phenotypic variability.[27] Both genes are members of the transforming growth factor-β receptor family.

HHT is the most common cause of pulmonary arteriovenous malformations (AVMs). Pulmonary AVMs occur in approximately 30% of affected individuals and may remain asymptomatic for many years.[28] Fistulous vascular communications in the lungs may be large and localized, or smaller, multiple, and diffuse. They are frequently bilateral and have a predilection for the lower lobes.[28] The usual communication is between the pulmonary artery and pulmonary vein; direct communication between pulmonary artery and left atrium is extremely rare. Desaturated blood in the pulmonary artery is shunted through the fistula into the pulmonary veins, bypassing the lungs, and entering the left side of the heart. This shunt may result in systemic arterial desaturation and cyanosis. The shunt across the fistula is of low pressure and resistance so that pulmonary arterial pressure is normal; cardiomegaly is not present. The electrocardiogram is normal.

The severity of pulmonary manifestations depends on the magnitude of the right-to-left shunting. Patients may present with dyspnea, exercise intolerance, and polycythemia. Hemoptysis is rare in children, but is the most common presenting symptom in adults. Physical findings include cyanosis, a

systolic or continuous bruit over the site of the fistula, and digital clubbing. Features of HHT occur in about 50% of patients or other family members and include recurrent epistaxis and gastrointestinal tract bleeding.[28] Recurrent epistaxis secondary to telangiectasia of the nasal septa and turbinates is the presenting sign in more than 50% of patients, and occurs in 95% at some point during the course of illness. Nosebleeds in patients with HHT, typically spontaneous and often nocturnal, have a mean age of onset of 12 years and a mean frequency of 18 episodes per month.[29]

Chest radiographs may show oval or round, homogeneous, nodular opacities from a few millimeters to several centimeters in diameter owing to large fistulas. Pulmonary angiography with contrast enhancement usually reveals an artery entering the fistula and a vein leaving it (Fig. 12-8).[28] Multiple fistulas may be visualized on fluoroscopy as abnormal pulsations or on MRI. Selective pulmonary arteriography may be required to confirm site, extent, and distribution of fistulas and can confirm the diagnosis in virtually all cases.

In addition to pulmonary complications, patients with HHT may have AVMs of the brain. Brain and systemic abscesses are potentially serious complications in patients with

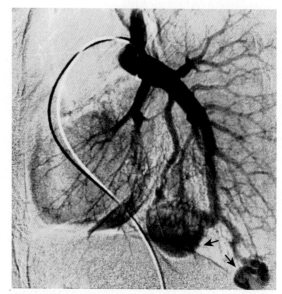

Figure 12-8. Pulmonary angiography shows two pulmonary arteriovenous malformations with a common feeding artery (*arrow*).

HHT. Brain abscess can be the initial presentation in a patient with previously asymptomatic pulmonary AVM. Forty percent of patients with pulmonary AVMs may present with central nervous system manifestations, such as transient dizziness, diplopia, aphasia, motor weakness, or seizures. These findings may result from cerebral thrombosis, abscess, or paradoxical embolic events.[28] Gastrointestinal bleeding secondary to telangiectasia occurs in 40% of patients, although rarely in children. AVMs also may manifest in the gastrointestinal tract, but are more typically seen in the liver. Hepatic AVMs, possibly more common in female patients, can lead to complications such as hemorrhage, portal hypertension, and cirrhosis (Table 12-3).

Pulmonary hypertension in association with HHT may involve the *ALK-1* mutation resulting in vascular dilation and occlusion of small pulmonary arteries more typical of primary pulmonary hypertension. External manifestations, including perioral and intraoral telangiectasia and facial and hand involvement, generally occur during the third or fourth decade. Abnormal nail-fold capillaries also may be seen.

Other complications include high-output congestive heart failure and portosystemic encephalopathy from hepatic AVMs. Disseminated intravascular coagulopathy has been reported in 50% of patients with documented HHT.

Current treatment includes pulmonary artery embolization using coils and other intravascular devices.[30] Multiple embolizations may be necessary in some patients because new fistulas may develop after successful treatment of earlier ones. Although embolization is the initial treatment of choice, large, solitary, or localized pulmonary AVMs may require lobectomy or wedge resection, which usually results in complete resolution of the symptoms.[30] In most instances, fistulas are widespread such that surgery is impossible. If there is a communication between the pulmonary artery and the left atrium, it can be obliterated by division and suture.

Klippel-Trénaunay-Weber Syndrome

Klippel-Trénaunay-Weber syndrome, or angio-osteodystrophy, is a noninheritable disorder that consists of the triad of cutaneous vascular malformation, venous varicosities, and bony or soft tissue overgrowth.[19] The cause of Klippel-Trénaunay-Weber syndrome is unknown, and diagnosis is based on clinical features. Affected patients typically present with a unilateral, lower extremity, extensive "geographic" capillary malformation (port wine stain) at birth that may or may not be associated with congenital ipsilateral extremity overgrowth (Fig. 12-9). Thick-walled venous varicosities typically become apparent ipsilateral to the vascular malformation after the child begins to ambulate. The deep venous system may be absent, hypoplastic, or obstructed, resulting in lymphedema. Lymphedema and osteohypertrophy tend to occur later, resulting in limb length or girth asymmetry. Pain can result from associated chronic venous insufficiency, cellulitis, superficial thrombophlebitis, and deep vein thrombosis.[31]

The diagnostic work-up should include dermatologic and orthopedic evaluations and clinical and radiographic limb length measurement, Doppler ultrasonography, arteriography, venography, and possibly CT or MRI and lymphography to assess the extent and distribution of anomalous vasculature. Uncommonly, urogenital and intestinal complications can develop and should be investigated symptomatically.

Pulmonary involvement is rare; however, recurrent pulmonary thromboembolic events are well described and may occur in 22% of

Table 12-3	Diagnostic Criteria of Hereditary Hemorrhagic Telangiectasia (HHT)

HHT is diagnosed in an individual who meets three or more of the following criteria*

Spontaneous, recurrent epistaxis; nocturnal nosebleeds heighten concern

Mucocutaneous telangiectasias (tongue, lips, oral cavity, fingers, and nose)

Internal arteriovenous malformations (pulmonary, cerebral, hepatic, gastrointestinal, spinal)

First-degree relative with HHT according to these criteria

*Diagnosis is possible or suspected when two are present and unlikely when less than two.

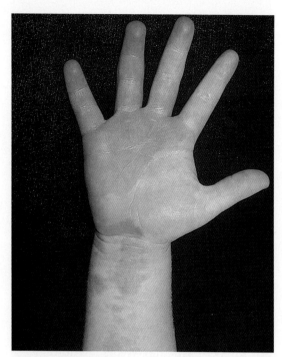

Figure 12-9. Port-wine stains clearly visible on right hand of a child affected with Klippel-Trénaunay-Weber syndrome. (See Color Plate)

affected patients. Pulmonary embolism in Klippel-Trénaunay-Weber syndrome has been described in children, but its mechanism is unclear.[32] Recurrent disease may be complicated by chronic thromboembolic pulmonary hypertension and small vessel pulmonary arterial hypertension.[33]

Consideration should be given to estrogen avoidance, aggressive deep vein thrombosis prophylaxis in patients undergoing surgical procedures, and anticoagulation where appropriate. In high-risk patients, venographic evaluation of the pelvic and abdominal venous anatomy may be warranted, and suprarenal filter placement should be considered.[34]

Surgical correction or palliation is often difficult. Leg length differences should be treated with orthotic devices to prevent the development of spinal deformities. One avenue of research into Klippel-Trénaunay-Weber syndrome has focused on the role of vasoactive factors. The angiogenic factor VG5Q has been described more recently in patients with Klippel-Trénaunay-Weber syndrome and may relate to the pulmonary-vascular complications associated with Klippel-Trénaunay-Weber syndrome.[35]

Cutis Laxa (Generalized Elastolysis)

Congenital cutis laxa is a rare disorder of generalized elastolysis. The clinical picture is characterized by inelastic, loose, hanging skin more marked in flexural areas, giving the appearance of premature aging.[36] The disease is inherited most commonly in a severe autosomal recessive form, or as a benign autosomal dominant form. There is often systemic organ involvement in patients with the autosomal recessive form. Cardiopulmonary abnormalities are common and are the main determinants of the prognosis and life expectancy.

Pulmonary emphysema resulting from a loss of elastic tissue in the lungs is very common.[37] Cor pulmonale and right-sided heart failure generally caused by pulmonary involvement are often seen in infancy. Other reported pulmonary complications include pneumothorax, pulmonary fibrosis, recurrent pulmonary infections, bronchiectasis, and tracheobronchomegaly. Various cardiovascular abnormalities, including aortic aneurysm, hypoplasia and stenosis of the pulmonary arteries, and pulmonary valve stenosis, have been reported in patients with this form of congenital cutis laxa. Several studies suggest a biochemical defect in elastin in cutis laxa.

Ehlers-Danlos Syndrome

EDS is a heterogeneous group of inherited disorders characterized by abnormalities in connective tissue. Affected children appear normal at birth, but skin hyperelasticity, fragility of the skin and blood vessels, and joint hypermobility develop. The basic defect is a quantitative deficiency of collagen.[38] EDS historically has been classified into 10 clinical forms, although more recent efforts have tried to simplify the taxonomy.

Type IV EDS, the most severe form, manifests with thin, translucent, fragile skin; prominent underlying venous network; and easy bruising. Joint hypermobility is less marked compared with the more common EDS subtypes, and is usually confined to the digits (Fig. 12-10). Distinctive gaunt

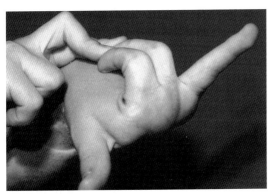

Figure 12-10. Joint hypermobility in Ehlers-Danlos syndrome type I.

facial and limb features reflect diminished subcutaneous fat. The diagnosis is based on the cutaneous features; physiognomy; and history of arterial, intestinal, or uterine rupture, which can manifest as an acute abdomen.

Type IV EDS (ecchymotic or arterial) may have autosomal dominant or autosomal recessive inheritance. Its precise incidence is unknown. Point mutations in the *Col3A1* gene that result in the production of a defective collagen have been identified.

Type IV EDS may have pulmonary involvement. Histochemical studies of lung tissue in EDS have revealed markedly decreased type III collagen; fibroblasts cultured from the abnormal lung produce less than normal type III procollagen relative to type I procollagen. Electron microscopy analysis of lung specimens has shown dilated endoplasmic reticulum of the fibroblasts with normal collagen. Pulmonary complications have been described in patients with type I EDS, including spontaneous pneumothorax from bullous lung disease and severe panacinar emphysema, but most cases reported in the literature are associated with type IV EDS.[39] Recurrent pneumothoraces may result in bullous disease and ultimately cavitary lesions. EDS-related weakness of the pulmonary arterial wall has resulted in rupture and hemoptysis, and spontaneous dissection of the aorta may occur. Tracheobronchomegaly similar to that in Mounier-Kuhn syndrome has been reported in a child with EDS.[40] An unusual pulmonary manifestation of EDS consisting of parenchymal cysts and fibrous

and fibro-osseous nodules also has been described.[41] These manifestations may be related to an abnormal attempt at repair of parenchymal or vascular tears. Recurrent congenital diaphragmatic hernia in young children also has been reported.[42]

Treatment of EDS-related pulmonary disease includes standard management of pneumothoraces with thoracotomy tubes, pleurodesis, and bullectomy where indicated.[43] Although no good data exist on the lung mechanics of this patient population, if mechanical ventilatory support is required, excessive tidal volumes or ventilatory rates may predispose to pneumothorax and should be avoided. Patients with type IV EDS tend to die prematurely of complications associated with arterial rupture.

Pseudoxanthoma Elasticum

Pseudoxanthoma elasticum is a rare, autosomal recessive or autosomal dominant inherited disorder characterized by progressive calcification of elastic tissue.[44] The skin, eyes, and cardiovascular system are most commonly affected, but secondary complications can develop in the lungs. Pseudoxanthoma elasticum has varied clinical presentations even within the same family. Skin lesions begin indolently during the second or third decade and are often described as "plucked chicken skin" (Fig. 12-11). Rubbery, yellow coalescing papules are most often seen on the sides of the neck, axilla, inguinal folds, and perineum. Affected skin may develop comedones or calcify or both. Involvement of the connective tissue of the media and intima of the arterial walls has been implicated in premature atherosclerosis. Ocular findings include a reddish brown extension from the optic disk called an "angioid streak," which is due to rupture of Bruch membrane, and a degenerative chorioretinitis. Angioid streaks have been reported in 13-year-old patients, although they typically do not occur until the third decade of life.[39] This change is generally asymptomatic, but visual loss can occur later in life.

Although rare, pulmonary complications tend to be secondary to aberrant deposition of calcium in the elastic fibers of the

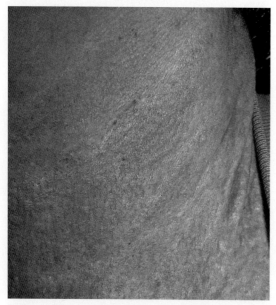

Figure 12-11. Pseudoxanthoma elasticum, showing typical "plucked chicken" grouped yellowish papules and prominent skin folds on the neck. Lesions are usually most apparent on the neck or in the axillary region; the latter may be confused with Fox-Fordyce disease, but this is confined to the axilla and does not have the soft slackness of the skin that is a feature of pseudoxanthoma elasticum. (See Color Plate)

internal elastic lamina of some arteries, arterioles, and venules, which leads to narrowing of vessel lumens.[44] Arterial calcification involving the coronary arteries or cerebral vasculature generally manifests in adulthood, but intermittent claudication and angina have occurred in adolescence.[41] Hypertension secondary to renal artery stenosis also can be seen. There is no effective treatment, although laser therapy may help prevent retinal hemorrhage.

Xanthoma Disseminatum and Erdheim-Chester Disease

Xanthoma disseminatum is a rare proliferative disorder characterized by multiorgan infiltration of non-Langerhans cell histiocytes. The classic clinical triad is cutaneous xanthomas, xanthomas of mucous membranes, and diabetes insipidus.[45] Skin lesions manifest as coalescent, yellow-red papules and plaques with accentuation in the flexures, such as the neck and axilla. The cause of xanthoma disseminatum is unknown, and treatment generally is unsatisfactory.

Upper respiratory involvement has been reported most commonly in the buccal mucosa, larynx, and pharynx, but few reports describe in detail involvement of the lower respiratory tract.[46] One young patient with xanthoma disseminatum has been reported with progressive dyspnea and distinctive skin lesions on the eyelids, neck, and axilla, and digital clubbing. Chest radiographs revealed hyperaeration and segmental atelectasis. High-resolution CT scan of the chest showed diffuse thickening of the tracheobronchial wall with bilateral lower lobe bronchiectasis. Bronchoscopy confirmed xanthomatous infiltration.[47]

Xanthoma disseminatum runs a chronic course, and the lesions may regress spontaneously. Obstructing lesions of the upper airway can be managed with surgical or laser excision or tracheostomy, but small lower airway involvement denotes a poor prognosis.

Erdheim-Chester disease is a rare nonfamilial, proliferative non-Langerhans cell histiocytosis with multisystem involvement. Erdheim-Chester disease is very rare in children. The long bones are the classic locus of involvement; however, other systems can be involved, including the lungs, kidneys, liver, spleen, central nervous system, and pericardium.[48] The cause is unknown.

Approximately 20% of patients with Erdheim-Chester disease have lung involvement. These patients present with dyspnea, and chest radiographs reveal interstitial disease with interlobar septal thickening and centrilobar nodular opacity.[49] Pulmonary function tests show a restrictive pattern with decreased diffusion capacity. Characteristic lung histopathology includes the accumulation of histiocytes with variable amounts of fibrosis and a variable lymphoplasmacytic infiltrate in a lymphangitic distribution.[50] Immunostains are diagnostically useful, showing immunopositivity for CD68 and factor XIIIa and immunonegativity for CD1a. Birbeck granules are uniformly absent ultrastructurally.[51]

Therapy is anecdotal, and the response is unpredictable. Nonsteroidal immunosuppressants such as cyclosporine, interferon, and chemotherapy and radiotherapy also have been attempted with limited results.

Chapter 12—Pulmonary Manifestations of Dermatologic Diseases 267

Hermansky-Pudlak Syndrome

Hermansky-Pudlak syndrome (HPS) is an autosomal recessive inherited disorder characterized by oculocutaneous albinism, platelet dysfunction with prolonged bleeding times, and lysosomal accumulation of ceroid-like lipofuscin in the reticuloendothelial system, resulting in granulomatous colitis and pulmonary fibrosis in some cases. Affected patients can exhibit a range of cutaneous pigmentary dilution from frank albinism resembling oculocutaneous albinism type I to a pale tan hue with lentigenes and freckling.[52] The severity of ocular involvement is directly correlated with the degree of cutaneous albinism and can include nystagmus, decreased visual acuity, and photophobia. Epistaxis is the most common manifestation of bleeding diathesis, although patients may first note difficulties after dental or surgical procedures. Renal failure, cardiomyopathy, and bacterial infections also have been described.

Hermansky and Pudlak described this disorder in 1959. Mutations in one of four human genes (HPS-1, HPS-2, HPS-3, HPS-4) are now known to cause HPS. HPS-1 is the most common mutation, and there is a carrier frequency of 1 in 18 in northwest Puerto Rico. HPS-1 encodes a lysosomal trafficking protein.

HPS is diagnosed based on a combination of the above-described clinical features and laboratory abnormalities including a prolonged bleeding time with normal platelet count, prothrombin time/partial thromboplastin time, and fibrinogen levels. Platelet function is abnormal owing to storage pool deficiencies of adenosine diphosphate and serotonin. Accumulation of ceroid-like material in macrophages can be identified on peripheral smear. Patients with oculocutaneous albinism and bleeding tendencies may be referred for genetic linkage analysis.

Pulmonary disease, which is common in HPS patients, usually begins in the third or fourth decade of life and manifests with chronic nonproductive cough and progressive dyspnea.[53] It follows a functional restrictive lung disease process similar to idiopathic pulmonary fibrosis. The incidence of pulmonary disease is twice as high in

women as in men. Histologically, diffuse septal and peribronchial stromal fibrosis is seen. Accumulation of the telltale ceroid-like lipofuscin in alveolar macrophages is the putative cause of this fibrosis.

Findings on chest radiograph include reticulonodular interstitial pattern, perihilar fibrosis, and pleural thickening. High-resolution CT reveals septal thickening, ground-glass opacities, and peribronchovascular thickening (Fig. 12-12).[53] Age older than 30 and presence of HPS-1 mutations portend more severe pulmonary involvement, and high-resolution CT findings correlate well with decreasing pulmonary function as measured by the percentage of forced vital capacity.

Because the pulmonary fibrosis in HPS is an irreversible, progressive process, symptomatic treatment is the only option. Pirfenidone, an antifibrotic agent, seems to slow the progression of pulmonary fibrosis in HPS patients who have significant residual lung function.[54] Intravenous or intramuscular desmopressin injections have improved platelet aggregation in some patients with HPS. The patient's response to desmopressin should be evaluated before elective surgical procedures. The report of a child with the characteristic findings of HPS, which often goes unrecognized because of the discrete nature of the cutaneous and hemorrhagic manifestations, highlights the importance of establishing this diagnosis because of the risk not only of hemorrhage, but also of granulomatous colitis and long-term pulmonary fibrosis.[55]

Erythema Multiforme

"Erythema multiforme" is a confusing term that has come to encompass a spectrum of disorders ranging from the typically benign, localized erythema multiforme minor, generally confined to the skin, to the more severe Stevens-Johnson syndrome (SJS) and toxic epidermal necrolysis (TEN). Some literature includes erythema multiforme major within this group of mucocutaneous multisystem reaction disorders.

SJS/TEN is a multisystem inflammatory dermatosis that most commonly results from a hypersensitivity response to a medication.

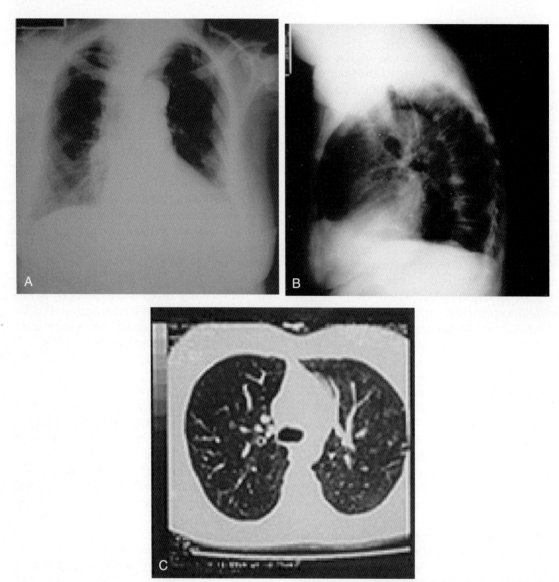

Figure 12-12. A and **B**, Chest radiograph in patient with Hermansky-Pudlak syndrome shows a diffuse bilateral emphysema and a streaking suggestive of interstitial lung disease. (**B**). **C**, This is confirmed by the appearance of ground-glass opacities with high-resolution CT examination, compatible with imaging pulmonary features described in albino patients with Hermansky-Pudlak syndrome.

Medications associated with SJS/TEN include sulfonamides; penicillin antibiotics; antiseizure medications (phenytoin); and nonsteroidal anti-inflammatory agents such as ibuprofen, pyrazolones, piroxicam, and salicylates. Less commonly, SJS/TEN can be associated with infections caused by herpes simplex virus and *Mycoplasma pneumoniae*. SJS/TEN has a prodrome of an upper respiratory illness with associated fever, cough, and malaise, for which children often receive therapy with antibiotics, antipyretics, or both. During or up to 2 weeks beyond the prodrome, abrupt mucocutaneous symptoms appear. The skin may be tender and has discrete erythematous symmetric macules that evolve into blisters. These blisters may remain localized or progress into more extensive epidermal necrosis and loss (Fig. 12-13). SJS by definition has two or more mucous membranes affected, with hemorrhagic crusting of the lips being the most characteristic finding. Purulent conjunctivitis is typical and may help distinguish SJS/TEN from the nonexudative ocular changes seen in Kawasaki syndrome, which can be in the clinical

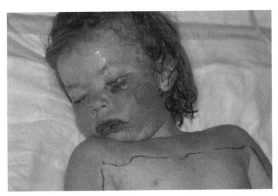

Figure 12-13. Extensive skin necrosis in Stevens-Johnson syndrome and toxic epidermal necrolysis. (See Color Plate)

differential diagnosis. Anogenital involvement with blisters and erosions is common. Lymphadenopathy, occasional arthralgias, hepatitis, nephritis, and myocarditis are rarely seen.

SJS/TEN has no ethnic or gender predilection. Although the exact mechanism has not been elucidated, cytokines released by activated mononuclear cells and keratinocytes by the offending medication or infection may contribute to apoptosis of epidermal cells and constitutional symptoms in a genetically predisposed individual.

Pulmonary complications are atypical in SJS/TEN.[56] One prospective evaluation found that early pulmonary complications occurred in 27% of cases and usually involved bronchial mucosal sloughing. Other respiratory complications that have been described include hemoptysis and expectoration of bronchial mucosal casts, pulmonary edema, patchy bronchopneumonic infiltrates, and chronic bronchiolitis obliterans.[57]

Clinical respiratory manifestations consist of cough, hoarseness, hemoptysis, and dyspnea. Interstitial infiltrates and diffuse loss of bronchial epithelium in the proximal airways may be seen on bronchoscopy. Bronchial biopsies confirmed epidermal necrosis with a mixed mononuclear inflammatory infiltrate. In one more recent study, 90% of patients with early pulmonary complications ultimately required ventilatory support, and 40% died of complications associated with respiratory failure.[58]

Treatment of SJS/TEN is controversial. Immediate cessation of suspected medications,

treatment of potential infectious triggers, and supportive therapy are the mainstays. The role of systemic corticosteroids and intravenous immunoglobulin is unclear. Numerous more recent reports have supported the use of intravenous immunoglobulin in adults and children with evolving SJS/TEN if started early in the course in the absence of renal risk factors.[59]

Mastocytosis

Mastocytosis is a disorder of mast cells and can develop at any age. It usually appears in the first weeks to months of life. The cause is unknown. In young children, the disease involves increased mast cells in the skin, but rarely other organs. In older children (>10 years old at diagnosis) and adults, it is more likely to be a systemic disease. Mast cells contain histamine and other inflammatory mediators, which when triggered are released into the skin, blood, and other organs. Cutaneous mastocytosis is characterized by the degree of skin involvement. Involvement can be confined to the skin or may involve other organ systems, including the lungs. The most common types in children are solitary mastocytomas, urticaria pigmentosa, and diffuse cutaneous mastocytosis.

Solitary mastocytomas are collections of mast cells with a single or multiple (usually five or fewer individual) orange-brown to red-brown plaques or nodules ranging from 0.5 to 3.5 cm in diameter. They typically appear within 3 months after birth. They may develop a peau d'orange, or an orange peel-like, texture. The clue to diagnosis is Darier sign, which is the development of a wheal and flare after firm stroking of a lesion with the dull edge of a pen or fingernail. The stroking leads to mast cell degranulation and histamine release. The lesion typically develops a raised, white wheal in the center and then a surrounding bright red flare within several minutes (Fig. 12-14). Mastocytoma in children typically is self-limited and involves only the skin.[60]

If there is enough histamine release, some patients may develop systemic symptoms, including nausea, diarrhea, abdominal pain, flushing, pruritus, hypotension,

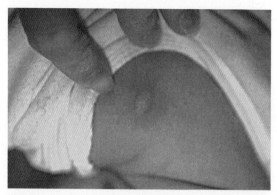

Figure 12-14. Urtication secondary to stroking of a mastocytoma (i.e., positive Darier sign). (See Color Plate)

and bronchospasm. Rarely, enough histamine is released to cause anaphylaxis and death. The treatment of choice is administration of oral antihistamines, such as diphenhydramine. Epinephrine can be given in acute situations. Lesions typically involute over 8 to 10 years.

Urticaria pigmentosa also occurs in infancy and is present in some patients at birth. Brown spots are typically present by age 6 months in most patients and may involve mucous membranes. They appear as hyperpigmented to red-brown, minimally elevated macules, papules, and plaques ranging in size from 0.5 to 1.5 cm in a random distribution. Typically, the scalp, palms, soles, and sun-exposed areas are spared. Lesions may become bullous in patients younger than 2 years old. Darier sign is positive, and patients may complain of flushing, pruritus, or dermatographism. Symptoms typically improve over time, and 50% of patients have resolution of lesions by adolescence. Extracutaneous involvement is uncommon.

Diffuse cutaneous mastocytosis is rare and more commonly associated with systemic symptoms of histamine release. This form involves diffuse infiltration of mast cells in the skin, and patients may be at risk for systemic disease. Skin may appear normal or have a thickened, red-brown appearance. Extensive blistering is common in infancy. Darier sign is difficult to elucidate in this type because of the extensive skin involvement. The disease is usually present by age 3 years and spontaneously resolves in most patients during early childhood, although dermatographism often persists. Systemic symptoms are more common with this subtype, including pruritus, wheezing, dyspnea, hypotension, tachycardia, bronchospasm, and syncope, and even death.

The diagnosis can be made with a careful history, physical examination, and the pathognomonic Darier sign on examination. Skin biopsy is confirmatory and shows collections of mast cells in the dermis. Diagnosis can be confirmed further by measuring serum tryptase, another mast cell mediator, or urine histamine and its metabolites. Bone involvement may appear on radiographs, but does not correlate with systemic involvement and may be self-limited.[61] Affected patients may show abnormalities in peripheral blood, such as anemia, leukocytosis, and hypereosinophilia.

With the exception of diffuse cutaneous mastocytosis, pulmonary involvement in any of these forms of mastocytosis generally is not seen. Pulmonary complications have been rarely reported in patients with urticaria pigmentosa and systemic mastocytosis.[62] Radiographic evidence of lung involvement in diffuse cutaneous mastocytosis occurs in 16% to 43%, and may include reticulonodular opacities, nodules, and cysts (Fig. 12-15).[63]

Treatment includes avoiding triggers of histamine release when possible. These triggers include sudden weather changes, hot beverages, hot baths, insect stings, mechanical irritation, and certain infections. Drugs known to induce symptoms include, but are not limited to, alcohol, nonsteroidal anti-inflammatory agents, aspirin, polymyxin B, vancomycin, morphine, codeine, and some local and general anesthetics. Anesthesiologists should be informed of the condition before any surgical procedures to avoid histamine-releasing agents. In addition, a nonsedating H_1 blocker can be used for systemic symptoms. More severe symptoms may require a classic (sedating) H_1 blocker or H_2 blockers (good for gastrointestinal symptoms), or both. In rare cases of gastrointestinal symptoms, oral sodium cromolyn can be used. There is some evidence that treatment with high-potency topical steroids can reduce the reactivity of mastocytomas. If they are causing significant systemic symptoms, solitary mastocytomas

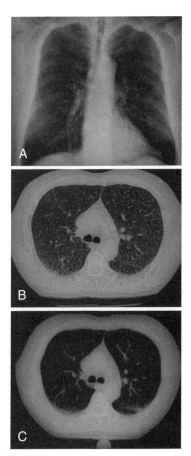

Figure 12-15. A, Chest radiograph shows diffuse fine reticular interstitial infiltration pattern of both lungs. **B,** CT scan of thorax shows faint cystic and nodular lesions of lung interstitium and mediastinal adenopathy at the time before interferon-α. **C,** After 6 months of treatment with interferon-α, interstitial lesions of the lung markedly improved on CT.

can be surgically excised. Automatic injection devices containing epinephrine (Epi-Pens) are recommended for patients with extensive disease, although all patients and their parents should be counseled about this possible complication.

Dyskeratosis Congenita

Dyskeratosis congenita (DKC) is a rare inherited condition characterized by cutaneous reticulated hyperpigmentation, nail dystrophy, premalignant leukoplakia of the oral mucosa, and progressive pancytopenia. The inheritance pattern of most cases of DKC is X-linked recessive, but autosomal

dominant and recessive patterns have been reported. The autosomal dominant form of DKC usually lacks the classic skin findings. It also is associated with idiopathic pulmonary fibrosis. The mutant gene is *DKC1* (located at Xq28) in the families studied.

The mucocutaneous features of DKC typically develop between age 5 and 15 years with abnormal skin pigmentation with tan-to-gray hyperpigmented or hypopigmented macules and patches. The typical distribution is on the upper trunk, neck, and face (involvement of sun-exposed areas). Mucosal leukoplakia typically occurs on the buccal mucosa and can affect the tongue and oropharynx. The leukoplakia may become verrucous, and ulceration may occur. Other mucosal sites may be involved (e.g., esophagus, urethral meatus, glans penis, lacrimal duct, conjunctiva, vagina, anus). There is an increased incidence of malignant neoplasms, squamous cell carcinoma of the skin, mouth, nasopharynx, esophagus, rectum, vagina, and cervix.

Pulmonary disease is present in 20% of patients with DKC. Affected patients had reduced diffusing capacity for carbon monoxide or a restrictive defect on pulmonary function testing. Pulmonary complications are the second most common cause of death in patients with DKC, about half occurring in patients who undergo bone marrow transplant. Yabe and colleagues[64] reported a 9-year-old boy who was diagnosed at age 2 years. Autopsy results showed a mixed inflammatory cell infiltrate of bronchioles and alveoli with interstitial fibrosis. Utz and associates[65] also reported two male patients, 28 years old and 48 years old, who were diagnosed at age 10 years. Lung biopsy specimens from both patients showed usual interstitial pneumonitis. The first patient had a bone marrow transplant 12 years before biopsy and died 4 months after the transplant. The second patient did not undergo bone marrow transplant or corticosteroids and died 6 months after biopsy.

The pathologic pattern for patients with a clinical diagnosis of idiopathic pulmonary fibrosis or cryptogenic fibrosing alveolitis reveals architectural destruction, fibrosis often with honeycombing, scattered fibroblastic foci, patchy distribution, and

272   Pulmonary Manifestations of Pediatric Diseases

involvement of the periphery of the acinus or lobule. The prognosis of adults with usual interstitial pneumonitis is poor, with most patients dying within 5 years of diagnosis. Children given a diagnosis of idiopathic pulmonary fibrosis or cryptogenic fibrosing alveolitis often live much longer and have a nonprogressive course, suggesting that they do not have usual interstitial pneumonitis.

References

1. Samman PD: The yellow-nail syndrome: Dystrophic nails associated with lymphedema. Trans St Johns Hosp Dermatol Soc 50:132, 1964.
2. Nordkild P, Kromann-Andersen H, Struve-Christensen E: Yellow-nail syndrome—the triad of yellow nails, lymphedema, and pleural effusions: A review of the literature and a case report. Acta Med Scand 219:221-227, 1986.
3. Govaert P, et al: Perinatal manifestations of maternal yellow nail syndrome. Pediatrics 89:1016-1018, 1992.
4. Paradisis M, Van Asperen P: Yellow nail syndrome in infancy. J Paediatr Child Health 33:454-457, 1997.
5. Bokszczanin A, Levinson AI: Coexistent yellow nail syndrome and selective antibody deficiency. Ann Allergy Asthma Immunol 91:496-500, 2003.
6. DeCoste SD, Imber MJ, Baden HP: Yellow-nail syndrome. J Am Acad Dermatol 22:608-611, 1990.
7. Beer DJ, Pereira W, Snider GL: Pleural effusion associated with primary lymphedema: A perspective on the yellow nail syndrome. Am Rev Resp Dis 117:595-599, 1978.
8. Solal-Celigny P, Cormier Y, Fournier M: The yellow-nail syndrome: Light and electron microscopic aspects of the pleura. Arch Pathol Lab Med 107:183-185, 1983.
9. Sacco O, et al: Yellow-nail syndrome and bilateral cystic lung disease. Pediatr Pulmonol 26:429-433, 1998.
10. Müller R-P, et al: Roentgenographic and clinical signs in yellow-nail syndrome. Lymphology 12:257-261, 1979.
11. McNicholas WT, Quigley C, FitzGerald MX: Upper lobe bronchiectasis in the yellow nail syndrome: Report of a case. Ir J Med Sci 153:394-395, 1984.
12. Brofman JD, et al: Yellow nails, lymphedema and pleural effusion: Treatment of chronic pleural effusion with pleuroperitoneal shunting. Chest 97:743-745, 1990.
13. Tan WC: Dietary treatment of chylous ascites in yellow nail syndrome. Gut 30:1622-1623, 1989.
14. Gutmann DH, et al: The diagnostic evaluation and multidisciplinary management of neurofibromatosis 1 and neurofibromatosis 2. JAMA 278:51-57, 1997.
15. Ward BA, Gutmann DH: Neurofibromatosis 1: From lab bench to clinic. Pediatr Neurol 32:221-228, 2005.
16. Unger PD, Geller SA, Anderson PJ: Pulmonary lesions in patients with neurofibromatosis. Arch Pathol Lab Med 108:654-657, 1984.
17. Webb WR, Goodman PC: Fibrosing alveolitis in patients with neurofibromatosis. Radiology 122:289-293, 1977.
18. Aughenbaugh GL: Thoracic manifestations of neurocutaneous disease. Radiol Clin North Am 22:741-756, 1984.
19. Behrman RE, et al, eds: Nelson's Textbook of Pediatrics, 16th ed. Philadelphia, WB Saunders, 2005.
20. Roach ES, Delgado MR: Tuberous sclerosis. Dermatol Clin 13:151-161, 1995.
21. Bissler JJ, et al: Sirolimus for angiomyolipoma in tuberous sclerosis complex or lymphangioleiomyomatosis. N Engl J Med 358:140-151, 2008.
22. Bowen J, Beasley SW: Rare pulmonary manifestations of tuberous sclerosis in children. Pediatr Pulmonol 23:114-116, 1997.
23. Vicente MP, Pons M, Medina M: Pulmonary involvement in tuberous sclerosis. Pediatr Pulmonol 37:178-180, 2004.
24. Ryu JH, et al: The NHLBI lymphangiomyomatosis registry: Characteristics of 230 patients at enrollment. Am J Resp Crit Care Med 173:105-111, 2006.
25. Franz DN, et al: Mutational and radiographic analysis of pulmonary disease consistent with lymphangioleiomyomatosis and micronodular pneumocyte hyperplasia in women with tuberous sclerosis. Am J Resp Crit Care Med 164:661-668, 2001.
26. Westermann CJ, et al: The prevalence and manifestations of hereditary hemorrhagic telangiectasia in the Afro-Caribbean population of the Netherlands Antilles: A family screening. Am J Med Genet 116A:324-328, 2003.
27. Letteboer TG, et al: Genotype-phenotype relationship in hereditary hemorrhagic telangiectasia. J Med Genet 43(4):371-377, 2006.
28. Kjeldsen A, et al: Prevalence of pulmonary arteriovenous malformations (PAVMs) and occurrence of neurological symptoms in patients with hereditary haemorrhagic telangiectasia (HHT). J Intern Med 248:255-262, 2000.
29. Assar A, et al: The natural history of epistaxis in hereditary hemorrhagic telangiectasia. Laryngoscope 101:977-980, 1991.
30. Guttmacher AE, Marchuk DA, White RI Jr: Hereditary hemorrhagic telangiectasia. N Engl J Med 333:918-924, 1995.
31. Lee A, et al: Evaluation and management of pain in patients with Klippel-Trenaunay syndrome: A review. Pediatrics 115:744-749, 2005.
32. Huiras EE, et al: Pulmonary thromboembolism associated with Klippel-Trenaunay syndrome. Pediatrics 116:e596-e600, 2005.
33. Ulrich S, et al: Klippel-Trenaunay syndrome with small vessel pulmonary arterial hypertension. Thorax 60:971-973, 2005.
34. Gianlupi A, et al: Recurrent pulmonary embolism associated with Klippel-Trenaunay-Weber syndrome. Chest 115:1199-1212, 1999.
35. Tian XL, et al: Identification of an angiogenic factor that when mutated causes susceptibility of KT syndrome. Nature 427:640-657, 2004.
36. Uitto J: Elastic fibers in cutaneous disease. Curr Concepts Skin Dis 6:19-23, 1985.
37. Agha A, et al: Two forms of cutis laxa presenting in newborn. Acta Paediatr Scand 76:775-780, 1978.
38. Yeowell HN, Pinnell SR: The Ehlers-Danlos syndromes. Semin Dermatol 12:229, 1993.
39. Dowton SB, et al: Respiratory complications of Ehlers-Danlos syndrome type IV. Clin Genet 50:510-514, 1996.
40. Cavanaugh MJ, Cooper DM: Chronic pulmonary disease in a child with the Ehlers-Danlos syndrome. Acta Paediatr Scand 65:679-684, 1976.

41. Murray RA, et al: Rare pulmonary manifestation of Ehlers-Danlos syndrome. J Thorac Imaging 10: 138-141, 1995.
42. Lin I, et al: Recurrent congenital diaphragmatic hernia in Ehlers-Danlos syndrome. Cardiovasc Interv Radiol 29:920-923, 2006.
43. Safdar Z, O'Sullivan M, Shapiro JM: Emergency bullectomy for acute respiratory failure in Ehlers-Danlos syndrome. J Intensive Care Med 19:349-351, 2004.
44. Christen-Zach S, et al: Pseudoxanthoma elasticum: Evaluation and diagnostic criteria based on molecular data. Br J Dermatol 155:89, 2006.
45. Mishkel MA, et al: Xanthoma disseminatum: Clinical, metabolic, pathologic, and radiologic aspects. Arch Dermatol 113:1094-1100, 1977.
46. Moloney JR: Xanthoma disseminatum: Its otolaryngological manifestations. J Laryngol Otol 93:201-210, 1979.
47. Ozcelik U, et al: Xanthoma disseminatum: A child with respiratory system involvement and bronchiectasis. Pediatr Pulmonol 39:84-87, 2005.
48. Chung JH, et al: Pulmonary involvement in Erdheim-Chester disease. Respirology 10:389-392, 2005.
49. Kenn W, et al: Erdheim-Chester disease: Evidence for a disease entity different from Langerhans cell histiocytosis? Three cases with detailed radiological and immunohistochemical analysis. Hum Pathol 31:734-739, 2000.
50. Egan AJ, et al: Erdheim-Chester disease: Clinical, radiologic, and histopathologic findings in five patients with interstitial lung disease. Am J Surg Pathol 23:17-26, 1999.
51. Allen TC, et al: Pulmonary and ophthalmic involvement with Erdheim-Chester disease: A case report and review of the literature. Arch Pathol Lab Med 128:1428-1431, 2004.
52. Gahl WA, et al: Genetic defects and clinical characteristics of patients with a form of oculocutaneous albinism (Hermansky-Pudlak syndrome). N Engl J Med 338:1258-1264, 1998.
53. Avila NA, et al: Hermansky-Pudlak syndrome: Radiography and CT of the chest compared with pulmonary function tests and genetic studies. AJR Am J Roentgenol 179:887-892, 2002.
54. Gahl WA, et al: Effect of pirfenidone on the pulmonary fibrosis of Hermansky-Pudlak syndrome. Mol Genet Metab 76:234-242, 2002.
55. Vanhooteghem O, et al: Hermansky-Pudlak syndrome: A case report and discussion. Pediatr Dermatol 15:374-377, 1998.
56. Lebargy F, et al: Pulmonary complications in toxic epidermal necrolysis: A prospective clinical study. Intensive Care Med 23:1237-1244, 1997.
57. Yatsunami J, et al: Chronic bronchiolitis obliterans associated with Stevens-Johnson syndrome. Intern Med 34:772-775, 1995.
58. Metry DW, Jung P, Levy M: Use of intravenous immunoglobulin in children with Stevens Johnson syndrome and toxic epidermal necrolysis: Seven cases and review of the literature. Pediatrics 112(6 Pt 1):1430-1436, 2003.
59. Heide R, Tank B, Oranje AP: Mastocytosis in childhood. Pediatr Dermatol 19:375-383, 2002.
60. McElroy EA, Phyliky RL, Li C: Systemic mast cell disease associated with the hypereosinophilic syndrome. Mayo Clin Proc 73:47-50, 1998.
61. Huang TY, Yam LT, Li CY: Radiological features of systemic mast-cell disease. Br J Radiol 60:765-770, 1987.
62. Schmidt M, et al: Pulmonary manifestations of systemic mast cell disease. Eur Respir J 15:623-625, 2000.
63. Kelly AM, Kazerooni EA: HRCT appearance of systemic mastocytosis involving the lungs. J Thorac Imaging 19:52-55, 2004.
64. Yabe M, et al: Fatal interstitial pulmonary disease in a patient with dyskeratosis congenita after allogeneic bone marrow transplantation. Bone Marrow Transplant 19:389-392, 1997.
65. Utz JP, et al: Usual interstitial pneumonia complicating dyskeratosis congenita. Mayo Clin Proc 80:817-821, 2005.

CHAPTER 13

Pulmonary Manifestations of Parasitic Diseases

SHERMAN J. ALTER AND NELSON L. TURCIOS

Protozoa 274
  Malaria 274
  Amebiasis 276
Nematodes 280
  Ascariasis 280
  Hookworm 281
  Strongyloidiasis 282
  Toxocariasis 285

Trematodes 287
  Paragonimiasis 287
Cestodes 290
  Echinococcosis 290
Other Parasites Causing Pulmonary Disease 292
Summary 292
  References 293

Respiratory diseases are important causes of morbidity and mortality among children throughout the world. Although diseases attributed to parasitic infection are uncommon for many physicians in temperate climates, these infections remain important conditions that must be addressed. Because of the influx of immigrants from developing countries and the volume of global travel, including children, physicians should have a basic understanding of respiratory illnesses attributed to parasitic infections.

The spectrum of syndromes related to parasitic respiratory infection is quite large. Diagnosis of a parasitic infection should be classified through the recognition of identifiable host characteristics, underlying medical conditions, and specific clinical manifestations. The etiology of acute respiratory infections caused by parasitic agents can be suggested, however, through knowledge of the specific geographic locale of the ill child or the location from which the child has arrived (Table 13-1).[1,2] Clinical presentations, findings on imaging studies, or individual laboratory results can differentiate infection among particular parasitic organisms. Underlying immunodeficiency should suggest infection with certain organisms, such as *Strongyloides stercoralis* or *Toxoplasma*

gondii. In patients from appropriate geographic locations with respiratory symptoms and elevated peripheral eosinophil counts, infection with *Ascaris lumbricoides*, hookworm, *S. stercoralis,* or *Toxocara* species should be considered. This chapter reviews parasitic diseases that have pulmonary manifestations.

Protozoa

Malaria

Epidemiology
Malaria is endemic throughout the tropical areas of the world; one half of the world's population lives in areas where malaria occurs. From a global perspective, there are approximately 300 to 500 million infections per year, resulting in approximately 1 million deaths (Fig. 13-1). Most of these deaths occur in children.[3]

Etiology
The *Anopheles* mosquito transmits the parasite (Fig. 13-2). Various *Plasmodium* species—*Plasmodium falciparum, Plasmodium vivax, Plasmodium ovale,* and *Plasmodium malariae*—are responsible for human malaria. Of these four,

Table 13-1	Etiologies of Pulmonary Infiltrates Based on Geographic Distribution of Infecting Parasite					
	GEOGRAPHIC DISTRIBUTION					
ORGANISM	**AF**	**AM**	**AS**	**E**	**OC**	**WS**
Helminthic						
Ascariasis						X
Capillariasis hepatica	X	X	X	X		
Dirofilariasis						X
Echinococcosis	X	X	X	X	X	
Filariasis	X	X	X			
Gnathostomiasis			X*			
Hookworm						X
Paragonimiasis	X	X	X	X	X	
Schistosomiasis†	X	X	X			
Strongyloidiasis						X
Toxocariasis						X
Trichinellosis (*Trichinella spiralis*)						X
Protozoan						
Amebiasis						X
Cryptosporidiosis						X
Malaria (*Plasmodium falciparum*)	X	X	X	X	X	
Toxoplasmosis						X

*Rare in other geographic locales.
†Infiltrate early in disease, Katayama disease.
AF, Africa; AM, Americas; AS, Asia; E, Europe; OC, Oceania; WS, widespread.
Modified from Martin G: Approach to the patient in the tropics with pulmonary disease. In Guerrant RL, ed: Tropical Infectious Diseases, vol 2, 2nd ed. Philadelphia, WB Saunders, 2006, pp 1544-1553.

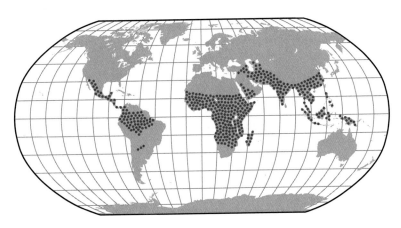

Figure 13-1. Geographic distribution of malaria (*dots*). The infection is distributed widely in many tropical and subtropical climates. *Plasmodium vivax* is the most prevalent WORLDWIDE type of malaria. *Plasmodium ovale* is especially prevalent in tropical West Africa. Infection with *Plasmodium falciparum* has the highest mortality rate. (*Adapted from Martinez S, et al. Thoracic manifestations of tropical parasitic infections: a pictorial review. Radiographics 25: 135-155, 2005.*)

only *P. falciparum* causes pulmonary disease. The disease onset is almost always within 1 year of exposure.

Clinical Manifestations

Shortness of breath and cough are the main respiratory symptoms in conscious patients; some also report chest tightness. Dyspnea often starts abruptly and progresses rapidly over a few hours, causing life-threatening hypoxia in patients with falciparum malaria.[4]

Pathogenesis

The pathogenesis of malarial lung disease is attributed to a diffuse alveolar injury resulting in a capillary leak syndrome and acute pulmonary edema. This noncardiogenic pulmonary edema is associated with normal or low capillary wedge pressures without evidence of left ventricular dysfunction.[5] Hypoalbuminemia and high-level parasitemia are risk factors associated with the development of pulmonary disease. Pathologic

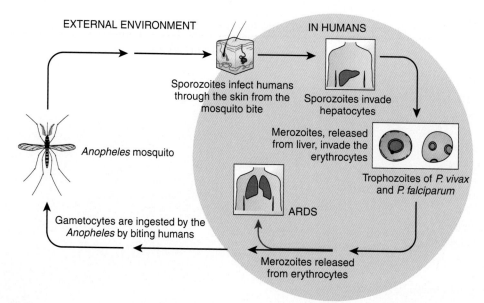

EXTERNAL ENVIRONMENT | IN HUMANS

Sporozoites infect humans through the skin from the mosquito bite

Sporozoites invade hepatocytes

Anopheles mosquito

Merozoites, released from liver, invade the erythrocytes

Trophozoites of *P. vivax* and *P. falciparum*

ARDS

Gametocytes are ingested by the *Anopheles* by biting humans

Merozoites released from erythrocytes

Figure 13-2. Life cycle of *Plasmodium* species (*P. falciparum, P. vivax, P. ovale,* and *P. malariae*). ARDS, acute respiratory distress syndrome. *(Adapted from Martinez S, et al. Thoracic manifestations of tropical parasitic diseases: a pictorial review. Radiographics 25:135-155, 2005.)*

findings may include features of acute respiratory distress syndrome in some individuals; this is thought to be secondary to sequestered malaria parasites in the lung, inducing an inflammatory cascade. This mechanism mainly involves cytokines, neutrophils, and endothelial adhesion molecules. Substantial evidence implicates the neutrophil as central to the pathogenesis of microvascular lung injury, which results in increased capillary permeability and subsequent pulmonary edema.

Diagnosis

Radiographic and computed tomography (CT) findings may suggest noncardiogenic pulmonary edema. Pleural effusion, diffuse interstitial edema, and lobar consolidation may be seen.[6,7] Laboratory assessments may show anemia and leukocytosis. A peripheral thick blood smear has high sensitivity for detecting parasitemia. A peripheral thin blood smear is better for species differentiation and staging of parasite development in *P. falciparum*.

Treatment

Effective treatment strategies for falciparum malaria depend on the pattern of parasite drug resistance in the geographic area where the infection is acquired and the severity of disease (Table 13-2).[8,9] The website for the Centers for Control and Prevention

should be reviewed to identify areas of chloroquine resistance. Severe malaria, such as that complicated by pulmonary disease, warrants therapy with parenteral medications. In addition to patient management in a critical care unit, the mortality rate is high. For physicians in nonmalarial areas, malaria always should be considered in the differential diagnosis of a sick patient who has traveled to a malaria-endemic area.

Amebiasis

Etiology and Epidemiology

Approximately 1% of the world's population is infected with *Entamoeba histolytica*. After malaria and schistosomiasis, amebiasis is the third most common cause of mortality from parasitic diseases. Although pleuropulmonary disease in *E. histolytica* infection is uncommon, it can occur in 15% of individuals with an amebic liver abscess.[10]

Pathogenesis

After a host ingests cysts in contaminated food or drink, pathogenic amebic trophozoites invade the colonic wall and disseminate hematogenously to the liver (Fig. 13-3). Less commonly, infection may occur after aspiration.[11] Disease onset may be either acute or chronic. Diarrhea is frequently absent. As an

Table 13-2	Drugs to Treat Parasitic Lung Infections		
INFECTION	**DRUG**	**PEDIATRIC DOSE**	**ADULT DOSE**
Malaria (*Plasmodium falciparum*—in areas of chloroquine resistance)			
Oral (*only* in uncomplicated or mild disease)			
Drugs of choice	Atovaquone/proguanil	<5 kg: not indicated	2 adult tabs bid *or*
		5-8 kg: 2 pediatric tabs once daily × 3 days	4 adult tabs once daily × 3 days
		9-10 kg: 3 pediatric tabs once daily × 3 days	
		11-20 kg: 1 adult tab once daily × 3 days	
		21-30 kg: 2 adult tabs once daily × 3 days	
		31-40 kg: 3 adult tabs once daily × 3 days	
		>40 kg: 4 adult tabs once daily × 3 days	
	or		
	Quinine sulfate	30 mg/kg/day in 3 doses × 3-7 days	650 mg q8h × 3-7 days
	plus		
	Doxycycline	4 mg/kg/day in 2 doses × 7 days	100 mg bid × 7 days
	or plus		
	Tetracycline	6.25 mg/kg qid × 7 days	250 mg qid × 7 days
	or plus		
	Clindamycin	20 mg/kg/day in 3 doses × 7 days	20 mg/kg/day in 3 doses × 7 days
Alternatives	Mefloquine	15 mg/kg followed 12 hr later by 10 mg/kg	750 mg followed 12 hr later by 500 mg
	Artesunate	4 mg/kg/day × 3 days	4 mg/kg/day × 3 days
	plus		
	Mefloquine	15 mg/kg followed 12 hr later by 10 mg/kg	750 mg followed 12 hr later by 500 mg
Malaria (*P. falciparum*—chloroquine-susceptible)			
Oral			
Drug of choice	Chloroquine phosphate	10 mg base/kg (maximum 600 mg base), then 5 mg base/kg at 24 hr and 48 hr	1 g (600 mg base), then 500 mg (300 mg base) 6 hr later, then 500 mg (300 mg base) at 24 hr and 48 hr
Parenteral (all *Plasmodium*)			
Drugs of choice	Quinidine gluconate	10 mg/kg loading dose (maximum 600 mg) in normal saline over 1-2 hr, followed by continuous infusion of 0.02 mg/kg/min until PO therapy can be started	10 mg/kg loading dose (maximum 600 mg) in normal saline over 1-2 hr, followed by continuous infusion of 0.02 mg/kg/min until PO therapy can be started
	or		
	Quinine dihydrochloride	20 mg/kg loading dose in 5% dextrose over 4 hr, followed by 10 mg/kg over 2-4 hr q8h (maximum	20 mg/kg loading dose in 5% dextrose over 4 hr, followed by 10 mg/kg over 2-4 hr q8h (maximum

(Continued)

Table 13-2	Drugs to Treat Parasitic Lung Infections—*Cont'd*		
INFECTION	**DRUG**	**PEDIATRIC DOSE**	**ADULT DOSE**
Alternative	Artemether	1800 mg/day) until PO therapy can be started	1800 mg/day) until PO therapy can be started
		3.2 mg/kg IM, then 1.6 mg/kg daily × 5-7 days	3.2 mg/kg IM, then 1.6 mg/kg daily × 5-7 days
Ascariasis (*Ascaris lumbricoides—* roundworm)			
Drug of choice	Albendazole	400 mg once	400 mg once
	or		
	Mebendazole	100 mg bid × 3 days or 500 mg once	100 mg bid × 3 days or 500 mg once
	or		
	Ivermectin	150-200 μg/kg once	150-200 μg/kg once
Hookworm (*Ancylostoma duodenale, Necator americanus*)			
Drug of choice	Albendazole	400 mg once	400 mg once
	or		
	Mebendazole	100 mg bid × 3 days or 500 mg once	100 mg bid × 3 days or 500 mg once
	or		
	Pyrantel pamoate	11 mg/kg/day (maximum 1 g) × 3 days	11 mg/kg/day (maximum 1 g) × 3 days
Strongyloidiasis (*Strongyloides stercoralis*)			
Drug of choice	Ivermectin	200 μg/kg/day × 2 days	200 μg/kg/day × 2 days
Alternatives	Albendazole	400 mg bid × 7 days	400 mg bid × 7 days
	or		
	Thiabendazole	50 mg/kg/day in 2 doses × 2 days (maximum 3 g/day)	50 mg/kg/day in 2 doses × 2 days (maximum 3 g/day)
Amebiasis (*Entamoeba histolytica*)			
Severe intestinal or extraintestinal disease	Metronidazole	30-50 mg/kg/day in 3 doses × 7-10 days	750 mg tid × 7-10 days
	or		
	Tinidazole	50 mg/kg/day (maximum 2 g) × 5 days	2 g once daily × 5 days
In treating extraintestinal disease follow with	Iodoquinol	30-40 mg/kg/day (maximum 2 g) in 3 doses × 20 days	650 mg tid × 20 days
	or		
	Paromomycin	25-35 mg/kg/day in 3 doses × 7 days	25-35 mg/kg/day in 3 doses × 7 days
Alternative	Diloxanide furoate	20 mg/kg/day in 3 doses × 10 days	500 mg tid × 10 days
Toxocariasis (visceral larva migrans)			
Drug of choice	Albendazole	400 mg bid × 5 days	400 mg bid × 5 days
	or		
	Mebendazole	100-200 mg bid × 5 days	100-200 mg bid × 5 days

Table 13-2	Drugs to Treat Parasitic Lung Infections—*Cont'd*			
INFECTION	**DRUG**	**PEDIATRIC DOSE**	**ADULT DOSE**
Echinococcosis (*Echinococcus granulosus*—hydatid cyst)			
Drug of choice	Albendazole	15 mg/kg/day (maximum 800 mg) × 1-6 mo	400 mg bid × 1-6 mo
	Patients may benefit from surgical resection or percutaneous drainage of cysts		
Echinococcosis (*Echinococcus multilocularis*)	Surgical excision is only available means of cure for this infection. In nonresectable cases, treatment with albendazole or mebendazole is recommended		
Paragonomiasis (*Paragonimus westermani*—lung fluke)			
Drug of choice	Praziquantel	75 mg/kg/day in 3 doses × 2 days	75 mg/kg/day in 3 doses × 2 days
Alternative	Bithionol	30-50 mg/kg on alternate days × 10-15 doses	30-50 mg/kg on alternate days × 10-15 doses

Modified from Drugs for parasitic infections. Med Lett Drugs Ther 1-12, August 2004.

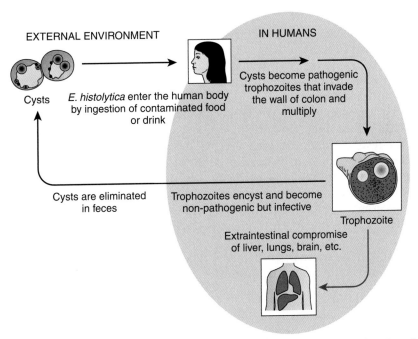

Figure 13-3. Life cycle of *Entamoeba histolytica.* (*Adapted from Martinez S, et al. Thoracic manifestations of tropical parasitic diseases: a pictorial review. Radiographics 25:135-155, 2005.*)

amebic liver abscess enlarges, adhesions may develop between the liver surface and the diaphragm. A sterile sympathetic pleural effusion may develop above the abscess. Alternatively, infection may spread through lymphatics or via the bloodstream and extend through the diaphragm after abscess rupture with empyema formation. The rupture frequently evokes severe pain in the right chest, back, or shoulder. Fever, hypoxemia, and circulatory collapse may follow. Classic "anchovy paste" can be obtained from an amebic hepatic abscess or from expectorate that has traveled through a hepatobronchial fistula.[12]

Clinical Manifestations

Physical findings in children with pulmonary amebiasis include toxic appearance and tachypnea with crackles and frequent findings of consolidation in the right lung base. Tender hepatomegaly and evidence of pericardial involvement may be noted.

Diagnosis

In any individual from an area endemic for *E. histolytica,* a right-sided pulmonary infiltrate or pleural effusion of obscure origin should suggest underlying amebic liver abscess in the differential diagnosis.[13] Chest radiography and CT may show right-sided basal consolidation, frequently with cavitations, and elevation of the right hemidiaphragm. An amebic empyema and pleural thickening are commonly noted. Abdominal CT and ultrasound are likely to show the associated liver abnormalities.

Stool examination is of limited diagnostic utility, with cysts being noted in only 15% to 33% of patients with extraintestinal amebiasis. It is possible that a patient with amebic forms identified in the stool may have pleuropulmonary disease of another etiology. Sputum stain or analysis of fluid obtained via bronchoalveolar lavage may identify trophozoites after rupture into a bronchus. Serologic analysis can be helpful in making the diagnosis in suspect cases in individuals from nonendemic areas of the world. Antibodies are detected in almost all cases. Although liver function tests can be normal, mild anemia and leukocytosis are noted in most infected patients.[14]

Treatment

Most patients with pulmonary amebiasis respond favorably over days following therapy with a tissue-active amebicide. Metronidazole or tinidazole is recommended (see Table 13-2). This therapy should be followed by a course of iodoquinol or paromomycin in dosages effective to treat concurrent asymptomatic intestinal amebiasis as well.

Nematodes

Ascariasis

Etiology and Epidemiology

Infection with the roundworm *Ascaris lumbricoides* is highly prevalent throughout the world. It is estimated that at any one point in time more than 1 billion individuals have disease caused by *Ascaris*. The highest prevalence is in developing countries, especially in regions of Africa, Asia, and Central and South America.[15] The organism reproduces prodigiously. An adult worm can produce 20 to 25 million eggs.[16] *Ascaris* eggs are quite hardy because of a thick proteinaceous coat, rendering them resistant to many environmental threats.

The frequency and intensity of *Ascaris* infections are greatest among children.[17] Children unintentionally ingest *Ascaris* eggs, which can be found in materials that are contaminated with human feces. Fully embryonated eggs that have matured under suitable environmental conditions become infective. Under the influence of gastric acid and bile salts, eggs hatch in the intestine, and larvae are liberated. They molt within the intestine into second-stage larvae and then travel to the liver. Larvae may traverse to the pulmonary vasculature, penetrate the alveoli, and develop into third-stage larvae (Fig. 13-4). After a period of 3 weeks, the organisms ascend the tracheobronchial tree, are swallowed, and return to the intestinal lumen. These develop into adult worms. After 2 to 3 months within the intestine, a worm is capable of producing thousands of eggs a day. Rarely, extremely heavy hematogenous dissemination (versus transpulmonary migration) of *Ascaris* eggs and larvae can manifest with cough, wheezing, and dyspnea associated with eosinophilia.

Clinical Manifestations

During lung migration by larvae, a nonproductive cough and fever commonly occur. Patients may complain of chest discomfort during coughing episodes or with deep breathing. Tachypnea is infrequent. Crackles or wheezing is noted in about half of patients, but evidence of consolidation is generally absent. An associated rash, frequently urticarial, can occur during this period. Pulmonary symptoms typically abate within 5 to 10 days.[17]

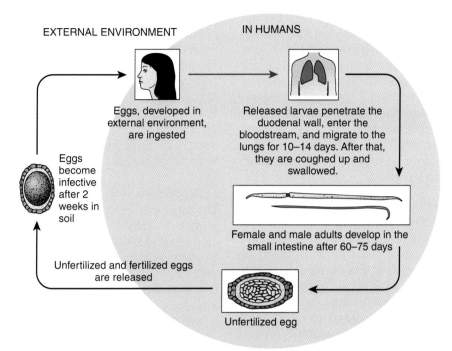

Figure 13-4. Life cycle of *Ascaris lumbricoides*. (*Adapted from Martinez S, et al. Thoracic manifestations of tropical parasitic diseases: a pictorial review. Radiographics 25:135-155, 2005.*)

The period of pulmonary migration of the parasite is associated with striking peripheral eosinophilia. It increases in magnitude several days and subsequently diminishes over several weeks. Individuals exposed to a large burden of the parasite can present with Löffler syndrome consisting of transient pulmonary infiltrates and eosinophilia. Ascariasis is the most commonly identified etiology of Löffler pneumonitis.[15]

Diagnosis

Chest radiography frequently shows either round or oval migratory infiltrates in both lung fields. The infiltrates can range from a few millimeters to several centimeters in size, and may become confluent in perihilar areas. Findings on chest films are more likely to be present in subjects with elevated blood eosinophils (>10%). The infiltrates usually clear completely after several weeks.[18,19]

Pulmonary ascariasis should be considered in individuals presenting with Löffler syndrome. Occasionally, eosinophils and eosinophilia-derived Charcot-Leyden crystals can be identified in sputum or bronchoalveolar fluid. Larvae also can be found in gastric aspirates. Stool evaluation for *Ascaris* eggs can confirm intestinal ascariasis. It may take 40 days after transpulmonary migration, however, for worms to deposit eggs within the intestine. The absence of *Ascaris* eggs in stool during an acute pulmonary disease followed by detection of eggs 2 to 3 months later would support the diagnosis of ascariasis. Ascariasis should be differentiated from infections caused by either hookworm or *Strongyloides*, which can manifest with similar findings of pneumonitis and peripheral eosinophilia.[20] Antibody titers to *Ascaris* and elevated IgE levels are found in infected patients.

Treatment

Benzimidazole drugs, such as albendazole and mebendazole, are effective first-line therapy against many helminths, including *A. lumbricoides* (see Table 13-2). Ivermectin is apparently equal in efficacy, but it has not been extensively studied in children weighing less than 15kg (see Table 13-2).[8]

Hookworm

Etiology

Human hookworms include two nematode (roundworm) species, *Ancylostoma duodenale* and *Necator americanus*. A smaller group of hookworms infecting animals can invade and parasitize humans (*Ancylostoma ceylanicum*) or can penetrate the human skin (causing cutaneous larva migrans) but do not develop any further (*Ancylostoma braziliense, Ancylostoma caninum, Uncinaria stenocephala*). Occasionally, *A. caninum* larvae may migrate to the human intestine causing eosinophilic enteritis; this may happen when larvae are ingested, rather than through skin invasion.[15]

Epidemiology

The burden of hookworm infection is considerable in children. There is a steady increase in the numbers of individuals infected as they get older, with a peak or plateau in adolescence or early adulthood.[21] High rates of hookworm transmission occur in the world's coastal regions, where sandy, moist soils, and temperature are optimal for viability of larvae. Eggs passed in the stool hatch into larvae. The released rhabditiform larvae grow in feces or soil, and become infective. These can survive 3 to 4 weeks in favorable environmental conditions. On contact with the human host, the larvae penetrate the skin and are carried through the venous circulation to the heart and lungs. Within 10 days of skin penetration, larvae invade the pulmonary alveoli, and ascend the bronchial tree to the pharynx, where they are swallowed. After reaching the small intestine, the larvae mature into adults, attach to the intestinal wall and are eliminated within 1 to 2 years. *N. americanus* always requires a transpulmonary migration phase. However, after penetration of the host skin, some *A. duodenale* larvae can become dormant (in the intestine or muscle).[15] *A. duodenale* also can infect by mouth when larvae are swallowed and develop into adult forms, without undergoing the lung migration.

Clinical Manifestations

The major clinical manifestations in humans infected with hookworms are related to chronic blood loss at the site of intestinal attachment of the adult worms. Because women and children have lower iron stores, they are most vulnerable to effects of hookworm-related intestinal blood loss. Severe anemia can be accompanied by cardiopulmonary symptoms. Respiratory symptoms consisting of chest discomfort, cough, and occasional wheezing can be seen during pulmonary migration of the larvae. Gastrointestinal and nutritional/metabolic symptoms also may occur. A history of a local pruritic, erythematous, papular rash ("ground itch") occurring during initial penetration by the filariform larvae can be elicited from some individuals with respiratory disease.

Diagnosis

Findings on chest radiography in patients with the pneumonitis of hookworm infection are less evident than the findings noted in patients with pulmonary ascariasis. Transient round or irregularly shaped infiltrates may be seen in both lung fields. Sometimes a nodular infiltrate may become confluent.[22]

Microscopic identification of eggs in a concentrated stool specimen is the most common method for diagnosing hookworm infection. In areas where concentration procedures are unavailable, a direct wet mount examination of the specimen is adequate for detecting moderate to heavy infections.[17]

Treatment

A single dose of a benzimidazole agent, either albendazole or mebendazole, is effective in removing hookworms from the intestine (see Table 13-2). Antihelminthic treatment combined with respiratory support in cases with pulmonary disease result in rapid improvement. Within a community, proper sanitation and the wearing of footwear are important in the control of hookworm infections.[21] Antihelminthic deworming of children may offer important health-related benefits to the population.

Strongyloidiasis

Infection with the nematode *S. stercoralis*, unlike that with other helminths, may occur as autoinfection with massive parasite invasion of the host (hyperinfection syndrome or disseminated strongyloidiasis) that may be fatal. This complication is more frequent in malnourished or immunosuppressed individuals. Although the parasite exists worldwide, infection is primarily encountered in individuals living in endemic tropical and subtropical areas of the world. Infection is sporadic in the United States, with the highest rates of infection in individuals residing in Appalachia or in southeastern states. The infection occurs more frequently in rural areas and in lower socioeconomic groups. The infection can persist for years to decades, and is often seen in immigrants one or more years after entry in the United States.

Etiology

S. stercoralis has its entire life cycle within the human (Fig. 13-5).[23] Infected individuals pass *S. stercoralis* larvae in their stools; these parasites may develop into free-living adults in the soil or may change into infective filariform larvae, which must penetrate the skin of a host in order to continue their life cycle. After penetration, they spread hematogenously to the lungs. Organisms ascend the trachea, are swallowed, and are transported to the intestine, where they complete their life cycle. Only adult female worms inhabit the intestine, depositing their eggs, which hatch into noninfectious first-stage (L1) larvae. In some individuals, larvae undergo morphologic changes into filariform (infective) larvae; these larvae are capable of infecting the same individual, resulting in autoinfection. In children and adults chronically infected

with *S. stercoralis*, worm burden increases markedly because of the completion of this autoinfection cycle within the host.

Epidemiology

Humans are the primary hosts of *S. stercoralis*. Transmission of infection and its endemicity depend on suitable soil, climatic conditions, and poor sanitary habits. Close contact and poor personal hygiene are important because the prevalence of infection is much higher in institutions for the mentally handicapped. Host factors such as nutrition and immune status may have a crucial role in the development of the hyperinfection syndrome.

Pathogenesis

Acute infection with *Strongyloides* larvae can elicit a cutaneous eruption at the site of skin penetration. A Löffler-like syndrome with eosinophilia may be noted during migration of the larvae through the lungs. Eosinophilia also may occur when adult worms burrow into the intestinal mucosa. Disseminated strongyloidiasis is a complex pathologic entity owing to larval invasion and injury of internal organs such as the liver, heart, pancreas, kidneys, and central nervous system. It may be accompanied by gram-negative bacteremia.

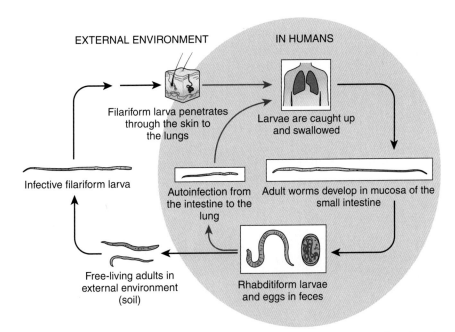

EXTERNAL ENVIRONMENT   IN HUMANS

Filariform larva penetrates through the skin to the lungs

Larvae are caught up and swallowed

Infective filariform larva

Autoinfection from the intestine to the lung

Adult worms develop in mucosa of the small intestine

Free-living adults in external environment (soil)

Rhabditiform larvae and eggs in feces

Figure 13-5. Life cycle of *Strongyloides stercoralis*. (*Adaptped from Martinez S, et al. Thoracic manifestations of tropical parasitic diseases: a pictorial review. Radiographics 25:135-155, 2005.*)

Clinical Manifestations

Signs and symptoms of strongyloidiasis occur in only a small proportion of infected individuals or in individuals with the hyperinfection syndrome. Because of the autoinfection phenomenon, many patients have a chronic infection, and symptoms may continue for years. Hyperinfection is the most serious and potentially fatal manifestation. Symptoms fall into three broad categories: cutaneous, pulmonary, and intestinal. These can be present during acute and chronic disease, and during hyperinfection syndrome.

The acute disease is often recognized by its cutaneous manifestations followed by pulmonary and intestinal symptoms. The hallmark of cutaneous symptoms is pruritus at the site of larval entry, usually at the foot or ankle. Within a week or so, the migration of larvae into the tracheobronchial tree causes itching of the throat, dry cough, and Löffler-like pneumonia with eosinophilia. This is followed by intestinal manifestations that include epigastric abdominal pain and distention and diarrhea. Acute infection is followed by the stage when the symptoms may be recurrent or continuous as the patient enters the chronic stage of the disease.

Although occurring less commonly in children than in adults, the hyperinfection syndrome is disseminated strongyloidiasis from massive autoinfection, resulting in an overwhelming larval burden and widespread dissemination to the lungs and other organ systems (Fig. 13-6).[24] Severe pulmonary and extrapulmonary systemic symptoms result. Although this syndrome can occur without a predisposing cause, it is usually associated with conditions of defective cellular immunity, such as lymphoma, Hodgkin disease, organ transplantation, and acquired immunodeficiency syndrome.[24] Malnourished and debilitated individuals are at increased risk, especially if they are receiving systemic steroids. Overwhelming infection also can occur after treatment with cytotoxic medications or corticosteroids. Pulmonary manifestations are increasing cough and dyspnea along with odorless mucopurulent or blood-tinged sputum. These manifestations may be accompanied by shock owing to gram-negative septicemia. Hypoxemia, respiratory failure, and acute respiratory distress syndrome may be seen. Frequently, even with effective therapy, the prognosis in patients with pulmonary strongyloidiasis and acute respiratory distress syndrome is poor. Individuals presenting with an overwhelming pulmonary infection may have findings of secondary bacterial or fungal infection.[23]

Diagnosis

The chest radiograph is normal in most infected patients. Alveolar infiltrates in either a lobar or a segmental distribution are seen in most patients with symptomatic pulmonary strongyloidiasis.[25] Less often, diffuse infiltrates are noted. In patients with hyperinfection, changes on chest radiograph that range from focal to diffuse alveolar infiltrates, abscesses, and cavitations to pleural effusions may be noted.[25] Eosinophilia is often absent in hyperinfection syndrome; as a result, this is considered a poor prognostic indicator.

Definitive diagnosis of *Strongyloides* infection relies on identification of first-stage rhabditiform larvae in the feces of an infected individual. However, because the female *S. stercoralis* releases few eggs, multiple stool specimens may be required, each concentrated by the use of various techniques may be required. A sensitive blood-agar plate

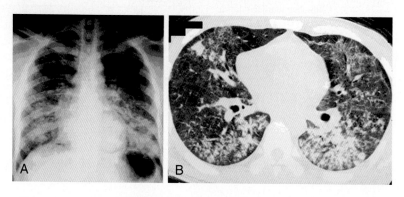

Figure 13-6. Strongyloidiasis in an 18-year-old man with hemoptysis. **A,** Chest radiograph shows extensive bilateral patchy areas of consolidation. **B,** High-resolution CT scan more clearly delineates the areas of consolidation. Bronchoalveolar lavage revealed larvae of *Strongyloides stercoralis*.

method useful for detecting larvae in various clinical specimens also has been described. Alternatively, the number of larvae recovered from feces can be amplified by allowing them to undergo the heterogonic cycle in Baermann cultures. Serologic analysis also may be helpful in the diagnosis of strongyloidiasis. Sputum or bronchoalveolar lavage may show larvae or, rarely, eggs.[26] Sputum analysis and culture may note evidence of secondary bacterial or fungal infection. Duodenal aspirates looking for parasites may be helpful in some cases. Lung biopsy may reveal larvae or findings documenting secondary infection.

Treatment

Because of the risk of hyperinfection, all individuals found to harbor *Strongyloides* should be treated, even in the absence of symptoms. The treatment goal is to eliminate all the worms; repeated treatment is sometimes needed. The two agents of choice for the treatment of strongyloidiasis are thiabendazole and ivermectin. Thiabendazole is administered at a dose of 25mg/kg twice a day (maximum 3g/day) for 2 days, or for 2 to 3 weeks for hyperinfection syndrome (if started early). Ivermectin (200μg/kg/day for 1 to 2 days) is also effective in the treatment of gastrointestinal tract disease. However, ivermectin has not been extensively studied in children. Safety profiles have not been established for children weighing less that 15kg (see Table 13-2).[8] Nonetheless, because of its greater efficacy, some clinicians still prefer it as first-line treatment for strongyloidiasis.

Toxocariasis

Toxocariasis is a worldwide soil-transmitted zoonotic infection that causes two main diseases in humans: visceral larva migrans (VLM), which can involve many organs and characteristically causes peripheral eosinophilia, hepatosplenomegaly, and pneumonitis, and ocular larva migrans. Humans are incidental hosts and not necessary for the life cycle of the *Toxocara*. VLM results from the inflammatory response to the migration of immature, second-stage larvae through the viscera of the host.

Etiology

Two species of *Toxocara* are primarily responsible for most cases of VLM: *Toxocara canis* and *Toxocara cati,* which are transmitted from dogs and cats, respectively. Other *Toxocara* species have been implicated in human infection, including *Toxocara leonine,* from dogs and foxes, and *Baylisascaris procyonis,* from raccoons.

Epidemiology

Toxocara are found worldwide in domesticated and wild dogs and cats. Infection with *Toxocara* is more prevalent than realized because many individuals do not express the complete VLM syndrome. Domestic animals, especially young ones, in urban and rural environments may harbor the parasite. *T. canis* is a common parasite of dogs found throughout the world. In fact, an estimated 20% of dogs in the United States excrete *T. canis,* and almost all juvenile raccoons excrete *B. procyonis.* Puppies are particularly dangerous because transplacental transmission results in 77% to 100% of puppies becoming infected. By the time the animals are 3 weeks old, mature egg-laying worms can be present. Adult female worms pass 200,000 unembryonated eggs per day onto the soil in the feces of the infected animal. Under suitable soil conditions, the eggs become embryonated and infectious in 2 to 3 weeks. Dogs and cats often defecate in areas where children play. Under optimal soil conditions, the deposited thick-shell embryonated eggs of *T. canis* and *T. cati* can survive for months to years.[28] Most infections occur in children with a history of pica and close contact with dogs and cats or in individuals who have accidentally ingested contaminated soil. Animals are not directly infectious because of the time lag before the eggs become infectious. Ocular larva migrans commonly occurs in older children or young adults, rarely with systemic manifestations.

Pathogenesis

After ingestion by dogs or cats, infective eggs hatch in the upper alimentary tract. The second-stage larvae migrate through the intestinal walls and into the bloodstream and then into the liver and lungs of the infected animal. From the lungs, the larvae mature by migrating through the tracheobronchial tree and passing into the upper alimentary tree. There, the mature worm can begin laying eggs, which pass out in the feces to begin the cycle anew.

In humans, the initial stages of infection are identical: Infectious second-stage larvae hatch in the small intestine and begin migrating through bloodstream and lymphatics to various tissues, including the liver, heart, lungs, brain, and eyes. Before the larvae can complete their transtracheal passage and maturation to adult worms, however, host defenses block further migration of the larvae by encasing them within an eosinophilic granulomatous reaction. The pathogenesis of VLM is the direct result of the immunologic response of the body to the dead and dying larvae. Multiple eosinophilic abscesses may develop in the infected tissues. The larvae remain alive, infective, and antigenic for an indefinite period. The local inflammatory reaction appears as an eosinophilic granuloma, and an open lung biopsy of a granulomatous lesion often shows *Toxocara* larvae. Host antibodies are generated against excretory-secretory antigens of the larvae.[29] A group of glycoprotein antigens has been identified that contain protease, acetylcholinesterase, and eosinophil-stimulating activity.[30]

Clinical Manifestations

Any child with fever of unknown origin and peripheral eosinophilia should be suspected to have VLM until proved otherwise. VLM is most common in young children because they have a greater opportunity of ingesting the infectious eggs while in playgrounds. Children are also less likely to follow good hygiene practices. The classic case occurs in a boy younger than 5 years with a history of pica and exposure to dogs. The extent of signs and symptoms depends on the number and location of granulomatous lesions and the host's immune response. The initial symptoms may include fever, anorexia, headache, lethargy, sleep and behavior disorders, cough, wheeze, cervical adenitis, and hepatomegaly. More recently, so-called "covert toxocariasis" has been implicated as responsible for a clinical presentation that occurs after long-term exposure of migrating juvenile larval forms. Some individuals are

totally asymptomatic or have symptoms and signs related to specific organ dysfunction.

In VLM, the specific signs and symptoms depend on the organ affected. Liver invasion is an early event; hepatomegaly of varying degrees is almost always present. With more severe involvement, various combinations of abdominal pain, arthralgias, myalgias, weight loss, intermittent fever, pulmonary disease, and neurologic disturbance may be seen. The immediate hypersensitivity response to the larvae manifests as symptoms of VLM. It is an environmental risk factor not only for asthma,[31] but also for seizure disorder, functional intestinal disease, urticaria, eosinophilic and reactive arthritis, and angioedema.

The natural course of VLM may be quite prolonged. The initial stage of the illness lasts several weeks, beginning with low-grade fevers and nonspecific symptoms and progressing to eosinophilia and hepatomegaly. Recurrent episodes of asthma or pneumonia may occur. Over the next few weeks, intermittent high fevers occur along with the major manifestations of the disease. Recovery may take 1 to 2 years, during which time the eosinophilia resolves along with the hepatomegaly. The pulmonary infiltrates resolve more rapidly.

Ocular larva migrans usually occurs in older children and is typically manifested as unilateral visual impairment. The degree of impairment relates to the specific area of involvement. Blindness is common.

Diagnosis

The pulmonary involvement secondary to toxocariasis has been reported in 20% to 80% of infected children. Cough, if present, is generally nonproductive. Wheezing is the most frequent finding on chest examination, although rhonchi and crackles also have been described. Because of the wheezing, some patients are diagnosed initially with asthma. There is no typical chest radiograph appearance. Descriptions of imaging studies range from patchy alveolar disease with pseudonodular infiltrates on CT, to diffuse interstitial pneumonitis, to an asymptomatic pulmonary mass. A pattern similar to miliary tuberculosis has been reported in severe cases. The varied patterns seen on imaging studies may reflect whether direct larval invasion of lung tissue or a hypersensitivity reaction to larval antigens is the primary pathologic process present in a particular patient. Although pulmonary symptoms are generally mild, acute respiratory failure has been reported from *Toxocara* infection.

Neutrophilia occurs during the first few days, but rapidly gives way to the eosinophilia characteristically seen in this disease. Eosinophilia can range up to 50% to 90% of the total white blood cell count. Leukocytosis is generally present, with extreme values of greater than 100,000 cell/mm^3 occasionally reported. *T. canis* also may produce PIE syndrome (pulmonary infiltrates and eosinophilia).

Other laboratory findings may be helpful in supporting a diagnosis of VLM. Serum IgE levels are greater than 900 IU/mL in 60% of patients tested. Hypergammaglobulinemia is often reported, characterized by elevations of one or all of the immunoglobulins. Because of cross-reactivity between larval and blood group antigens, many patients develop high anti-A and anti-B isohemagglutinin titers, which persist for months after the initial infection. Bronchoalveolar lavage may also show eosinophilia.

A presumptive diagnosis of VLM rests on clinical signs and symptoms, history of exposure to puppies, laboratory findings (including eosinophilia), and the detection of antibodies to *Toxocara*. Antibody detection is the only means of confirming a clinical diagnosis of VLM or covert toxocariasis. The currently recommended serologic test for toxocariasis is enzyme-linked immunosorbent assay (ELISA) using the larval excretory-secretory antigens to detect the host's antibodies. If a titer greater than 1:32 is considered positive, the diagnostic sensitivity is approximately 78%, with a specificity of greater than 93%. A measurable titer does not indicate current clinical *T. canis* infection, however. Because antibodies against *Toxocara* are present for years, an antigen-capture ELISA has been developed to separate acute from dormant infection. A few individuals tested have positive ELISA titers that apparently reflect the prevalence of asymptomatic toxocariasis. The diagnosis of toxocariasis does not rest on identification of the parasite. Because the larvae do not develop into adults in humans, a stool examination would not detect any *Toxocara* eggs.[28] Evidence of coexisting parasitic diseases, such as detecting *Ascaris* and *Trichuris* eggs in feces, indicates fecal exposure, however, increasing the probability of *Toxocara* involvement in the tissues.

Treatment

For symptomatic pulmonary toxocariasis, therapy with either albendazole or mebendazole twice daily for 5 days is recommended (see Table 13-2).[8] Corticosteroids have been used in patients with severe pulmonary involvement, possibly to treat the hypersensitivity component of the disease. Otherwise, treatment is symptomatic.

Trematodes

Paragonimiasis

Etiology

Paragonimiasis, also known as lung fluke disease, is caused by the genus *Paragonimus*. There are more than 40 species, of which only a few are considered relevant to humans. Most human disease is caused by *Paragonimus westermani*. In humans, the organism primarily infects the lungs. Paragonimiasis is a zoonotic infection of carnivorous animals, including animals in the canine and feline families, which also serve as reservoir hosts. Endemic areas for human paragonimiasis are the Far East, Southeast Asia from India to Japan, Africa, and Latin America (Fig. 13-7).[32]

The life cycle of these flukes involves two intermediate hosts plus humans. The complex life cycle involves seven distinct phases: egg, miracidium, sporocyst, redia, cercaria, metacercaria, and adult (Fig. 13-8). Unembryonated eggs from individuals previously infected with *P. westermani* are excreted in the stool or expectorated in the sputum. The eggs embryonate and hatch in the external environment. These miracidia seek their first intermediate host, a snail, and penetrate its soft tissue. Miracidia go through several developmental stages inside snails and eventually later give rise to many cercariae, which emerge from the snail. The cercariae invade the second intermediate host, a crustacean such as a crab or crayfish, where they encyst and become metacercariae, the infective stage for the mammalian host.

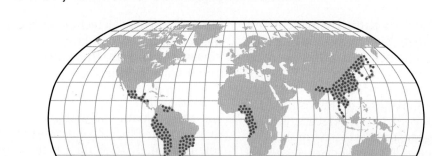

Figure 13-7. Geographic distribution of *Paragonimus* species (*dots*). (*Adapted from Martinez S, et al. Thoracic manifestations of tropical parasitic diseases: a pictorial review. Radiographics 25:135-155, 2005.*)

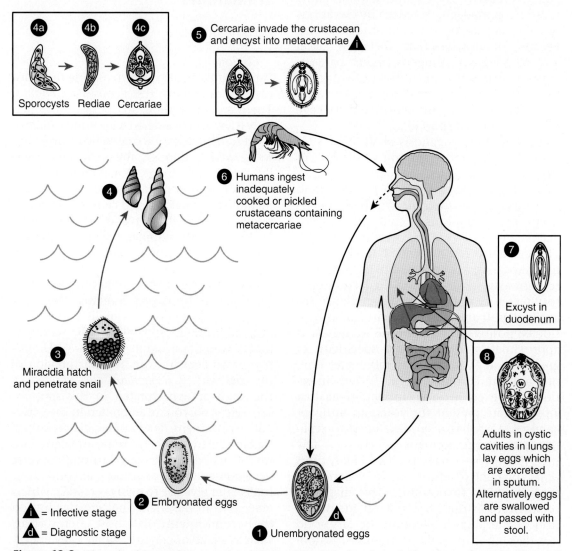

Figure 13-8. Life cycle of *Paragonimus westermani*. (*Adapted from Martinez S, et al. Thoracic manifestations of tropical parasitic diseases: a pictorial review. Radiographics 25:135-155, 2005.*)

Human infection with *P. westermani* occurs by eating raw or inadequately cooked or pickled crab or crayfish that harbor metacercariae of the parasite. The parasites excyst in the duodenum, penetrate through the intestinal wall into the peritoneal cavity, and cross the diaphragm into the lungs, where they become encapsulated and develop into adults. Within the lung, parasites migrate to the small bronchioles and trigger an acute inflammatory process. This process results in necrosis of lung parenchyma and formation of a fibrous capsule in which adult worms and ova are noted. These cystic areas frequently can communicate with additional bronchioles or bronchi.[22,33] Worms can invade other organs and tissues, such as the brain and striated muscles. When this invasion occurs, however, completion of the life cycle is not achieved because the eggs laid cannot exit these sites. Individuals infected as children may have infections that persist for 20 years. Animals such as pigs, dogs, and various feline species also can harbor *P. westermani*.

As the life cycle of the fluke suggests, it can cause pulmonary and extrapulmonary disease. The pathogenesis of pulmonary disease is a result of parasite and host factors. The lesions are a result of direct mechanical damage by the flukes or their eggs or by toxins released by the fluke. The host response adds to the damage in the lungs when the host immune response assumes the form of eosinophilic infiltration and the subsequent development of a cyst of host granulation tissue around the flukes. Besides the adult flukes, the cyst also contains eggs and Charcot-Leyden crystals. The cysts develop in the lung parenchyma close to the bronchioles. The release of cyst contents can cause bronchopneumonia, and the cyst wall may fibrose and become calcified.

Pulmonary paragonimiasis has acute and chronic stages with different clinical manifestations. The main clinical manifestations of paragonimiasis are respiratory symptoms and eosinophilia. When the flukes reach the lungs, the patient can have cough, dyspnea, or chest tightness or chest pain, and systemic symptoms of fever, malaise, and night sweats. The patient may recall being sick days or weeks before the current illness, with fever, diarrhea, and abdominal pain. Chills and urticarial rash may occur, leading to the diagnosis of a viral syndrome. A peripheral smear at this time would show eosinophilia.

The diagnosis of paragonimiasis is often not made in the acute stage of the disease. The chronic stage usually follows 2 to 4 weeks later. Most patients look well, and the disease may resemble chronic bronchitis or bronchiectasis, with a persistent cough frequently worse in the morning hours that starts out dry and becomes productive and profuse. The sputum may range from brown or rust in color to frank hemoptysis. Hemoptysis can be frequent and fatal. Low-grade fever along with vague pleuritic chest pain may be present. In uncomplicated pulmonary paragonimiasis, the chest examination may be normal, although progressive infection may have detectable crackles, or digital clubbing with chronic infection. Pulmonary paragonimiasis can be complicated by lung abscess, pneumothorax, pleural adhesions, empyema, and interstitial pneumonia. Extrapulmonary locations of the adult worms result in more severe manifestations, especially when the brain is involved.[22,34]

A normal chest radiograph is obtained in 21% of infected individuals.[34] In others, pleuropulmonary findings include migratory, frequently inconspicuous infiltrates that modify their appearance over time. Later, chest films may show fixed single or multiple, patchy round opacities, noted either in the periphery or in the lung bases (Fig. 13-9). The pathognomonic radiographic

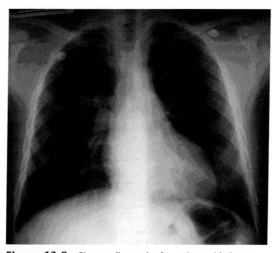

Figure 13-9. Chest radiograph of a patient with *Paragonimus westermani* infection shows patchy round opacities.

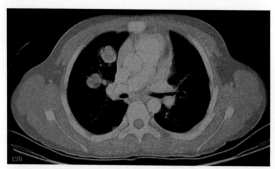

Figure 13-10. Chest CT scan of a patient with *Paragonimus westermani* infection shows nodules.

picture shows a ring shadow with a crescent-shaped opacity along one side of the border. Calcifications of cystic lesions are seen until healing occurs. Signs include pleural effusions, pleural thickening, or hydropneumothorax; pleural effusions are reported in 5% to 71% of patients with *P. westermani* infections. Contrast-enhanced CT scan of the chest may show single or multiple nodules (Fig. 13-10) or fluid-filled cysts, occasionally accompanied by burrow tracts, which are better visualized after the acute consolidation resolves.[35]

Diagnosis

Diagnosis is based on microscopic demonstration of eggs in stool or sputum, but these are not present until after 2 to 3 months of infection. Ova may frequently be detected when hemoptysis occurs. Bronchoalveolar lavage occasionally may reveal ova. Concentration techniques may be necessary in patients with light infections. Pleural fluid may show increased eosinophils with rare ova. Only one third of infected patients have eggs detected in the stool.[34] Lung

biopsy may allow diagnostic confirmation and species identification when an adult or developing fluke is recovered.

Treatment

Praziquantel, given three times daily for 2 days, is the therapy of choice (see Table 13-2). Infected individuals may transiently have worsening of radiographic features in the lung after treatment. Patients do not have concomitant exacerbation of respiratory symptoms, however.

Cestodes

Echinococcosis

Human echinococcosis (hydatidosis, or hydatid disease) is caused by the larval stages of cestodes (tapeworms) of the genus *Echinococcus*. *Echinococcus granulosus,* the most frequent hydatid disease in humans, causes cystic disease. *E. granulosus* occurs practically worldwide, and more frequently in rural, grazing areas where dogs ingest organs from infected animals. *Echinococcus multilocularis* occurs in the Northern Hemisphere, including central Europe and the northern parts of Europe, Asia, and North America (Fig. 13-11). *E. multilocularis* causes alveolar echinococcosis.

The adult *E. granulosus* resides in the small bowel of the definitive canine hosts (Fig. 13-12). Other carnivores also may act as a host. Gravid proglottids release eggs that are passed in the feces. After ingestion by a suitable intermediate host, such as sheep grazing on contaminated ground, the egg hatches in the small bowel and releases an

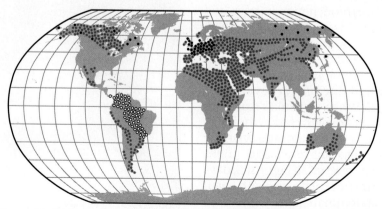

Figure 13-11. Geographic distribution of hydatid disease from *Echinococcus granulosus* (solid *dots*), Echinococcus multilocularis (black dots), and Echinococcus vogeli (grey dots). E. granulosus *is the most common of the* Echinococcus species. (*Adapted from Martinez S, et al. Thoracic manifestations of tropical parasitic diseases: a pictorial review. Radiographics 25:135-155, 2005.*)

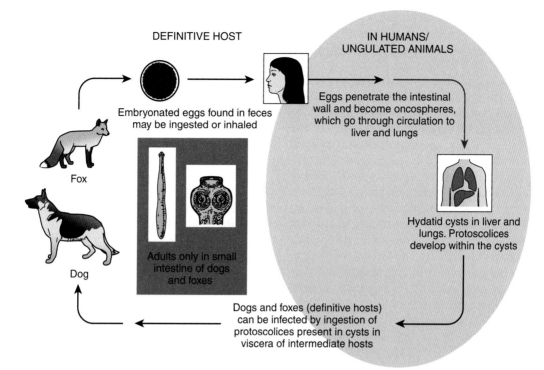

DEFINITIVE HOST

IN HUMANS/
UNGULATED ANIMALS

Embryonated eggs found in feces
may be ingested or inhaled

Eggs penetrate the intestinal
wall and become oncospheres,
which go through circulation to
liver and lungs

Fox

Dog

Adults only in small
intestine of dogs
and foxes

Hydatid cysts in liver and
lungs. Protoscolices
develop within the cysts

Dogs and foxes (definitive hosts)
can be infected by ingestion of
protoscolices present in cysts in
viscera of intermediate hosts

Figure 13-12. Life cycle of *Echinococcus* species. (*Adapted from Martinez S, et al. Thoracic manifestations of tropical parasitic infections: a pictorial review. Radiographics 25:135-155, 2005.*)

oncosphere. This oncosphere penetrates the intestinal wall and migrates through the circulatory system into various organs, especially the liver and lungs, and develops into a gradually enlarging cyst capable of producing protoscolices and daughter cysts. Ingesting the cyst-containing viscera of the infected intermediate host infects the definitive host. After ingestion, the protoscolices evaginate, attach to the intestinal mucosa, and develop into adult organisms. The same life cycle occurs with *E. multilocularis,* although the definitive hosts vary (foxes and, to a lesser extent, other animals, including dogs). Humans become intermediate hosts through contact with a definitive host (usually a domesticated dog) or ingestion of contaminated water or produce.[36,37] Humans ingest eggs, with resulting release of oncospheres in the intestine and the development of cysts in various organs.

E. granulosus infection may occur with silent infection for many years before the enlarging cysts cause symptoms in the affected organs. When the parasite traverses the intestinal wall and reaches the portal venous system and gut lymphatics, the liver serves as an initial line of defense and is the most frequently involved

organ in human hydatid disease. Multilocular cysts form in the liver and clinically can result in abdominal pain, a mass in the hepatic area, and biliary duct obstruction.

Pulmonary involvement by *Echinococcus* occurs by two routes. Transdiaphragmatic incursion into the lung is reported in 0.6% to 16% of cases of hepatic echinococcal disease. Cyst adherence to the diaphragm or seeding of the pulmonary parenchyma produces chest pain, cough, and hemoptysis. Rupture of the cysts into the pleural space can produce fever, urticaria, eosinophilia, and anaphylactic shock, and cyst dissemination. Other organs (brain, bone, heart) also can be involved, with resulting symptoms. *E. multilocularis* affects the liver as a slow-growing, destructive mass with occasional metastatic lesions into the lungs.

Hematogenous dissemination of the organism directly to the lungs is most common in children.[37] Many hydatid cysts acquired in childhood remain asymptomatic, with the diagnosis made incidentally on a chest radiograph. Cysts may be located in any lobes, but most are noted in the lower lobes. Symptomatic childhood disease can manifest with a sudden cough paroxysm, hemoptysis, or vague chest discomfort. After rupture of a pulmonary cyst, expectoration of parasites, cyst fluid, or membranes can be seen. Bacterial superinfection of a ruptured pulmonary cyst is common.[38]

Abdominal radiograph and ultrasound can document hepatic involvement. Calcification of hepatic hydatid cysts is seen in 20% to 30% of cases. CT has a high specificity in the diagnosis of unilocular or multilocular hydatid cysts, with or without calcifications. Uncomplicated pulmonary cysts appear radiographically as well-defined round, oval, or polycyclic cysts measuring 1 to 20 cm in diameter.[39] Large cavitary lesions with air-fluid levels may be seen. Occasionally, cystic growth may cause bronchial erosion with air flow introduced between the cyst and bronchiole; this can be seen as a thin, radiolucent crescent in the upper part of the cyst. After expectoration, retained membranes or remaining solid components can be recognized within the collapsed cystic areas. CT can clarify further many of these findings noted on chest x-rays.

The diagnosis of echinococcosis relies mainly on findings by ultrasound or other imaging techniques supported by positive serologic tests. In seronegative patients with hepatic image findings compatible with echinococcosis, ultrasound-guided fine needle biopsy may be useful to confirm the diagnosis. Precautions must be taken during aspiration to control allergic reactions or prevent secondary seeding in the event of leakage of hydatid fluid or protoscolices.[40,41]

Surgery is the most common form of treatment for echinococcosis, although removal of the parasite mass is usually not 100% effective. After surgery, medication may be necessary to keep the cyst from recurring. The drug of choice for treatment of echinococcosis is albendazole (*E. granulosus*). Some reports have suggested the use of albendazole or mebendazole for *E. multilocularis* infections (see Table 13-2).

Other Parasites Causing Pulmonary Disease

Toxoplasma gondii, an intracellular protozoan parasite, may cause lung infection in immunocompromised individuals, particularly those with underlying human immunodeficiency virus infection or after organ transplantation.

Clinical manifestations of pulmonary toxoplasmosis include fever, dyspnea, and cough.[42] Imaging of the chest typically shows reticulonodular infiltrates. The clinical presentation in an immunocompromised individual can mimic that of pneumonitis caused by *Pneumocystis jiroveci* (formerly *Pneumocystis carinii*).

Filarial infection (*Brugia malayi, Wuchereria bancrofti, Brugia timori*) can present with a clinical picture known as tropical pulmonary eosinophilia, caused by the microfilaria stage in the lungs.[43,44] This clinical presentation is uncommon during childhood, however. Clinical findings in individuals with filariasis include mild fever, weight loss, and lymphadenopathy. Chest radiographs reveal small (<5mm), indistinct, frequently migratory nodular opacities throughout all lung fields. Eosinophilia is noted and may be strikingly elevated with counts up to 50%. In the appropriate clinical setting, a singular "coin lesion" noted on chest radiograph might be representative of infection with *Dirofilaria immitis,* the dog heartworm (Figs. 13-13 and 13-14).[45] Many cases were seen in the southeastern United States, but increasingly cases are being diagnosed in other areas of the country as the disease spreads in dogs into these areas. Eosinophilia is rare in individuals with dirofilariasis.

Schistosomiasis caused by the trematodes *Schistosoma mansoni, Schistosoma japonica,* and *Schistosoma haematobium* is common throughout the world with the exception of the United States. During early infection with these parasites, when transpulmonary migration occurs, patients may present with an acute febrile illness associated with peripheral blood eosinophilia and diffuse nodular infiltrates in chest radiographs (Katayama fever).[46] Such a clinical presentation can be confused with miliary tuberculosis. The patient's clinical status and findings on chest films may worsen in infected individuals given effective therapy against the parasite. These findings might be reflective of an allergic alveolitis.[46]

Summary

The human lower respiratory tract can be affected by numerous parasitic agents. Infections occur in adults and children. In individuals with parasitic pulmonary disease,

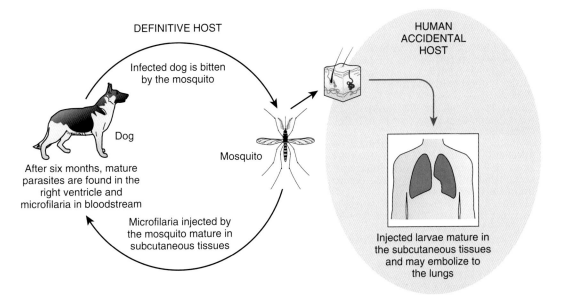

Figure 13-13. Life cycle of *Dirofilaria immitis*. (*Adapted from Martinez S, et al. Thoracic manifestations of tropical parasitic infections: a pictorial review. Radiographics 25:135-155, 2005.*)

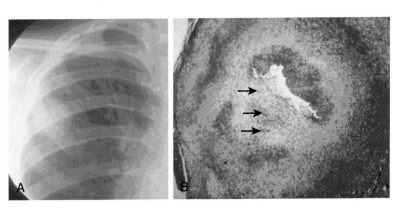

Figure 13-14. Dirofilariasis in an asymptomatic 14-year-old girl with a solitary pulmonary nodule. **A,** Chest radiograph shows a nodule with soft tissue opacity in the right upper lung. **B,** Photomicrograph obtained after surgical resection shows an infarcted peripheral vessel surrounded by necrotic lung tissue. Some remnants of the parasites are present in the lumen (*arrows*). (Masson stain, original magnification 40×.) (See Color Plate)

clinical manifestations and findings on imaging may be nonspecific and can present a diagnostic challenge. Most parasitic infections of the lung would be expected to occur in individuals from endemic tropical or subtropical areas of the world, but immigration and ease of travel might permit an infected individual to present to a clinician unfamiliar with these diseases. It is important to have an understanding of the epidemiology, clinical features, and approach to therapy in children with parasitic infections of the lung.

References

1. Martin G: Approach to the patient in the tropics with pulmonary disease. In Guerrant RL, ed: Tropical Infectious Diseases, vol 2, 2nd ed. Philadelphia, WB Saunders, 2006, p 1544.

2. Wilson CM: Respiratory distress caused by parasites. Pediatr Ann 22:443-446, 1994.
3. Guerin PJ, et al: Malaria: Current status of control, diagnosis, treatment and a proposed agenda for research and development. Lancet Infect Dis 2:564-573, 2002.
4. Redd SC, et al: Usefulness of clinical case definitions in guiding therapy for African children with malaria or pneumonia. Lancet 340:1140, 1992.
5. Shann F: The management of severe malaria. Pediatr Crit Care Med 4:489-498, 2003.
6. Taylor WR, White NJ: Malaria and the lung. Clin Chest Med 23:457-468, 2002.
7. Gachot B, et al: Acute lung injury complicating imported *Plasmodium falciparum* malaria. Chest 108:746-749, 1995.
8. Moon TD, Oberhelman RA: Antiparasitic therapy in children. Pediatr Clin North Am 52:917-948, 2005.
9. Drugs for parasitic infections. Med Lett Drugs Ther 1-12, August 2004.
10. Kubitschek KR, et al: Amebiasis presenting as pleuropulmonary disease. West J Med 142:203, 1985.
11. Shamsuzzaman SM, Hashiguchi Y: Thoracic amebiasis. Clin Chest Med 23:479-492, 2002.

12. Ibarta-Perez S, Selman-Lam M: Diagnosis and treatment of amebic empyema. Am J Surg 134:283-287, 1977.
13. Adams EB, MacLeod IN: Invasive amebiasis, II: Amebic liver abscess and its complications. Medicine 56:325-334, 1977.
14. Ravdin JI: Amebiasis. Clin Infect Dis 20:1453-1466, 1995.
15. Sarinas PSA, Chitkara RK: Ascariasis and hookworm. Semin Resp Infect 12:130-137, 1997.
16. Chan MS, et al: The evolution of potential global morbidity attributable to intestinal nematode infections. Parasitology 109:373-387, 1994.
17. Hotez PJ: Pediatric geohelminth infections: Trichuriasis, ascariasis, and hookworm. Semin Pediatr Infect Dis 11:236-244, 2000.
18. Martinez S, et al: Thoracic manifestations of tropical parasitic infections: A pictorial review. Radiographics 25:135-155, 2005.
19. Chitkara R, Krishna G: Parasitic pulmonary eosinophilia. Semin Resp Crit Care Med 27:171-184, 2006.
20. Hotez PJ: Nematode infections. In Jenson HB, Baltimore RS, eds: Pediatric Infectious Diseases, 2nd ed. Philadelphia, WB Saunders, 2002, p 504.
21. Hotez PJ, et al: Hookworm infection. N Engl J Med 351:799-807, 2004.
22. Barrett-Connor E: Parasitic pulmonary disease. Am Rev Respir Dis 126:558-563, 1982.
23. Liu LX, Weller PF: Strongyloidiasis and other intestinal nematode infections. Infect Dis Clin North Am 7:655-682, 1993.
24. Keiser PB, Nutman TB: *Strongyloides stercoralis* in the immunocompromised population. Clin Microbiol Rev 17:208-217, 2004.
25. Woodring JH, Halfhill H: Clinical and imaging features of pulmonary strongyloidiasis. South Med J 89:10-19, 1996.
26. Kramer MR, et al: Disseminated strongyloidiasis in AIDS and non-AIDS immunocompromised hosts: Diagnosis by sputum and bronchoalveolar lavage. South Med J 83:1226-1229, 1990.
27. Despommier D: Toxocariasis: Clinical aspects, epidemiology, medical ecology, and molecular aspects. Clin Microbiol Rev 16:265-272, 2003.
28. Maizels RM, Holland MJ: Parasite immunology: Pathways for expelling intestinal helminthes. Curr Biol 8:R711-R714, 1998.
29. Sharghi N, Schantz P, Hotez PJ: Toxocariasis: An occult cause of childhood neuropsychological deficits and asthma. Semin Pediatr Infect Dis 11:257-260, 2000.
30. Oteifa NM, Moustafa MA, Elgozamy BM: Toxocariasis as a possible cause of allergic diseases in children. J Egypt Soc Parasitol 28:365-372, 1998.
31. Kagawa FT: Pulmonary paragonimiasis. Semin Resp Infect 12:149-158, 1997.
32. Singh TS, Mutum SS, Razaque MA: Pulmonary paragonimiasis: Clinical features, diagnosis and treatment of 39 cases in Manipur. Trans R Soc Trop Med Hyg 80:967-971, 1986.
33. Maclean JD, Cross J, Mabanty S: Liver, lung, and intestinal fluke infections. In Guerrant RL, Walker DH, Weller PF, eds: Tropical Infectious Diseases. Philadelphia, Churchill Livingstone, 2006.
34. Im JG, et al: Pleuropulmonary paragonimiasis: Radiologic findings in 71 patients. AJR Am J Roentgenol 159:39-43, 1992.
35. Lewall DB: Hydatid disease: Biology, pathology, imaging and classification. Clin Radiol 52:863-874, 1998.
36. Tanowitz HB, Weiss LM, Wittner M: Tapeworms. Curr Infect Dis Rep 3:77-84, 2001.
37. Jaray M, et al: Hydatid disease of the lungs: Study of 386 cases. Am Rev Respir Dis 146:185-189, 1992.
38. Balikan JP, Mudarris FF: Hydatid disease of the lungs: A roentgenologic study of 50 cases. AJR Am J Roentgenol 122:692-707, 1974.
39. Dixon JB: Echinococcosis. Comp Immunol Microbiol Infect Dis 20:87-94, 1997.
40. Elburjo M, Gani EA: Surgical management of pulmonary hydatid cysts in children. Thorax 50:396-398, 1995.
41. Pomeroy C, Filice GA: Pulmonary toxoplasmosis: A review. Clin Infect Dis 14:863-870, 1992.
42. Boggild AK, Keystone JS, Kain KC: Tropical pulmonary eosinophilia: A case series in a setting of non-endemicity. Clin Infect Dis 39:1123-1128, 2004.
43. Chitkara MK, Krisha G: Parasitic pulmonary eosinophilia. Semin Resp Crit Care Med 27:171-184, 2006.
44. Kuzucu A: Parasitic diseases of the respiratory tract. Curr Opin Pulm Med 12:212-221, 2006.
45. Schwartz E: Pulmonary schistosomiasis. Clin Chest Med 23:433-443, 2002.
46. Doherty JF, et al: Katayama fever: an acute manifestation of schistosomiasis. BMJ 313:1071-1072, 1996.

Useful Websites

Centers for Disease Control and Prevention, National Center for Infectious Diseases, Division of Parasitic Diseases. Available at: www.cdc.gov/ncidod/dpd/.
Karolinska Institute: Parasitic disease resources. Available at: www.mic.ki.se/Diseases/C03.html.
Radiology Department, Uniformed Services University. Available at: http://tmcr.usuhs.mil/toc.htm.

CHAPTER 14

Pulmonary Manifestations of Genetic Diseases

BETH A. PLETCHER

Congenital Anomalies 295
  Overview of Prenatal Lung Development 295
  Lung Agenesis and Pulmonary Hypoplasia 296
  Congenital Diaphragmatic Hernia 300
  Segmentation Defects and Heterotaxy 305
  Cystic Adenomatoid Malformations 306
  Bronchogenic Cysts and Other Cystic
    Lesions 308
  Pulmonary Sequestration 309
  Bronchobiliary Fistulas 310
  Congenital Lobar Emphysema 310
  Tracheoesophageal Fistula and Tracheal
    Agenesis 311
  Pulmonary Lymphangiectasia and Other
    Diseases of the Lymphatic Tree 311
  Pulmonary Arteriovenous Malformations and
    Hemangiomas 314
  α_1-Antitrypsin Deficiency 315

**Bronchiectasis, Primary Ciliary Dyskinesia,
  and Kartagener Syndrome** 316
Spontaneous Pneumothorax 320
Inborn Errors of Metabolism 320
Pulmonary Arterial Hypertension 322
Pulmonary Fibrosis 327
Pulmonary Embolism 327
Cystic Fibrosis 329
  CFTR 329
  Mutations in *CFTR* and Their
    Consequences 330
  Screening and Diagnosis 330
  Clinical Manifestations 331
  Lung Disease 332
  Symptomatic Treatment 333
  Curative Therapy 335
Miscellaneous Genetic Conditions 335
Summary 336
  References 338

Many different pulmonary manifestations are seen in conjunction with genetic disorders. Pulmonary findings have been noted with some cytogenetic conditions, many single gene or mendelian disorders, and numerous inborn errors of metabolism. In addition, congenital lung anomalies are common, occurring as isolated anomalies and as part of multiple anomaly syndromes. Recognition of pulmonary problems in patients with genetic disorders may lead to prompt treatment and intervention, which ultimately might translate into improved outcome.

Congenital Anomalies

Overview of Prenatal Lung Development

Lung morphogenesis can be subdivided into distinct periods on the basis of the morphologic characteristics of the tissue (Table 14-1).

Embryonic Period

Prenatal lung development begins during the embryonic stage of fetal development, at 4 weeks gestation, with lung buds emerging from the ventral side of the foregut, which is lined by endodermally derived epithelium. The trachea is separated from the primitive esophagus beginning at week 5. Secondary bronchi then form, three on the right and two on the left, which ultimately form the five lobes of the lungs. Developmental anomalies occurring during this period of development may include tracheal, laryngeal, and esophageal atresia; tracheal stenosis; pulmonary agenesis; tracheoesophageal fistulas (TEFs); and bronchial malformations.

Pseudoglandular Period

The pseudoglandular stage is so called because of the distinct glandular appearance of the lung from 6 to 16 weeks of gestation. During this period, branching of the airways

Table 14-1	Morphogenetic Periods of Human Lung Development	

PERIOD	GESTATIONAL AGE (WK)	STRUCTURAL EVENTS
Embryonic	3-6	Lung buds, trachea, main stem, lobar, and segmental bronchi
Pseudoglandular	6-16	Subsegmental bronchi, terminal bronchioles, acinar tubules, mucous glands, cartilage, smooth muscle
Canalicular	16-26	Respiratory bronchioles, acinus formation and vascularization, type I and type II cell differentiation
Saccular and alveolar	26-36 (saccular); 36 to maturity (alveolar)	Dilation and subdivision of alveolar saccules, increase of gas-exchange surface area, further growth and alveolarization, maturation of alveolar-capillary network

continues, and formation of the terminal bronchioles and primitive acinar structures is completed by the end of this period. Surfactant proteins A, B, and C are first detected during this stage. Bronchial arteries arise from the aorta and form along the epithelial tubules. Various congenital defects may arise during this stage of lung development, including tracheobronchomalacia, pulmonary sequestration, cystic adenomatoid malformation, ectopic lobes, cyst formation, and congenital pulmonary lymphangiectasia. The pleuroperitoneal canal also closes early in the pseudoglandular period. Failure to close the pleural cavity, often accompanied by herniation of the abdominal contents into the chest (congenital diaphragmatic hernia [CDH]), leads to lung hypoplasia.

Canalicular Period

The canalicular stage occurs at 16 to 26 weeks of gestation. It is characterized by the formation of acinar structures in the distal tubules, thinning of the mesenchyme, and formation of the capillary bed. By the end of this period, the terminal bronchioles have divided to form two or more respiratory bronchioles, and each of these has divided into multiple acinar tubules, forming the primitive alveolar ducts and pulmonary acini. At the end of this stage in infants, gas exchange can be supported after birth. Abnormalities of lung development occurring during this period include pulmonary hypoplasia (caused by diaphragmatic hernia or compression by thoracic or abdominal masses and prolonged rupture of membranes causing oligohydramnios) and renal agenesis, in which amniotic fluid production is impaired.

Saccular and Alveolar Periods

Saccular and alveolar periods occur at 26 to 36 weeks and 36 weeks through adolescence. Increased thinning of the respiratory epithelium and pulmonary mesenchyme, further growth of the lung acini, and development of the distal capillary network characterize these stages. In the periphery of the acinus, maturation of type II epithelial cells occurs in association with increasing numbers of lamellar bodies and increased synthesis of surfactant phospholipids. Pulmonary arteries enlarge and elongate in close relationship to the increased growth of the lung. After birth, alveoli expand a bit, but, more importantly, lung growth remains active throughout the first 10 years of life. There is a sixfold increase in the number of alveoli during postnatal life.[1]

Before birth, fetal respiratory movements allow lung fluid that is constantly produced to efflux into the amniotic fluid. These respiratory efforts promote further lung development and strengthen the muscles of respiration. As discussed in the next section, prenatal circumstances that prevent adequate respiratory movements before birth (i.e., oligohydramnios, thoracic cage abnormalities, or neuromuscular disease) may lead to life-threatening pulmonary hypoplasia.[1]

Lung Agenesis and Pulmonary Hypoplasia

Primary pulmonary hypoplasia is occasionally reported as an isolated finding and has been described in many sibships, suggesting autosomal recessive inheritance in at least some cases.[2] This serves as a reference point for some families who have given birth to one child with pulmonary hypoplasia because risks for recurrence may be 25% in subsequent pregnancies.

Tracheal atresia accompanied by bilateral agenesis of the lungs is most likely to arise as an isolated defect, possibly secondary to a vascular event occurring very early in the embryonic period. Variable degrees of pulmonary agenesis have been reported in many sibships, however, with and without consanguinity.[3] Developmental anomalies of the lungs also have been described in association with other birth defects, as part of at least one possible mendelian disorder,[4] and as an occasional finding in a microdeletion syndrome (Table 14-2).

More often, pulmonary hypoplasia identified at birth in association with severe respiratory distress is found to be secondary to another underlying defect or disorder. These primary problems can be divided into three broad categories: (1) renal problems leading to oligohydramnios, (2) skeletal dysplasia resulting in thoracic cage limitation and pulmonary insufficiency, and (3) neuromuscular disorders leading to pulmonary hypoplasia owing to poor respiratory efforts *in utero.*

Any renal abnormality, developmental or obstructive, leading to decreased urine output *in utero* with concomitant oligohydramnios has the potential to cause pulmonary hypoplasia (see Chapter 6). The degree of oligohydramnios and length of time the fetus is exposed to limitation of movement likely determine the severity of pulmonary hypoplasia and potential for long-term survival. Most instances of oligohydramnios are not genetically determined, but instead are secondary to prolonged rupture of membranes. Late loss of amniotic fluid with a relatively short duration of fetal constriction is less likely to cause significant respiratory compromise. In contrast, prolonged, severe oligohydramnios secondary to renal agenesis or sirenomelia results in the Potter sequence with severe pulmonary hypoplasia and neonatal death.

In between these two extremes are variable findings and prognoses associated with decreased amniotic fluid volume. A common isolated birth defect in male fetuses, posterior urethral valves, may result in oligohydramnios, bladder distention, hydronephrosis, and ultimately renal damage. In severe cases, the bladder distention leads to anterior abdominal wall musculature hypoplasia and

Table 14-2	Genetic Conditions Associated with Primary Pulmonary Hypoplasia		
SYNDROME	**CLINICAL FEATURES**	**MODE OF INHERITANCE**	**GENE OR LOCUS IF KNOWN**
Total anomalous pulmonary venous return (scimitar syndrome)[4]	Right lung hypoplasia Pulmonary hypertension Total anomalous pulmonary venous return Dextrocardia	Autosomal dominant with incomplete penetrance (40% penetrant)	Locus = 4q12
Anophthalmia and pulmonary hypoplasia (Matthew-Wood syndrome)[5]	Anophthalmia Pulmonary hypoplasia (with or without diaphragmatic hernia)	Possible autosomal recessive	Unknown
Velocardiofacial syndrome (22q11.2 deletion syndrome)	Pierre-Robin sequence Velopharyngeal insufficiency Cardiac defects (especially septal or aortic arch) Unilateral pulmonary dysgenesis T cell defects Hypocalcemia Learning disabilities Psychosis	Autosomal dominant with many new or de novo deletions	Locus = 22q11.2; cytogenetic microdeletion

renal failure (prune-belly syndrome). These boys also may have respiratory compromise that tends to correlate with the duration and severity of the oligohydramnios.

Suboptimal urine output associated with many genetic conditions may be seen with varying degrees of pulmonary hypoplasia at birth. Table 14-3 lists some of these syndromes. Bilateral or unilateral renal agenesis may occur as an isolated (nonhereditary) defect during early fetal development.

In some instances, skeletal dysplasias with associated thoracic anomalies can result in secondary pulmonary hypoplasia. In addition to severe and universally fatal skeletal dysplasias, such as achondrogenesis, osteogenesis imperfecta type 2, a few short-rib polydactyly syndromes, and thanatophoric dysplasia, there are many less severe skeletal dysplasias that may result in pulmonary compromise and respiratory difficulties at or shortly after birth. The long-term prognosis for each depends on the extent of the pulmonary hypoplasia and ability for the lungs to grow within the confines of the thoracic cage over time. Table 14-4 lists some of the skeletal

Table 14-3	Genetic Conditions Associated with Renal Problems and Secondary Pulmonary Hypoplasia		

SYNDROME	CLINICAL FEATURES	MODE OF INHERITANCE	GENE OR LOCUS IF KNOWN
Hereditary renal agenesis	Pulmonary hypoplasia Renal agenesis Other genitourinary anomalies Potter facies Secondary equinovarus	Autosomal dominant (general recurrence risk of 1% in isolated cases—if parents have two normal kidneys)	Gene = *PAX2*; locus = 5q11.2-q11.3
Autosomal recessive polycystic kidney disease (incidence 1:16,000 live-born infants)	Pulmonary hypoplasia Enlarged cystic kidneys with interstitial fibrosis Hepatic and pancreatic cysts Potter facies	Autosomal recessive	Gene = *PKHD1*
Meckel syndrome (Meckel-Gruber syndrome)	Pulmonary hypoplasia Polycystic kidneys with or without renal agenesis Occipital encephalocele Postaxial polydactyly	Autosomal recessive	Gene = *MKS1* on 17q; locus = 11q13 (*MKS2*); 8q24 (*MKS3*)
Nephronophthisis type 2	Pulmonary hypoplasia Hyperechogenic kidneys with cortical microcysts and tubulointerstitial nephritis	Autosomal recessive	Unknown
Genitopatellar syndrome	Pulmonary hypoplasia Polyhydramnios (not oligohydramnios) Microcephaly, CNS defects Cardiac septal defects Multicystic kidneys Hydronephrosis Joint flexion deformities Mental retardation	Autosomal recessive	Unknown

CNS, central nervous system.

Table 14-4	Nonlethal Skeletal Dysplasias Associated with Pulmonary Hypoplasia

SYNDROME	CLINICAL FEATURES	MODE OF INHERITANCE	GENE OR LOCUS IF KNOWN
Camptomelic dysplasia	Pulmonary hypoplasia Cystic hygroma, lymphedema Acromelia with short bowed limbs, clubfoot, splayed toes Polycystic kidneys	Autosomal recessive versus autosomal dominant	Gene = *SOX*
Asphyxiating thoracic dystrophy (Jeune syndrome) (incidence 1:100,000-130,000 live-born infants)	Pulmonary hypoplasia or insufficiency Long, narrow thorax with rib and clavicular anomalies Polydactyly Hepatic, renal, and pancreatic cysts	Autosomal recessive	Unknown
Autosomal recessive spondylocostal dysostosis (Jarcho-Levin syndrome)	Pulmonary insufficiency Vertebral and rib anomalies with a crablike chest Short neck with normal limbs	Autosomal dominant	Gene = *DLL3* at 19q13; *MESP2*; *LFNG*
Spondylocostal dysostosis with anal atresia and urogenital anomalies	Pulmonary hypoplasia X-ray findings similar to Jarcho-Levin syndrome Single umbilical artery Internal and external genitourinary anomalies Hydronephrosis	Autosomal recessive	Unknown
Spondyloepiphyseal dysplasia congenita	Pulmonary insufficiency secondary to restrictive lung disease Barrel chest with platyspondylisis Scoliosis, kyphosis, lordosis Pectus carinatum Coxa vara and clubfeet Myopia and retinal detachment Cleft palate Hypotonia	Autosomal dominant	Gene = *COL2A1*
Rhizomelic chondrodysplasia punctata type 1	Pulmonary insufficiency Rhizomelic limb shortening with epiphyseal calcifications Coronal vertebral clefts and kyphoscoliosis Microcephaly with seizures, mental retardation, or cortical atrophy Sensorineural hearing loss Congenital cataracts Often lethal before age 2 years	Autosomal recessive	Gene = *PEX7*

dysplasias associated with respiratory difficulties at birth, but with the possibility of long-term survival.

Severe neuromuscular disorders associated with lack of fetal movement (fetal akinesia) may cause a host of problems in addition to pulmonary hypoplasia. Prenatal history is often significant for polyhydramnios (believed to be secondary to decreased fetal swallowing), joint contractures, and clubfeet. Whether the fetal akinesia is secondary to an inherent muscle or peripheral nerve problem, or instead a central nervous system problem, the clinical presentations are similar. Severe, congenital

forms of inborn errors of metabolism, myopathies, or neuropathies may be clinically indistinguishable, unless specific diagnostic tests are done. Table 14-5 summarizes genetic conditions with neuromuscular underpinnings that may result in secondary pulmonary hypoplasia.

Congenital Diaphragmatic Hernia

CDH is a common anomaly and frequently associated with secondary pulmonary hypoplasia. CHD is seen in approximately 1 in

Table 14-5 Neuromuscular Conditions Associated with Pulmonary Hypoplasia

SYNDROME	CLINICAL FEATURES	MODE OF INHERITANCE	GENE OR LOCUS IF KNOWN
Pena-Shokeir syndrome (fetal akinesia deformation sequence)	Pulmonary hypoplasia Generalized joint contractures with clubfeet Polyhydramnios Intrauterine growth restriction Facial dysmorphism Small thorax and thin ribs Hydrocephaly with or without cerebellar hypoplasia 30% are stillborn Frequently lethal in neonatal period	Autosomal recessive (about 50% of cases). Empirical recurrence risks for siblings may be close to 10-15%	Unknown—may represent many different genetic syndromes causing suboptimal fetal movement
Multiple pterygium syndrome (Escobar variant)[6]	Pulmonary hypoplasia Eventration of diaphragm Reduced facial movements Severe joint contractures with pterygia (webbing) of joints and neck Pathognomonic indentations over elbows and knees Reduced muscle mass Genitourinary anomalies	Autosomal recessive	Gene = CHRNG
Stuve-Wiedemann syndrome	Pulmonary hypoplasia Pulmonary hypertension Short neck; short stature Dysphagia Thin ribs, osteoporosis Progressive scoliosis Short, thick long bones Flexion contractures of fingers, elbows, and knees Clubfeet Hypotonia Normal intelligence	Autosomal recessive	Gene = LIFR

Table 14-5	Neuromuscular Conditions Associated with Pulmonary Hypoplasia—*Cont'd*		
SYNDROME	**CLINICAL FEATURES**	**MODE OF INHERITANCE**	**GENE OR LOCUS IF KNOWN**
Marden-Walker syndrome	Pulmonary hypoplasia	Autosomal recessive	Unknown
	Prenatal and postnatal growth restriction		
	Microcephaly with CNS malformations		
	Hypotonia and decreased muscle mass		
	Fixed facial expression with dysmorphism		
	Joint contractures, clubfeet		
	Radioulnar synostosis		
	Scoliosis, kyphosis		
	Renal microcysts and dysplasia		
	Cryptorchidism		
Spinal muscular atrophy type 1[7]	Pulmonary hypoplasia (in about ¼ of infants with spinal muscular atrophy type 1)	Autosomal recessive. Carried by about 1:40 otherwise healthy individuals	Gene = *SMN1*
	Above due to prenatal onset of hypotonia		
	Joint contractures		
	Feeding difficulties		
Perinatal lethal Gaucher disease	Pulmonary hypoplasia	Autosomal recessive	Gene = *GBA* (enzyme acid β-glucosidase)
	Severe fetal hydrops (30% stillborn)		
	Polyhydramnios		
	Fetal akinesia		
	Hypertonia; joint contractures		
	Microcephaly		
	Facial dysmorphism		
	Small thorax		
	Cardiomegaly		
	Collodion skin		
	Usually lethal by age 3 mo		

CNS, central nervous system.

2000 live-born infants. This birth defect occurs as an isolated event and in association with more than 15 genetic syndromes (Table 14-6). CDH also is seen with numerous cytogenetic deletion and duplication syndromes as one of many congenital anomalies; 15% of infants with CDH have a structural or numeric cytogenetic abnormality. Prenatal or postnatal detection of a CDH would require a thorough evaluation to look for dysmorphic features or additional birth defects that may be diagnostic of a specific syndrome.

CDH arises early in gestation when the pleuroperitoneal membranes fail to seal the pleuroperitoneal canal completely. Of CDHs, 80% are left-sided and result in abdominal viscera sliding up into the pleural cavity (Fig. 14-1).[10] Postnatal survival reportedly ranges from 39% to 95% after repair of CDH. This large variation in mortality depends largely on the severity of the resulting pulmonary hypoplasia and abnormal pulmonary vasculature. If extracorporeal membrane oxygenation is required, the prognosis is not favorable. The overall outcome of CDH is recognized to be worse when it is found in association with certain syndromes, such as Fryns syndrome.[9] A recurrence risk for sibs of a child with an isolated CDH, based on empiric data, is approximately 2%.[11]

Table 14-6	Genetic Conditions Associated with Congenital Diaphragmatic Hernia		
SYNDROME	**CLINICAL FEATURES**	**MODE OF INHERITANCE**	**GENE OR LOCUS IF KNOWN**
Congenital diaphragmatic hernia 1	Diaphragmatic hernia alone	Autosomal dominant	Gene = ?NR2FZ; locus = 15q26.1-q26.2
Congenital diaphragmatic hernia 2	Diaphragmatic hernia alone	Autosomal recessive	Locus = 8p23.1
Congenital diaphragmatic hernia 3	Diaphragmatic hernia alone	Autosomal dominant	Gene = ZFPM2 (8q22.3)
Anterior diaphragmatic hernia	Anterior diaphragmatic hernia	X-linked or multifactorial M > F	Unknown
Cornelia de Lange syndrome (Brachmann-de Lange syndrome)	Diaphragmatic hernia Prenatal growth restriction Abnormal cry at birth Microcephaly and classic facial dysmorphism Congenital heart defects Oligodactyly and other limb defects Mental retardation	Autosomal dominant	Gene = NIPBL
Fryns syndrome	Diaphragmatic hernia Large for gestational age Coarse facies with excess hair Small thorax Distal limb and nail hypoplasia Gastrointestinal, genitourinary, and CNS malformations Often stillborn or die as neonates	Autosomal recessive. Two recognized microdeletions	Microdeletions = 15q26.2 and 8p23.1
Meacham syndrome	Diaphragmatic hernia Pulmonary hypoplasia Pulmonary rhabdomyomatous dysplasia Congenital heart defects Males with ambiguous genitalia or sex reversal	Unknown versus de novo autosomal dominant	Unknown
Simpson-Golabi-Behmel syndrome	Diaphragmatic hernia Lung segmentation defects Prenatal and postnatal overgrowth Bulldog facies; macroglossia Accessory nipples; 13 rib pairs Cardiac and gastrointestinal defects Large, cystic kidneys Umbilical hernia Polydactyly, syndactyly Clubfoot Embryonal tumors	X-linked recessive versus X-linked semidominant	Gene = GPC3

Table 14-6	Genetic Conditions Associated with Congenital Diaphragmatic Hernia—*Cont'd*		
SYNDROME	**CLINICAL FEATURES**	**MODE OF INHERITANCE**	**GENE OR LOCUS IF KNOWN**
Focal dermal hypoplasia (Goltz syndrome)	Diaphragmatic hernia Ocular, dental, gastrointestinal, and genitourinary defects Syndactyly, polydactyly Cutaneous linear or patchy atrophy; papillomas with or without telangiectasias Absent or hypoplastic nails	X-linked dominant (lethal in males)	Unknown
Autosomal recessive cutis laxa	Diaphragmatic hernia Prenatal and postnatal growth restriction Cutis laxa Emphysema and cor pulmonale Gastrointestinal and genitourinary diverticula Joint laxity Arterial tortuosity Aneurysms Hernias Decreased elastin fibers in dermis	Autosomal recessive	Unknown
Epidermolysis bullosa with diaphragmatic hernia	Diaphragmatic hernia Epidermolysis bullosa Reported infants died shortly after birth	Autosomal recessive	Unknown
Syndromic microphthalmia (MIDAS syndrome [microphthalmia, dermal aplasia, sclerocornea])	Diaphragmatic hernia Unilateral or bilateral microphthalmia Linear skin defects on face and neck Cardiac defects Genital with or without anal anomalies CNS malformations	X-linked dominant (lethal in males). Also X chromosome microdeletion	Gene = *HCCS* (Xp22.3)
Syndromic anophthalmia with mild facial dysmorphism and normal intrauterine growth	Diaphragmatic hernia Pulmonary dysplasia even in absence of diaphragmatic defect Bilateral anophthalmia Cardiac and genitourinary anomalies Blepharophimosis with unusual eyebrows (trichoglyphic) Large, low-set ears	Autosomal recessive	Gene = *STRA6* (15q24.1)
Thoracoabdominal syndrome (X-linked midline defects including pentalogy of Cantrell)	Diaphragmatic hernia Cleft lip with or without cleft palate Cardiac defects Omphalocele; ventral hernias Hydrocephaly, anencephaly Renal agenesis, hypospadias	X-linked recessive or X-linked dominant	Locus = Xq25-q26

(Continued)

Table 14-6	Genetic Conditions Associated with Congenital Diaphragmatic Hernia—*Cont'd*		
SYNDROME	**CLINICAL FEATURES**	**MODE OF INHERITANCE**	**GENE OR LOCUS IF KNOWN**
Donnai-Barrow syndrome (diaphragmatic hernia, exomphalos, absent corpus callosum, hypertelorism, myopia, and sensorineural deafness)	Diaphragmatic hernia Abnormal ears Sensorineural deafness Myopia, ocular defects Cardiac defects Ventral abdominal wall defects Agenesis of the corpus callosum	Autosomal recessive	Unknown
Omphalocele, diaphragmatic hernia, and radial ray defects	Diaphragmatic hernia Omphalocele Single umbilical artery Radioulnar synostosis with thumb anomalies Facial dysmorphism Abnormal ears Scoliosis	Probable autosomal recessive	Unknown
Diaphragmatic defects, limb deficiencies, and ossification defects of the skull	Diaphragmatic hernia Omphalocele Limb deficiencies with syndactyly Cranial ossification defects	Autosomal recessive versus autosomal dominant with gonadal mosaicism	Unknown
Denys-Drash syndrome (Wilms tumor and pseudohermaphroditism or true hermaphroditism)	Diaphragmatic hernia Ambiguous genitalia (M or F) Gonadal dysgenesis (M or F) Gonadoblastoma Nephropathy, nephritic syndrome leading to renal failure Wilms tumor	Autosomal dominant (overlaps with WAGR and Frasier syndrome)	Gene = *WT1* (11p13)
Agonadism with multiple internal malformations (PAGOD syndrome [pulmonary hypoplasia, hypoplasia of the pulmonary artery, agonadism, omphalocele, diaphragmatic defects and dextrocardia])	Diaphragmatic hernia Omphalocele Female external genitalia without internal gonads Dextrocardia Cardiac defects Hypoplasia of lung even without diaphragmatic defect	Autosomal recessive	Unknown
Perlman syndrome (renal hamartomas, nephroblastomatosis, and fetal gigantism)	Diaphragmatic hernia Prenatal overgrowth Polyhydramnios Facial dysmorphism Visceromegaly Hyperinsulinism Renal hamartomas Nephroblastomatosis Wilms tumor	Autosomal recessive	Unknown

Table 14-6	Genetic Conditions Associated with Congenital Diaphragmatic Hernia—*Cont'd*		
SYNDROME	**CLINICAL FEATURES**	**MODE OF INHERITANCE**	**GENE OR LOCUS IF KNOWN**
Pallister-Killian syndrome (mosaic tetrasomy 12p)	Diaphragmatic hernia Coarse facies with a prominent forehead and micrognathia Sparse eyebrows, large ears Short, webbed neck Cardiac and genitourinary defects Ventral wall defects Polydactyly Profound mental retardation and seizures Stillbirth and neonatal mortality common	Cytogenetic	Mosaic tetrasomy 12p in skin fibroblasts (often not seen in lymphocytes)
Emanuel syndrome (supernumerary derivative 22 chromosome)	Diaphragmatic hernia Prenatal growth restriction Microcephaly Preauricular tags and sinuses Cleft palate Cardiac, genitourinary, and anal defects Mental retardation	Cytogenetic (results from 3:1 segregation from a parent who is a balanced carrier of an 11q23-22q11 translocation)	Supernumerary chromosome—a derivative 22 with part of 11q attached
Deletion 1q32.3-q42.3[8]	Diaphragmatic hernia	Cytogenetic	Deletion = 1q32.3-1q42.3
Deletion 8p23.1[9]	Fryns phenotype Congenital diaphragmatic hernia 2	Cytogenetic	Microdeletion = 8p23.1
Deletion 15q26.1[9]	Fryns phenotype Diaphragmatic hernia	Cytogenetic	Microdeletion = 15q26.2

CNS, central nervous system; F, female; M, male; WAGR, Wilms tumor, aniridia, genitourinary abnormalities, and mental retardation.

Isolated CDH is generally believed to be a sporadic occurrence, although autosomal dominant and autosomal recessive pedigrees have been described. Several loci and putative predisposition genes have been found in cases of CDH, with cytogenetic deletions, duplications, and translocations often uncovering a CDH locus (see Table 14-6).

Segmentation Defects and Heterotaxy

During the embryonic stage, the right and left bronchial buds begin to grow, subsequently dividing into secondary bronchi. Normally, the right lung bud divides into three segments, and the left lung bud divides into two segments. Rarely, segmentation or lobulation defects occur and may or may not be associated with other visceral heterotaxies. Nearly

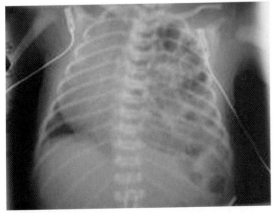

Figure 14-1. X-ray shows left sided diaphragmatic hernia with loops of bowel in the left hemithorax.

80% of children with right isomerism (bilateral right lung) have asplenia, leading to a risk for overwhelming pneumococcal sepsis. A similar proportion with left isomerism (bilateral left lung) has multiple small spleens (polysplenia). A few genetic syndromes have been associated with these types of defects (Table 14-7).

Cystic Adenomatoid Malformations

Cystic adenomatoid malformation of the lungs is a developmental abnormality that results from overgrowth of the terminal respiratory bronchioles modified by intercommunicating cysts. Cystic adenomatoid malformation encompasses variably sized cysts that, as they enlarge, compress adjacent lung tissue (Fig. 14-2). The reported incidence is 1 in 25,000 to 35,000. It is useful to divide these cystic lesions into large cyst and small cyst types. The changes that have long been associated with the "adenomatoid" type now are recognized in various conditions with large airway obstruction and are more accurately called "pulmonary hyperplasia."

Large Cyst Type (Stocker Type 1)

The type 1, or large cyst lesion usually manifests in early infancy with progressive respiratory distress as the cystic region expands

Table 14-7	Genetic Conditions Associated with Lung Segmentation Defects with or without Heterotaxy		

SYNDROME	CLINICAL FEATURES	MODE OF INHERITANCE	GENE OR LOCUS IF KNOWN
Smith-Lemli-Opitz syndrome (RSH syndrome) (Incidence 1:20,000-40,000)	Incomplete lobulation of lung with or without lung hypoplasia	Autosomal recessive	Gene = *DHCR7* (enzyme is 7-dehydrocholesterol reductase)
	Prenatal growth restriction		
	Failure to thrive		
	Microcephaly, epicanthal folds		
	Broad alveolar ridges		
	Cardiac defects		
	Hypospadias and other genitourinary defects		
	Two to three toe syndactyly and polydactyly		
	Foot anomalies		
	Mental retardation, seizures		
	CNS defects		
Pallister-Hall syndrome (hypothalamic hamartoblastoma, hypopituitarism, imperforate anus, and postaxial polydactyly)	Abnormal lung lobulation	Autosomal dominant. Most cases are sporadic	Gene = *GLI3* (7p13)
	Intrauterine growth restriction		
	Microphthalmia, abnormal ears		
	Buccal frenula, cleft lip/palate		
	Cardiac, genitourinary, and anal defects		
	Polydactyly, syndactyly		
	CNS hypothalamic hamartoblastoma with pituitary hypoplasia		
Simpson-Golabi-Behmel syndrome	See Table 14-5	See Table 14-5	See Table 14-5
Asplenia with cardiovascular anomalies (Ivemark syndrome)	Right isomerism (bilateral right lung)	Autosomal recessive	Locus = 11q13
	Asplenia		
	Severe cardiac defects (TAPVR)		
	Midline liver		
	Malrotation of the gut		

Table 14-7	Genetic Conditions Associated with Lung Segmentation Defects with or without Heterotaxy—*Cont'd*		
SYNDROME	**CLINICAL FEATURES**	**MODE OF INHERITANCE**	**GENE OR LOCUS IF KNOWN**
Situs inversus viscerum	Left isomerism (bilateral left lung)	Autosomal recessive	Locus = 7p21
	Polysplenia		
	Intrauterine growth restriction		
	Cardiac defects (PAPVR)		
Severe Rubinstein-Taybi syndrome (chromosome 16p13.3 deletion)[12]	Abnormal lung lobulation	Cytogenetic. Contiguous gene syndrome, as opposed to a point mutation or nondeletion Rubinstein-Taybi syndrome	Microdeletion = 16p13.3; deletion size 400 kb to 3 Mb
	Accessory spleens		
	Cardiac defects, especially hypoplastic left heart		
	Renal agenesis		
	Neonatal seizures		

CNS, central nervous system; PAPVR, partial anomalous pulmonary venous return; TAPVR, total anomalous pulmonary venous return.

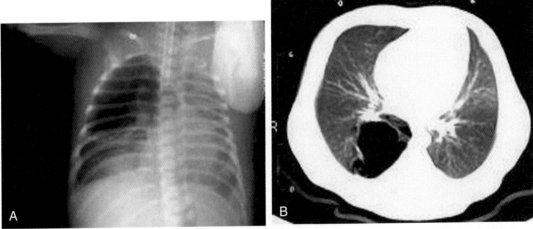

Figure 14-2. A, X-ray shows right upper lung cystic area filled with air after resorption of fluid from congenital cystic adenomatoid malformation. **B,** CT scan shows septated cystic adenomatoid malformation in right upper lobe.

by air trapping with compression of adjacent lung tissue and ultimately mediastinal shift. Occasionally, these lesions are so large that growth of the normal lung tissue is impaired, resulting with pulmonary hypoplasia related to this space-occupying lesion. It is the most common type of cystic adenomatoid malformation and has the best prognosis because these malformations are usually localized and affect only part of one lobe. Cysts are usually larger than 2 cm in diameter. They are lined by respiratory epithelium and have a wall resembling bronchioles with small amounts of smooth muscle, but no glands. Some of these lesions may contain mucigenic epithelium. Increased risks for neoplasias, most commonly bronchioloalveolar carcinoma, have been a rationale for the early surgical resection of these lesions even when there are no clinical symptoms. This relationship is presumed to be related to neoplastic change in the mucigenic epithelium, which frequently is found as a minor component of the large cyst type of cystic adenomatoid malformation.[22]

Small Cyst Type (Stocker Type 2)

The small cyst lesion has been recognized widely in areas of lung in which there is airway obstruction during development, such as bronchial atresia, isolated and with systemic arterial connection and extralobar sequestration. On pathologic examination, these lesions show typical and distinctive features with regional replacement of the lung parenchyma by microcystic maldevelopment. Mucigenic epithelium is rare. Depending on the size and degree of pulmonary compromise, infants may or may not be symptomatic at birth. A small percentage may be asymptomatic until later in childhood and often manifest with recurrent pneumonia or chest pain. Cystic adenomatoid malformations are usually isolated occurrences and are not thought to be genetically determined.

Bronchogenic Cysts and Other Cystic Lesions

Foregut cysts are closed epithelium-lined sacs developing abnormally in the thorax from the respiratory tract and primitive developing gut. When these structures differentiate toward airway and contain hyaline cartilage plates in the wall, they are called "bronchogenic cysts," whereas structures developing toward the gut are termed "enterogenous cysts." Bronchogenic cysts are the most common cysts in infancy, although many do not manifest until adolescence or adulthood. Most are situated in the middle mediastinum close to the carina, but do not communicate with the trachea or bronchi. Less frequently, they are adjacent to the esophagus. They are usually single, unilocular cystic structures that are filled with fluid or mucus, and more

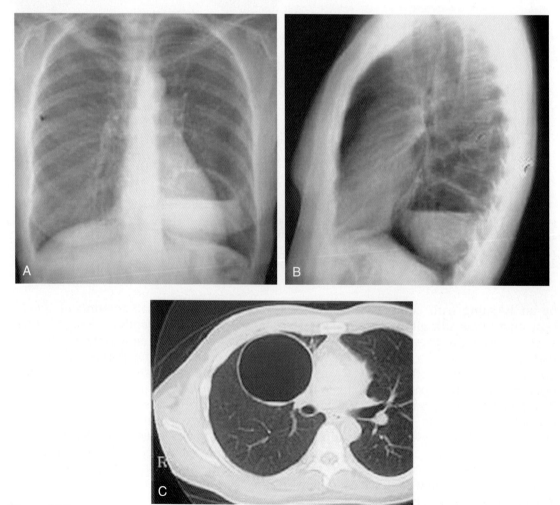

Figure 14-3. A and **B,** X-rays show thin-walled cyst in left lower lobe with air-fluid level. **C,** CT scan shows right upper lobe bronchogenic cyst.

commonly are located on the right (Fig. 14-3). Because of inadequate drainage, such cysts may be associated with recurrent infections and may appear as a consolidation or area of atelectasis on chest x-ray. Bronchogenic cysts also may be found within the lung hilum and parenchyma. When located within the lung, they are identical in their gross and histologic appearance to cysts in the mediastinum.

Similarly located cysts with enteric-type mucosa, usually gastric or esophageal and without cartilage plates within their wall, are enteric duplication cysts. Esophageal cysts are more common. They are intramural and do not involve the mucosa. Gastro-enteric cysts characteristically are not connected to the esophagus. In infants, they are a common cause of a posterior mediastinal mass. Neurenteric cysts are posterior mediastinal lesions, also lined by enteric-type mucosa, and with a pedicle that extends into the spinal canal. They are virtually always associated with vertebral defects in the region of this communication. Rarely, congenital cystic lesions may be seen in conjunction with genetic syndromes. There is a specific autosomal recessive disorder described with multiple peripheral lung cysts or fibrocystic pulmonary dysplasia as the primary feature (Table 14-8).

Pulmonary Sequestration

Bronchopulmonary sequestration, sometimes referred to simply as "pulmonary sequestration," is a rare congenital malformation of the lower respiratory tract. It consists of a nonfunctioning mass of lung tissue that receives its vascular supply from the systemic rather than pulmonary circulation, and it

Table 14-8 Genetic Conditions Associated with Pulmonary Cysts

SYNDROME	CLINICAL FEATURES	MODE OF INHERITANCE	GENE OR LOCUS IF KNOWN
Cystic disease of the lung	Cystic pulmonary lesions Recurrent lung infections Spontaneous pneumothorax in the neonate	Autosomal recessive (especially common in Yemenite and other non-Ashkenazi Jews)	Unknown
Proteus syndrome (encephalocraniocutaneous lipomatosis)	Cystic pulmonary lesions Macrocephaly Hemihypertrophy with localized overgrowth Variable cutaneous lesions, including lymphangiomas, lipomas, epidermal nevi, hemangiomas High risk of thrombosis Kyphoscoliosis CNS malformations	Autosomal dominant (some cases may be due to somatic mosaicism for a gene mutation)	Gene = PTEN (only some cases)
Down syndrome (trisomy 21)	Characteristic subpleural cysts[13] Facial dysmorphism Short, broad neck Cardiac, gastrointestinal, and genitourinary defects Brachydactyly, clinodactyly Single palmar crease	Cytogenetic	Extra copy of chromosome 21

CNS, central nervous system.

lacks communication with the tracheobronchial tree and alveoli. Sequestrations are classified anatomically. The intralobar variant, also known as intrapulmonary sequestration, is contained within otherwise normal lung and lacks its own pleura, and the veins normally drain into the pulmonary system. It is usually found in the posterior basal segment of the left lower lobe (Fig. 14-4). The less common extralobar sequestration, also known as extrapulmonary sequestration, is located outside the normal lung and has its own visceral pleura, and the venous drainage, although variable, is commonly through the azygos system. These lesions generally receive a systemic arterial supply from the descending thoracic aorta. They are commonly found beneath the left lower lobe. A rare variant of sequestration is bronchopulmonary-foregut malformation. With this anomaly, the sequestered lung tissue is connected to the gastrointestinal tract. Histologically, a pulmonary sequestration is composed of cystic lung tissue of embryonic origin. Rarely symptomatic at birth, pulmonary sequestration may appear as a cystic or solid infiltrate on chest x-ray. A pulmonary sequestration may become infected, with fistulas occasionally tracking into functional lung tissue or the gastrointestinal tract. Surgical resection of a pulmonary sequestration is generally recommended, and there are no strong genetic factors predisposing to the development of pulmonary sequestration.

Bronchobiliary Fistulas

Bronchobiliary fistulas often manifest with recurrent pulmonary infections and concomitant atelectasis during early life. Rarely, the diagnosis may not be made until after the second year of life. A bronchobiliary fistula represents a direct, congenital connection between the bronchus of the right middle lobe and the left hepatic duct. When the diagnosis of bronchobiliary fistula is made, surgery is clearly indicated. These are isolated occurrences with no recognized genetic associations.

Congenital Lobar Emphysema

Congenital lobar emphysema (CLE) is a developmental anomaly of the lower respiratory tract that is characterized by hyperinflation

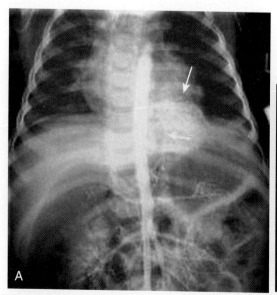
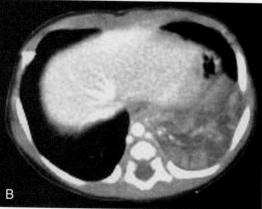

Figure 14-4. A, X-ray shows intralobar pulmonary sequestration (*longer arrow*) with anomalous artery arising from aorta (*shorter arrow*). **B,** CT scan shows large pulmonary sequestration on the left with arterial blood supply coming from aorta.

of one or more pulmonary lobes. Other terms for CLE include "congenital lobar overinflation," "congenital large hyperlucent lobe," and "infantile lobar emphysema." CLE is an uncommon cause of respiratory distress in infants. It has a marked predilection for the left upper lobe. The most frequently identified cause of CLE is obstruction of the developing airway, which occurs in about 25% of cases. Airway obstruction can be intrinsic or extrinsic, with the former more common. This leads to a "ball-valve" effect, whereby a greater volume of air enters the affected lobe during inspiration than leaves during expiration, producing air trapping. Intrinsic obstruction is often caused by defects in the bronchial wall, such as deficiency of bronchial cartilage. Intraluminal obstruction caused by meconium or mucous plugs, granulomas, or mucosal folds can result in partial obstruction of a lower airway. Extrinsic compression may be caused by vascular anomalies, such as a pulmonary artery sling or anomalous pulmonary venous return, or intrathoracic masses.

CLE is often associated with hyperinflation of the affected lung leading to compression of adjacent lung tissue and respiratory distress. Although most cases of CLE are isolated occurrences, affected siblings and an affected mother and daughter have been described. CLE also has been seen in association with cerebral (berry) aneurysms, cerebral calcifications, and cirrhosis in three brothers.[14] The appropriate treatment of CLE in newborns with respiratory distress is surgical resection of the affected lobe. Conservative management is reasonable in infants who have no or minimal symptoms.

Tracheoesophageal Fistula and Tracheal Agenesis

TEF is a common congenital anomaly of the respiratory tract, with an incidence of about 1 in 3,500 live births. TEF typically occurs with esophageal atresia. Esophageal atresia and TEF are classified according to their anatomic configuration. Type A consists of a proximal esophageal blind pouch, with the distal esophagus connecting directly to the trachea, and accounts for approximately 85% of cases. TEF occurs without esophageal atresia (H-type fistula) in only 5% of cases. These defects result from failure of the tracheoesophageal ridges to fuse fully during early embryonic life, with incomplete separation of the esophagus from the trachea.[1] One third of infants born with a TEF have additional birth defects. TEFs may be seen as part of multiple anomaly associations and in numerous mendelian disorders (Table 14-9).

The clinical presentation of TEF depends on the presence or absence of esophageal atresia. In cases with esophageal atresia (95%), polyhydramnios occurs in approximately two thirds of pregnancies. Infants with esophageal atresia become symptomatic immediately after birth, with excessive secretions resulting in drooling, choking, respiratory distress, and the inability to feed. A fistula between the trachea and distal esophagus often leads to gastric distention and reflux of gastric contents through the TEF resulting in aspiration pneumonia. Children with H-type TEFs may present early if the defect is large, with coughing and choking associated with feeding as the milk is aspirated through the fistula. Smaller defects of this type may not be symptomatic in the newborn period. These patients typically have a prolonged history of mild respiratory distress associated with feedings or recurrent pneumonias. Treatment consists of surgical ligation of the fistula; patients with esophageal atresia require esophageal anastomosis.

Pulmonary Lymphangiectasia and Other Diseases of the Lymphatic Tree

Congenital pulmonary lymphangiectasias may be either secondary to prenatal obstruction of the pulmonary lymphatic or venous drainage or a primary defect. Primary pulmonary lymphangiectasias may be limited to the lung itself, or may manifest as part of more generalized lymphangiectasia. They are frequently, but not always, associated with a chylothorax and may result in

Table 14-9	Genetic Conditions Associated with Tracheoesophageal Fistulas		
SYNDROME	**CLINICAL FEATURES**	**MODE OF INHERITANCE**	**GENE OR LOCUS IF KNOWN**
Tracheoesophageal fistula with or without esophageal atresia	Tracheoesophageal fistula Esophageal atresia	Autosomal dominant versus multifactorial	Unknown and deletion = 17q22-q23.3
X-linked VACTERL association with hydrocephalus	Tracheoesophageal fistula Hydrocephalus Vertebral malformations Anal atresia Cardiac and genitourinary defects Radial dysplasia and thumb anomalies	X-linked versus autosomal recessive	Unknown
VATER association	Tracheal agenesis (occasional) Tracheoesophageal fistula Single umbilical artery Vertebral defects Anal atresia Cardiac and renal defects Radial dysplasia and thumb anomalies	Isolated cases (may find similar defects in children with Fanconi anemia, which is autosomal recessive)	Unknown. Fanconi genes (group A, C, D1, E, F and G)[15]
Hemifacial microsomia (Goldenhar syndrome) (incidence 1:3000-5000)	Tracheoesophageal fistula (5%) Facial asymmetry, microsomia Epibulbar dermoids Microtia Conductive hearing loss Cardiac, vertebral, and renal defects CNS malformations	Multifactorial versus autosomal dominant	Locus = 14q32; possible locus = 22q11.2
CHARGE syndrome	Tracheoesophageal fistula Anal atresia or stenosis External ear malformations Sensorineural with or without conductive deafness Ocular colobomas Choanal atresia Cleft lip with or without cleft palate Cardiac and renal defects Genital anomalies	Autosomal dominant	Gene = CHD7
Posterior cleft larynx	Common tracheoesophagus Posterior cleft larynx	Autosomal recessive	Unknown
Opitz-Frias syndrome (hypertelorism with esophageal abnormality and hypospadias)	Tracheoesophageal fistula Pulmonary hypoplasia Hypertelorism with telecanthus	Autosomal dominant and X-linked	Locus = 5p13-p12 (duplication); 13q32.3—ter (deletion); Xp22—p11.2 (deletion)

		MODE OF	GENE OR LOCUS
SYNDROME	**CLINICAL FEATURES**	**INHERITANCE**	**IF KNOWN**
	Cleft lip with or without cleft palate		
	Cardiac, genitourinary, and renal defects		
	Hernias		
	CNS defects with mental retardation		
Feingold syndrome (oculodigitoesophagoduodenal syndrome)	Tracheoesophageal fistula	Autosomal dominant	Gene = *MYCN* (2p24.1)
	Polyhydramnios		
	Microcephaly		
	Facial asymmetry		
	Hearing loss		
	Patent ductus arteriosus		
	Vocal cord paralysis		
	Asplenia or polysplenia		
	Hypoplasia of middle phalanx of fingers 2 and 5		
	Syndactyly		
	Learning disabilities or mental retardation		
McKusick-Kaufman syndrome	Tracheoesophageal fistula (occasional)	Autosomal recessive	Gene = *MKKS* (20p12). Allelic with Bardet-Biedl syndrome type 6
	Pulmonary hypoplasia		
	Females with hydrometrocolpos		
	Cardiac, genitourinary, and renal malformations		
	Polydactyly, syndactyly		
Syndromic microphthalmia 3	Esophageal atresia	Autosomal dominant	Gene = *SOX2* (3q26.3-q27)
	Microphthalmia, anophthalmia		
	Microcephaly		
	Cardiac, vertebral, genitourinary, and CNS defects		
Multiple gastrointestinal abnormalities	Tracheoesophageal fistula	Autosomal recessive	Unknown
	Duodenal atresia		
	Hypoplasia of pancreas, gallbladder, biliary ducts, and intestines		
	Hypospadias		

Table 14-9   Genetic Conditions Associated with Tracheoesophageal Fistulas—*Cont'd*

CNS, central nervous system.

secondary pulmonary hypoplasia. Although most pulmonary lymphangiectasias are isolated occurrences, primary pulmonary lymphangiectasias have been reported in siblings and as part of several genetic syndromes (Table 14-10). Lymphatic hypoplasia of varied distribution underlies the yellow nail syndrome, and pulmonary lymphatic hyperplasia is part of Klippel-Trénaunay-Weber syndrome (see Chapter 12).

| Table 14-10 | Genetic Conditions Associated with Pulmonary Lymphangiectasia |

SYNDROME	CLINICAL FEATURES	MODE OF INHERITANCE	GENE OR LOCUS IF KNOWN
Congenital pulmonary lymphangiectasia	Pulmonary lymphangiectasia Polyhydramnios Hydrothorax, chylothorax Facial edema Ascites Hypertelorism Recurrent respiratory infections Frequently lethal in neonatal period	Autosomal recessive	Unknown
Persistence of müllerian derivatives with lymphangiectasia and postaxial polydactyly	Pulmonary lymphangiectasia Polyhydramnios Facial dysmorphism Short neck Ventricular septal defect Narrow thorax Intestinal lymphangiectasia Protein-losing enteropathy Genitourinary anomalies in males including residual müllerian duct structures (uterus and fallopian tubes)	Autosomal recessive	Unknown
Lymphedema-hypoparathyroidism syndrome	Pulmonary lymphangiectasia Short stature Cataracts, ptosis, telecanthus Mitral valve prolapse Nephropathy Hypoparathyroidism	Autosomal recessive versus X-linked recessive	Unknown

Pulmonary Arteriovenous Malformations and Hemangiomas

Pulmonary arteriovenous malformations (PAVMs) may manifest at birth or occasionally can develop postnatally. AVMs represent direct arterial-to-venous communications without intervening capillary networks. They are frequently asymptomatic, but are a significant cause of morbidity and mortality, especially if located in the central nervous system, spinal cord, or internal organs. AVMs can result in acute bleeding that may be difficult to control. For most individuals with pulmonary AVMs, however, they remain asymptomatic throughout their lives. Pulmonary AVMs occur as frequently in females and males. They are seen in individuals of all ethnicities. Several genetic conditions are associated with multiple pulmonary AVMs and a high likelihood of vascular symptoms and mortality. Individuals from these high-risk families require increased surveillance because they may have internal and external AVMs, including pulmonary lesions (Table 14-11).

Other vascular lesions, such as hemangiomas, also may arise congenitally, but generally carry less medical risk than AVMs. Superficial capillary hemangiomas are extremely common lesions noted at birth that often fade with time. Larger cavernous hemangiomas are sometimes associated with bleeding, infections, or ulceration, but are rarely life-threatening. Although frequently cosmetically problematic, hemangiomas usually do

SYNDROME	CLINICAL FEATURES	MODE OF INHERITANCE	GENE OR LOCUS IF KNOWN
HHT (Osler-Weber-Rendu) type 1	Pulmonary AVMs (in lower lobes)	Autosomal dominant	Gene = *ENG* (9q34.1)
	Other internal organ AVMs		
	Congestive heart failure (high-output)		
	Polycythemia		
	Digital clubbing		
	Telangiectasias (face, tongue, lips, conjunctiva, finger tips)		
	Epistaxis (most common presentation)		
	Gastrointestinal bleeding		
	Embolic complications		
	Cirrhosis of liver		
	Migraine headaches		
HHT (Osler-Weber-Rendu) type 2	Same as HHT type 1, but with slightly fewer pulmonary AVMs	Autosomal dominant	Gene = *ACVRL1* (12q11-q14)
HHT (Osler-Weber-Rendu) type 3	Same as HHT type 1	Autosomal dominant	Locus = 5q31
HHT (Osler-Weber-Rendu) type 4	Same as HHT type 1, but with fewer nosebleeds and telangiectasias	Autosomal dominant	Locus = 7p14
Juvenile polyposis HHT syndrome	Pulmonary AVMs	Autosomal dominant	Gene = *SMAD4* (18q21.1)
	Other vascular features of HHT		
	Juvenile gastrointestinal polyps with rectal bleeding		

AVM, arteriovenous malformation; HHT, hereditary hemorrhagic telangiectasia.

not require surgical or medical treatment. Isolated internal hemangiomas also may never pose serious medical risks. Pulmonary hemangiomas do occur, however, and may be identified incidentally. One genetic condition that is associated with multiple internal hemangiomas and other angiomas is von Hippel–Lindau syndrome. This syndrome is an autosomal dominant condition resulting in development of benign and sometimes malignant lesions. Although pulmonary hemangiomas are seen in some individuals with von Hippel–Lindau syndrome, the classic lesions seen are: cerebellar or spinal cord hemangioblastomas, pancreatic and renal cysts, retinal angiomas, and pheochromocytomas. Renal cell carcinoma is a common malignancy in von Hippel–Lindau syndrome. Recognition of this serious genetic condition enables aggressive screening measures and provides patients and their families with important medical and familial risk information. The *VHL* gene has been well characterized, and at-risk individuals may

choose to undergo molecular testing to determine their own status. Pulmonary AVMs and hemangiomas are discussed further in Chapter 12.

α_1-Antitrypsin Deficiency

α_1-Antitrypsin is a member of the serine proteinase inhibitor family and functions to inhibit the activity of proteolytic enzymes with a serine residue within the active site. α_1-antitrypsin deficiency is an autosomal recessive condition associated with early-onset obstructive pulmonary disease in childhood and adulthood. It is seen in about 1 in 5000 to 7000 whites residing in North America; 1 in 1500 to 3000 Scandinavians are affected.[16] Although emphysema is rarely diagnosed in childhood, the diagnosis of α_1-antitrypsin deficiency is sometimes made in infants with cholestatic jaundice and elevated liver function tests. In adulthood, the liver disease may progress to fibrosis and cirrhosis. Avoidance of environmental triggers, such as smoke, dust, and fumes, may delay the onset of lung disease in at-risk children and teens; this information should be included in counseling of children diagnosed with α_1-antitrypsin deficiency. Parents should be cautioned that even passive exposure to smoke poses significant health risks to affected children.

Although there is no cure for α_1-antitrypsin deficiency, a specific therapy is available and currently consists of α_1-antitrypsin protein replacement. Intravenous infusions of purified α_1-antitrypsin can increase the level of α_1-antitrypsin and antineutrophil elastase activity in the lung epithelial lining fluid of affected individuals. In the future, therapies such as this may become available to patients before alveolar destruction occurs and symptoms of chronic obstructive pulmonary disease become apparent.

The diagnosis of α_1-antitrypsin deficiency is made by measuring the plasma concentration of α_1-antitrypsin in an infant, child, or adult with clinical signs of the condition. If the concentration is less than 50% of normal, consideration should be given to performing a Protease Inhibitor (PI) analysis either by isoelectric focusing or molecular mutation analysis to confirm the diagnosis. Most affected individuals are homozygous for the Z allele. Compound heterozygotes with a Z allele and a milder S allele may develop lung disease when exposed to cigarette smoke, but generally do not have liver involvement.

For couples who have an affected child, risks to future children are on the order of 25%. When an individual is diagnosed with α_1-antitrypsin deficiency, siblings should be offered testing for their own medical information. When a prospective parent is known to carry one or two abnormal α_1-antitrypsin alleles, his or her partner might wish to undergo PI typing to determine their joint reproductive risks.

Bronchiectasis, Primary Ciliary Dyskinesia, and Kartagener Syndrome

"Bronchiectasis" is the pathologic term for bronchial destruction, bronchial dilation, and accumulation of infected secretions, which occurs most often in the setting of chronic lung infections. Although cystic fibrosis (CF) is the most frequent genetic condition associated with bronchiectasis, primary and secondary immunodeficiencies and ciliary dysfunction also may result in chronic pulmonary infections and lung tissue destruction, especially in dependent areas of the lung. Because more than two thirds of children with non–CF-related bronchiectasis have evidence of an immune defect, primary ciliary dyskinesia, or recurrent aspiration, evaluation of patients with this finding should include immunologic and other diagnostic studies to rule out these other etiologies.[17] Several genetic syndromes with bronchiectasis as a major feature have been described that are associated with a primary immunodeficiency (Table 14-12).

Kartagener described a curious combination of situs inversus, chronic sinusitis, and bronchiectasis, which subsequently became known as the Kartagener triad. The term "Kartagener syndrome" was later adopted when additional features of rhinitis, nasal polyps, chronic otitis media, and reduced fertility were recognized. Kartagener syndrome is now considered the most severe clinical expression of a spectrum of abnormalities of ciliary motility caused by defective cilia in several parts of the body that renders ciliary function ineffective. This entity has been termed "immotile-cilia syndrome," "dyskinetic cilia syndrome," and, more appropriately, "primary ciliary dyskinesia" (PCD).[18]

The large airways and contiguous structure, such as nares, paranasal sinuses, and middle ear, are lined by a ciliated, pseudostratified columnar epithelium. Ciliated cells contain approximately 200 cilia. Each normal cilium contains an array of longitudinal microtubules, consisting of nine doublets arranged in an outer circle around a central pair. A network of structural proteins provides linkages to maintain the 9+2 pattern of microtubules in healthy cilia. The protein nexin links the outer microtubular doublet, creating a circumferential network, and radial spokes connect the outer microtubular doublets with a central sheath of protein that surrounds the central tubules. Dynein is attached to the microtubules as distinct inner and outer "arms" thought to participate in the supply of energy for microtubular

Table 14-12	Genetic Conditions Associated with Bronchiectasis Resulting from an Immunodeficiency		

SYNDROME	CLINICAL FEATURES	MODE OF INHERITANCE	GENE OR LOCUS IF KNOWN
Ataxia-telangiectasia	Bronchiectasis Immune defects with thymus hypoplasia and decreased T cells, defective B cell differentiation, lymphopenia Recurrent sinopulmonary infections Short stature Cutaneous and conjunctival telangiectasias Cerebellar ataxia and cerebellar atrophy, dysarthria, seizures Hypogonadism Sensitivity to ionizing radiation Risks for leukemia with or without lymphoma Increased AFP and CEA Decreased IgA, IgE, and IgG2	Autosomal recessive. Heterozygotes may be at increased risk for certain neoplasias	Gene = *ATM* (11q22.3)
Bloom syndrome	Bronchiectasis Prenatal and postnatal growth restriction Microcephaly Facial dysmorphism Malar hypoplasia Polydactyly, syndactyly, with or without clinodactyly Sun sensitivity Facial telangiectasias Cutaneous hyperpigmentation and hypopigmentation IgA, IgG, and IgM deficiency Impaired lymphocyte response Recurrent life-threatening infections Increased risk for malignancy Cytogenetic instability with increased sister chromatid exchanges	Autosomal recessive. Almost ⅓ of reported cases are in Ashkenazi-Jewish population	Gene = *RECQL3* (15q26.1)
Young syndrome (Barry-Perkins-Young syndrome)	Bronchiectasis Congenital cystic lung disease Recurrent sinopulmonary infections Azoospermia owing to obstructed vas deferens Normal bronchial cilia on EM	Autosomal recessive. Should be differentiated from congenital absence of vas deferens owing to mutations in *CFTR* (cystic fibrosis) gene	Unknown. Distinct from *CFTR*

AFP, α-fetoprotein; CEA, carcinoembryonic antigen; EM, electron microscopy.

sliding through adenosine triphosphatase activity (Fig. 14-5). Ciliary motion occurs within an aqueous layer of airway surface liquids and is divided into two phases: an effective stroke phase that sweeps forward, and a recovery phase during which the cilia bend backward and extend into the starting position for the stroke phase.

PCD has been reported in many ethnic groups without racial or gender predilection.

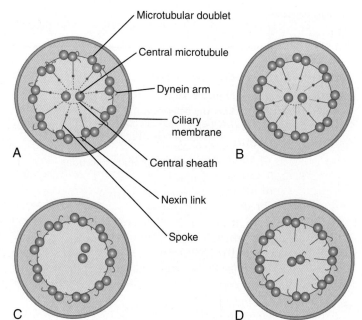

Figure 14-5. A, Normal cilia contain nine outer microtubular doublets around a central pair. **B,** Dynein arms control beats within cilia; outer dynein arms are related to beat frequency, and inner arms affect the beat waveform. **C,** Radial spoke defect. **D,** Microtubular transposition abnormality, both clear, cilia structural variants. (*Adapted from Turcios, NL, Your patient may have primary ciliary dyskinesia. J Respir Dis Pediatr 3:99, 2001.*)

In most families, PCD seems to be transmitted by an autosomal recessive pattern of inheritance; however, rare instances of autosomal dominant or X-linked inheritance patterns have been reported. The incidence of PCD is 1 in 15,000 to 20,000 births. The incidence of situs inversus is random within affected families, suggesting that this phenotype is not genetically determined. The numerous ultrastructural phenotypes suggest genetic heterogeneity. PCD seems to be caused by mutations in at least three different genes. Not all individuals who carry two copies of these gene mutations have the visceral abnormalities, which greatly complicates diagnostic testing and genetic counseling of these families. More recent advances in molecular genetics have identified mutations that can be tracked in certain families.

Bronchiectasis may develop in young individuals, but is never present at birth; no individual is born with full-blown Kartagener syndrome. Although individuals with PCD, which includes Kartagener syndrome, are plagued by recurrent sinopulmonary infections and chronic otitis media, they do not have any recognized immunologic problem. Their infections are tied to structurally defective cilia, resulting in inability to clear

secretions, with a buildup of mucus and bacteria in the respiratory tract.

The clinical manifestations vary among PCD patients and depend on age. The diagnosis of PCD should be considered in term newborns with respiratory distress or persistent atelectasis/pneumonia with symptoms resembling "wet lung" and no obvious predisposing risk factors. The former presumably reflects the importance of functional cilia in clearing lung liquid shortly after birth.

Infants and older children with PCD may present with atypical asthma that is nonresponsive to treatment or with an increased number of respiratory infections associated with chronic cough and expectoration of mucopurulent sputum over time. The classic presentation of PCD includes chronic rhinosinusitis, recurrent serous otitis media (often requiring multiple interventions, such as repeated courses of antibiotics and placement of myringotomy tubes), and recurrent pneumonia. Nasal polyps and agenesis of the frontal sinuses also are common in childhood. *Situs inversus* is a useful sign when PCD is being considered, but as described earlier, is present only in approximately 50% of patients with PCD.

The symptoms in adolescents and adults are similar to the symptoms in older children, but otitis media seems to be less prominent. Infertility is common in affected adults, especially in men owing to immotile sperm—a modified cilium. Fatigue and headaches are common complaints and may be related to chronic sinusitis, although the headaches may persist even during infection-free periods.

Cylindrical or saccular bronchiectasis may occur, even in childhood, usually affecting the middle and lower lobes and the lingula. Patients with bronchiectasis have auscultatory crackles and may have wheezes that mimic asthma. Common findings on chest x-ray and computed tomography (CT) scan are a moderate degree of hyperinflation, peribronchial thickening, atelectasis, and bronchiectasis. Digital clubbing is uncommon in patients younger than 18 years old.

Complete *situs inversus* may be an incidental and clinically insignificant finding in half of patients with PCD. Heterotaxy or *situs ambiguus* results from failure of left-to-right differentiation and occurs in about 1 in 17 PCD patients. This condition may be associated with anomalies such as cardiac defects, asplenia, and polysplenia. The presence of asplenia may add to the risk for infection in an already immunocompromised host.

Studies have shown that nasal nitric oxide is extremely low in PCD patients and may be useful for screening for PCD. The final diagnosis of any of the PCDs, including Kartagener syndrome, rests on electron microscopic evaluation of respiratory cilia. Scraping of the anterior aspect of the inferior nasal turbinate or biopsy of the bronchial epithelium at the time of bronchoscopy may provide an adequate sample for ultra-structural analysis. The most frequent electron microscopic finding in patients with PCD is absence of, or abnormalities in, the dynein arms; about 1 in 10 ciliary samples has obvious abnormalities in the central pair of microtubules or in the radial spokes.

Management of patients with PCDs includes many of the same therapies used for children with CF who have secondary ciliary dysfunction. Table 14-13 outlines many of the genes and loci recognized to be associated with bronchiectasis and PCD.

Table 14-13	Primary Ciliary Dyskinesia with or without Situs Abnormalities		
SYNDROME	**CLINICAL FEATURES**	**MODE OF INHERITANCE**	**GENE OR LOCUS IF KNOWN**
Kartagener syndrome, Siewert syndrome (situs inversus, bronchiectasis, and sinusitis)	Bronchiectasis Dyskinetic cilia Immotile sperm Decreased fertility in males and females Recurrent sinopulmonary infections Dextrocardia Situs inversus Asplenia Absent or abnormal dynein arms of sperm and respiratory cilia on EM	Autosomal recessive	Gene = *DNAI1* (9p21-p13); *DNAH5* (5p15-p14); locus = 7p21
PCD 1	Bronchiectasis Dyskinetic cilia Recurrent rhinosinusitis Chronic ear infections Situs inversus (only in 20%) Dynein arm defect on EM	Autosomal recessive	Gene = *DNAI1* (9p21-p13). Allelic with Kartagener
PCD 2	Same as PCD 1	Autosomal recessive	Locus = 19q13.3-qter

(Continued)

Table 14-13	Primary Ciliary Dyskinesia with or without Situs Abnormalities—*Cont'd*		

SYNDROME	CLINICAL FEATURES	MODE OF INHERITANCE	GENE OR LOCUS IF KNOWN
PCD 3	Same as PCD1	Autosomal recessive	Gene = *DNAH5* (5p15-p14). Allelic with Kartagener
PCD 4	Same as PCD1	Autosomal recessive	Locus = 15q13.1-q15.1
PCD 5	Same as PCD1	Autosomal recessive	Locus = 16p12.2-p12.1
PCD 6	Same as PCD1	Autosomal recessive	Gene = *TXNDC3* (17p14)
Dyskinetic cilia owing to defective radial spokes	Chronic sinopulmonary infections Immotile sperm Absence of ciliary axoneme radial spokes on EM	Autosomal recessive	Unknown
Dyskinetic cilia owing to transposition of ciliary microtubules	Chronic sinopulmonary infections Evidence of transposition of the first doublet microtubule on EM	Autosomal recessive	Unknown
Hypohydrotic ectodermal dysplasia with hypothyroidism and ciliary dyskinesia	Recurrent pulmonary infections Hypohydrotic ectodermal dysplasia Primary hypothyroidism Abnormalities of ciliary microtubules on EM	Autosomal recessive	Unknown
X-linked retinitis pigmentosa with recurrent respiratory infections	Recurrent pulmonary infections Retinitis pigmentosa Normal male fertility Inner dynein arm deficiency, incomplete microtubules, and ciliary disorientation on EM	X-linked recessive	Gene = *RPGR* (Xp21.1)

EM, electron microscopy; PCD, primary ciliary dyskinesia.

Spontaneous Pneumothorax

Spontaneous pneumothorax is usually an acute, sometimes life-threatening event, occurring in otherwise healthy individuals. Spontaneous pneumothorax occurs more often in tall, thin men and can be seen in individuals with certain underlying connective tissue disorders. Familial spontaneous pneumothorax can be inherited as an autosomal dominant condition associated with subpleural blebs and bullae, or can be a sporadic (nongenetic) occurrence. Table 14-14 summarizes genetic associations with spontaneous pneumothoraces. For any child, teen, or adult with a spontaneous pneumothorax, a focused physical examination and targeted family history may help to uncover evidence of a connective tissue disorder or a heritable trait.

Inborn Errors of Metabolism

Although one would not typically associate inborn errors of metabolism with pulmonary problems, many storage and biochemical disorders cause respiratory complications. Because most of these conditions are systemic, virtually all organs may be involved to a greater or lesser degree. Interstitial or restrictive lung disease can be seen in some lysosomal storage disorders. Pulmonary hypertension or pulmonary hypoplasia may be identified with

SYNDROME	CLINICAL FEATURES	MODE OF INHERITANCE	GENE OR LOCUS IF KNOWN
Marfan syndrome	Spontaneous pneumothorax Pulmonary blebs Rarely emphysema Disproportionate tall stature Long, narrow face Severe myopia Risk for retinal detachment Mitral valve prolapse Aortic root dilation and risk for aortic dissection Pectus deformity Kyphosis or scoliosis Arachnodactyly Joint hypermobility Pes planus	Autosomal dominant. At least ¼ due to new or de novo gene mutations	Gene = FBN1 (15q21.1)
Primary spontaneous pneumothorax	Spontaneous pneumothorax Subpleural blebs and bullae (randomly distributed throughout lungs in familial instances) More common in tall, thin men	Autosomal dominant	Gene = FLCN (17p11.2)
Birt-Hogg-Dube syndrome (fibrofolliculomas with trichodiscomas and acrochordons)	Spontaneous pneumothorax Lung cysts Hair follicle hamartomas Skin tags Renal tumors	Autosomal dominant	Gene = FLCN (17p11.2). Allelic with primary spontaneous pneumothorax
Ehlers-Danlos type IV	Spontaneous pneumothorax Pinched nose Premature tooth loss Mitral valve prolapse Spontaneous bowel and uterine rupture Uterine and bladder prolapse Easy bruising, prominent veins Poor scar formation, thin skin Distal interphalangeal joint hypermobility Acro-osteolysis	Autosomal dominant	Gene = COL3A1 (2q31)
Autosomal recessive Ehlers-Danlos type VII	Neonatal pneumothorax Short stature Micrognathia Blue sclera Myopia Gingival hyperplasia Hypodontia and abnormal teeth Hernias Visceral rupture Short limbs and digits Significant joint laxity Skin laxity and fragility Easy bruising Doughy, redundant skin	Autosomal recessive	Gene = ADAMTS2 (5q23)

other inborn errors of metabolism. Organic acidemias, aminoacidopathies, cholesterol ester storage diseases, disorders of glycosylation, and peroxisomal disorders have been found to have pulmonary complications. Table 14-15 highlights some commonly recognized inborn errors of metabolism associated with pulmonary symptoms.

Pulmonary Arterial Hypertension

Although pulmonary hypertension frequently results from other systemic problems, idiopathic pulmonary arterial hypertension (previously termed "primary pulmonary

| **Table 14-15** | Inborn Errors of Metabolism Associated with Pulmonary Manifestations |

METABOLIC DISORDER	ENZYME DEFICIENCY	CLINICAL FEATURES	INHERITANCE	GENE OR LOCUS
Mucopolysaccharidosis type IH/S (Hurler-Scheie syndrome)	α-L-iduronidase. Lysosomal storage disorder—mucopolysaccharidosis	Restrictive lung disease Recurrent upper respiratory infections Short stature Corneal clouding Joint stiffness Dysostosis multiplex Hepatosplenomegaly Declining or normal IQ	Autosomal recessive	Gene = *IDUA* (4p16.3)
Gaucher disease (pulmonary findings associated with severe phenotype)	Acid β-glucosidase. Lysosomal storage disorder—sphingolipidosis	Interstitial lung disease Restrictive lung disease Pulmonary infiltrates (<1 in 20) Pulmonary hypertension Hepatosplenomegaly Bone pain, pathologic fractures Cutaneous hyperpigmentation Pancytopenia	Autosomal recessive. Highly variable expression and incomplete penetrance. Carrier frequency in Ashkenazi-Jewish population is about 1:14	Gene = *GBA* (1q21)
Fabry disease	α-galactosidase A. Lysosomal storage disorder—sphingolipidosis	Mild obstructive lung disease (may be mutation dependent) Mild short stature Corneal dystrophy Painful crises Strokes, seizures Angina, hypertension Left ventricular hypertrophy Abdominal pain Renal failure Acroparesthesias Angiokeratomas	X-linked recessive	Gene = *GLA* (Xq22)

Table 14-15	Inborn Errors of Metabolism Associated with Pulmonary Manifestations—*Cont'd*			
METABOLIC DISORDER	**ENZYME DEFICIENCY**	**CLINICAL FEATURES**	**INHERITANCE**	**GENE OR LOCUS**
GM_1 gangliosidosis type I	Acid β-galactosidase. Lysosomal storage disorder—sphingolipidosis	Pulmonary infiltrates with foam cell vacuoles filled with fibrillar material	Autosomal recessive	Gene = *GLB1* (3p21.33)
		Respiratory insufficiency		
		Short stature		
		Short neck		
		Cherry-red spots (50%)		
		Gingival hypertrophy		
		Kyphoscoliosis		
		Hepatosplenomegaly		
		Visceral foamy histiocytes		
		Stiff joints		
		Dysostosis multiplex		
		Declining IQ		
Krabbe disease (globoid cell leukodystrophy)	Galactocerebroside β-galactosidase. Lysosomal storage disorder—sphingolipidosis	Respiratory failure	Autosomal recessive	Gene = *GALC* (14q31)
		Intra-alveolar and interstitial macrophages		
		Failure to thrive		
		Progressive neurologic deterioration, seizures		
		Hydrocephalus		
		Optic atrophy, blindness		
		Hyperirritability		
		Sensitive to sound		
		Peripheral neuropathy		
Farber disease	Acid ceramidase. Lysosomal storage disorder—sphingolipidosis	Respiratory insufficiency	Autosomal recessive	Gene = *AC* or *ASAH* (8p22-p21.3)
		Failure to thrive		
		Cherry-red spots		
		Hoarse cry		
		Irritability		
		Cognitive decline, motor delays		
		Lipogranulomatosis		
		Periarticular subcutaneous nodules		
		Painful, enlarged joints		
		Hepatosplenomegaly		
		Nephropathy		

(Continued)

Table 14-15	Inborn Errors of Metabolism Associated with Pulmonary Manifestations—*Cont'd*			
METABOLIC DISORDER	**ENZYME DEFICIENCY**	**CLINICAL FEATURES**	**INHERITANCE**	**GENE OR LOCUS**
Wolman disease	Acid cholesterol ester hydrolase. Lysosomal storage disorder—other	Pulmonary hypertension Failure to thrive Hepatosplenomegaly Hepatic fibrosis Malabsorption Adrenal calcifications	Autosomal recessive	Gene = *LIPA* (10q24-q25)
Glycogen storage disease type Ic/Id	Undefined, but due to a phosphate-pyrophosphate translocase defect. Glycogen storage disorder	Pulmonary hypertension Respiratory infections Hypoglycemia Growth delay Hepatomegaly Renal insufficiency Xanthomas Gout Lactic acidemia	Autosomal recessive	Locus = 11q23-q24
Zellweger syndrome (cerebrohepato-renal syndrome)	Genetic heterogeneity. Peroxisome biogenesis factors and peroxisomal membrane protein and peroxisome receptor. Peroxisomal disorder	Pulmonary hypoplasia Bell-shaped thorax Breech presentation Failure to thrive Facial dysmorphism Nerve deafness Corneal clouding Cataracts, glaucoma Cardiac defects Hepatomegaly Neonatal jaundice Hypospadias Hydronephrosis Stippled epiphyses Clubfeet Hypotonia, seizures CNS defects Elevated long-chain fatty acids and phytanic acid Death in first year of life	Autosomal recessive	Gene = *PEX1* (7q21); *PEX2* (8q); *PEX3* (6q); *PEX5* (chr 12); *PEX6* (6p); *PEX12*; *PEX14* (chr 1); *PEX26*; locus = 7q11
Congenital disorder of glycosylation type Ih (carbohydrate-deficient glycoprotein)	Dolichyl-P-glucose: Glc-1-Man-9-GlcNAc-2-PP-dolichyl-α-3-glucosyltransferase. Carbohydrate-deficient glycoprotein disorder	Pulmonary hypoplasia Intrauterine growth restriction Feeding difficulties Low factor XI, protein C, and antithrombin III Protein-losing enteropathy	Autosomal recessive	Gene = *ALG8* (11pter-p15.5)

Table 14-15		Inborn Errors of Metabolism Associated with Pulmonary Manifestations—*Cont'd*		
METABOLIC DISORDER	**ENZYME DEFICIENCY**	**CLINICAL FEATURES**	**INHERITANCE**	**GENE OR LOCUS**
Multiple Acyl-CoA dehydrogenase deficiency (glutaric aciduria type II)	Electron transfer flavoprotein-ubiquinone oxidoreductase. Electron transfer disorder—mitochondrial fatty oxidation pathway	Severe diarrhea Hepatomegaly Hypoalbuminemia Ascites and edema Assorted anomalies Pulmonary hypoplasia Respiratory distress Facial dysmorphism Neonatal acidosis Jaundice Hypoglycemia Hepatomegaly Hypotonia Renal cysts and other genitourinary defects Glutaric aciduria	Autosomal recessive	Gene = *ETFA* (15q23-q25); *ETFB* (19q13.3); *ETFDH* (4q32-qter)
Homocystinuria	Cystathionine β-synthase. Amino acid disorder—methionine pathway	Pulmonary embolism Other thromboses Pectus deformities Ectopia lentis Mitral valve prolapse Arachnodactyly Kyphoscoliosis Osteoporosis Joint contractures Seizures, strokes Learning disabilities or mild mental retardation Elevated plasma and urinary homocystine	Autosomal recessive. About half are responsive to vitamin B_6	Gene = *CBS* (21q22.3)
Lysinuric protein intolerance	Amino acid transporter. Defect in transport of dibasic amino acids in the intestine, liver, and kidneys. Amino acid disorder—amino acid transport	Alveolar proteinosis Subpleural cysts Acinar nodules Thick pleural interstitial septa Protein intolerance Failure to thrive Malabsorption Hepatomegaly Cirrhosis Osteopenia	Autosomal recessive. More common in Finnish population	Gene = *SLC7A7* (14q11.2)

CNS, central nervous system.

hypertension") can occur as a mendelian disorder (autosomal dominant and autosomal recessive) and as part of other well-described genetic syndromes. There seems to be a relationship between systemic vascular development and idiopathic pulmonary arterial hypertension in some, but not all, of these conditions. An *IPAH* gene has been identified in selected families, which codes for the BMPR2 protein, which resides on chromosome 2 within band q33. Table 14-16 presents genetic conditions associated with idiopathic pulmonary arterial hypertension. See Chapter 4 for further information.

Table 14-16 Genetic Conditions Associated with Primary Pulmonary Hypertension

SYNDROME	CLINICAL FEATURES	MODE OF INHERITANCE	GENE OR LOCUS IF KNOWN
PPH	PPH	Autosomal dominant. About 6% of cases of PPH are genetic. Females more often affected than males	Gene = *BMPR2* (2q33)
	PFTs with restrictive pattern		
	Arterial hypoxemia		
	RVH and failure		
	Increased pulmonary arterial pressure and pulmonary vascular resistance		
	Arterial fibrosis and medial hypertrophy		
	Thrombosis		
Autosomal recessive PPH	Same as PPH	Autosomal recessive	Unknown
Familial persistent pulmonary hypertension of the newborn	Neonatal pulmonary hypertension	Autosomal recessive	Susceptibility gene = *CPS1* (T1405N polymorphism)
	Abnormal pulmonary lobules		
	Increased muscular wall in arterioles		
	Lethal in infants		
Lymphedema and cerebral arteriovenous anomaly	PPH	Autosomal dominant	Unknown
	AVM		
	Cranial bruit		
	Lymphedema		
Familial pulmonary capillary hemangiomatosis	PPH	Autosomal recessive	Unknown
	Pulmonary capillary hemangiomatosis		
Familial cirrhosis	PPH	Autosomal recessive	Gene = *KRT8* (12q13); *KRT18* (12Q13)
	Congenital or childhood cirrhosis		
	Esophageal varices		
	Edema		
	Liver with panlobular swelling, fibrosis, and micronodular cirrhosis		
	Increased hepatic copper		

SYNDROME	CLINICAL FEATURES	MODE OF INHERITANCE	GENE OR LOCUS IF KNOWN
VATER-like defects with pulmonary hypertension, laryngeal webs, and growth deficiency	Pulmonary hypertension Short stature Blue sclera Cardiac defects Laryngeal webs Pectus excavatum Rib and vertebral anomalies Absent kidney Polydactyly	Autosomal recessive	Unknown
Rowley-Rosenberg syndrome	Pulmonary hypertension Growth deficiency Muscle atrophy Decreased adipose tissue RVH and cor pulmonale Aminoaciduria Increased plasma unesterified fatty acids	Autosomal recessive	Unknown

AVM, arteriovenous malformation; PFT, pulmonary function test; PPH, primary pulmonary hypertension; RVH, right ventricular hypertrophy.

Pulmonary Fibrosis

Idiopathic pulmonary fibrosis is usually a sporadic occurrence, often identified in adults. Approximately 2% of patients are identified to have a familial form of the disease. In addition, several genetic syndromes have pulmonary fibrosis as part of the clinical picture. Table 14-17 summarizes some syndromes associated with pulmonary fibrosis.

Pulmonary Embolism

Thromboembolic events, including pulmonary embolism, are uncommon in pediatric patients. As individuals age, the risk of developing a deep vein thrombosis and subsequent pulmonary embolism increases. The incidence of pulmonary embolism is decreased in children compared with adults. The incidence of pulmonary embolism may be increasing, however, as a result of prolonged survival of children with chronic diseases and increased use of central venous catheters. In teenagers, pleuritic chest pain seems to be the most common presenting complaint. Other complaints include dyspnea, cough, and hemoptysis. Unexplained persistent tachypnea can be an important indication of pulmonary embolism in pediatric patients. More than 95% of children with venous thromboembolic disease have at least one underlying clinical condition. Central venous catheters are the most frequent clinical risk factor. Other underlying clinical conditions associated with pediatric thromboembolic disease are congenital heart disease, infection, surgery, malignancy, kidney disease, trauma, immobility, systemic lupus erythematosus, sickle cell disease, antiphospholipid syndrome, ventriculoatrial shunts, and medications, including estrogens and asparaginase.

Although most thrombi occur in otherwise low-risk individuals, patients with genetic disorders that increase their risk for thrombosis are considered to have thrombophilia. For many years, it has been known that

Table 14-17 Genetic Conditions Associated with Pulmonary Fibrosis

SYNDROME	CLINICAL FEATURES	MODE OF INHERITANCE	GENE OR LOCUS IF KNOWN
Idiopathic pulmonary fibrosis (Hamman-Rich disease)	Idiopathic pulmonary fibrosis Alveolar inflammation Digital clubbing Increased risk for alveolar cell carcinoma	Autosomal dominant. Most are sporadic	Susceptibility gene = *SPA1* polymorphism 6A(4); locus = 4q31 with possible candidate gene *ELMOD2*; 8p21
Hermansky-Pudlak syndrome (albinism with hemorrhagic diathesis and pigmented reticuloendothelial cells)	Interstitial pulmonary fibrosis Restrictive lung disease Oculocutaneous albinism Nystagmus, low vision Epistaxis Inflammatory bowel disease Platelet dysfunction Absent platelet dense bodies	Autosomal recessive. Carrier frequency in Puerto Rico is about 1:20, a little higher in the northwest region of the country	Gene = *HPS1* (10q23.1-q23.2); *AP3B1* (5q14.1); *HPS3* (3q24); *HPS4* (22q11.2-q12.2); *HPS5* (11p15-p13); *HPS6* (10q24.3); *DTNBP1* (6p22.3); locus = 19q13
Pulmonary alveolar microlithiasis	Progressive pulmonary fibrosis Intra-alveolar calcifications PFTs with restrictive lung changes Chest x-ray with "sandstorm" appearance	Autosomal recessive. About $^2/_3$ are sporadic and $^1/_3$ familial	Gene = *SLC34A2* (4p15.31-p15.2)
X-linked dyskeratosis congenita	Pulmonary fibrosis Restrictive lung disease Short stature Cytopenias, bone marrow failure Recurrent infections Risks for squamous cell carcinomas and other malignancies Optic atrophy Leukoplakia, dental caries Nail dystrophy Skin atrophy and reticulated pigmentation Sparse hair Cirrhosis Hypospadias, cryptorchidism Renal anomalies	X-linked recessive	Gene = *DKC1* (Xq28)
Autosomal dominant dyskeratosis congenita	Same as X-linked dyskeratosis congenita	Autosomal dominant	Gene = *TERC* (3q21-q28)

PFT, pulmonary function test.

deficiencies of protein S, protein C, or anti-thrombin are thrombophilic. More recently, the Arg506-to-Gln506 mutation in factor V (commonly known as factor Leiden) has been identified and found to confer an eightfold increased risk for thrombosis in individuals heterozygous for the disorder. This risk is much higher when factor Leiden is present in the homozygous state. Factor Leiden is present in about 5% of the white population. Similarly, a common mutation in the pro-thrombin gene is the factor II polymorphism known as 20210G→A, present in about 2% of whites, which causes a modest increased risk for deep vein thrombosis and pulmonary embolism. Individuals who carry one copy of the factor V Leiden mutation *and* one prothrombin mutation have a much more significant risk of developing a deep vein thrombosis or pulmonary embolism or both.

In addition to the thrombotic risks noted with homocystinuria as outlined in Table 14-14, there are a few genetic conditions that are thrombogenic. Sporadic protein S, protein C, or antithrombin III deficiencies are often noted during episodes of thrombosis. Occasionally, these deficiencies may be transmitted through the family as autosomal dominant traits. In these cases, the family history may be very compelling, with multiple affected individuals in several generations, with individuals having more than one thrombotic event over their lifetime. Protein S deficiency is seen in about 1 in 50 individuals with deep vein thrombosis. Infants who are homozygous for protein C or anti-thrombin III mutations are at incredibly high risk for neonatal thrombosis and pulmonary embolism, and may die in the newborn period if untreated. Recognition of patients with strong family histories of thrombosis may allow for (1) better preoperative and postoperative planning, (2) ordering of appropriate diagnostic studies, (3) discussion of risk factors, and possibly (4) referral to a hematologist for discussion of therapeutic options and management strategies.

Cystic Fibrosis

CF occurs wherever Europeans have settled. CF has been reported in significant numbers of African-Americans, however, and natives of Middle Eastern countries, India, and Pakistan. More recent data from the CF Foundation Patient Registry suggest an incidence of 1 in 3000 white births, 1 in 6000 Hispanic births, and 1 in 10,000 African-American births. CF is caused by mutations in a single gene, known as the cystic fibrosis trans-membrane regulator (*CFTR*), which functions as a chloride channel on the apical membranes of epithelial cells lining the airways, pancreatic ducts, sweat ducts, intestines, biliary tree, and vas deferens.

CFTR

The absence or underfunctioning of *CFTR* in CF patients is the basis for the cellular defects, and explains some, but not all, of the various organ dysfunctions in CF. In addition to its function as an apical chloride channel, *CFTR* regulates other apical membrane conductance pathways. Numerous other cellular functions have been ascribed to *CFTR*: It downregulates transepithelial sodium transport, in particular, the epithelial sodium channel, which accounts for increased sodium absorption in CF airways; it also regulates calcium-activated chloride channels and potassium channels, and may serve important functions in exocytosis and the formation of molecular complexes in the plasma membrane. In airway epithelial cells of patients with CF, chloride impermeability caused by abnormal or absent *CFTR* and increased sodium absorption caused by the epithelial sodium channel dysfunction cause a twofold increase in the transepithelial potential difference. More recent data suggest that *CFTR* also transports HCO_3^- or regulates its transport through epithelial cell membranes.

The role of *CFTR* in epithelial cells seems to extend well beyond chloride permeability. In human CF, and in mice with targeted deletions of the *CFTR* gene, the absence of *CFTR* influences the expression of several other gene products, including proteins important in inflammatory responses, maturational processing, ion transport, and cell signaling. These other proteins are potential modifiers of the CF phenotype and may help explain the substantial differences in clinical severity among patients with the same mutations in *CFTR*.

Mutations in *CFTR* and Their Consequences

The *CFTR* gene encompasses approximately 180,000 base pairs on the long arm of chromosome 7. The protein contains 1480 amino acids. More than 1500 disease-associated mutations have been described in the coding sequence, messenger RNA splice signals, and other regions. These mutations can be classified on the basis of the mechanism by which they are believed to cause disease (Fig. 14-6). The most common mutation, known as *ΔF508*, is present in approximately 70% of defective *CFTR* alleles and in 90% of patients with CF in the United States, and is categorized as inadequately processed (class II defect). *CFTR* with the *ΔF508* mutation is missing a phenylalanine (F) residue at position 508. The defective protein retains substantial chloride channel function in cell-free lipid membranes, but when synthesized by the normal cellular machinery, the protein is rapidly recognized as misfolded and is quickly degraded. This degradation occurs well before *CFTR* can reach its crucial site of action at the cell surface. Similar to *ΔF508*, several other clinically important mutations (e.g., *N1303K*, *G85E*, and *G91R*) lead to misfolded *CFTR* proteins that are prematurely degraded.

About 5% to 10% of *CFTR* mutations result in premature truncation or nonsense alleles, designated by "X"; with *G542X*, *CFTR* is not synthesized (class I defect). As a result of a genetic founder effect, specific *CFTR* mutations are particularly common among individuals of Ashkenazi Jewish descent. Other *CFTR* mutations encode properly processed, full-length *CFTR* protein that lacks normal ion channel activity. The *G551D* mutation (class III) is believed to possess little or no chloride channel function *in vivo* because of abnormal function of a nucleotide-binding domain, resulting in defective regulation. The *A455E* mutation (class IV) retains partial *CFTR* ion channel activity, a feature that probably explains the less severe pulmonary phenotype. Other mutation classes include reduced numbers of *CFTR* transcripts (class V) and defective *CFTR* stability at the cell surface (class VI).

Screening and Diagnosis

Most U.S. states and several countries screen newborns for CF by measuring immunoreactive trypsinogen, a pancreatic enzyme precursor, in dried blood spots. Asymptomatic newborns identified by neonatal screening have elevated blood immunoreactive trypsinogens, most likely secondary to pancreatic ductular obstruction and leakage of enzyme into the circulation. This screening test has a substantial false-positive rate, however, and as such, cannot be used as a confirmation of a diagnosis of CF. Instead, the diagnosis of CF is best confirmed by performing a genotype or a sweat test.

Genotyping that reveals two known CF-causing mutations confirms the diagnosis. Molecular tests can readily detect a specific mutation, and some vendors can sequence the entire gene. Among the more than 1500 recognized mutations, however, many are "private" mutations that occur in only a single family. A patient in whom two CF mutations are not identified by commercial genotyping still can have CF.

The diagnosis also can be made when the sweat chloride concentration is greater than

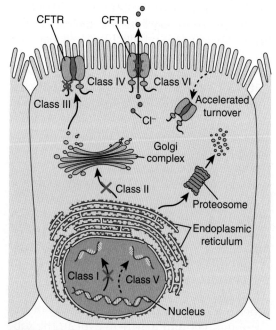

Figure 14-6. *CFTR* mutations classes I through VI. (*Adapted from Rowe SM, Miller S, Sorcher EJ: Cystic fibrosis. N Engl J Med 352:1992-2001, 1998, 2005.*)

60 mEq/L in the presence of typical clinical features (chronic pulmonary disease, pancreatic insufficiency, or both). A family history (sibling or first cousin who has CF) significantly increases the index of suspicion for CF in a symptomatic child or infant with an elevated immunoreactive trypsinogen on newborn screening, and should immediately prompt diagnostic testing. The sweat test is very reliable and is an excellent discriminant for CF, if it is performed by experienced personnel, and the samples are handled carefully to avoid evaporation or contamination. About 5% of patients who have CF exhibit sweat chloride values less than 60 mEq/L. The sweat test is performed by iontophoresis of pilocarpine into the skin to stimulate sweating. Sweat is collected for chloride quantification by titrimetric analysis. Technical errors tend to produce elevated values, so a "positive" result must always be confirmed by a second sweat test or *CFTR* molecular analysis. If neither of these procedures is diagnostic, another test of *CFTR* function, such as measurement of the nasal potential difference, should be performed. There is a small subset of patients (often adults) who have atypical clinical manifestations, a normal or borderline sweat test result, and equivocal *CFTR* molecular results (zero or one mutation identified) in whom a definite diagnosis cannot be made.

Prenatal diagnosis of CF can be accomplished in pregnancies known to be at increased risk because of a positive family history, or through routine antenatal screening programs. In cases where the genotype of the parents is known, the diagnosis of CF can be confirmed or excluded by direct mutation analysis performed on fetal cells obtained by chorionic villus sampling after 10 weeks' gestation, or cultured amniotic fluid cells performed between 15 and 18 weeks gestation. There is currently no biochemical assay for the protein gene product.

In pregnancies not known to be at increased risk for CF, the diagnosis is sometimes suggested by prenatal ultrasound findings, including a hyperechoic bowel pattern suggestive of intestinal obstruction. Meconium peritonitis secondary to small bowel perforation *in utero* also can be detected by prenatal ultrasound. Only 7% of such cases are associated with CF, however.

Clinical Manifestations

Many clinical findings prompt consideration of the diagnosis of CF (Fig. 14-7). After birth, because of the presence of the high protein concentration in meconium, newborns with CF can present with meconium ileus or meconium plug syndrome. About 15% of patients who have CF present in the neonatal period with meconium ileus (obstruction of the distal ileum or proximal colon with inspissated meconium). Meconium ileus is virtually diagnostic of CF, so the patient should be treated presumptively as having CF until a valid sweat test or genotype can be obtained. Meconium plug syndrome, in which there is transient distal colonic obstruction, also may be the presenting manifestation of CF. A few affected infants present with prolonged obstructive jaundice, presumably secondary to obstruction of extrahepatic bile ducts by thick bile along with intrahepatic bile stasis.

An increased concentration of electrolytes in the sweat may result in hyponatremic or hypochloremic dehydration secondary to salt depletion, or hypokalemic metabolic alkalosis secondary to chronic salt loss. CF should always be considered in any child who presents with dehydration and severe hypoelectrolytemia that is not accounted for by gastrointestinal losses. Because of their high ratio of surface area to volume, infants who have CF are prone to heat prostration.

During infancy and beyond, a common presentation of CF is failure to thrive. Any child who fails to gain weight despite a good appetite, and especially if the child produces frequent, bulky, foul-smelling, oily stools, should be evaluated for CF. These children may develop abdominal cramps after feeding and begin to refuse food, with resultant decreased oral intake that worsens the malnutrition. There also may be excessive flatus. These symptoms are usually the result of pancreatic insufficiency (failure of the pancreas to produce sufficient digestive enzymes), which impairs the breakdown and absorption of fats and protein. Affected infants also may present with hypoproteinemia with or without edema, anemia, and manifestations of deficiency of the fat-soluble vitamins A, D, E, and K, which are poorly absorbed in the

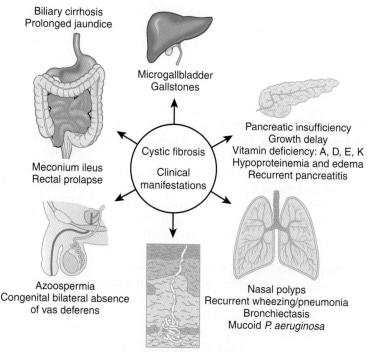

Biliary cirrhosis
Prolonged jaundice

Microgallbladder
Gallstones

Pancreatic insufficiency
Growth delay
Vitamin deficiency: A, D, E, K
Hypoproteinemia and edema
Recurrent pancreatitis

Cystic fibrosis

Clinical
manifestations

Meconium ileus
Rectal prolapse

Azoospermia
Congenital bilateral absence
of vas deferens

Nasal polyps
Recurrent wheezing/pneumonia
Bronchiectasis
Mucoid *P. aeruginosa*

Hyponatremic/Hypochloremic
Dehydration
Chronic metabolic alkalosis

Figure 14-7. Clinical manifestations of cystic fibrosis.

presence of severe steatorrhea. In patients with CF who are malnourished, connective tissue quality may be poor and support for the rectum may be inadequate; this, combined with abnormal stools, may lead to rectal prolapse. The association of rectal prolapse with CF is so strong that this finding alone is an indication for obtaining a sweat test. Another gastrointestinal manifestation of CF is idiopathic pancreatitis.

Nasal polyps occur frequently in patients with CF and may be present at a very early age. Occasionally, opacification of all the paranasal sinuses on radiography suggests the diagnosis of CF.

Men with CF are frequently infertile because of glandular obstruction of the vas deferens *in utero*, which causes involution of the wolffian duct, vas deferens, and associated structures. *CFTR* mutations also can cause infertility in otherwise normal men as a result of the CF variant, called congenital bilateral absence of the vas deferens. Similarly, obstruction of bile canaliculi frequently causes hepatic damage and, in some patients, overt cirrhosis.

In approximately 50% of CF patients, the diagnosis is first considered because of pulmonary symptoms. Although the lower respiratory tract is almost invariably involved, manifestations may not appear until months or years after birth. CF should be considered in every patient with recurrent pneumonia, refractory asthma, bronchiectasis, and empyema. Isolation of mucoid *Pseudomonas* from the lung should prompt diagnostic investigation for CF.

The diagnosis of CF also can be considered in the absence of clinical features. An individual with an affected sibling has a 1 in 4 chance of having the disease. First cousins of a CF patient have about a 1 in 120 chance of having the disease.

Lung Disease

Pulmonary involvement in CF accounts for much of the morbidity and almost all of the mortality from CF. Although the lungs are histologically normal at birth, patients soon acquire bacterial infections that are difficult to eradicate. In the first year of life, many types of bacteria, including enteric organisms, can be recovered from the lungs of an infant with CF, but later in childhood, two organisms predominate: *Staphylococcus aureus* and *Pseudomonas aeruginosa*. *Staphylococcus* colonization comes and goes; methicillin-resistant S. *aureus* is being seen increasingly at some CF centers. *Pseudomonas* eventually colonizes the lungs of most CF patients, reaching a prevalence of 80% by age 18 years. *P. aeruginosa* specifically adapts to the pulmonary microenvironment in patients with CF through the formation of macrocolonies (or biofilms) and the production of a capsular polysaccharide (an alginate product) that inhibits penetration by antimicrobial agents and confers the mucoid phenotype. Acquisition of the mucoid phenotype has been associated with accelerated decline of pulmonary function. Later in life, some patients acquire a *Burkholderia cepacia* infection, which is associated with poor lung function and poor prognosis.

Pulmonary inflammation is another major cause of the decline in respiratory function in patients with CF and may precede the onset of chronic infection. An exaggerated and sustained inflammatory response to bacterial and viral pathogens, characterized by neutrophil-dominated airway inflammation, is an accepted feature of lung disease in CF. Inflammation is present even in clinically stable patients with mild lung disease and in young infants diagnosed through newborn screening.

Elevated levels of interleukin-8, interleukin-6, tumor necrosis factor-α, and leukotriene B$_4$, along with reduced levels of anti-inflammatory cytokines and proteases, have been found in the airways of patients with CF. An elevated ratio of arachidonic acid to docosahexaenoic acid was found in mucosal scrapings from patients with CF compared with scrapings from normal individuals and from patients with inflammatory bowel disease; the altered ratio cannot be explained by a systemic inflammatory process alone. These and other inflammatory mediators, such as mannose-binding protein and α_1-antitrypsin, influence the progression of lung disease.

Symptomatic Treatment

Knowledge about the functional basis of CF has led to many new strategies for curative treatment, but at present, treatment for the most part remains symptomatic. Prevention of bacterial lung infection is considered a primary objective in CF treatment. Epidemiologic studies have suggested that transmission of *P. aeruginosa* and other pathogens occurs either by direct patient-to-patient contact or from various environmental reservoirs. Improved hygiene measures and segregation regimens have been implemented in several CF centers to limit cross-infection.

Improved antibiotic treatment regimens targeting CF-specific respiratory tract infections are regarded as the main reason for the increasing life expectancy of patients with CF that has been achieved over the last decades. Although most patients are initially colonized with S. *aureus*, the rate of S. *aureus* infection in patients with CF decreases with age, whereas the rate of *P. aeruginosa* increases, rendering this latter microorganism the major pathogen in this disease. After an initial transient colonization period with nonmucoid strains, untreated patients generally become chronically infected with mucoid strains of *P. aeruginosa*. Even with intensive antibiotic regimens, mucoid *P. aeruginosa* cannot be eradicated, probably because of poor penetration of antimicrobials into anaerobic sputum plugs and rapid development of mutant strains, which show enhanced resistance to antibiotics.

To minimize adverse effects and to achieve optimal airway concentrations of antibiotics, the inhalation route has been used for patients with CF. Long-term use of inhaled tobramycin has had positive effects in improving lung function and reducing exacerbations in patients who have moderate to severe lung disease with airways chronically infected with *P. aeruginosa*.

The results have been released of clinical trials using azithromycin to treat patients older than 6 years of age with CF who also were chronically infected with *P. aeruginosa*. The azithromycin group experienced benefit in pulmonary function, decreased pulmonary exacerbations, reduction in the use of oral antibiotics, decreased hospitalizations, and weight gain compared with the placebo group. The mechanism of action is unknown; however, the benefits of long-term azithromycin therapy in patients with CF are thought to be due primarily to a decreased inflammatory reaction associated with bacterial infections. Azithromycin should be considered for CF patients who are older than 6 years of age and who are chronically colonized with *P. aeruginosa*.

Currently, the strategy to combat pulmonary *P. aeruginosa* infection in patients with CF is early antibiotic treatment. In the early phase of *P. aeruginosa* colonization, antibiotics may prevent or delay the shift to chronic mucoid infection. The combination of inhaled tobramycin, colistin, or aztreonam with oral ciprofloxacin, or inhaled tobramycin or inhaled colistin alone has been used to treat early *P. aeruginosa* colonization.

Pulmonary exacerbations are common in patients with CF. Specific antibiotics are selected on the basis of a recent throat swab or sputum culture. Therapy with oral antibiotics is often used for mild exacerbations. Parenteral antibiotics are used in combination for the treatment of moderate to severe pulmonary exacerbations. Inhaled antibiotics are sometimes used in combination with parenteral antibiotics. Pulmonary exacerbations also have been associated with respiratory viral infections.

It is now widely acknowledged that an intense, neutrophil-dominated chronic airway inflammation plays a crucial role in the pathophysiologic sequence leading to parenchymal destruction and fibrosis. Theoretically, strategies for the treatment of CF-associated inflammation should include drugs that have direct effects on neutrophils and may block specifically proinflammatory mediators, or target neutrophil-specific activities. Although treatment with inhaled steroids theoretically should reduce inflammatory effects, results of a controlled study instead showed a beneficial effect, primarily in airway hyperreactivity, whereas clear improvement in pulmonary function and reducing exacerbations was not shown. Ibuprofen is the only other anti-inflammatory drug that has proven moderate benefit in

patients with mild lung disease as a prophylactic agent. The major disadvantage of ibuprofen relates to its narrow therapeutic window, which means that serum concentrations of the drug have to be carefully titrated in all patients. Low concentrations might increase neutrophil influx into the lung, and high concentrations are associated with an increased risk of gastrointestinal and renal toxicity.

Viscid airway secretions are characteristic of CF lung disease. Mucolytics such as N-acetyl cysteine have little effect on lung disease in patients with CF. By contrast, long-term use of dornase alfa has been reported to reduce sputum viscosity, modestly improves pulmonary function, and reduces the number of pulmonary exacerbations in patients with moderate to severe lung disease. Also, a short-term clinical trial using an inhaled 7% saline solution reported an improvement in lung function. Although hypertonic saline solution has the potential to cause bronchospasm in CF patients, this may be preventable by pretreating with a β_2-adrenergic inhaled bronchodilator.

Retained secretions play an important role in the pathophysiology of CF pulmonary disease. They physically obstruct the airways, aggravating infection and directly causing hyperinflation and ventilation/perfusion mismatching. They also contain high concentrations of inflammatory chemical mediators, which can cause bronchospasm and progressive parenchymal injury. Various airway clearance techniques are available. Conventional chest physiotherapy is the technique of chest percussion and postural drainage. Despite the absence of controlled studies, clinical experience supporting chest physiotherapy seems to be convincing. As patients become older and more independent, they frequently seek airway clearance methods that can be performed without assistance. Several alternative modalities have been developed, including active cycle breathing, positive expiratory pressure devices, high-frequency chest wall oscillator vest, the Flutter® valve, and intrapulmonary percussive devices.

Most patients with CF have bronchial hyperreactivity at least some of the time.

Bronchodilators have become a standard component of the therapeutic regimen. Short-acting β_2-adrenergic agents are the most commonly prescribed. They are often used to provide symptomatic relief and, before chest physiotherapy, to facilitate airways clearance. Long-acting aerosolized β_2-adrenergic agonists combined with inhaled steroids also may be helpful in patients with CF and asthma. Anticholinergic bronchodilators, such as ipratropium, may be beneficial for some patients with CF. Some patients apparently benefit from combination therapy of a β-adrenergic agonist and an anticholinergic agent.

Physical activity augments airway clearance by forcing deep breathing and, for many individuals, producing bronchodilation and facilitating cough and airway clearance. In addition, appropriate physical exercise enhances cardiovascular fitness, increases functional capacity, and improves quality of life. For these reasons, with the exception of patients whose clinical condition precludes it, all patients with CF should be encouraged to exercise. Aerobic activities, such as swimming, jogging, and cycling, are the most commonly recommended forms of exercise.

Curative Therapy

Insight into the cellular consequences of defective *CFTR* suggests a role for tailored therapies, a predominant theme in clinical research on CF. Robotic drug screening of more than 1 million random compounds has led to the discovery of compounds that correct the *ΔF508* abnormality by restoring the mutant protein to its normal position at the cell surface (partially restoring chloride channel function). The more recently elucidated crystal structure of nucleotide-binding domain 1 localizes the crucial phenylalanine 508 residue to a loop on the external surface of the domain. Because of this structure, drug screening laboratories can test the specificity of *ΔF508*-correcting compounds by cocrystallization with the *CFTR* protein. Curcumin, a nontoxic compound and the major constituent of the spice tumeric, has been shown to correct *ΔF508* processing in many *in vitro* model systems and prolong life in mice that are homozygous for the *ΔF508*

mutation. New compounds that correct this fundamental processing abnormality in *CFTR* should undergo clinical testing in the near future.

Many agents also have been shown to suppress premature stop codons in *CFTR* (class I) mutations, including the surprising finding that ribosomally active drugs, such as gentamicin, may be capable of correcting premature stop codons in human subjects. High-throughput screening programs specifically designed to identify drugs that activate residual *CFTR* activity (class III and IV mutations) also have been successful.

Luminal chloride secretion of airway epithelial cells occurs through *CFTR* and alternative chloride channels. An increased activity of the alternative epithelial chloride channel in the lower airways may compensate for reduced or absent *CFTR* function and potentially improve clinical status in CF patients. Two components are currently in clinical trials that have been shown to stimulate chloride secretion through this pathway: denufosol and peptide drug Moli1901.

Important advances have improved understanding of the role of the *CFTR* protein in the progression of suppurative pulmonary failure in CF. These discoveries are ushering in a new era of translational research that incorporates specific therapeutic targets and new cellular pathways. Progress in research on CF will continue to rely on an improved understanding of *CFTR* function and its relationship to mucociliary clearance, airway secretion, and other ion channels. Clinical advances directed at the correction of *CFTR* function predict an optimistic future for patients with CF and their families. Discussion about pancreatic, nutritional, and gastrointestinal system manifestations and their complications is beyond the scope of this chapter. The reader may wish to consult several more recent reviews to learn more about these other aspects of CF management.[19,20]

Miscellaneous Genetic Conditions

In addition to the many genetic conditions previously discussed, there are a few outliers that defy classification into specific categories of lung disease. Surfactant protein B (SP-B) deficiency has been recognized as a rare genetic cause of lung disease.[21] It is inherited as an autosomal recessive condition. It is encoded on a single gene (*SFTPB*) on chromosome 2. SP-B is primarily produced by alveolar type II epithelial cells. Pathology findings in lung tissue from SP-B-deficient infants include nonspecific interstitial fibrosis and alveolar type II epithelial cell hyperplasia. Characteristic electron microscopic findings include absence of lamellar bodies. Affected infants are typically full-term and generally present with symptoms and signs of surfactant deficiency, with chest radiographs resembling those of premature infants with respiratory distress syndrome. Although the lung disease in SP-B-deficient infants is often severe, affected infants may have initially mild symptoms not requiring mechanical ventilation. Their respiratory disease is progressive, however, and death usually results from hypoxic respiratory failure within 3 to 6 months, even with optimal medical management. Transient improvement may be seen in response to treatment with systemic steroid or exogenous surfactant; however, the only effective treatment is lung transplantation.

Surfactant protein C (SP-C) deficiency also is a rare autosomal recessive disorder associated with lung disease.[21] Clinical features in infants and adults with SP-C mutations have included chronic respiratory symptoms (tachypnea, cough, cyanosis in room air) and failure to thrive. The age of onset varies, with some infants developing respiratory distress immediately after birth, and other individuals remaining apparently asymptomatic well into adulthood. The lung disease in some children seems to be triggered or exacerbated by viral infections. The diagnosis should be considered in an infant with progressive forms of interstitial lung disease, particularly with biopsy findings interpreted as desquamative interstitial pneumonitis, chronic pneumonitis of infancy, or nonspecific interstitial pneumonitis. Electron microscopic findings also reveal absence of lamellar bodies. All SP-C mutations associated with human lung disease identified to date would result in the production of an abnormal protein that is likely to be misfolded.

ABCA3 deficiency is the most recently recognized inborn error of surfactant metabolism, but may eventually prove to be the most common genetic defect associated with surfactant production. The clinical phenotype is similar to that of SP-B deficiency, with death usually resulting from respiratory failure within 3 months of life. More research is needed to clarify the role of *ABCA3* in surfactant metabolism, its contribution to lung disease, and the potential roles of other ABC transporters in type II cell and surfactant metabolism.

Table 14-18 includes some supplemental conditions of clinical interest with specific pulmonary findings.

Summary

Myriad pulmonary complications have been identified in association with cytogenetic and mendelian disorders. Lung development in early embryonic life is a complex process that is closely tied to development of the gastrointestinal tract. Intrinsic or extrinsic factors that impair lung expansion within the fetal thorax may lead to significant pulmonary hypoplasia and subsequent respiratory distress at birth. The degree of pulmonary compromise often predicts long-term survival despite aggressive intervention at birth. Most pulmonary defects are isolated occurrences, but children born with lung anomalies should be evaluated for additional malformations and syndromic features. Identification of additional anomalies or the diagnosis of a specific syndrome may provide important long-term prognostic information, in addition to guidance for medical management. Making a syndromic diagnosis also may provide essential information to the parents and extended family about recurrence risks and may guide family planning decisions.

Multisystem disorders, which include lung findings, should alert the clinician to the possibility of a genetic condition or inborn error of metabolism. Gene mutations that affect ciliary function, impair collagen or other connective tissue synthesis, or result in vascular abnormalities also may affect pulmonary function. Thinking broadly about possible genetic conditions

Table 14-18	Genetic Conditions Associated with Miscellaneous Pulmonary Findings		
SYNDROME	**CLINICAL FEATURES**	**MODE OF INHERITANCE**	**GENE OR LOCUS IF KNOWN**
Tuberous sclerosis	Pulmonary lymphangiomatosis Cardiac rhabdomyoma Facial angiofibromas Hypopigmented "ash-leaf" spots Subependymal nodules and intracranial calcifications CNS giant cell astrocytomas Renal cysts Seizures Mental retardation	Autosomal dominant. New or de novo mutations in about 80% of patients with TSC1 and 60% of patients with TSC2	Gene = *TSC1* (9q34); *TSC2* (16p13.3); possible locus = 11q23; possible locus = 12q22-q24
Diffuse panbronchiolitis	Micronodular pulmonary lesions Chronic pulmonary disease Sinobronchial infections	Autosomal dominant susceptibility locus with shared haplotypes in affected East Asian patients	Locus = 6p21.3 (most telomeric portion of HLA-B locus)
Familial Mediterranean fever	Pleuritis Episodic fevers Pericarditis Hepatosplenomegaly Abdominal pain and peritonitis Nephrotic syndrome Renal amyloidosis	Autosomal dominant or autosomal recessive. Seen with increased frequency among Sephardic and Armenian Jews	Gene = *MEFV* (16p13)
Hereditary pancreatitis	Hemorrhagic pleural effusions Pancreatitis Recurrent fevers Portal or splenic vein thrombosis Diabetes	Autosomal dominant	Gene = *PRSS1* (7q35); *SPINK1* (5q32); *CFTR* (7q31.2) rare heterozygotes with pancreatitis, but the same gene seen with cystic fibrosis, which is identified in homozygotes
Familial dysautonomia (hereditary sensory and autonomic neuropathy type III or Riley-Day syndrome)	Breath-holding spells Recurrent aspiration Failure to thrive Alacrima Decreased lingual fungiform papillae Gastroesophageal reflux and cyclic vomiting Hypertension Autonomic dysfunction Episodic fevers Hypotonia Hyporeflexia Acrocyanosis Absent flare with intradermal injection of histamine	Autosomal recessive. Seen almost exclusively in Ashkenazi Jews	Gene = *IKBKAP* (9q31)

CNS, central nervous system.

that might be linked to pulmonary disease enables physicians to care for patients better. This approach to diagnosis helps clinicians identify essential subspecialists and prevents patients from embarking on a medical odyssey that children and adults with complex or puzzling symptoms frequently face.

As gene discoveries continue, and molecular technologies advance at lightning speed, it is likely that mutation analysis and gene sequencing will become more readily available to patients with suspected genetic syndromes. The cost of such testing at this time is often prohibitive and of limited clinical utility. It is reasonable, however, that with advances in gene therapy and the advent of personalized medicine, in the near future, identification of specific gene mutations will be closely tied to therapeutic strategies. This approach to pulmonary disease would surely improve the quality of life for many children and adults, leading to risk reduction for pulmonary complications and enhanced pulmonary function.

References

1. Sadler TW: The respiratory system. In Langman's Medical Embryology, 9th ed. Baltimore, Lippincott Williams & Wilkins, 2004, p 275.
2. Langer R, Kaufman HJ: Primary (isolated) bilateral pulmonary hypoplasia: A comparative study of radiologic findings and autopsy results. Pediatr Radiol 16:175-179, 1986.
3. Mardini MK, Nyhan WL: Agenesis of the lung: Report of four patients with unusual anomalies. Chest 87:522-527, 1985.
4. Bleyl S, et al: Familial total anomalous pulmonary venous return: A large Utah-Idaho family. Am J Med Genet 52:462-466, 1994.
5. Seller MJ, et al: Two sibs with anophthalmia and pulmonary hypoplasia (the Matthew-Wood syndrome). Am J Med Genet 62:227-229, 1996.
6. Thompson EM, et al: Multiple pterygium syndrome: Evolution of the phenotype. J Med Genet 24:733-749, 1987.
7. Leistikow EA, et al: Migrating atelectasis in Werdnig-Hoffman disease: Pulmonary manifestations in two cases of spinal muscular atrophy type 1. Pediatr Pulm 28:149-153, 1999.
8. Youssoufian H, et al: Association of a new chromosomal deletion [del (1)(q32q42)] with diaphragmatic hernia: Assignment of a human ferritin gene. Hum Genet 78:267-270, 1988.
9. Slavotinek A, et al: Fryns syndrome phenotype caused by chromosome microdeletions at 15q26.2 and 8p23.1. J Med Genet 42:730-736, 2005.
10. Sadler TW: Body cavities. In Langman's Medical Embryology, 9th ed. Baltimore, Lippincott Williams & Wilkins, 2004, p 211.
11. Pober BR, et al: Infants with Bochdalek diaphragmatic hernia: Sibling precurrence (sic) and monozygotic twin discordance in a hospital-based malformation surveillance program. Am J Med Genet 138A:81-88, 2005.
12. Bartsch O, et al: Evidence for a new contiguous gene syndrome, the chromosome 16p13.3 deletion syndrome alias-severe Rubinstein-Taybi syndrome. Hum Genet 120:179-186, 2006.
13. Gyves-Ray K, et al: Cystic lung disease in Down syndrome. Pediatr Radiol 24:137-138, 1994.
14. Kahn E, et al: Berry aneurysms, cirrhosis, pulmonary emphysema, and bilateral symmetrical cerebral calcifications: A new syndrome. Am J Med Genet Suppl 3:343-356, 1987.
15. Alter BP, Rosenberg PS, Brody LC: Clinical and molecular features associated with biallelic mutations in FANCD1/BRCA2. J Med Genet 44:1-9, 2007.
16. Campbell EJ: Alpha-1-antitrypsin deficiency: Incidence and detection program. Respir Med 94 Suppl C:18-21, 2000.
17. Li AM, et al: Non-CF bronchiectasis: Does knowing the aetiology lead to changes in management? Eur Respir J 26:8-14, 2005.
18. Noone PG, et al: Primary ciliary dyskinesia. Am J Respir Crit Care Med 169:459-467, 2004.
19. Turcios NL: Cystic fibrosis: An overview. J Clin Gastroenterol 39:307-317, 2005.
20. Rowe SM, Miller S, Sorcher EJ: Cystic fibrosis. N Engl J Med 352:1992-2001, 2005.
21. Nogee LM: Genetic mechanisms of surfactant deficiency. Biol Neonate 85:314-318, 2004.
22. Langston C: New concepts in the pathology of congenital lung malformations. Semin Pediatr Surg 12:17-37, 2003.

Web-Based Resources

Gene Clinics and Gene Reviews. Available at: http://www.geneclinics.org.
Online Mendelian Inheritance in Man (OMIM). Available at: http://www.ncbi.nlm.nih.gov.

Index

Page numbers followed by *f* indicates figures and followed by *t* indicates table.

A

Accessory inspiratory muscles, 185, 186*t*
ACE. *See* Angiotensin-converting enzyme
Acetylcholine, 185
Acquired immunodeficiency syndrome, 284
Acquired tracheobronchomalacia, 20
ACR. *See* American College of Rheumatology
ACS. *See* Acute chest syndrome
Activated partial thromboplastin time, 129
Acute chest syndrome (ACS), 147, 148–150
Acute idiopathic polyradiculitis, 190
Acute lung injury (ALI), 131
Acute lupus pneumonitis (ALP), 202, 203*t*, 204*t*, 205, 206, 207
Acute lymphoblastic leukemia (ALL), 64, 135, 136, 137
Acute myeloid leukemia (AML), 135, 136, 138–139
Acute pancreatitis, 114
Acute renal failure, 130–131, 130*t*
Acute respiratory distress syndrome (ARDS), 114–116, 125, 131, 276*f*
Acute respiratory failure, 157
Acute respiratory infections, 29–41
Adjunctive corticosteroids, 34
Adrenal disorders, 172
Aerosol therapy/technology, 142–143
Agonadism, 304*t*
Airway(s)
    clearance of, 196–197
    compression of, 91, 92, 92*t*
    hyperreactivity of, 180
    inflammatory, 219
    intraparenchymal, 92
    malacia, 91
    mucosa, 20
    mucosal edema, 131
    rare diseases of, 210*t*
    reactive, disease with, 150
    vascular compression of, causes of, 89*t*
    viscid, 334
ALI. *See* Acute lung injury
Alkalinization, 126
Alkylating agents, 66*t*, 67, 162
ALL. *See* Acute lymphoblastic leukemia
Alloantigens, 73
ALP. *See* Acute lupus pneumonitis
ALTEs. *See* Apparent life-threatening events
Alveolar damage, 206
Alveolar hemorrhage, 155, 202, 247
Alveolar hyperplasia, 260
Alveolar period, of lung development, 296, 296*t*

Alveolar ventilation, 122
Amebiasis, 276–280, 278*t*
American Academy of Pediatrics, 16
American College of Rheumatology (ACR), JRA classification, 217
American Thoracic Society, on asthma, 105
AML. *See* Acute myeloid leukemia
ANAs. *See* Anti-nuclear antibodies
ANCA. *See* Antineutrophil cytoplasmic antibody(ies)
Ancylostoma braziliense, 282
Ancylostoma caninum, 282
Ancylostoma duodenale, 281, 282
Anemia, 127–128
    chronic, 147
    normochromatic normocytic, 127
Aneurysm thrombosis, 252
Aneurysmal dilation, 253
Angioedema, 286
Angiomyolipomas, 260
Angiotensin-converting enzyme (ACE), 8
Ankylosing spondylitis, 226–228
Antenatal chorioamnionitis, 6
Antenatal corticosteroids, 13
Anterior horn cell disorders, 189–190
Antibiotic therapy, 72, 192
Antibodies
    antineutrophil cytoplasmic, 243*f*
    anti-nuclear, 211
    antiphospholipid, 208
Antibody underproduction, 52*t*
Anticardiolipin antibodies, 208
Anticholinergic bronchodilators, 334
Antileukemia treatment, 139
Antimetabolites, 162
Antimicrobial sensitivity, 202
Antineutrophil cytoplasmic antibody(ies) (ANCA), 243–244, 243*f*, 244*f*, 248–251
Anti-nuclear antibodies (ANAs), 211
Antiphospholipid antibodies, 208
α₁-Antitrypsin deficiency, 315–316
Aortic stenosis, 88
Apparent life-threatening events (ALTEs), 99, 105–106
Arteriovenous malformations (AVMs), 262, 263, 314–315, 315*t*
Arthralgias, 124, 245*t*
Arthritis
    enthesitis-related, 227, 227*t*
    juvenile rheumatoid, 217–220
    reactive, 286
    rheumatoid, 218
    seronegative, 57
Ascariasis, 280–281
Ascaris eggs, 280
Ascaris lumbricoides, 274, 280, 281, 281*f*
ASD. *See* Atrial septal defect
Aseptic inflammatory process, 219

Ash-leaf macule, 260*f*, 337*t*
Aspergillosis, 40, 61
Assisted coughing, 197
Asthma, 179–180, 251, 254
    cardiac, 84
    and GERD, 105
    and obesity, 179–180
Ataxia telangiectasia, 58*t*, 59, 317*t*
Atrial septal defect (ASD), 81, 83*t*
Autoimmune cell cytopenias, 57
Autoimmune disorders, 62
Autosomal recessive cutis laxa, 303*t*
AVMs. *See* Arteriovenous malformations
Azathioprine, 207, 208, 226, 249

B

Bacterial pneumonia, 30–32, 31*t*
Bacterial sepsis, 149
BAL. *See* Bronchoalveolar lavage
Barium esophagogram, 90, 90*f*
Barium swallow, 103–104, 103*t*, 104*f*
Basophils, 54
Baylisascaris procyonis, 285
Beclomethasone, 16
Behçet disease, 251–252
Benzimidazole drugs, 281
Bicarbonate-carbonic acid system, 122
Bilevel positive airway pressure (BiPAP), 187, 189, 195
Biopsy(ies)
    bronchoscopic transbronchial, 248
    lung, 42, 216*f*
    open lung, 75
    transbronchial, 38
    transthoracic needle aspiration, 75
    in Wegener granulomatosis, 248
BiPAP. *See* Bilevel positive airway pressure
Birt-Hogg-Dube syndrome, 321*t*
Blalock-Taussig shunt, 94
Blau syndrome, 228
Bleomycin toxicity, 158, 158*t*, 159–162
Bloom syndrome, 317*t*
Bombesin-like peptides, 7
BOOP. *See* Bronchiolitis obliterans with organizing pneumonia
Botulism, 191–192
BPD. *See* Bronchopulmonary dysplasia
Breathing disorders, 127
Bronchial circulation, 80
Bronchial malformations, 295
Bronchial stenosis, 20
Bronchial-associated lymphoid tissues, 53
Bronchiectasis, 43, 316–319, 317*t*, 319*t*
Bronchiolar disease, 110
Bronchiolitis obliterans, 41

Bronchiolitis obliterans syndrome, 72
Bronchiolitis obliterans with organizing pneumonia (BOOP), 73, 109, 210, 226
Bronchiolitis, obliterative, 71–73
Bronchitis, 51
    plastic, 96
    recurrent, 90
    suppurative, 109
Bronchoalveolar lavage (BAL), 33, 72, 74, 75, 140, 153, 206
Bronchobiliary fistulas, 310
Bronchodilator therapy, 13
Bronchogenic cysts, 308–309, 308f
Bronchopulmonary dysplasia (BPD), 1
    antenatal corticosteroids, 13
    bombesin-like peptides, 7
    bronchodilator therapy, 13
    caffeine, 17
    cardiopulmonary function, 10–11
    cardiovascular monitoring/ oxygenation, 21
    chest radiograph, 9
    classic, 2f
    clinical course, 9–10
    clinical features, 9
    coordination of care/discharge planning, 21–22
    corticosteroids, 13
    definitions of, 2–4
    development/vision/hearing, 21
    diagnostic criteria, 3t
    diuretics, 12–13
    epidemiology, 4
    fluid management, 12
    fluid restriction, 14
    genetic factors, 7–8
    glottic/subglottic damage, 20
    growth, 19
    high-frequency oscillatory ventilation, 11, 14
    hyperoxia/oxidant stress, 5–6
    infection, 6–7
    inflammation, 7
    inhaled corticosteroids, 13, 16
    inhaled nitric oxide, 16–17
    management of, 11–13
    mechanical ventilation/ volutrauma, 6
    minimal ventilation, 14
    monitoring, 21
    neurodevelopment, 18–19
    nutrition, 7
        and fluid management, 12
    outcome, 17–20
    pathogenesis, 4–8
    pathology, 8–11
    physical examination, 9
    prenatal events, 5
    prevention, 13–17
    pulmonary function, 18
    respiratory care, 11–12
    respiratory infections, 18
    schematic representation of, 10f
    superoxide dismutase, 17
    systemic corticosteroids, 13, 15–16

Bronchopulmonary dysplasia (BPD) (Continued)
    tracheal stenosis/bronchial stenosis/granuloma formation, 20
    vitamin A, 15
Bronchoscopic transbronchial biopsy, 248
Bronchoscopy, 150
    flexible, 75, 91
Bronchospasm, 104
Brugia species, 292
Bruton tyrosine kinase, 51
Burkholderia cepacia, 61, 333
Burkitt lymphoma, 136

C
Café au lait macules, 258, 258f, 259t
Caffeine, 17
Calcium channel blockers, 225t
Campylobacter jejuni, 190
Canadian Pediatric Society, 16
Canalicular period, of lung development, 296, 296t
Cancer therapy, pulmonary complications of, 64–67
Candida, 40, 70
Candida albicans, 50, 54
Capillary permeability changes, 115
Carbon monoxide diffusion capacity, 109, 160, 209
Cardiac catheterization, 96
Cardiac dysrhythmias, 179
Cardiac involvement, in DMD, 194
Cardiac rhythm disturbances, 178
Cardiac sphincter, 102
Cardiopulmonary function, in BPD, 10–11
Cardiovascular circulation, 79–80
Cardiovascular lesions with increased work of breathing, 80–96
Cardiovascular monitoring/ oxygenation, 21
Cavitations, 124
Cellular immunity deficiencies, 53–59
Cercariae, 287, 288f
Cerebral palsy, 15
Cestodes, 290–292
CFTR. See Cystic fibrosis transmembrane regulator and gene
Charcot-Leiden crystals, 96, 281
CHARGE syndrome, 312t
Chemotherapeutic agents, 66–67, 66t. See also specific agent, e.g. Cyclophosphamide and Cytotoxic drugs
Chemotherapy, 63
    high-dose, with radiotherapy, 156
    lung toxicity of, 158–162
Chest radiograph, 9
    of infant, 9f
Chest wall mobility, 194–195
Chest wall restriction, 227
Childhood vasculitis, 242t
Chlamydia pneumoniae, 148–149

Chloroquine-associated retinopathy, 231
Chronic granulomatous disease, 61
Chronic interstitial edema, 87
Chronic lung disease, in HIV infection, 41–43
Chronic lung disease of infancy (CLDI), 1–27
Chronic obstructive pulmonary disease, 73
Chronic pulmonary venous hypertension, 86f
Chronic renal failure, 124–126, 124t
Chronic sickle cell lung disease, 150–151
Churg-Strauss syndrome, 242t, 250–251, 251t
Circulation
    bronchial, 80
    cardiovascular, 79–80
    lymphatic, 80
    mature pulmonary, 80
    pulmonary, 79–80
Cisplatin-doxorubicin regimen, with methotrexate, 142
Classic bronchopulmonary dysplasia, 2f
CLDI. See Chronic lung disease of infancy
Clostridium botulinum, 191
CMV. See Cytomegalovirus
Coarctation of aorta, 88–89
Cogan syndrome, 242t
Complement system/deficiencies, 61–62
Computed tomography (CT), 72, 146
Congenital anomalies, 100–102, 295–316
Congenital diaphragmatic hernia, 101, 300–305, 302t–305t
Congenital lobar emphysema, 310–311
Congenital lymphedema, 256
Congenital myotonic dystrophy, 193
Congestive heart failure, 84
COP. See Cryptogenic organizing pneumonia
Corticosteroids, 13, 39, 42, 231
    adjunctive, 34
    antenatal, 13
    in bronchopulmonary dysplasia, 13
    inhaled, 16
    in SLE, 208
    systemic, 15–16
Crohn disease, 108, 109
Cryoprecipitate, 157
Cryptococcus, 74
Cryptogenic organizing pneumonia (COP), 73, 155, 156
CT. See Computed tomography
Curative therapy, in genetic disorders, 335
Cushing syndrome, 172
Cutis laxa, 264
Cyanotic spells, 186
Cyclic neutropenia, 62
Cyclophosphamide, 162, 206, 207, 208, 213, 224, 233

Cyclophosphamide therapy, 223, 249
Cyclosporine, 71
Cylindrical bronchiectasis, 319
Cyst(s)
  bronchogenic, 308–309, 308f
  foregut, 308
  gastroenteric, 309
  parenchymal, 265
  pulmonary, 309t
  small, 308
Cystic adenomatoid malformations, 306–308
Cystic fibrosis, 112f, 171, 174, 174f, 316, 329–335
  clinical manifestations of, 331–332, 332f
  screening/diagnosis, 330–331
Cystic fibrosis transmembrane regulator and gene (CFTR), 317t, 329
  mutations of, 317t, 330, 330f, 332
Cystic kidneys, bilateral, 2
Cytomegalovirus (CMV), 31t, 35, 36, 54, 60t, 70
Cytotoxic drugs, 159–162

D

DAH. See Diffuse alveolar hemorrhage
Damage
  alveolar, 206
  drug-induced pulmonary, 158
  glottic/subglottic, 20
Defect(s)
  atrial septal, 81
  lung segmentation, 305–306, 306t
  T cell, 55t
  ventricular septal, 81
Deficiency(ies)
  antitrypsin, 315–316
  in cellular immunity, 53–59
  complement, 61–62
  dehydrogenase, 325t
  GM-CSF, 140–141, 142
  phagocyte number, 59–62
  vitamin, 12
Dehydrogenase deficiency, 325t
Denys-Drash syndrome, 304t
Dermatologic disease(s), with pulmonary manifestations, 256–273
  cutis laxa, 264
  dyskeratosis congenita, 271–272
  Ehlers-Danlos syndrome, 256, 264–265, 321t
  erythema multiforme, 267–269
  hereditary hemorrhagic telangiectasia, 256, 261–263, 263t
  Hermansky-Pudlak syndrome, 267, 328t
  Klippel-Trenaunay-Weber syndrome, 263–264
  mastocytosis, 269–271

Dermatologic disease(s), with pulmonary manifestations (Continued)
  neurofibromatosis type 1, 258–259
  pseudoxanthoma elasticum, 265–266
  tuberous sclerosis complex, 259–261, 260f
  xanthoma disseminatum/ Erdheim-Chester disease, 266
  yellow nail syndrome, 256–258
Desmopressin, 267
Development/vision/hearing, 21
Dexamethasone, 15, 16
Diabetes, 170–172
Diabetic ketoacidosis, 171
Dialysis-related hypoxemia, 121, 129–130, 130f
Diaphragmatic excursion, 65
Diffuse alveolar hemorrhage (DAH), 155
Diffuse panbronchiolitis, 337t
Diffusing capacity for carbon monoxide (DLCO), 109, 160, 209
DiGeorge syndrome, 57, 177
Dilated bronchial anastomotic vessels, 86
Dilated intercostals, 88
Dirofilaria immitis, 292
Disease(s). See also Endocrine/ metabolic disease(s); Neuromuscular disease(s); Parasite(s)/parasitic disease(s)
  affecting lung and kidney, 123–124, 123t
  Behçet, 251–252
  bronchiolar, 110
  chronic lung, 1–27, 41–43
  Crohn, 108, 109
  dermatologic, pulmonary manifestations of, 256–272
  Erdheim-Chester, 266
  gastroesophageal reflux, 99–106
  gastrointestinal, 98–117
  Gaucher, 301t, 322t
  graft-versus-host, 50, 155
  hematologic/oncologic, 135–163
  Hodgkin, 64, 135–137, 284
  idiopathic/sporadic pulmonary veno-occlusive, 87f
  immunosuppressive, 49–76
  inflammatory, 62
  inflammatory airway, 219
  inflammatory bowel, 57, 98, 108–111
  interstitial lung, 202
  Kawasaki, 241, 242t, 243
  kidney, 327
  Krabbe, 323t
  Kugelberg-Welander, 189
  mixed connective tissue, 212–215, 214t
  neonatal Graves, 176
  oncologic, 135–147, 154–163
  parenchymal, 109, 230
  pleural, 109
  primary immunodeficiency, 51
  pulmonary, 248

Disease(s) (Continued)
  rare airway, 210t
  reactive airway, 150
  renal, 121–132
  rheumatoid, 201–240
  sickle cell, 147–152
  sight-threatening ocular, 231
  Werdnig-Hoffman, 189
  Wolman, 324t
  xanthoma disseminatum, 266
Disorders. See also Genetic disorder(s), with pulmonary manifestations
  adrenal, 172
  anterior horn cell, 189–190
  autoimmune, 62
  breathing, 127
  growth hormone, 172
  hematologic, 147–154
  histiocytic, 152–154
  of muscles, 192–193
  of neuromuscular junctions, 191–192
  oncologic, 154–163
  of peripheral nerves, 190
  post-transplant lymphoproliferative, 67
  of reproductive system, 177
  sleep, 175, 193
Diuretics, 12–13
DLCO. See Diffusing capacity for carbon monoxide
DMD. See Duchenne muscular dystrophy
Donnai-Barrow syndrome, 304t
Doppler ultrasonography, 138
Dornase alfa, 334
Down syndrome, 309t
Drug(s)
  benzimidazole, 281
  cytotoxic, 140
  lung disease from, 159
  lupus from, 202, 211–212, 211t
  myelosuppressive, 73
  nonsteroidal anti-inflammatory, 202, 268
  for parasitic lung infections, 278t–279t
  for pediatric cancer treatment, toxicity of, 158t
  pulmonary damage from, 158
D-transposition of great arteries, 94
Duchenne muscular dystrophy (DMD), 184, 192–194
Dynein, 316
Dyskeratosis congenita, 271–272
Dystrophy
  congenital myotonic, 193
  Duchenne muscular, 184, 192–194

E

Early-onset pathologic pulmonary changes, 160f
Early-onset sarcoidosis, 232
EBV. See Epstein-Barr virus
Echinococcosis, 279t, 290–292
Echinococcus, 291

Echinococcus granulosus, 279t, 291, 292
Echinococcus multilocularis, 279t, 290, 292
Echocardiography, 113
Edema
 airway mucosal, 130
 angio, 286
 chronic interstitial, 87
 pulmonary, 81–83, 84, 125, 155
EDS. *See* Ehlers-Danlos syndrome
Ehlers-Danlos syndrome (EDS), 264–265, 321t
Eisenmenger syndrome, 85
Elastolysis, generalized, 264
ELBW. *See* Extremely-low-birth-weight infants
Electrophysiologic studies, 191
ELISA. *See* Enzyme-linked immunosorbent assay
ELISPOT. *See* Enzyme-linked immunospot assay
Emanuel syndrome, 305t
Emphysema
 congenital lobar, 310–311
 pulmonary, 264
Empyema, 257
Endocrine/metabolic disease(s), 170–181
 adrenal disorders, 172
 diabetes, 170–171
 growth hormone disorders, 172
 hyperthyroidism, 175–176
 hypothyroidism, 174–175, 181
 obesity-hypoventilation syndrome, 177–181
 pseudohypoaldosteronism, 172–174
 reproductive system, 177
End-of-life care, 199
Endoscopic retrograde cholangiopancreatography (ERCP), 116
Endothelins, 111–112
Entamoeba histolytica, 276, 278t, 279–280
Enthesitis-related arthritis, 227t
Enzyme-linked immunosorbent assay (ELISA), 287
Enzyme-linked immunospot assay (ELISPOT), 33
Eosinophilia, 251
Eosinophilic microabscesses, 251
Epidermolysis bullosa, 303t
Epigastric discomfort, 105
Epithelial Na+ channel mutations, 173–174
Epoprostenol, 215
Epstein-Barr virus (EBV), 59
ERCP. *See* Endoscopic retrograde cholangiopancreatography
Erdheim-Chester disease, 266
Erythema multiforme, 267–269
Erythema nodosum, 253
Erythrocyte sedimentation rate, 231
Escherichia coli, 62
ESFT. *See* Ewing sarcoma family of tumors
Esophageal atresia, 311
Esophageal dysmotility, 211t

Esophageal peristalsis, 99
Ethambutol, 34, 35
Ewing sarcoma, 64
Ewing sarcoma family of tumors (ESFT), 143–144
Exercise fitness, 181
Extracardiac shunts, 81
Extracorporeal membrane oxygenation, 301
Extralobar sequestration, 309
Extremely-low-birth-weight (ELBW) infants, 3
Extubation/decannulation, 197–198

F

Fabry disease, 322t
Failure
 acute renal, 130–131
 acute respiratory, 157
 chronic renal, 124–126
 congestive heart, 84
 respiratory muscle, 186t
Falciparum malaria, 274–275
Familial cirrhosis, 326t
Familial dysautonomia, 101f, 337t
Familial Mediterranean fever, 337t
Familial pulmonary capillary hemangiomatosis, 326t
Farber disease, 323t
Feingold syndrome, 313t
Fetal lung growth, kidney and, 121
Fibrinous pleuritis, 125
Fibroblast proliferation, 222
Fibrosarcoma, 147
Fibrosis
 cystic. *See* Cystic fibrosis
 extensive interstitial, 222
 pulmonary, 159, 161, 326t, 327, 328t
Flexible bronchoscopy, 75, 91
Flow-volume loops, 136
Focal dermal hypoplasia, 303t
Forced vital capacity (FVC), 186–187
Foregut cysts, 308
Fryns syndrome, 301, 302t
Full overnight polysomnography, 187
Functional asplenia, 151
Fungal infections, 40–41
FVC. *See* Forced vital capacity

G

Gangliosidosis, GM$_1$, 323t
Gastroenteric cysts, 309
Gastroesophageal reflux (GER), 98
Gastroesophageal reflux disease (GERD), 99–106
Gastroesophageal reflux-associated pulmonary involvement, 100f
Gastroesophageal sphincter, 102
Gastrointestinal bleeding, 262
Gastrointestinal disease, 98–117, 285
Gaucher disease, 301t, 322t
Gemcitabine, 162
Gene therapy, 59

Genetic disorder(s), with pulmonary manifestations, 295–338
 bronchiectasis, 43, 316–319, 317t, 319t
 congenital anomalies, 100–102, 295–316
 curative therapy, 335
 cystic fibrosis, 112f, 171, 174, 174f, 316, 329–335
 inborn errors of metabolism, 320–322, 322t
 miscellaneous genetic conditions, 335–336
 pulmonary arterial hypertension, 209t, 322–326
 spontaneous pneumothorax, 320, 321t
 symptomatic treatment, 333–335
GER. *See* Gastroesophageal reflux
GERD. *See* Gastroesophageal reflux disease
Glossopharyngeal breathing, 198
Glottic/subglottic damage, 20
Glucocorticoids, 220
Glucose tolerance, 171
Glutathione-S-transferase (GST), 5
Glycogen storage disease, 324t
Glycosylation, 171
 disorder of, 322t
GM-CSF deficiency, 140–141
Goodpasture syndrome, 124, 207, 243
Graft-versus-host disease (GVHD), 50, 155
Granuloma, 250
 in CLDI, 20
 noncaseating, 229
Graves disease, neonatal, 176
Growth hormone disorders, 172
GST. *See* Glutathione-S-transferase
Guillain-Barré syndrome, 190
GVHD. *See* Graft-versus-host disease

H

HAART. *See* Highly active antiretroviral therapy
Haemophilus influenzae, 31t, 50, 53, 149, 151
 type b, 30, 31
Hamman-Rich disease, 328t
Heart transplantation, 70
Heiner syndrome, 98, 106–108
Hematologic disorders, 147–154
Hematologic/oncologic diseases, 135–163
Hematopoietic stem cell transplantation, 154–156
Hemodialysis-related hypoxemia, 129–130
Hemoptysis, 205, 262, 269
Hemorrhage
 alveolar, 155, 202, 247
 diffuse alveolar, 155
 pulmonary, 245, 246
Hemosiderosis, 106, 107, 108f
Henderson-Hasselbalch equation, 122

Henoch-Schönlein purpura, 245, 246–247
Hepatoblastoma, 146
Hepatopulmonary syndrome, 111–114
Hereditary hemorrhagic telangiectasia (HHT), 256, 261–263, 263*t*
Hereditary pancreatitis, 337*t*
Hermansky-Pudlak syndrome (HPS), 267, 328*t*
Herpesvirus, 36
Heterotaxy, 305–306, 319
HFOV. *See* High-frequency oscillatory ventilation
HHT. *See* Hereditary hemorrhagic telangiectasia
High-dose chemotherapy/radiotherapy, 156
High-frequency oscillatory ventilation (HFOV), 11, 14
Highly active antiretroviral therapy (HAART), 28–30, 30*t*, 34–36, 40
High-potency topical steroids, 270
Histamine H_1/H_2 blockers, 270
Histamine release, 269
Histiocytic disorders of lung, 152–154
Histoplasma, 74
HIV. *See* Human immunodeficiency virus
Hodgkin disease, 64, 135–137, 284
Home oxygen therapy, 19
Homocystinuria, 325*t*
Hookworm, 281–282
HPS. *See* Hermansky-Pudlak syndrome
HPV. *See* Human papillomavirus
Human immunodeficiency virus (HIV), 28–48, 208
Human lung development, 296*t*
Human papillomavirus (HPV), 36
Hurler-Scheie syndrome, 322*t*
Hyaline membranes, 206
Hydrocortisone therapy, 15
Hydronephrosis, 297
Hydroxychloroquine, 226
Hydroxyurea, 151
Hypercalciuria, 229, 232
Hypereosinophilia, 270
Hyperglycemia, 15
Hyper-IgE syndrome, 60*t*, 61
Hyperinfection, 284
Hyperinsulinemia, 172
Hyperkalemia, 173
Hyperleukocytosis, 65, 139
Hyperoxia/oxidant stress, 5–6
Hyperreactivity of airways, 180
Hypersensitivity, immediate, 286
Hypertension, 15
    chronic pulmonary venous, 86*f*
    idiopathic pulmonary arterial, 95–96
    portal, 111
    portopulmonary, 111
    primary pulmonary, 322, 326, 326*t*
    pulmonary, 10, 151–152, 263, 320
    pulmonary arterial, 209*t*, 225*t*, 322–326
Hyperthyroidism, 175–176

Hypertrophy, medial smooth muscle, 215
Hypoalbuminemia, 125
Hypocalcemia, 177
Hypocapnia, 122
Hypocarbia, 6
Hypoparathyroidism, 177, 181
Hypoplasia
    focal dermal, 303*t*
    primary pulmonary, 297*t*
    pulmonary, 94, 296–300, 300*t*
    secondary pulmonary, 298*t*–299*t*
Hypopnea, 179
Hypothyroidism, 174–175, 181
Hypoventilation, 174
Hypoxemia, 37, 79, 94, 112, 113, 129–130, 130*f*, 139
Hypoxia, 175
Hypoxic vasoconstriction, 80

I

IBD. *See* Inflammatory bowel disease
Idiopathic pneumonitis syndrome, 155
Idiopathic pulmonary arterial hypertension, 95–96
Idiopathic pulmonary fibrosis, 326*t*
Idiopathic pulmonary-renal syndrome, 253
Idiopathic/sporadic pulmonary veno-occlusive disease, 87*f*
ILD. *See* Interstitial lung disease
Immune inflammatory response, 229
Immune reconstitution inflammatory syndrome (IRIS), 41, 42–43
Immunodeficiency syndromes, 58*t*, 60*t*
Immunoglobulin deficiencies, 50–53, 317*t*
Immunoglobulin production, 50–53
Immunomodulatory therapy, 215
Immunosuppressive agents, 68*t*, 211
Immunosuppressive diseases, 49–76
Inborn errors of metabolism, 320–322, 322*t*
Increased pulmonary venous pressure, 83–87, 83*t*, 85*t*
Increased venous admixture, 92–94
Indirect immunofluorescence, 244*f*
Induced lung disease, 159
Infant botulism, 191
Infection(s)
    acute respiratory, 29–41
    BPD, 6–7, 18
    chronic pulmonary, 42
    hyper, 284
    mycobacterial, 32–35
    nosocomial, 6
    opportunistic respiratory, 32*f*
    parasitic lung, 277*t*
    pneumocystis, 37–40
    pulmonary, 66
    respiratory, 18
    s. aureus, 32*f*
    urinary tract, 131
    viral, 35–37

Inflammation, 5, 7
    BPD, 7
    monophasic, 206
    pulmonary, 333
    vascular, 241
Inflammatory airway disease, 219
Inflammatory bowel disease (IBD), 57, 98, 108–111
Inflammatory disease, 62
Inflammatory microenvironment, 180
Inflammatory pseudotumor, 147
Influenza, 36
Inhaled bronchodilators, 42
Inhaled corticosteroids, 16
Inhaled nitric oxide, 16–17
Injury(ies)
    acute lung, 131
    kidneys, mechanical ventilation-induced, 131–132
    laryngeal, 20
    progressive parenchymal, 334
    transfusion-related acute lung, 156–157
Inspiratory muscle aids, 195–196
Intercostal muscle paralysis, 188
Interleukin-12, 142
Internal hemangiomas, 315
Interstitial lung disease (ILD), 202
Interstitial pneumonitis, 42
Intra-abdominal pressure, 131
Intrahepatic bile stasis, 331
Intraluminal impedance testing, 103*t*
Intraparenchymal airways, 92
Intrapulmonary bleeding, 107
Intravenous immunoglobulin (IVIG), 32
Intravenous methylprednisolone, 206
Intrinsic nitric oxide synthesis pathway, 111–112
Iontophoresis, 331
IRIS. *See* Immune reconstitution inflammatory syndrome
IVIG. *See* Intravenous immunoglobulin

J

JDMS. *See* Juvenile dermatomyositis
Jeune syndrome, 299*t*
JLS. *See* Juvenile localized scleroderma
Job syndrome, 61
Juvenile dermatomyositis (JDMS), 225–226
    characteristics of, 226*t*
Juvenile localized scleroderma (JLS), 220, 221, 221*t*
Juvenile myasthenia gravis, 191
Juvenile rheumatoid arthritis, 217–220
Juvenile systemic sclerosis, 220, 221, 222*t*

K

Kaposi sarcoma, 136
Kartagener syndrome, 316–319, 319*t*
Kasukawa criteria, 212
Kawasaki disease, 241, 242*t*, 243
Keratosis obturans, 257
Kidney. *See* Renal
Kidney disease, 327
Kidney injury, mechanical
    ventilation–induced, 131–132
Klebsiella aerobacter, 211
Klebsiella pneumoniae, 30, 31*t*
Klippel-Trenaunay-Weber
    syndrome, 263–264
Kommerell diverticulum, 89
Kostmann syndrome, 61
Krabbe disease, 323*t*
Kugelberg-Welander disease, 189

L

Lactate dehydrogenase (LDH), 37
Langerhans cell histiocytosis (LCH),
    152–154, 153*t*
Large left-to-right shunts, 81–87, 82*f*
    treatment of, 85
Laryngeal injury, with intubation, 20
Laryngeal nerves, 101
Laryngomalacia, 101
LCH. *See* Langerhans cell
    histiocytosis
LDH. *See* Lactate dehydrogenase
Left ligamentum arteriosum,
    89, 90
Left ventricular outflow obstruction,
    87–88
Lesions
    cardiovascular with increased
        work of breathing, 80–96
    noncalcified, 142
    plexiform lung, 83*f*
    renal, 261
    small cyst, 308
    vascular, 209
Leukocytosis, 217, 276
Leukostasis, 138
Liddle syndrome, 172
Lifelong prophylaxis, 40
LIP. *See* Lymphocytic interstitial
    pneumonia
Liver transplantation, 70–71
Löffler pneumonitis, 281
Löffler syndrome, 281
Lung(s). *See also* Pulmonary
    biopsy, 41, 75, 216*f*
    disease. *See* Lung disease
    and kidneys, physiologic
        connections between,
        121–123
    morphogenesis, 295
    segmentation defects of, 306*t*
    toxicity, 158–162, 158*t*
    transplantation, 63, 71–72
Lung disease, 332–333
    chronic, 41–43
    chronic sickle cell, 150–151
    genetic disorders, 332–333
    of infancy, 1–27
    interstitial, 202

Lung metastases, 144
Lupus
    drug-induced, 202, 211–212
    systemic. *See* Systemic lupus
        erythematosus
Lymphatic circulation, 80
Lymphedema, 326*t*
    congenital, 256
    primary, 257
Lymphoblastic lymphoma, 137*f*
Lymphocytes, 115
Lymphocytic interstitial pneumonia
    (LIP), 41–42, 42*f*, 216
Lymphoid interstitial pneumonitis,
    216*t*, 219
Lymphoma, 135, 284
    Burkitt, 136
    lymphoblastic, 137*f*, 138*f*
Lysinuric protein intolerance, 325*t*
Lysosomal trafficking protein, 267

M

M. bovis, 34
Macroaggregated albumin (MAA),
    113
Macrolide antibiotics, 72
Magnetic resonance
    cholangiopancreatography,
    116
Magnetic resonance imaging
    (MRI), 90
Malacia of airways, 91
Malaria, 274–276
Malignancies, 65*t*. *See also* Oncologic
    diseases
Malnutrition, and PCP, 38
Mannose-binding lectin (MBL), 61
Marden-Walker syndrome, 301*t*
Marfan syndrome, 321*t*
Mastocytosis, 269–271
Mature pulmonary circulation, 80
Maximum insufflation capacity
    (MIC), 187
Maximum voluntary ventilation,
    179
MBL. *See* Mannose-binding lectin
McKusick-Kaufman syndrome, 313*t*
Meacham syndrome, 302*t*
Measles, mumps, rubella vaccine
    (MMR), 36
Mebendazole, 282
Mechanical insufflation-
    exsufflation, 197
Mechanical ventilation and
    volutrauma, 6
Meckel syndrome, 298
Medial smooth muscle hypertrophy,
    215
Mediastinal adenopathy, 223
Mediastinal lymphadenopathy, 218
Medroxyprogesterone, 261
Meigs syndrome, 177
Mesalamine, 109
Metabolic acidosis, 122
Metabolism, inborn errors of, 320–322,
    322*t*–325*t*. *See also* Endocrine/
    metabolic disease(s)
Metacercariae, 287

Metastatic nodules, 142
Methotrexate, 162, 208
    cisplatin-doxorubicin regimen
        with, 142
    pneumonitis, 232–233
Methylprednisolone, 111, 206
MIC. *See* Maximum insufflation
    capacity
Micro-Ouchterlony technique,
    107
Microphthalmia syndrome, 303*t*
Microscopic polyangiitis, 242*f*, 243,
    249–250
Miliary tuberculosis, 32, 33*f*
Milk scan, 103*t*
Minimal ventilation, 14
Mixed connective tissue disease
    (MTCD), 212–215
    pulmonary manifestations of,
        214*t*
MMR. *See* Measles, mumps, rubella
    vaccine
Model End-Stage Liver Disease
    score, 111
Monocyte chemoattractant
    protein–1, 222
Mononeuritis multiplex, 251
Monophasic inflammation,
    206
Mounier-Kuhn syndrome, 265
MPO. *See* Myeloperoxidase
MRI. *See* Magnetic resonance
    imaging
MTCD. *See* Mixed connective tissue
    disease
MTP-PE. *See* Muramyl tripeptide
    phosphatidylethanolamine
Mucopolysaccharidosis, 322*t*
Mucosal barrier, 155
Mulberry tumors, 259
Multinucleated giant cells, 249*f*
Multiorgan dysfunction, 115
Muramyl tripeptide
    phosphatidylethanolamine
    (MTP-PE), 142
Muscles
    accessory inspiratory, 185
    hypertrophy, 70
    inspiratory, 195–196
    intercostal, 188
    respiratory, 185
        aids, 194
        dysfunction, 189*t*
        failure, 186*t*
        fatigue, 187–194
        function, 185–187
Muscular disease, 188
Mutations
    CFTR gene, 115
    epithelial Na^+ channel,
        173–174
Myasthenia gravis, 191
Mycobacterial infection,
    32–35
Mycoplasma pneumoniae, 148,
    190, 268
Myeloperoxidase (MPO), 244
Myelosuppressive drugs, 73
Myotonic dystrophy, 193
    neonatal, 193

N

N-acetyl cysteine, 150, 334
NADPH. *See* Nicotinamide adenine dinucleotide phosphate
Nasal polyps, 332
Nasopharyngeal washes, 74–75
Nasopharynx, 246
National Institutes of Health
　on asthma, 105
　and rituximab, 226
Natural killer (NK) cells, 53, 54, 55t–56t, 57
Necator americanus, 281
Neisseria meningitidis, 53
Nemaline myopathy, 101*f*
Nematodes, 280–287
　hookworm, 281–282
　N. americanus, 281
　strongyloidiasis, 282–285
　toxocariasis, 285–287
Neonatal Graves disease, 176
Neonatal hyperthyroidism, 176*f*
Neonatal intensive care units (NICUs), 4
Nephrocalcinosis, 12
Nephrotoxicity, 67
Neuroblastoma, 64, 145–146
Neurodevelopment in BPD, 3, 18–19
Neurofibromatosis type 1, 258–259
Neuromuscular disease(s), 184–200
　cardiac involvement, 194
　disorders of muscles, 192–193
　disorders of neuromuscular junction, 191–192
　disorders of peripheral nerves, 190
　end-of-life care, 199
　extubation/decannulation, 197–198
　management, 194–198
　muscular disease, 188
　outcomes, 198–199
　physiology, 184–185
　respiratory muscle fatigue, 187–194
　respiratory muscle function assessment, 185–187
　sleep evaluation in, 193–194
Neuropsychiatric disability, 258
Neutrophilia, 287
Neutrophils, 59
　influx, 334
　recruitment, 53
NHL. *See* Non-Hodgkin lymphoma
Nicotinamide adenine dinucleotide phosphate (NADPH), 61
NICUs. *See* Neonatal intensive care units
NK cells. *See* Natural killer cells
NK-T cells, 53–54, 57
Nocturnal noninvasive ventilation (NIV), 187
Noncalcified lesions, 142
Noncaseating granuloma, 229
Non-Hodgkin lymphoma (NHL), 64, 135–137, 138*f*
Noninfectious pulmonary complications, 79, 202, 203*t*
Non-invasive intermittent positive-pressure ventilation (NPPV), 194, 195*f*, 198

Nonirradiated blood products, 57
Non–Langerhans cell histiocytosis, 266
Nonlethal skeletal dysplasia, 299*t*
Nonsteroidal anti-inflammatory drugs, 202, 268
Nonsteroidal immunosuppressants, 266
Normal alveolar ventilation, 195–196
Normal cough, 197
Normochromatic normocytic anemia, 127
Nosocomial infection, 6
NPPV. *See* Non-invasive intermittent positive-pressure ventilation
Nutrition, 7
　BPD, 7

O

Obesity, and asthma, 179–180
Obesity-hypoventilation syndrome, 177–181
Obliterative bronchiolitis, 71–73
Ocular larva migrans, 285, 286
Oligohydramnios, 297
Omphalocele, 304*t*
Oncologic diseases, 135–147
　complications related to, 135–141, 154–163
Oophorectomy, 261
Open lung biopsy, 75
Opitz-Frias syndrome, 312*t*–313*t*
Opportunistic respiratory infections, 32*f*
Oropharyngeal discoordination, 100
Oropharynx, 246
Orthopnea, 136
Osler-Weber-Rendu syndrome, 261, 315*t*
Osteohypertrophy, 263
Osteopenia, 12
Osteosarcoma, 141–143
Oxidant stress, 201
Oxidative stress, 12
Oxygen steal, 139
Oxygenation, 150
Oxyhemoglobin desaturation, 196

P

PAH. *See* Pseudohypoaldosteronism; Pulmonary arterial hypertension; Pulmonary arterial pressure
Palivizumab prophylaxis, 36
Pallister-Killian syndrome, 305*t*
Pancreatitis, 114–117
　acute, 114
　clinical management, 116–117
　diagnostic approach, 116
　etiology, 114
　hereditary, 337*t*
　pathophysiology, 115–116
　pulmonary manifestations, 114–115
Paradoxical breathing, 186

Paragonimiasis, 287–290
Paragonimus, 287, 288*f*
Paragonimus westermani, 279*t*, 287–290, 288*f*, 290*f*
Parasite(s)/parasitic disease(s), 274–294
　cestodes, 290–292
　nematodes, 280–287
　protozoa, 274–280
　trematodes, 287–290
Parasitic lung infections, drugs for, 277*t*
Parenchymal cysts, 265
Parenchymal disease, 109, 230
Parry-Romberg syndrome, 220, 221*t*
Patchy pneumonia, 107
Patent ductus arteriosus (PDA), 81, 83*t*
PCD. *See* Primary ciliary dyskinesia
PCP. *See* *Pneumocystis* pneumonia
PDA. *See* Patent ductus arteriosus
Peak inspiratory pressure, 196
Pena-Shoeir syndrome, 300*t*
Pentamidine, 38
Percutaneous balloon angioplasty, 89
Peripheral eosinophilia, 286
Peritoneal dialysis, 125
Perlman syndrome, 304*t*
PET. *See* Positron emission tomography
PFTs. *See* Pulmonary function tests
Phagocyte number deficiencies, 59–62
Phosphodiesterase type 5 inhibitor, 225*t*
Pirfenidone, 267
Plasmodium species, 276*f*
Plastic bronchitis, 96
Pleural disease, 109
Pleural effusion, 84*f*
Pleural thickening, 160
Pleuritic chest pain, 128
Pleuroperitoneal shunting, 257
Pleuropulmonary blastoma (PPB), 146–147
Pleuropulmonary manifestations, 218
Plexiform lesion, 83*f*
Plexiform neurofibromas, 258
Pneumococcal conjugate vaccine, 35
Pneumococcal pneumonia, 224
Pneumococcal sepsis, 306
Pneumocystis infection, 37–40
　with other pathogens, 44
Pneumocystis jiroveci, 37, 42, 50, 54, 57, 59, 70, 211
Pneumocystis pneumonia (PCP), 29, 35*t*, 37*f*, 38
Pneumonia
　bacterial, 30–32
　bronchiolitis obliterans with organizing, 73, 210
　cryptogenic organizing, 155
　lymphocytic interstitial, 41–42, 42*f*, 216
　Mycoplasma, 148, 190, 267
　patchy, 107
　pneumococcal, 224

Pneumonia (*Continued*)
Pneumocystis, 29, 35*t*, 37*t*, 38
recurrent, 99
viral, 32*f*
Pneumonitis
bleomycin-induced, 161
interstitial, 42
Löffler, 281
lymphoid interstitial, 216*t*, 219
methotrexate, 232–233
resulting from antirheumatic
therapy, 232–233
Pneumothorax, 264, 320, 321*t*
Polymorphonuclear leukocytes, 223
Polymorphonuclear neutrophils,
157
Polysomnography, 103*t*, 104, 187
Portopulmonary-hypertension, 111
Port-wine stains, 263, 264*f*
Positron emission tomography
(PET), 136
Postdiphtheritic neuropathy, 190
Postextubation stridor, 20
Postmortem pleuropulmonary
evaluation, 219
Post-transplant lymphoproliferative
disorder (PTLD), 67
PPB. *See* Pleuropulmonary blastoma
PPHTN, 111
Prader-Willi syndrome, 179
Praziquantel, 290
Prenatal lung development,
295–296
Pressure
bilevel positive airway, 187, 189,
195
increased pulmonary venous,
85–87
intra-abdominal, 131
NPPV, 194, 195*f*, 198
peak inspiratory, 196
pulmonary arterial, 82*f*, 83*t*, 202
pulmonary microvascular, 125
pulmonary venous, 83–85,
83*t*, 85*t*
respiratory system, 180*f*
Primary ciliary dyskinesia (PCD),
316–319, 319*t*–320*t*
Primary immunodeficiencies, 50–62
with antibody underproduction,
52*t*
Primary lung neoplasms, 146–147
Primary lymphedema, 257
Primary pulmonary hypertension,
322, 326, 326*t*, 327*t*
Primary pulmonary hypoplasia,
297*t*
Primary pulmonary Langerhans cell
histiocytosis, 147, 153–154
Primary spontaneous
pneumothorax, 321*t*
Progesterone, 179
Progressive parenchymal injury, 334
Proinflammatory cytokines, 6
Prophylaxis, 35, 40, 59, 62, 71
Prostacyclins, 225*t*
Protein
intolerance, 325*t*
lysosomal trafficking, 267
surfactant, 336

Protozoa, 274–280
amebiasis, 276–280
malaria, 274–276
Proximal skin sclerosis, 220
Pseudoglandular period, of lung
development, 295–296, 296*t*
Pseudohypoaldosteronism (PAH),
170, 172–174
Pseudomonas, 50, 332, 333
Pseudomonas aeruginosa, 173, 174,
333, 334
Pseudoxanthoma elasticum,
265–266
PTLD. *See* Post-transplant
lymphoproliferative disorder
Pulmonary alveolar microlithiasis,
328*t*
Pulmonary alveolar proteinosis,
140–141, 140*f*
Pulmonary angiography, 262*f*
Pulmonary arterial hypertension
(PAH), 209*t*, 225*t*, 322–326
Pulmonary arterial pressure, 82*f*,
83*t*, 202
Pulmonary arteries, 82
Pulmonary arteriovenous
malformations, 314–315
Pulmonary calcification, 126
Pulmonary capillary blood, 122
Pulmonary circulation, 79–80
Pulmonary cysts, 309*t*
Pulmonary edema, 81–83, 84, 125,
155
Pulmonary embolism, 124*t*, 263,
327–328
Pulmonary emphysema, 264
Pulmonary fibrosis, 159, 161, 327,
328*t*
Pulmonary function tests (PFTs), 18,
98, 207
Pulmonary hemorrhage, 245, 246
Pulmonary hypertension, 10,
151–152, 263, 320
diagnostic classification, 95*t*
Pulmonary hypoplasia, 94, 296, 300
neuromuscular conditions
associated with, 300*t*–301*t*
Pulmonary infections, 66
Pulmonary inflammation, 333
Pulmonary leukostasis syndrome,
138–140
Pulmonary lymphangiectasia,
311–313, 314*t*
Pulmonary lymphatic drainage, 10
Pulmonary manifestations/
complications, 322*t*–325*t*.
See also specific disorders
of cardiac diseases, 79–97
of chronic lung disease of infancy,
1–22
of dermatologic diseases,
256–272
of endocrine/metabolic diseases,
170–181
of gastrointestinal diseases,
98–117
of genetic disorders, 295–336
of hematologic/oncologic
diseases, 154–163
of HIV infection, 28–43

Pulmonary manifestations/
complications (*Continued*)
of inborn errors of metabolism,
322*t*–325*t*
of neuromuscular diseases,
184–199
of non-HIV immunosuppressive
diseases, 49–76
of parasitic diseases, 274–293
of renal disease, 121–132
of rheumatoid disease, 201–233
of systemic vasculitis, 241–254
Pulmonary nodules, 142
Pulmonary paragonimiasis, 289
Pulmonary parenchyma, 252
Pulmonary sequestration, 309–310
Pulmonary valve, 91
Pulmonary vascular resistance,
81, 91
Pulmonary venous pressure, 83–85,
83*t*, 85*t*
Pulmonary-renal syndrome(s),
244–246, 245*f*, 245*t*
idiopathic, 253–254
Pyloric stenosis, 102

R
Radiation therapy/radiotherapy,
153, 161, 162–163
Rapid eye movement (REM) atonia,
178
Rare airway diseases in SLE, 210*t*
Rasburicase, 137–138
RDS. *See* Respiratory distress
syndrome
Reactive airway disease, 150
Reactive arthritis, 286
REM. *See* Rapid eye movement
Renal diseases, 121–132
Renal dysplasia, 2
Renal insufficiency, 126
Renal lesions, 261
Renal transplantation, 70
Reproductive system disorders, 177
Respiratory acidosis, 123*t*
Respiratory distress syndrome
(RDS), 1
Respiratory infections, 18
Respiratory muscle aids, 194
Respiratory muscle dysfunction,
189*t*
Respiratory muscle failure, 186*t*
Respiratory muscle fatigue,
187–194
Respiratory muscle function,
185–187
Respiratory syncytial virus (RSV), 35
Respiratory system pressure-volume
curves, 180*f*
Restrictive syndrome, 192
Rhabditiform larvae, 282
Rhabdomyosarcoma (RMS), 64, 144
Rheumatoid arthritis, 218
juvenile, 217–220
Rheumatoid disease(s), 201–240
ankylosing spondylitis, 226–228
juvenile dermatomyositis,
225–226

Rheumatoid disease(s) (*Continued*)
  juvenile rheumatoid arthritis, 217–220
  pneumonitis resulting from antirheumatic therapy, 232–233
  sarcoidosis, 228–232
  scleroderma, 220–224
  Sjögren syndrome, 215–216
  systemic lupus erythematosus, 124, 202–211, 205f, 210t
Rheumatology medications, and pneumonitis, 232–233
Rifampin, 34
Riley-Day syndrome, 101f, 337t
Rituximab, 72, 159t, 236
RMS. *See* Rhabdomyosarcoma
Rowley-Rosenberg syndrome, 327t
RSV. *See* Respiratory syncytial virus
Rubinstein-Taybi syndrome, 307t

S
Salbutamol, 13
Saline, inhaled, 334
Salivagram, 103t, 104
Sarcoidosis, 228–232
SCD. *See* Sickle cell disease
Schistosoma species, 292
SCID. *See* Severe combined immunodeficiency
Scleroderma, 220–224
Scleroderma-renal crisis, 213
SCT. *See* Stem cell transplant
Secondary immunodeficiencies, 62–73
Secondary organ dysfunction, 66
Secondary pulmonary hypoplasia, 298t–299t
Serologic diagnosis, 250
Seronegative arthritis, 57
Seronegative enthesitis, 227
Serositis, 217
Serratia marcescens, 61
Serum chitotriosidase, 231
Severe combined immunodeficiency (SCID), 50
Shrinking lung syndrome, 124, 209, 222
Sickle cell disease (SCD), 147–152
Sight-threatening ocular disease, 231
Simpson-Golabi-Behmel syndrome, 302t
Single unilocular cystic structures, 308
Sjögren syndrome, 215–216
SJS. *See* Stevens-Johnson syndrome
Skeletal dysplasias, 298
Skin rash, 243
Sleep apnea, 127, 178
Sleep hypoventilation, 188
  muscular disorders and, 193
Sleep-disordered breathing, 175
SMA. *See* Spinal muscular atrophy
Small cysts, 308
Small pulmonary artery, 94
Soft tissue sarcomas (STS), 144–145
Solid malignancies, 141

Solid tumors, 141–146
Spinal muscular atrophy (SMA), 184, 301t
Spontaneous pneumothorax, 320, 321t
Sputum, 74–75
Staphylococcus, 50
Staphylococcus aureus, 30, 31f, 60t, 61, 62, 67
  methicillin-resistant, 30
Stem cell transplant (SCT), 50, 72–73
Sternocleidomastoids, 185
Stevens-Johnson syndrome (SJS), 267–269
  extensive skin necrosis, 269f
Streptococcus pneumoniae, 30, 31t, 36, 50, 53, 57, 59, 62, 149, 150, 151
Streptococcus pyogenes, 62
Streptococcus viridans, 67
Strongyloides, 281, 283
Strongyloides stercoralis, 274, 282, 283, 283f, 284, 284f
Strongyloidiasis, 282–285
STS. *See* Soft tissue sarcomas
Stuve-Wiedemann syndrome, 300t
Subcutaneous fat, 265
Superior vena cava (SVC), 64, 136
  syndrome, 136–138
Superoxide dismutase, 17
Supplemental oxygen, 213
Suppurative bronchitis, 109
Surfactant protein, 336
Surgery, fundoplication, 106
Surgical palliation, 93
Sweat test, 331
Syndrome(s)
  acquired immunodeficiency, 284
  acute chest, 147, 148–150
  acute respiratory distress, 114–116, 125, 276f
  Birt-Hogg-Dube, 321t
  Blau, 227
  Bloom, 317t
  bronchiolitis obliterans, 72
  Churg-Strauss, 250–251, 251t
  Cogan, 242t
  defined immunodeficiency, 58t
  Denys-Drash, 304t
  DiGeorge, 57, 177
  Donnai-Barrow, 304t
  drug-induced lupus, 211t
  Ehlers-Danlos, 256, 264–265, 321t
  Eisenmenger, 85
  Emanuel, 305t
  Feingold, 313t
  Fryns, 301, 302t
  Goodpasture, 124, 207, 243
  Heiner, 98, 106–108
  hepatopulmonary, 111–114
  Hermansky-Pudlak, 267, 328t
  hyper-IgE, 60t, 61
  hyperleukocytosis, 65
  idiopathic pneumonitis, 155
  idiopathic pulmonary-renal, 253
  immune reconstitution inflammatory, 41, 42–43
  immunodeficiency, 58t, 60t
  Kartagener, 316–319, 319t

Syndrome(s) (*Continued*)
  Klippel-Trenaunay-Weber, 263–264
  Liddle, 172
  Löffler, 281
  Marfan, 321t
  McKusick-Kaufman, 313t
  Meacham, 302t
  Meckel, 298
  Meigs, 177
  Microphthalmia, 303t
  Mounier-Kuhn, 265
  obesity-hypoventilation, 177–181
  Opitz-Frias, 312t–313t
  Pallister-Killian, 305t
  Parry-Romberg, 220
  Perlman, 304t
  Prader-Willi, 179
  pulmonary leukostasis, 138–140
  pulmonary-renal, 244–246, 245f, 245t, 253
  respiratory distress, 1
  restrictive, 192
  Rowley-Rosenberg, 327t
  shrinking lung, 124, 209, 222
  Simpson-Golabi-Behmel, 302t
  Stevens-Johnson, 267–269
  Stuve-Wiedemann syndrome, 300t
  superior vena cava, 64, 136–138
  thoracoabdominal, 303t
  vasculitis, 243
  vena cava compression, 137f
  Wiskott-Aldrich, 57, 58t, 59
  yellow nail, 256–258
  Young, 317t
  Zellweger, 324t
Syndromic anophthalmia, 303t
Syndromic microphthalmia, 313t
Systemic corticosteroids, 15–16
Systemic lupus erythematosus, 124, 202–211, 203t–204t, 205f
  noninfectious complications of, 203t
  rare airway diseases, 210t
Systemic vasculitis (vasculitides), 241–254
  Behçet disease, 251–252
  Churg-Strauss syndrome, 242t, 250–251, 251t
  Henoch Schönlein purpura, 245, 246–247
  idiopathic pulmonary-renal syndrome, 253–254
  microscopic polyangiitis, 249–250
  pulmonary-renal syndromes, 244–246, 245f, 245t
  Takayasu arteritis, 241, 252–253
  Wegener granulomatosis, 121, 123–124, 242t, 247–249, 248t, 249f
Systemic ventricle obstruction, 87–89

T
T cell defects, 55t
Tachypnea, 217, 280
Takayasu arteritis, 241, 252–253

Tamoxifen, 261
TEFs. *See* Tracheoesophageal fistulas
Temporal arteritis, 241
TEN. *See* Toxic epidermal necrolysis
Tetralogy of Fallot, 92*f*, 93–94
Theophylline, 179
Therapy. *See also* Chemotherapy
    antibiotic, 192
        macrolide, 72
    bronchodilator, 13
    cancer, 64–67
    curative, 335
    gene, 59
    highly active antiretroviral, 28
    home oxygen, 19
    hydrocortisone, 15
    immunomodulatory, 215
    pneumonitis resulting from
        antirheumatic, 232–233
    radiation, 156, 161, 162–163
    transfusion, 152
Thoracentesis, 137
Thoracoabdominal syndrome, 303*t*
Thoracoscopy, 142, 207
Thromboembolism, 74
Thrombotic risks, 329
Thymoma, 64
Thyromegaly, 176
Thyrotoxicosis, 176
Tinidazole, 280
TLC. *See* Total lung capacity
TMP-SMX. *See* Trimethoprim-
    sulfamethoxazole
Tonsillectomy, 179
Total lung capacity (TLC), 217
Toxic epidermal necrolysis (TEN),
    267–269
Toxicity
    chemotherapy-induced lung,
        158–162
    lung, 158*t*
    renal, 70
Toxocara canis, 285, 287
Toxocara catis, 285
Toxocariasis, 285–287
Toxoplasma gondii, 274, 292
Tracheal agenesis, 311
Tracheal atresia, 297
Tracheal compression, 136–138
Tracheal stenosis, 247
Tracheobronchial glands, 63
Tracheobronchomalacia, 19–20
Tracheoesophageal fistulas (TEFs),
    295, 311, 312*t*
Tracheomalacia, 100
Transbronchial biopsy, 38
Transepithelial potential difference,
    329
Transfusion therapy, 152
Transfusion-related acute lung
    injury, 156–157
Transient neonatal myasthenia, 191

Transplant-related pulmonary
    complications, 67–73
Transthoracic Doppler
    echocardiography, 224
Transthoracic needle aspiration, 75
"Tree in bud" CT pattern, 110, 110*f*
Trematodes, 287–290
Tricuspid atresia, 93
Trimethoprim-sulfamethoxazole
    (TMP-SMX), 31*t*, 32, 39*t*, 40, 44
    prophylaxis with, 39, 211
Tuberculosis, 33*f*, 34, 42, 44,
    125–126, 233
Tuberous sclerosis, 259–261,
    260*f*, 337*t*
    complex, 259–261, 260*t*
Tumor necrosis factor, 233

U

Ulcerative colitis, 110
Ultrasonography, 116
Uncinaria stenocephala, 282
Upper motor neuron, 188–189
Ureaplasma urealyticum, 7
Urinary tract infection, 131
Urine output, suboptimal, 298
Urinothorax, 126–127
Urticaria pigmentosa, 270

V

Vaccines
    measles, mumps, rubella, 36
    pneumococcal conjugate, 36
Varicella-zoster virus, 36
Vascular anomalies, respiratory
    manifestations of,
    pathophysiology of, 91–92
Vascular compression of airway, 86*f*
Vascular endothelium, 59
Vascular inflammation, 241
Vascular lesions, 209
Vasculitis. *See also* Systemic
    vasculitis
    childhood, 242*t*
    definition of, 241–244
    syndromes, 243
VATER-like defects, 327*t*
Vena cava compression syndrome,
    137*t*
Venous thrombosis, 208
Ventilation
    alveolar, 122
    high-frequency oscillatory, 11, 14
    maximum voluntary, 179
    mechanical, 6
        glottic/laryngeal injury and, 20
    minimal, 14
    nocturnal noninvasive, 187

Ventilation (*Continued*)
    non-invasive intermittent
        positive-pressure, 194, 195*f*,
        198
    normal alveolar, 195–196
Ventricular septal defect (VSD), 81,
    83*t*
Very-low-birth-weight (VLBW)
    infants, 3
Video-assisted thoracoscopy, 207
Viral infections, 35–37
Viral pneumonia, 37*f*
Visceral larva migrans (VLM),
    285–287
Viscid airway secretions, 334
Vitamin A, 15
Vitamin deficiency, 12
VLBW. *See* Very-low-birth-weight
    infants
VLM. *See* Visceral larva migrans
Vomiting, versus reflux, 102–103,
    102*f*
von Hippel-Lindau syndrome, 315
VSD. *See* Ventricular septal defect

W

Wegener granulomatosis, 121,
    123–124, 242*t*, 247–249, 248*t*,
    249*f*
Weight loss, 179
Werdnig-Hoffman disease, 189
Wilms tumor, 145
Wiskott-Aldrich syndrome, 57
Wolman disease, 324*t*
World Health Organization stage,
    for lymphocytic interstitial
    pneumonia, 42
Wuchereria bancrofti, 292

X

Xanthoma disseminatum disease,
    266
X-linked agammaglobulinemia, 51
X-linked dyskeratosis congenita,
    328*t*

Y

Yellow nail syndrome, 256–258,
    257*f*
Young syndrome, 317*t*

Z

Zellweger syndrome, 324*t*